Fundamentals
of **Modern**
Bioprocessing

Fundamentals of **Modern Bioprocessing**

Sarfaraz K. Niazi
Therapeutic Proteins International LLC
Chicago, Illinois, USA

Justin L. Brown
Pennsylvania State University
University Park, Pennsylvania, USA

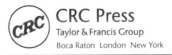
CRC Press
Taylor & Francis Group
Boca Raton London New York

CRC Press is an imprint of the
Taylor & Francis Group, an **informa** business

CRC Press
Taylor & Francis Group
6000 Broken Sound Parkway NW, Suite 300
Boca Raton, FL 33487-2742

First issued in paperback 2017

ISBN-13: 978-1-4665-8573-7 (hbk)
ISBN-13: 978-1-138-89329-0 (pbk)

Library of Congress Cataloging-in-Publication Data

Niazi, Sarfaraz, 1949- , author.
  Fundamentals of modern bioprocessing / Sarfaraz K. Niazi and Justin L. Brown.
  p. ; cm.
  Includes bibliographical references and index.
  ISBN 978-1-4665-8573-7 (alk. paper)
  1. Biochemical engineering. I. Brown, Justin L. (Justin Lee), 1980- , author. II. Title.
  [DNLM: 1. Biotechnology. 2. Biochemical Phenomena. 3. Chemical Engineering. TP 248.3]

TP248.3.N533 2015
660--dc23   2015016870

Visit the Taylor & Francis Web site at
http://www.taylorandfrancis.com

and the CRC Press Web site at
http://www.crcpress.com

To my grand proteins, Durdana, Aliyah, Noor, and Aminah

Sarfaraz K. Niazi

To my dear wife, Amanda

Justin L. Brown

CONTENTS

SECTION II   *Handbook of Bioprocessing*

PREFACE

Bioprocess engineering is a support specialty of biotechnology and chemical or agricultural engineering. It deals with the design and development of equipment and processes for the manufacturing of products such as food, feed, pharmaceuticals, therapeutic proteins, nutraceuticals, fine chemicals, and polymers and paper-utilizing biological catalyst materials as the primary production engine and their many modern variants. Bioprocess engineering encompasses, at various levels, the science of mathematics, biology, and industrial design and, on a more in-depth basis, the designs and operations of bioreactors, construction of biological catalysts, and facility designs to conform to regulatory agency requirements.

The scope of bioprocess engineering is vast, and it represents a highly sought-after program. In 2012, over 150 accredited institutions offered at least one course in bioprocess engineering, with thousands of students enrolling at both undergraduate and graduate levels. The popularity of bioprocess engineering comes from the practical qualification this academic training imparts to students, thereby enabling them to pursue lucrative careers. More recently, with the fast expansion of the application of bioprocess engineering in the manufacturing of healthcare products, the market for students with a bioprocess engineering background has increased and is projected to grow substantially faster than that in any other related engineering discipline. A recent approval of a biosimilar product in the United States has opened a pathway for bio-similar recombinant drugs in that country, while it is already open in the rest of the world; this will produce a stellar rise in the demand for qualified bioprocess engineers. Additional sectors where bioprocess engineering graduates are finding fresh career opportunities include the biofuels industry; for example, the technology of producing energy from biofuels includes the bioprocessing of ethanol, butanol, acetic acid, polymers, and other chemicals that have traditionally been produced from fossil fuels such as oil, coal, and natural gas.

A survey of job openings for bioprocess engineers on www.simplyhired.com yielded over 1000 open positions with average starting salaries over $70,000. The U.S. food industry is currently employing 20,000 engineers from all disciplines, exceeds $400 billion in annual sales, and represents over 25% of all nondurable goods produced. Each of these provides potential career opportunities for well-trained engineers with the knowledge, interest, skills, and commitment to be a part of this diverse and increasingly important field. Bioprocess engineers are employed in the food industry, multinational corporations, biotechnology companies, government agencies, private consulting firms, and agricultural commodity processors.

Most bioprocess engineers now find job opportunities that had traditionally gone to chemical engineers, and those with only a few years of experience will find stable high-paying jobs. However, the teaching of bioprocess engineering faces a challenge because of a serious gap between what the market needs and what is currently taught at most institutions. As people who have been academics for decades and now equally industrialists, we are able to understand the reason for this flaw. While most academicians keep up with the science, they are not necessarily fully appreciative of what the industry needs, more particularly in the fields where the needs are changing very fast. This is a universal phenomenon. What the industry needs is a professional who can fit into a commercial development and manufacturing environment.

This book is written specifically to meet the needs of students in the field of bioprocessing and discusses both theory underlying bioprocessing and potential practical uses of their qualification. As a result, the book is divided into two sections: Section I pertains to engineering fundamentals of bioprocessing and Section II is basically a handbook of bioprocessing, with practical advice and steps.

Section I	Engineering Fundamentals of Bioprocessing
Chapter 1	Frontiers of Bioprocessing: A forward-looking view to introducing the scope and applications of bioprocessing, particularly pointing out applications of basic scientific disciplines and the expanding areas of new career opportunities.
Chapter 2	Introduction to Molecular Biology: As the focus of this book is on biological manufacturing, molecular biology studies become important for understanding both the basic engine of production, which is now likely to be a recombinant entity, and the biological entities produced. A keen understanding of molecular biology is required for every bioprocess engineer. In this chapter, we introduce the fundamentals that are essential for the engineering aspect of the practice of the profession.
Chapter 3	Introduction to Biochemistry: The fundamentals of biochemistry form the core of the development of the manufacturing engine—how does a living entity metabolize nutrients and convert them into a variety of products. Understanding biochemistry is important for the appropriate selection of manufacturing entities and their optimization cycles and the creation of a financially practical model of manufacturing.
Chapter 4	Introduction to Cellular Biology and Microbiology: Microbiology is the third leg of science required to fully understand the scope of bioprocessing; in all instances, microbes, cells, yeasts, and tissue cells are the starting point of a bioprocess; a detailed understanding of microbiological aspects is additionally required to understand the value and need to prevent contamination of manufacturing batches, which is the most important consideration in managing commercial production.
Chapter 5	Reaction Stoichiometry, Thermodynamics, and Kinetics: A mathematical understanding of heat transfer, reaction kinetics, and free energy of reactions is needed to adequately plan and simulate various fermentation systems; this chapter refreshes the basic principles used for these calculations.
Chapter 6	Kinetics of Enzymes and Cell Growth: Modeling of fermentation processes or upstream management and the kinetics of various enzymes, as well as their impact on cell growth, are studied; the rate constants associated with these reactions and change are utilized to optimize the conditions.
Chapter 7	Data Management: Presentation of data requires clear understanding of what constitutes a data point, the nature of data conversions, and data extrapolation; presentation forms the basis of reports relating to bioprocess operations.

(Continued)

Examining the choice of textbooks, both current and about a decade old, available to students, one may notice that the textbooks continue to teach bioprocessing in a traditional theoretical way. For example, a bioprocess engineer must be fluent in various regulatory requirements, including the requirements of good manufacturing practice; he or she should also be totally familiar with the landscape of disposable processing systems and be able to use the most efficient tools for data collection and analysis. A keen understanding of digital data collection and manipulation in light of the strict regulatory requirements is also needed. Obviously, these additional requirements do not dilute the prerequisite requirement of a sound basic understanding of mathematics, physics, and chemistry. We are sure that teachers of bioprocess engineering will take this advice by adopting a more dynamic and current curriculum; there is a fine line between *what the students should know* and *what the students ought to know*. It is for this reason this book has a title that reflects its plan and utility. This book is about *fundamental* principles, the core of understanding the discipline, particularly for those who may not have extensive training in engineering and mathematical sciences; reading this book does not require any advanced knowledge of any specific field of knowledge. This book is intended to train engineers who are ready to start a productive career. The second key term in the title of the book is *modern*, and that is where this book differentiates itself from all other texts available. The book emphasizes current and future career opportunities and is geared to prepare students to begin their career fully prepared with the knowledge of the *fundamental* tools.

Fundamentals of Modern Bioprocessing is a textbook, a handbook, and, above all, a teaching manual for both the principles and applications of bioprocessing. It will be very difficult and perhaps unmanageable to cover all applications of bioprocess engineering in one volume; fortunately, the basic principles remain the same, regardless of the industry because of the unitary nature of the systems used—a biological catalyst and its many modern variants.

We have chosen one of the highest-value fields of bioprocess engineering—biological manufacturing of drugs and vaccines—to be a major subtopic to demonstrate the application of the principles provided in this book. Those with greater exposure to other disciplines will soon find that the common teaching platforms provided here are the same as those needed for training new manpower for numerous and varied industries.

On a bigger scale, all bioprocesses have two stages and components in common: there is a catalyst (a biological source) that is used to conduct an upstream process (of converting a chemical source into desired product), followed by a downstream process to purify or isolate the target product from the upstream process. In some instances, the processes are conducted under a highly rigid environment, for example, when drugs are made; at other times, it is done in open air, for example, when treating wastewater effluent. However, even this big picture is becoming obsolete in light of the disciplines of bioinformatics, which we have described in great detail in Chapter 1.

In addressing the modernity of bioprocessing, this book presents a detailed description of the fastest growing area in the field of bioprocessing—the use of disposable components, which is superior to the currently used stainless steel components. All aspects of design, component selection, regulatory concerns, and practicality of adopting disposable systems for bioprocessing are described.

Sarfaraz K. Niazi
Therapeutic Proteins International, LLC
Chicago, Illinois

Justin L. Brown
Pennsylvania State University
Pennsylvania

ACKNOWLEDGMENTS

A book of this size cannot be produced without the recognition and arduous support of the publisher. The untiring encouragement and support of Michael Slaughter, executive editor, bioengineering, biotechnology (engineering, medical, clinical), mechanical engineering (outside the United States), CRC Press/Taylor & Francis Group LLC, in creating the plan for this book and his continuous motivation to us to complete the manuscript on a timely basis, were exemplary. Laurie Oknowsky, project coordinator at Taylor & Francis Group, provided the essential discipline and push that every author needs; she was able to nudge us when we needed it the most.

Last, but not the least, we are thankful to scores of our scientific and professional colleagues and particularly those whom we came to know through the landmark literature in the field but never met them. We may have quoted their work thinking subconsciously that this is all in the public domain; we hope they will excuse us for taking this liberty, as it would be impossible to recognize them properly. An elaborate bibliography does not necessarily replace this obligation of properly acknowledging their work. Although we have extensively benefited from published works, the errors, whatsoever remaining, are altogether ours. We would appreciate readers bringing any errors to our attention so that we may correct them in future editions of the book. This communication may be sent to SKN at Niazi@niazi.com or JLB at jlbbio@engr.psu.edu.

We would be remiss if we did not acknowledge the continuous support, loyalty, and love of our wives, Anjum and Amanda, without whose dedication to our academic ambitions we would not have been able to complete this work, nor many other works in the past.

AUTHORS

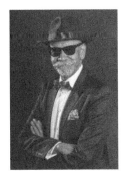

Sarfaraz K. Niazi, PhD, is the founding executive chairman of Therapeutic Proteins International, LLC, a world class developer and manufacturer of biosimilar and interchangeable recombinant biologics, located in the heart of Chicago. Dr. Niazi began his career teaching pharmacy at the University of Illinois, where he was a tenured professor, before entering the pharmaceutical industry with Abbott International, where he became a Volwiler fellow; he left Abbott International to establish his own consulting business to develop recombinant drugs, with a passion to make them affordable. In 2003, Dr. Niazi established Therapeutic Proteins International, which remains the only integrated U.S. company of its kind to date. To make biosimilar drugs affordable and to manufacture them in the United States, he reinvented the bioprocessing technology that has been in use for centuries; his inventions are protected by dozens of U.S. and worldwide patents. His other inventions include new drugs, new dosage forms, biosimilarity testing, wine aging, water purification, automobile safety, and no-fly hats; many of his inventions are used widely across the world, and this has earned him the highest civilian award, the Star of Distinction from the Government of Pakistan, for his contribution of royalty-free technologies to help millions in the developing world. Dr. Niazi has written over 40 major books, including textbooks, handbooks, technical treatise, poetry books, foreign language poetry translations, and philosophical treatise; he has published over 100 research publications and many more research abstracts. He authored the first *Handbook of Biogeneric Therapeutic Proteins* in 2005. He has delivered hundreds of lectures on a variety of subjects including science, philosophy, religion, health care, rhetoric and contemporary solutions, and societal transformation. He is also a licensed practitioner of patent law in the United States, and in this capacity, he helps scientists in the developing world on a voluntary basis to secure their inventions in the United States. He has been widely recognized for his contributions to science and literature, including the BioProcess International award for single-use bioreactors for bacterial systems manufacturing in 2012 and the 2014 Global Generics and Biosimilar Award of Innovation of the Year sponsored by Honeywell. His inventions, philanthropy, and passion for science, literature, music, and photography have been widely written about in newspapers and magazines, such as *Forbes*, *Chicago Tribune*, and *Crain's Chicago Business*. Dr. Niazi continues to serve on the faculty of several major universities around the world.

Professional website: http://www.theraproteins.com
Website: http://www.niazi.com
LinkedIn: https://www.linkedin.com/pub/sarfaraz-k-niazi/18/24/592
Wikipedia: http://en.wikipedia.org/wiki/Sarfaraz_K._Niazi
Twitter: @moustaches

Selection of Works by Sarfaraz K. Niazi

Textbook of Biopharmaceutics and Clinical Pharmacokinetics. New York: John Wiley & Sons, 1979.

The Omega Connection. Oakbrook, IL: Esquire Press, 1982.

Adsorption and Chelation Therapy. Oakbrook, IL: Esquire Press, 1987

Attacking the Sacred Cows: The Health Hazards of Milk. Oakbrook, IL: Esquire Press, 1988.

Endorphins: The Body Opium. Oakbrook, IL: Esquire Press, 1988.

Nutritional Myths: The Story No One Wants to Talk About. Oakbrook, IL: Esquire Press, 1988.

Wellness Guide. Lahore, Pakistan: Ferozsons Publishers, 2002.

Love Sonnets of Ghalib: Translations, Explication and Lexicon. Lahore, Pakistan: Ferozsons Publishers, 2002.

Filing Patents Online. Boca Raton, FL: CRC Press, 2003.

Pharmacokinetic and pharmacodynamic modeling in early drug development. In: Smith, C.G., and O'Donnell, J.T. (eds.), *The Process of New Drug Discovery and Development* (2nd Ed.). New York: CRC Press, 2004.

Handbook of Biogeneric Therapeutic Proteins: Manufacturing, Regulatory, Testing and Patent Issues. Boca Raton, FL: CRC Press, 2005.

Handbook of Preformulation: Chemical, Biological and Botanical Drugs. New York: Informa Healthcare, 2006.

Handbook of Bioequivalence Testing. New York: Informa Healthcare, 2007.

Handbook of Pharmaceutical Manufacturing Formulations, Sterile Products. Volume 6, Second Edition. New York: Informa Healthcare, 2009.

Handbook of Pharmaceutical Manufacturing Formulations, Compressed Solids. Volume 1, Second Edition. New York: Informa Healthcare, 2009.

Handbook of Pharmaceutical Manufacturing Formulations, Uncompressed Solids. Volume 2, Second Edition. New York: Informa Healthcare, 2009.

Handbook of Pharmaceutical Manufacturing Formulations, Liquid Products. Volume 3, Second Edition. New York: Informa Healthcare, 2009.

Handbook of Pharmaceutical Manufacturing Formulations, Semisolid Products. Volume 4, Second Edition. New York: Informa Healthcare, 2009.

Handbook of Pharmaceutical Manufacturing Formulations, Over the Counter Products. Volume 5, Second Edition. New York: Informa Healthcare, 2009.

Textbook of Biopharmaceutics and Clinical Pharmacokinetics. Hyderabad, India: The Book Syndicate, 2010.

Wine of Passion: Love Poems of Ghalib. Lahore, Pakistan: Ferozsons Publishers, 2010.

Disposable Bioprocessing Systems. Boca Raton, FL: CRC Press, 2012.

Handbook of Bioequivalence Testing (2nd Ed.). New York: Informa Healthcare, 2014.

There is No Wisdom: Selected Love Poems of Bedil. Translations from Farsi, D., Niazi, S.K., and Tawoosi, M. Lahore, Pakistan: Ferozsons Publishers, 2015.

Wine of Love: Complete Translations of Urdu Persian Love Poems of Ghalib. Lahore, Pakistan: Ferozsons Publishers, 2015.

Biosimilars and Interchangeable Biological Products—From Cell Lines to Commercial Launch, Volume 1: Strategic Elements. Boca Raton, FL: CRC Press, 2015.

Biosimilars and Interchangeable Biological Products—From Cell Lines to Commercial Launch, Volume 2: Tactical Elements. Boca Raton, FL: CRC Press, 2015.

With Brown, J.L. *Fundamentals of Modern Bioprocessing*. Boca Raton, FL: CRC Press, 2015.

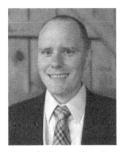 **Justin L. Brown, PhD**, is currently an assistant professor of biomedical engineering at The Pennsylvania State University. Prior to joining the faculty at The Pennsylvania State University, Dr. Brown spent seven years at the University of Virginia, where he earned his PhD in 2008 in biomedical engineering and completed an NIH-sponsored fellowship in cellular and molecular biology. During his tenure at the University of Virginia, Dr. Brown carried out research related to novel biomaterial synthesis and novel scaffold design for the regeneration of damaged or diseased bone tissue and explored the ability of substrate polarity and geometry to alter signal transduction in osteoblast progenitor cells. His research interests are in exploring the signaling cascades and phenotype progression of mesenchymal stem cells on biomaterial interfaces fabricated into novel geometries. Dr. Brown's research blends a reductionist approach toward generating novel biomaterial geometries coupled with a high-throughput systems approach to studying the cellular response to each independent scaffold parameter. He has acquired government funding through the NIH, industry funding through a collaboration with Titan Spine LLC, and foundation funding through the Grace Woodward Foundation for his research efforts. Dr. Brown has published numerous articles on biomaterials and musculoskeletal regenerative medicine. Additionally, he has published several book chapters, the most notable being "Bone Tissue Engineering" in the third edition of *Biomaterials Science: An Introduction to Materials in Medicine* (Academic Press, 2013). At Penn State, he has taught two courses required of undergraduates pursuing the biochemical option in biomedical engineering, bioengineering transport phenomena, and reaction kinetics of biological systems. Additionally, Dr. Brown has developed a graduate course that explores current research in regenerative medicine.

Section I

Engineering Fundamentals of Bioprocessing

1

Frontiers of Bioprocessing

LEARNING OBJECTIVES

1. Understand the definition of Bioprocessing.
2. Recognize the scope that Bioprocessing encompasses.
3. Envision how Bioprocessing will enhance daily life.

1.1 DEFINING BIOPROCESSING

The discipline of *bioprocess engineering* comprises three components: the *bio*, the *process*, and the *engineering*. The *bio* component is what comes out of biotechnology innovations. A couple of decades ago, this meant a biological catalyst or engine that had the potential of producing a myriad of useful products; now biotechnology has begun to yield surprisingly diversified products, widely expanding the scope of bioprocess engineering. The *process* part involves converting a biotechnological discovery into a practical method (process), such as an upstream process, a microarray, or a mold for growing stem cells. Process development requires extensive use of scientific and engineering principles. The *engineering* component is responsible for operating a process to an optimal commercial level.

Bioprocess engineering is therefore the application of the engineering knowledge to the fields of medicine and biology. The bioengineer must be well grounded in biology and have engineering knowledge that is broad, drawing upon electrical, chemical, mechanical, and other engineering disciplines ranging from the provision of artificial means to assist defective body functions—such as hearing aids, artificial limbs, and supportive or substitute organs—to achieving biosynthesis of animal or plant products, such as from fermentation processes.

Medical engineering concerns the application of engineering principles to medical problems, including the replacement of damaged organs, instrumentation, and the systems of health care, including diagnostic applications of computers.

Optimization engineering includes the application of engineering principles to the problems of biological production and to the external operations and environments that influence this production.

Bionics is the study of living systems so that the knowledge gained can be applied to the design of physical systems.

Biochemical engineering includes fermentation engineering, which is the application of engineering principles to microscopic biological systems that are used to create new products by synthesis, such as the production of protein from suitable raw materials.

Human systems engineering concerns the application of engineering, physiology, and psychology to optimize the human–machine relationship.

Environmental engineering, also called bioenvironmental engineering, is a field concerned with the application of engineering principles to the control of the environment for the health, comfort, and safety of human beings. It includes the field of life-support systems for the exploration of outer space and the ocean.

Bioprocess engineering borrows from each of the above sciences to create a system that consistently produces a biologic product of commercial value. To understand the nature of work involved in a bioprocess engineering job, we must first fully understand the biotechnological concepts behind a process. For example, if you are responsible for optimizing a fermentation process to produce a recombinant protein, then you must fully understand (if not become an expert) the science behind recombinant manufacturing.

1.1.1 Biotechnology Connection of Bioprocessing

Biotechnology Industry Organization (www.bio.org) defines biotechnology as, "Biotechnology, the combination of biology and technology, includes biologic applications, diagnostic tools and businesses that improve everyday life by providing solutions to some of life's most vexing problems." Since 1982 (when biotechnology took a dramatic turn), hundreds of millions of people have been helped by about 200 biotechnology drugs and vaccines with many more in the pipeline treating diseases that were just a couple of decades ago considered untreatable, from auto-immune deficiency syndrome to Alzheimer's disease to stroke prevention. Prevention of diseases like cancer appears possible within a short time. Many enzymes used to make food products are likely to be produced by recombinant techniques, as are the ingredients in most of the processed foods. Newer generations of oils without trans fats and cholesterol are now available that reduce incidence of heart disease; *golden rice* fortified with vitamins and allergen-free foods is now common, as are safer meats.

Today, over 2,500 biologics are used to fight nearly 200 different animal diseases. To make animal products safe, products are made to keep animals free of infectious bacteria, for example, *Escherichia coli* O157:H7, and to identify animals with deoxyribonucleic acid (DNA) tagging to trace outbreaks of disease; BSE (bovine serum encephalitis)-resistant bovine species are also being cloned. New plastics made with corn and other plants rather than petroleum serve ecology, as are the plants that consume carbon dioxide rather than exude it to control environment warming. New fuels for automobiles would come from soybeans and other crops, as would biodegradable grease and industrial lubricants. Bacteria are used to clean up oil spills and other contaminants. Energy consumption in production is reduced drastically, and crop yields are enhanced and crops made resistant to disease, for example, virus-resistant cotton plants. Today, farmers in 18 countries are growing more than 167 million acres of crops improved through biotechnology helping feed the world population at a lower cost than ever before. Fiber made from goat's milk is used as body armor, and mustard plant is modified to serve as *sentinel plants*, to warn against chemical or biological warfare agents. DNA typing and testing is now routinely settling the criminal investigation and paternity suites. What more is about to come is only limited by our imagination—such is the power of biotechnology.

What we need to understand today is the projection on the impact of biotechnology in the future in light of fast-changing sciences that are bound to impinge on this technology. The Rand Corporation, funded by the Central Intelligence Agency, makes an excellent projection of this scenario in a recent report. According to this report, life in 2015 will be revolutionized by the growing effect of multidisciplinary technology across all dimensions of life: social, economic, political, and personal. The report identifies biotechnology, nanotechnology, and materials technology as the technologies that will make the most impact.

Biotechnology, in the near future, will enable us to identify, understand, manipulate, improve, and control living organisms, which obviously includes human beings as well. Smart materials, agile manufacturing, and nanotechnology will change the way we produce devices while expanding their capabilities. These technologies may also be joined by what is called long shot or *wild cards* such as novel nanoscale computers, molecular manufacturing, and self-assembly.

Biotechnology will soon begin to revolutionize life: disease, malnutrition, food production, pollution, life expectancy, quality of life, crime, and security will be significantly addressed, improved, or augmented. Some advances could be viewed as accelerations of human-engineered evolution of plants, animals, and in some ways even humans with accompanying changes in the ecosystem.

Biotechnology and materials advances are likely to continue producing revolutionary surgical procedures and systems that will significantly reduce hospital stays and cost and increase effectiveness. New surgical tools and techniques and new materials and designs for vesicle and tissue support will continue to reduce surgical invasiveness and offer new solutions to medical problems. Techniques such as angioplasty may continue to eliminate whole classes of surgeries; others such as laser perforations of heart tissue could promote regeneration and healing. Advances in laser surgery could refine techniques and improve human capability (e.g., LASIK® eye surgery to replace glasses), especially as costs are reduced and experience spreads.

Hybrid imaging techniques will improve diagnosis, guide human and robotic surgery, and aid in basic understanding of body and brain function. Finally, collaborative information technology (e.g., telemedicine) will extend specialized medical care to remote areas and aid in the global dissemination of medical quality and new advances.

The research and development costs for drug development are currently extremely high and may even be unsustainable, with averages of approximately $800 million/drug brought to market. These costs may drive the pharmaceutical industry to invest heavily in technology advances with the goal of long-term viability of the industry. Combined with genetic profiling, drug development tailored to genotypes, chemical simulation and engineering programs, and drug testing simulations may begin to change pharmaceutical development from a broad application trial-and-error approach to custom drug development, testing, and prescription based on a deeper understanding of subpopulation response to drugs. This understanding may also rescue drugs previously rejected because of adverse reactions in small populations of clinical trials. Along with the potential for improving success rates, reducing trial costs, and opening new markets for narrowly targeted drugs, tailoring drugs to subpopulations will also have the opposite effect of reducing the size of the market for each drug. Thus, the economics of the pharmaceutical and health industries will change significantly if these trends come to fruition. Note that patent protection is not uniformly enforced across the globe for the pharmaceutical industry. As a result, certain regions (e.g., Asia) may continue to focus on the production of non-legacy (generic) drugs, and other regions (e.g., the United States, the United Kingdom, and Europe) will continue to pursue new drugs in addition to such low-margin pharmaceuticals.

Appendix 1A provides a listing of major milestones in the field of biotechnology.

1.1.2 History of Bioprocessing

Before World War II, the field of bioengineering was essentially unknown, and little communication or interaction existed between the engineer and the life scientist. A few exceptions, however, should be noted. The agricultural engineer and the chemical engineer, involved in fermentation processes, have always been bioengineers in the broadest sense of the definition since they deal with biological systems and work with biologists. The civil engineer, specializing in sanitation, has applied biological principles in the work. Mechanical engineers have worked with the medical profession for many years in the development of artificial limbs. Another area of mechanical engineering that falls in the field of bioengineering is the air-conditioning field. In the early 1920s, engineers and physiologists were employed by the American Society of Heating and Ventilating Engineers to study the effects of temperature and humidity on humans and to provide design criteria for heating and air-conditioning systems.

Today, there are many more examples of interaction between biology and engineering, particularly in the medical and life-support fields. In addition to an increased awareness of the need for communication between the engineer and the associate in the life sciences, there is an increasing recognition of the role the engineer can play in several of the biological fields, including human medicine, and, likewise, an awareness of the contributions biological science can make toward the solution of engineering problems.

Much of the increase in bioengineering activity can be credited to electrical engineers. In the 1950s, bioengineering meetings were dominated by sessions devoted to medical electronics. Medical instrumentation and medical electronics continue to be major areas of interest, but biological modeling, blood-flow dynamics, prosthetics, biomechanics (dynamics of body motion and strength of materials), biological heat transfer, biomaterials, and other areas are now included in conference programs.

Bioengineering developed out of specific desires or needs: the desire of surgeons to bypass the heart, the need for replacement organs, the requirement for life support in space, and many more. In most cases, the early interaction and education were a result of personal contacts between a physician, or a physiologist, and an engineer. Communication between the engineer and the life scientist was immediately recognized as a problem. Most engineers who wandered into the field in its early days probably had an exposure to biology through a high-school course and no further work. To overcome this problem, engineers began to study not only the subject matter but also the methods and techniques of their counterparts in medicine, physiology, psychology, and biology. Much of the information was self-taught or obtained through personal association and discussions. Finally, recognizing a need to assist in overcoming the communication barrier as well as to prepare engineers for the future, engineering schools developed courses and curricula in bioengineering.

1.2 CURRENT AND EMERGING TRENDS IN BIOPROCESS ENGINEERING

The scope of bioprocessing is tightly connected with biotechnology developments. Given below is a summary of these trends, followed by details on various fast-expanding disciplines.

- Biotechnology has a close relationship with developments in other technology sectors like information technology and nanotechnology that will converge along with genomic medicine.
- Diagnostic techniques (e.g., DNA chips and biosensor devices) will grow substantially with applications in genomic medicine, nutrigenomics, food safety, environmental monitoring, and biodefense.
- Genomic medicine will make diagnosis of disease more predictive, diets become more preventive of disease, and personalized medicines made available.
- Development of regenerative medicine with understanding of stem cells and neurological systems will make replacement of tissues to a more biologically based method for the repair and regeneration of tissues.
- More than two-third of new drugs discovered will be of biologic origin.
- Biofuels and bioplastics will resolve current shortages of both from renewable biomass such as crops and trees.
- Gene silencing will be used to avert diseases.
- Neuroprosthetics using brain signals like artificial limbs will be possible
- Genetically modified crops will resolve worldwide food shortage.
- Biopharmaceuticals will be widely produced in plants.
- Marker-assisted selection will revolutionize breeding for plants and animals.
- Metabolic engineering will manipulate microbial cells to bypass cell process.
- Biosensing technology needed for security purposes will allow appearance of real time lab on a chip capability.
- Antiviral therapeutics will become more widely used to avert epidemics and also in biodefense.
- Better understanding of multigene functions and regulation will lead to molecular regulation at a network level.
- The U.S. Department of Defense push to produce drugs on demand will result in multiple genetic modifications in a single organism to produce multiple products.

- Chemical genetics will allow better understanding of protein function in living organisms.
- There will be worldwide harmonization of standards of biotechnology-derived products.

1.2.1 Bioinformatics

Bioinformatics, parallel to the science of biophysics and biochemistry, is a branch of biological science that deals with the study of methods for storing, retrieving, and analyzing biological data, such as nucleic acid (DNA/RNA) and protein sequence, structure, function, pathways, and genetic interactions. It generates new knowledge that is useful in such fields as drug design and development of new software tools to create that knowledge. Bioinformatics also deals with algorithms, databases and information systems, web technologies, artificial intelligence and soft computing, information and computation theory, structural biology, software engineering, data mining, image processing, modeling and simulation, discrete mathematics, control and system theory, circuit theory, and statistics. Commonly used software tools and technologies in this field include Java, XML, Perl, C, C++, Python, R, MySQL, SQL, CUDA, MATLAB®, and Microsoft Excel.

Important subdisciplines within bioinformatics and computational biology include the following:

- The development and implementation of tools that enable efficient access to, and use and management of, various types of information.
- The development of new algorithms (mathematical formulas) and statistics with which to assess relationships among members of large data sets. For example, methods to locate a gene within a sequence, predict protein structure and/or function, and cluster protein sequences into families of related sequences.

The primary goal of bioinformatics is to increase the understanding of biological processes. What sets it apart from other approaches, however, is its focus on developing and applying computationally intensive techniques to achieve this goal. Examples include pattern recognition, data mining, machine learning algorithms, and visualization. Major research efforts in the field include sequence alignment, gene finding, genome assembly, drug design, drug discovery, protein structure alignment, protein structure prediction, prediction of gene expression and protein–protein interactions, genome-wide association studies, and the modeling of evolution.

Over the past few decades, rapid developments in genomic and other molecular research technologies and developments in information technologies have combined to produce a tremendous amount of information related to molecular biology.

Common activities in bioinformatics include mapping and analyzing DNA and protein sequences, aligning different DNA and protein sequences to compare them, and creating and viewing three-dimensional (3D) models of protein structures. There are two methods of modeling a biological system, static or dynamic. In static systems, sequencing proteins, nucleic acids, and peptides, along with their interaction in microarray and networks, are included. In dynamic methods, structures of proteins, nucleic acids, ligands, and peptides are elucidated; also included in dynamic methods is the systems biology that includes reaction fluxes and variable concentration of metabolites along with multi-agent-based modeling to capture cellular events such as signaling, transcription, and reaction dynamics.

1.2.1.1 Sequence Analysis

Sequence analysis comes under bioinformatics. Since phage Φ-X174 was sequenced in 1977, the DNA sequences of thousands of organisms have been decoded and stored in databases. This sequence information is analyzed to determine genes that encode polypeptides (proteins), RNA genes, regulatory sequences, structural motifs, and repetitive sequences. A comparison of genes within a species or between different species can show similarities between protein functions, or relations between species (the use of molecular systematics to construct phylogenetic trees). With the growing amount of data, it long ago became impractical to analyze DNA sequences manually. Today, computer programs such as basic logical alignment search tool are used daily to search sequences from more than 260,000 organisms, containing over 190 billion nucleotides. These programs can compensate for mutations (exchanged, deleted, or inserted bases) in the DNA sequence, to identify sequences that are related, but not identical. A variant of this sequence alignment is used in the sequencing process itself. The so-called shotgun sequencing technique (which was used, e.g., by The Institute for Genomic Research to sequence the first bacterial genome, *Haemophilus influenzae*) does not produce entire chromosomes. Instead, it generates the sequences of many thousands of small DNA fragments (ranging from 35 to 900 nucleotides long, depending on the sequencing technology). The ends of these fragments overlap and, when aligned properly by a genome assembly program, can be used to reconstruct the complete genome. Shotgun sequencing yields sequence data quickly, but the task of assembling the fragments can be quite complicated for larger genomes. For a genome as large as the human genome, it may take many days of CPU time on large-memory, multi-processor computers to assemble the fragments, and the resulting assembly will usually contain numerous gaps that have to be filled in later. Shotgun sequencing is the method of choice for virtually all genomes sequenced today, and genome assembly algorithms are a critical area of bioinformatics research.

1.2.1.2 Gene Annotation

Another aspect of sequence analysis is annotation. This involves computational gene finding to search for protein-coding genes, RNA genes, and other functional sequences within a genome. Not all of the nucleotides within a genome are part of genes. Within the genomes of higher organisms, large parts of the DNA do not serve any obvious purpose. This so-called junk DNA may, however, contain unrecognized functional elements. Bioinformatics helps to bridge the gap between genome and proteome projects—for example, in the use of DNA sequences for protein identification.

In the context of genomics, annotation is the process of marking the genes and other biological features in a DNA sequence. The first genome annotation software system was designed in 1995 by Dr. Owen White, who was part of the team at The Institute for Genomic Research that sequenced and analyzed the first genome of a free-living organism to be decoded, the bacterium *H. influenzae*. Dr. White built a software system to find the genes (fragments of genomic sequence that encode proteins), to find the transfer RNAs, and to make initial assignments of function to those genes. Most current genome annotation systems work similarly, but the programs available for the analysis of genomic DNA, such as the GeneMark program trained and used to find protein-coding genes in *H. influenzae*, are constantly changing and improving.

1.2.1.3 Computational Evolutionary Biology

Evolutionary biology is the study of the origin and descent of species, as well as their change over time. Informatics has assisted evolutionary biologists in several key ways; it has enabled researchers to

- Trace the evolution of a large number of organisms by measuring changes in their DNA, rather than through physical taxonomy or physiological observations alone.
- Compare entire genomes, which permits the study of more complex evolutionary events, such as gene duplication, horizontal gene transfer, and the prediction of factors important in bacterial speciation.
- Build complex computational models of populations to predict the outcome of the system over time.
- Track and share information on an increasingly large number of species and organisms.

The area of research within computer science that uses genetic algorithms is sometimes confused with computational evolutionary biology, but the two areas are not necessarily related.

1.2.1.4 Analysis of Gene Expression

The expression of many genes can be determined by measuring mRNA levels with multiple techniques including microarrays, expressed cDNA sequence tag sequencing, serial analysis of gene expression tag sequencing, massively parallel signature sequencing, RNA-seq, also known as *whole transcriptome shotgun sequencing*, or various applications of multiplexed in situ hybridization. All of these techniques are extremely noise-prone and/or subject to bias in the biological measurement, and a major research area in computational biology involves developing statistical tools to separate signal from noise in high-throughput gene expression studies. Such studies are often used to determine the genes implicated in a disorder: one might compare microarray data from cancerous epithelial cells to data from non-cancerous cells to determine the transcripts that are upregulated and downregulated in a particular population of cancer cells.

1.2.1.5 Analysis of Regulation

Regulation is the complex orchestration of events starting with an extracellular signal such as a hormone and leading to an increase or decrease in the activity of one or more proteins. Bioinformatics techniques have been applied to explore various steps in this process. For example, promoter analysis involves the identification and study of sequence motifs in the DNA surrounding the coding region of a gene. These motifs influence the extent to which that region is transcribed into mRNA. Expression data can be used to infer gene regulation: one might compare microarray data from a wide variety of states of an organism to form hypotheses about the genes involved in each state. In a single-cell organism, one might compare stages of the cell cycle, along with various stress conditions (heat shock, starvation, etc.). One can then apply clustering algorithms to that expression data to determine which genes are co-expressed. For example, the upstream regions (promoters) of co-expressed genes can be searched for overrepresented regulatory elements.

1.2.1.6 Analysis of Protein Expression

Protein microarrays and high-throughput mass spectrometry can provide a snapshot of the proteins present in a biological sample. Bioinformatics is very much involved in making sense of protein microarray and high-throughput mass spectrometry data; the former approach faces similar problems as with microarrays targeted at mRNA, the latter involves the problem of matching large amounts of mass data against predicted masses from protein sequence databases, and the complicated statistical analysis of samples where multiple, but incomplete, peptides from each protein are detected.

1.2.1.7 Analysis of Mutations in Cancer

In cancer, the genomes of affected cells are rearranged in complex or even unpredictable ways. Massive sequencing efforts are used to identify previously unknown point mutations in a variety of genes in cancer. Bioinformaticians continue to produce specialized automated systems to manage the sheer volume of sequence data produced, and they create new algorithms and software to compare the sequencing results to the growing collection of human genome sequences and germ line polymorphisms. New physical detection technologies are employed, such as oligonucleotide microarrays to identify chromosomal gains and losses (called comparative genomic hybridization) and single-nucleotide polymorphism arrays to detect known point mutations. These detection methods simultaneously measure several hundred thousand sites throughout the genome, and when used in high throughput to measure thousands of samples, they generate terabytes of data per experiment. Again the massive amounts and new types of data generate new opportunities for bioinformaticians. The data are often found to contain considerable variability, or noise, and thus, hidden Markov model and change-point analysis methods are being developed to infer real copy number changes.

Another type of data that require novel informatics development is the analysis of lesions found to be recurrent among many tumors.

1.2.1.8 Comparative Genomics

The core of comparative genome analysis is the establishment of the correspondence between genes (orthology analysis) or other genomic features in different organisms. It is these intergenomic maps that make it possible to trace the evolutionary processes responsible for the divergence of two genomes. A multitude of evolutionary events acting at various organizational levels shape genome evolution. At the lowest level, point mutations affect individual nucleotides. At a higher level, large chromosomal segments undergo duplication, lateral transfer, inversion, transposition, deletion, and insertion. Ultimately, whole genomes are involved in processes of hybridization, polyploidization, and endosymbiosis, often leading to rapid speciation. The complexity of genome evolution poses many exciting challenges to developers of mathematical models and algorithms, who have recourse to a spectrum of algorithmic, statistical, and mathematical techniques, ranging from exact, heuristics, fixed parameter, and approximation algorithms for problems based on parsimony models to Markov chain Monte Carlo algorithms for Bayesian analysis of problems based on probabilistic models.

Many of these studies are based on the homology detection and protein families computation.

1.2.1.9 Modeling Biological Systems

Systems biology involves the use of computer simulations of cellular subsystems (such as the networks of metabolites and enzymes which comprise metabolism, signal transduction pathways, and gene regulatory networks) to both analyze and visualize the complex connections of these cellular processes. Artificial life or virtual evolution attempts to understand evolutionary processes via the computer simulation of simple (artificial) life forms.

1.2.1.10 High-Throughput Image Analysis

Computational technologies are used to accelerate or fully automate the processing, quantification, and analysis of large amounts of high-information-content biomedical imagery. Modern image analysis systems augment an observer's ability to make measurements from a large or complex set of images, by improving accuracy, objectivity, or speed. A fully developed analysis system may completely replace the observer. Although these systems are not unique to biomedical imagery, biomedical imaging is becoming more important for both diagnostics and research. Some examples are as follows:

- High-throughput and high-fidelity quantification and subcellular localization (high-content screening, cytohistopathology, bioimage informatics)
- Morphometrics
- Clinical image analysis and visualization
- Determining the real-time air-flow patterns in breathing lungs of living animals
- Quantifying occlusion size in real-time imagery from the development of and recovery during arterial injury
- Making behavioral observations from extended video recordings of laboratory animals
- Infrared measurements for metabolic activity determination
- Inferring clone overlaps in DNA mapping, for example, the Sulston score

1.2.1.11 Prediction of Protein Structure and Function

Proteomics is the study of protein function and genes. Developments in this field are highly dependent on bioinformatics: genetic code combination and sequencing, just like the hierarchical programming in computer languages.

Protein structure prediction is another important application of bioinformatics. The amino acid sequence of a protein, the so-called primary structure, can be easily determined from the sequence on the gene that codes for it. In the vast majority of cases, this primary structure uniquely determines a structure in its native environment. (Of course, there are exceptions, such as the bovine spongiform encephalopathy—also known as mad cow disease—prion.) Knowledge of this structure is vital in understanding the function of the protein. For lack of better terms, structural information is usually classified as one of secondary, tertiary, and quaternary structure. A viable general solution to such predictions remains an open problem. As of now, most efforts have been directed toward heuristics that work most of the time.

One of the key ideas in bioinformatics is the notion of homology. In the genomic branch of bioinformatics, homology is used to predict the function of a gene: if the sequence of gene A, whose function is known, is homologous to the sequence of gene B, whose function is unknown, one could infer that B may share A's function. In the structural branch of bioinformatics, homology is used to determine which parts of a protein are important in structure formation and interaction with other proteins. In a technique called homology modeling, this information is used to predict the structure of a protein once the structure of a homologous protein is known. This currently remains the only way to predict protein structures reliably.

One example of this is the similar protein homology between hemoglobin in humans and the hemoglobin in legumes (leghemoglobin). Both serve the same purpose of transporting oxygen in the organism. Though both of these proteins have completely different amino acid sequences, their protein structures are virtually identical, which reflects their near identical purposes. Other techniques for predicting protein structure include protein threading and de novo (from scratch) physics-based modeling.

1.2.1.12 Molecular Interaction

Efficient software is available today for studying interactions among proteins, ligands, and peptides. Types of interactions most often encountered in the field include protein–ligand (including drug), protein–protein, and protein–peptide.

Molecular dynamic simulation of movement of atoms about rotatable bonds is the fundamental principle behind computational algorithms, termed *docking algorithms* for studying molecular interactions.

1.2.1.13 Docking Algorithms

In the last two decades, tens of thousands of protein 3D structures have been determined by X-ray crystallography and protein nuclear magnetic resonance spectroscopy (protein nuclear magnetic resonance spectroscopy). One central question for the biological scientist is whether it is practical to predict possible protein–protein interactions only based on these 3D shapes, without doing protein–protein interaction experiments. A variety of methods have been developed to tackle the protein–protein docking problem, though it seems that there is still much work to be done in this field.

1.2.1.14 Software and Tools

Software tools for bioinformatics range from simple command-line tools to more complex graphical programs and stand-alone web services available from various bioinformatics companies or public institutions. Many free and open source software tools have existed and continued to grow since the 1980s. The combination of a continued need for new algorithms for the analysis of emerging types of biological readouts, the potential for innovative in silico experiments, and freely available open code bases have helped to create opportunities for all research groups to contribute to both bioinformatics and the range of open source software available, regardless of their funding arrangements. The open source tools often act as incubators of ideas, or community-supported plug-ins in commercial applications. They may also provide de facto standards and shared object models for assisting with the challenge of bioinformation integration.

The range of open source software packages includes titles such as Bioconductor, BioPerl, Biopython, BioJava, BioRuby, Bioclipse, EMBOSS, Taverna workbench, and UGENE. To maintain this tradition and create further opportunities, the non-profit Open Bioinformatics Foundation has supported the annual Bioinformatics Open Source Conference (BOSC) since 2000.

The simple object access protocol- and representational state transfer-based interfaces have been developed for a wide variety of bioinformatics applications allowing an application running on one computer in one part of the world to use algorithms, data, and computing resources on servers in other parts of the world. The main advantages derive from the fact that end users do not have to deal with software and database maintenance overheads.

Basic bioinformatics services are classified by the European Bioinformatics Institute into three categories: SSS (sequence search services), MSA (multiple sequence alignment), and BSA (biological sequence analysis). The availability of these service-oriented bioinformatics resources demonstrates the applicability of web-based bioinformatics solutions, and ranges from a collection of stand-alone tools with a common data format under a single, stand-alone, or web-based interface to integrative, distributed, and extensible bioinformatics workflow management systems.

1.2.1.15 Bioinformatics Workflow Management Systems

A bioinformatics workflow management system is a specialized form of a workflow management system designed specifically to compose and execute a series of computational or data manipulation steps, or a workflow, in a bioinformatics application. Such systems are designed to

- Provide an easy-to-use environment for individual application scientists themselves to create their own workflows.
- Provide interactive tools for the scientists enabling them to execute their workflows and view their results in real time.
- Simplify the process of sharing and reusing workflows between the scientists.
- Enable scientists to track the provenance of the workflow execution results and the workflow creation steps.

Currently, there are at least three platforms giving this service: Galaxy, Taverna, and Anduril.

1.2.2 Tissue Engineering

Tissue engineering is the use of a combination of cells, engineering and materials methods, and suitable biochemical and physiochemical factors to improve or replace biological functions. While it was once categorized as a subfield of biomaterials, having grown in scope and importance, it can be considered as a field in its own right.

While most definitions of tissue engineering cover a broad range of applications, in practice the term is closely associated with applications that repair or replace portions of or whole tissues (i.e., bone, cartilage, blood vessels, bladder, skin, and muscle). Often, the tissues involved require certain mechanical and structural properties for proper functioning. The term has also been applied to efforts to perform specific biochemical functions using cells within an artificially created support system (e.g., an artificial pancreas or a bioartificial liver). The term *regenerative medicine* is often used synonymously with tissue engineering, although those involved in regenerative medicine place more emphasis on the use of stem cells to produce tissues.

Implanting *bioartificial* organ has begun to show promise with successes in artificial bladders and windpipes, achieved in June 2011. Scientists around the world are using similar techniques with the goal of building more complex organs.

Human stem cells are part of the body's system for building and repairing itself. Human embryonic stem cells are pluripotent and can thus be used to generate many cell types present in the human body. In addition, the cells are highly expandable, which enables large numbers to be produced prior to differentiation into the cell type required. They begin as a blank slate, but are able to become specialized cells specific to particular tissues or organs like the windpipe. In recent years, scientists have made great advances in understanding how stem cells can differentiate in this way. Much of the tissue engineering is based on the use of stem cells.

EMD Millipore is developing a platform of scalable, disposable production solutions based on its Mobius® CellReady bioreactor to enable more effective and efficient manufacture of cell-based therapies.

In recent years, the use of a simple ink-jet technology for cell printing has triggered tremendous interest and established the field of biofabrication. In laboratories, we have seen exciting demonstrations of printing 2D tissue like skins and 3D structures such as artery and kidney; however, there are still many challenges to overcome before the technology can be used clinically to generate transplantable organs. Printing of preformed stem cell spheroids may also enable 3D tissue to be built up more quickly. After printing, the well plate is inverted to allow cells to gravity aggregate and begin dividing.

1.2.3 Eugenics and Cloning

Cloning humans is not improbable, though highly controversial. Significant ethical, moral, religious, privacy, and environmental debates and protests are already being raised in such areas as genetically modified foods, cloning, and genomic profiling even though advances in artificially producing genetically identical organisms through cloning for engineered crops, livestock, and research animals are on the way.

The Human Genome Project and Celera Genomics have released drafts of the human genome. The drafts are undergoing additional validation, verification, and updates to weed out errors, sequence interruptions, and gaps. Whereas most think that human cloning will not be a reality, companies like Clonaid (www.clonaid.com) are charging ahead with human cloning.

1.2.4 Genomics

In 2003, the Institute of Biological Energy Alternatives (Rockville, MD) reported generating a synthetic genome by whole genome assembly: ΦX174 bacteriophage from synthetic nucleotides, the first successful experiment to create virus totally in situ. Assembly of the complete infectious genome of bacteriophage from a single pool of chemically synthesized oligonucleotides has raised many questions and challenged religious beliefs.

DNA analysis machines and chip-based systems have brought these techniques to many and will accelerate the proliferation of genetic analysis capabilities, improve drug search, and enable development of biological sensors. The genomes of plants (ranging from important food crops such as rice and corn to production plants such as pulp trees) and animals (ranging from bacteria such as *E. coli*, through insects and mammals) will continue to be decoded and profiled. To the extent that genes dictate function and behavior, such extensive genetic profiling would provide an ability to better diagnose human health problems, design drugs tailored for individual problems and system reactions, better predict disease predispositions, and track disease movement and development across global populations, ethnic groups, and other genetic pools. Note that a link between genes and function is generally accepted, but other factors such as the environment and phenotype play important modifying roles. Genetic profiling could also have a significant effect on security, policing, and law. DNA identification may complement existing biometric technologies (e.g., retina and fingerprint identification) for granting access to secure systems (e.g., computers, secured areas, or weapons), identifying criminals through DNA left at crime scenes, and authenticating items such as fine art. Genetic identification will likely become more commonplace tools in kidnapping, paternity, and fraud cases.

Biosensors (some genetically engineered) may also aid in detecting biological warfare threats, improving food and water quality testing, monitoring health continuously, and studying medical laboratory analyses. Such capabilities could fundamentally change the way health services are rendered by greatly improving disease diagnosis, understanding predispositions, and improving monitoring capabilities. Such profiling may be limited by technical difficulties in decoding some genomic segments and in understanding the implications of the genetic code. Our current technology has decoded nearly all of the entire human gene sequence. More important, although there is a strong connection between an organism's function and its genotype, we still have large gaps in understanding the intermediate steps in copying, transduction, isomer modulation, activation, immediate function, and this function's effect on larger systems in the organism.

Cloning and genetic modification also raise biodiversity concerns. Standardization of crops and livestock has already increased food supply vulnerabilities to diseases that can wipe out larger areas of production. Genetic modification may increase our ability to engineer responses to these threats, but the losses may still be felt in the production year unless broad-spectrum defenses are developed. In addition to food safety, the ability to modify biological organisms holds the possibility of engineered biological weapons that circumvent current or planned countermeasures. On the other hand, genomics could aid in biological warfare defense (e.g., through improved understanding and control of biological function both in and between pathogens and target hosts as well as improved capability for engineered biosensors). Advances in genomics, therefore, could advance a race between threat engineering and countermeasures.

1.2.5 Genetically Modified System

The science of genetic engineering involves manipulation, modification, and recombination of DNA or other nucleic acid molecules to modify an organism capable of producing protein drugs such as human insulin, human growth hormone, and hepatitis B vaccine making, it possible to provide life-saving therapies to billions at an affordable cost. These developments in genetic engineering have been well established, while the traditional techniques for genetic manipulation such as cross-pollination, selective breeding, and irradiation continue to be employed. The focus of genetic engineering remains set on food crops, production plants, insects, and animals, wherein desirable properties such as taste, composition, fat content, disease resistance, improved shelf life (e.g., the Flavr Savr tomato), herbicide tolerant, improved growth in poor soil condition, and nutrition fortification can be achieved. Beyond systemic disease resistance, in vivo pesticide production has already been demonstrated (e.g., in corn) and could have a significant effect on pesticide production, application, regulation, and control with targeted release.

In genetically modified animals such as cows where mammary glands might be engineered to produce pharmaceuticals and therapeutic organic compounds, other organisms could be engineered to produce or deliver therapeutics (e.g., the so-called prescription banana). If accepted by the population, such improved production and delivery mechanisms could extend the global production and availability of these therapeutic agents.

The plants may be engineered to artificially produce new products. Trees, for example, will be engineered to optimize their growth and tailor their structure for particular applications such as lumber, wood pulp for paper, fruiting, or carbon sequestering (to reduce global warming) while reducing waste by-products. Plants might be engineered to produce biopolymers for engineering applications with lower pollution and without using oil reserves. Biofuel plants could be tailored to minimize polluting components while producing additives needed by the consuming equipment.

Genetic engineering of microorganisms such as *E. coli* and Chinese hamster ovary (CHO) cells is widely used to produce hundreds of endogenous proteins and antibodies and has been used responsibly for mass production of drugs like insulin and thus saving millions of lives. The recombinant DNA (rDNA) production methods allow the genes of one species to be transplanted into another species (gene coding). Thus, gene coding for the expression (production) of a desired protein (usually human) could be inserted into a host prokaryotic (e.g., bacteria) or eukaryotic (e.g., mammalian) cell in such a manner that the host cell would then express (yield) usable (commercially) quantities of the desired protein. These techniques are also used for producing large quantities of monoclonal antibodies (i.e., antibodies arising from a single lymphocyte).

The choice of an expression system for the high-level production of recombinant proteins depends on many factors. These include cell growth characteristics, expression levels, intracellular and extracellular expression, posttranslational modifications, and biological activity of the protein of interest, as well as regulatory issues in the production of therapeutic proteins. In addition, the selection of a particular expression system requires a cost breakdown in terms of process, design, and other economic considerations. The relative merits of bacterial, yeast, insect, and mammalian expression systems have been examined in detail in Chapter 9 in the book. For bioprocess engineering purpose, the construction of a genetically modified system is in the domain of biotechnologists, while its large-scale deployment remains the responsibility of the bioprocess engineer.

Other animal manipulations could include modification of insects to impart desired behaviors, provide tagging (including GMC tagging), or prevent physical uptake properties to control pests in specific environments to improve agriculture and disease control.

The newest wave in genetic modification comes to humans now. Research is fast progressing on modifying human genes to avert diseases that have been identified as the causative factors. Gene therapy stands for addressing genetic deficiencies or for modulating physical processes such as beneficial protein production or control mechanisms for cancer. Advances in genetic profiling will improve our understanding and selection of therapy techniques and provide breakthroughs with significant health benefits. While cloning of humans may still be far, the use of genetic modification to treat hereditary conditions (i.e., sickle-cell anemia) through in vitro techniques or other mechanisms is more plausible.

Genetically modified "knock-out" animals (animals with selected DNA sequences removed from their genome) are providing scientists additional tools to study the effect of the removed sequence on the animal; they also enable subsequent analysis of the interaction of those functions or components with the animal's entire system. Although knockouts are not always complete, they provide another important tool to confirm or refute hypotheses regarding complex organisms.

1.2.6 DNA Microchips

Mutation or alteration in a particular gene's DNA often results in certain diseases, but this is very difficult to test because most large genes have many regions where mutations can occur. For example, researchers believe that mutations in the genes *BRCA1* and *BRCA2* cause as many as 60% of all cases of hereditary breast and ovarian cancers. But there is not one specific mutation responsible for all of these cases. Researchers have already discovered over 800 different mutations in *BRCA1* alone.

The DNA microchip is a new tool used to identify mutations in genes like *BRCA1* and *BRCA2*. The chip, which consists of a small glass plate encased in plastic, is manufactured somewhat like a computer microchip. On the surface, each chip contains thousands of short, synthetic, single-stranded DNA sequences, which together add up to the normal gene in question.

A DNA microarray (also commonly known as DNA chip or biochip) is a collection of microscopic DNA spots attached to a solid surface. Scientists use DNA microarrays to measure the expression levels of large numbers of genes simultaneously or to genotype multiple regions of a genome. Each DNA spot contains picomoles (10–12 mol) of a specific DNA sequence, known as probes (or reporters or oligos). These can be a short section of a gene or other DNA element that are used to hybridize a cDNA or cRNA (also called *antisense RNA*) sample (called *target*) under high-stringency conditions. Probe–target hybridization is usually detected and quantified by the detection of fluorophore-, silver-, or chemiluminescence-labeled targets to determine relative abundance of nucleic acid sequences in the target.

Since an array can contain tens of thousands of probes, a microarray experiment can accomplish many genetic tests in parallel. Therefore, arrays have dramatically accelerated many types of investigation. In standard microarrays, the probes are synthesized and then attached via surface engineering to a solid surface by a covalent bond to a chemical matrix (via epoxy-silane, amino-silane, lysine, polyacrylamide, or others). The solid surface can be a glass or a silicon chip (e.g., the Affymetrix® chip) or microscopic beads instead of large solid support (e.g., the Illumina® chip). Microarrays can also be constructed by the direct synthesis of oligonucleotide probes on solid surfaces. DNA arrays are different from other types of microarray only in that they either measure DNA or use DNA as part of its detection system.

DNA microarrays can be used to measure changes in the expression levels, to detect single nucleotide polymorphisms, or to genotype or targeted resequencing. The main applications of DNA microarrays are in the field of gene expression profiling, comparative genomic hybridization, gene identification (of organisms in food, mycoplasms in cell culture, or pathogens), chromatin immunoprecipitation, single nucleotide polymorphism detection, and alternative splicing detection. Another type of microarray is fusion gene microarray that can detect fusion transcripts, for example, from cancer specimens. The genome tiling arrays consist of overlapping probes designed to densely represent a genomic region of interest, sometimes as large as an entire human chromosome. The purpose is to empirically detect the expression of transcripts or alternatively splice forms, which may not have been previously known or predicted.

Microarrays can be fabricated using a variety of technologies, including printing with fine-pointed pins onto glass slides, photolithography using pre-made masks, photolithography using dynamic micromirror devices, ink-jet printing, or electrochemistry on microelectrode arrays.

1.3 MATERIALS ADVANCES

The adage that the need is the mother of invention is broadly displayed in the development of newer materials to address specific needs of technology, biotechnology being no exception. As the Industrial Era arrived, man began to process finer metals, steel and copper being one of the earliest forms that date back to the Stone Age. Ceramics also find their dating back to several millennia. Man improvised tools and utensils that he could carve or mold with limited skills and methods. Fire was the only means of working out materials, man learned very early. Excavations across the globe attest to the ingenuity of man in adapting his skills to his needs. Wood, cotton, wool, leather, and felts came to his rescue to protect him from inclement weather, and the art he learned to make pottery went into building brick homes and rain-resistant roofs over the head. Man was able to heat treat materials and otherwise weave, knit, or compress materials that last a long time until the sciences of physics and chemistry came to his rescue.

The first major breakthrough in material sciences came with the discovery of plastic—a result of polymerization of chemicals. The space program produced materials like Kevlar® and an entire industry go with it. Today, we cannot go around in a room and find dozens ol objects that could not have been possible without the discovery of plastic. A major utilization of plastics that changed bioprocessing significantly is the use of disposable systems. Over the past 20 years, we have become totally dependent on these molded pieces that we can use only once and discard. However, the use of plastics spread so quickly that it adversely affected the environment from the consumer refuse that contained an enormous quantity of plastic—it was cheap, was easily molded, and would not degrade. Environmental awareness has begun to abet the deleterious effects of plastics, and greater uses are found in building equipment, instruments, and systems from plastic that have reduced the cost of manufacturing significantly. This book contains a detailed description of the disposable systems used in bioprocessing.

1.4 NANOSCALE ADVANCES

The bioprocess engineer of tomorrow will become obsolete quickly if he or she did not keep up with the advances in nanosciences. Nanotechnology (sometimes shortened to "nanotech") is the manipulation of matter on an atomic and molecular scale. Generally, nanotechnology works with materials, devices, and other structures with at least one dimension sized from 1 to 100 nm. Quantum mechanical effects are important at this quantum-realm scale. With a variety of potential applications, nanotechnology is a key technology for the future, and governments have invested billions of dollars in its research. Through its National Nanotechnology Initiative, the United States has invested $3.7 billion. The European Union has invested $1.2 billion and Japan $750 million.

Nanotechnology is very diverse, ranging from extensions of conventional device physics to completely new approaches based upon molecular self-assembly, from developing new materials with dimensions on the nanoscale to direct control of matter on the atomic scale. Nanotechnology entails the application of fields of science as diverse as surface science, organic chemistry, molecular biology, semiconductor physics, microfabrication, and so on.

Nanotechnology is defined by the U.S. government's National Nanotechnology Initiative to be "science, engineering and technology conducted at the nanoscale, which is about 1 to 100 nanometers." The concept of nanotechnology can be attributed initially to a talk by the noted physicist Richard Feynman titled "There's Plenty of Room at the Bottom," presented at the California Instituted of Technology on December 29, 1959. Dr. Feynman envisioned a future where scientists would be able to manipulate individual atoms and molecules. The term nanotechnology was first used by Professor Norio Taniguchi in reference to ultraprecise machining in 1974. Examining the scale of nanotechnology, we can see that it corresponds to things nearly as small as a single atom, Francium has a diameter of approximately 0.7 nm, on up to things nearly as large as the smallest cellular organism, *Mycoplasma* are approximately 200 nm in length.

Nanotechnology introduces interesting behaviors in fields ranging from chemistry to biology. For instance, the flagellum, the appendage some bacteria use for locomotion, is on the nanoscale in size. Because the flagellum is on the nanoscale, the Reynolds number (which describes the ratio of inertial and viscous forces) reduces to near zero; indicating a viscous-dominated system. With no inertial forces, every motion is reversible and has no time dependence. This necessitates the flagellum spiral like a corkscrew. This corkscrew motion is reversible and allows the bacteria to propel themselves in a viscous-dominated environment, whereas a more intuitive paddle motion would result in the bacteria moving slightly in one direction and then back the same amount in the other direction.

Bioprocessing has already, and will continue to see many advances thanks to nano-technology. However, the *nano* is often applied a bit more liberally in fields associated with bioprocessing. More often, *nano* refers to anything from 1 μm to 1 nm. This slightly larger scale may not have the nuances of nanotechnology in chemistry and physics, but is still a range with great applicability to biology. Proteins, nucleic acids, and most intracellular organelles fall into this broader *nano* range. The manipulation of proteins, nucleic acids, and organelles is of far greater value to bioprocessing than the manipulation of single atoms. Already fields within bioprocessing ranging from pharmaceuticals to tissue engineering have seen great advances due to this broader *nano* technology.

1.5 BIOPROCESSING FOR CHEMICAL AND BIOLOGIC PRODUCT MANUFACTURING

Man has done well utilizing other life forms to his own advantage. From the taming of the cattle to making recombinant therapeutic proteins using the CHO cells, the history of man interacting with nature is full of great and exciting surprises, genius exploitation, and pursuit to find solutions to problems faced by mankind in nature. The first wave of this interaction began very early when man fermented food articles to make bread, wine, cheese, and yogurt long before he had any knowledge of the invisible, microbial world. The thesis that technology does not necessarily depend on science is well proven here. The next wave arrived when man learned the scientific basis of biological world and began manufacturing drugs and other essential components from biological tissues; the discovery of penicillin opened the way for this research; the process of fermentation then routinely manufactured antibiotics. The third wave of technologic and scientific break-through came in the late 1970s and 1980s when the new technology related to cell culture, fusion, bioprocessing, and genetic engineering took roots in the industry. Today, prokaryotes, eukaryotes, algae, glycophytes, and halophytes are all likely to contribute to products of the future. The techniques of DNA manipulation, monoclonal antibody preparation, tissue culture, protoplast fusion, protein engineering, immobilized enzymes, cell catalysis, antisense DNA, and so on are helping mankind find solutions to his problems, from what began with a glass of brewed grape juice that made man feel good and it is now proving good for mankind.

A bioproduct is best described by its chemical composition or structure and its function or application. Proteins, organic acids, and lipids are typical structure classes, while the application can include food and feed additives, pharmaceuticals, detergents, chemical intermediates, or agriculturally used products, for example, insecticides and herbicides. The process designer faces a dilemma in the initial stage of the development because the particular structure of the molecule causes some constraints, and also the product's function causes other constraints. The process needs to be designed around the structure and the function of the product. For example, a therapeutic protein and an industrially used enzyme might have very similar structures and might be produced by the same organism but they have totally different functions. Resulting production processes will be very different. Therefore, when discussing bioproduct classes, one has to keep in mind both the chemical structure and the final application. Organic alcohols and ketones are mainly produced in anaerobic fermentations, from inexpensive carbon-energy sources such as glucose, starchy materials, molasses, or sucrose-containing materials. Examples are the production of ethanol using *Saccharomyces* or *Zymomonas ssp.*, and acetone and butanol or *z*-propanol using *Clostridium ssp.* Organic acids are used, for instance, as intermediates or as food additives. The three major organic acids produced via a bioprocess are citric, lactic, and gluconic acid. Citric acid is produced by fermentation using *Aspergillus niger.* The gluconic acid fermentation also uses *A. niger* or *Gluconobacter suboxydans*, while lactic acid is produced via different *Lactobacillus* species. Metabolic engineering creates a new opportunity to improve the production of other organic acids, such as pyruvic acid (see Chapter 6). Amino acids are the building blocks of proteins and are connected via peptide bonds. The bioproduction of single amino acids started in the 1950s using *Corynebacterium glutamicum*; later *E. coli* was also applied. Amino acids are used as food additives (flavor enhancer, sweetener), feed additives, and in pharmaceuticals. The industrially most important amino acids are L-glutamic acid and L-lysine that are produced from molasses and starch hydrolysates, and the chemically synthesized racemic DL-methionine. Nucleic acids are used as therapeutics, for example, DNA vaccines, and in gene therapy. Short interference RNA molecules also have a large future commercial potential as therapeutics and diagnostics. Short interference RNA molecules interfere with messenger RNA and can as such be applied for the silencing of specific genes. Additionally, these molecules can also interfere with genes and suppress a gene's expression. Aptamers, another pharmaceutically interesting group of biochemicals, are small DNA, RNA, or peptide molecules that bind with high specificity and affinity to DNA, RNA, or proteins. Antibiotics with a frequent use in human and animal health are produced in fungal fermentation. Penicillin G and V (*Penicillium chrysogenum*), cephalosporin (*Cephalosporium* spp.), and streptomycin (*Streptomyces griseus*) belong to the major antibiotics. A number of vitamins are produced in bioprocesses, for example, vitamins A, C, E, and the B vitamins. *Propionibacterium* or *Pseudomonas* spp. are used to ferment glucose or molasses to obtain vitamin B_{12}, while vitamin B_2 (riboflavin) is produced by *Ashbya gossypii, Candida* spp., and genetically engineered *Bacillus subtilis. Eremothecium ashbyii* also can be used, as described in Chapter 8. Biodegradable biopolymers are plastics derived from renewable material. A common form is the polyhydroxyalkanoates accumulated as storage material in bacteria. The most common biopolymer is polyhydroxybutyrate that is produced at large scale from glucose using recombinant *E. coli.* Dextran and xanthan are industrially produced microbial polysaccharides. Xanthan is obtained from glucose or starch using the bacterium *Xanthomonas campestris* as biocatalyst. Dextran is produced from sucrose by *Leuconostoc, Acetobacter*, and other genera. Polysaccharides can be used as thickening, gelatinizing, or suspending agents in food and pharmaceuticals. Cyclodextrins are produced by enzymatic conversion of starch. Carotenoids are natural pigments (yellow or red color). Different carotenoids are produced in different microorganisms. *Blakeslea trispora*, for example, is used to obtain β-carotene; xanthophylls are produced by bacteria and algae. Here, oils are often used as carbon source. Pesticides, especially insecticides, are a relatively new group of bioproducts. The most prominent example is from *Bacillus thuringiensis*, which produces an endotoxin selectively effective against a group of insects. The world production in 2003 was around 13,000 tons. The group of lipids includes fats, oils, waxes, phospholipids, and steroids. Glycerol and fatty acids are important building blocks. Prostaglandins, leukotrienes, and thromboxane are commercially produced lipids. Proteins are characterized by four levels of structure: the primary structure (linear amino acid sequence); the secondary, hydrogen-bonded structure (alpha helix and beta sheet); the tertiary structure (folding pattern of hydrogen-bonded and disulfide-bonded structures); and the quaternary structure (formation of homo- and hetero-multimeric complexes by individual protein molecules). Proteins are of interest predominantly because of their function that depends on a correctly formed structure. However, there are an increasing number of performance proteins of interest because of their physical properties. Proteins have two major applications, as industrial enzymes and as therapeutic and diagnostic proteins. Industrial enzymes are often produced from inexpensive carbon sources by filamentous fungi, such as *Aspergillus*, *Fusarium*, *Pichia*, and *Saccharomyces ssp.*, and bacteria, mainly *E. coli*. Proteases, lipases, amylases, and cellulases are produced in large amounts at low prices and are applied as washing detergents and in the food, feed, leather, and textile industry. The emergence of the biofuels industry will have a major impact on the need for more of these enzymes at large scale. Therapeutic and diagnostic proteins are of higher value but are produced in very small amounts, using mainly mammalian cell culture but also bacteria and fungi. They require complex downstream processing. Typical groups of therapeutic proteins are vaccines, monoclonal antibodies, and hormones such as insulin, glucagon, and the human growth hormone. Cytokines are a diverse group of regulatory proteins. From this group, interferons are used to treat autoimmune diseases and cancer; interleukins are used to treat asthma, cancer, and HIV treatment; and erythropoietin is used as a growth factor. A large but special field of bioprocessing is the bioleaching of metals, mainly copper, gold, and uranium from low-grade ores and mining wastes using acidophilic, chemolithotrophic iron- and sulfur-oxidizing microbes. The bacteria used for biomining, such as *Thiobacillus* and *Acidothiobacillus*, extract the metals from large heaps of sulfidic ore, for example, several hundred thousand tons of copper per year.

To focus more on the immediate tasks entrusted to a bioprocess engineer, we need to review the most common manufacturing processes.

1.5.1 Alcoholic Beverage

Alcoholic beverages include any fermented liquor, such as wine, beer, or distilled spirit, that contains ethyl alcohol, or ethanol (CH_3CH_2OH), as an intoxicating agent. Alcoholic beverages are fermented from the sugars in fruits, berries, grains, and other ingredients such as plant saps, tubers, honey, and milk and may be distilled to reduce the original watery liquid to a liquid of much greater alcoholic strength. Beer is the best-known member of the malt family of alcoholic beverages, which also includes ale, stout, porter, and malt liquor. It is made from malt, corn, rice, and hops. Beers range in alcoholic content from about 2% to about 8%. Wine is made by fermenting the juices of grapes or other fruits such as apples (cider), cherries, berries, or plums. Winemaking begins with the harvest of the fruit, the juice of which is fermented in large vats under rigorous temperature control. When fermentation is complete, the mixture is filtered, aged, and bottled. Natural, or unfortified, grape wines generally contain from 8% to 14% alcohol; these include wines such as Bordeaux, Burgundy, Chianti, and Sauterne. Fortified wines, to which alcohol or brandy has been added, contain 18%–21% alcohol; such wines include sherry, port, and muscatel.

The making of distilled spirits begins with the mashes of grains, fruits, or other ingredients. The resultant fermented liquid is heated until the alcohol and flavorings vaporize and can be drawn off, cooled, and condensed back into a liquid. Water remains behind and is discarded. The concentrated liquid, called a distilled beverage, includes liquors such as whiskey, gin, vodka, rum, brandy, and liqueurs, or cordials. They range in alcoholic content usually from 40% to 50%, though higher or lower concentrations are found.

1.5.2 Biofuel

Biofuel consists of two major categories of fuels—bioethanol and biodiesel; therefore, there are two different procedures of producing biofuel from biomass. The methods followed have a strong impact on the end results that are achieved. There are two key reactions that are involved in the production of bioethanol, one is hydrolysis and the other is fermentation.

The traditional way of producing bioethanol would be to mix sugar, water, and yeast bacteria, which are then allowed to ferment in warm environment. Gradually the mixture becomes a liquid that has an approximate of 15% alcohol. As and how the alcohol percentage increases, the yeast consumes itself in the process and dies out eventually which stops the process altogether. Then, the liquid mash that is created is distilled and purified to get approximately 99.5% bioethanol. Thus, this process of fermentation is a series of chemical reactions wherein the simple sugars are converted into ethanol. Yeast or bacteria, which feed on the sugars, cause the reaction and thus fermentation occurs. Ethanol and carbon dioxide are produced as and how the yeast consumes the sugar. There is a simple formula that represents the process of simplified fermentation reaction, which is as follows:

$$C_6H_{12}O_6 \left(glucose\right) \rightarrow 2CH_3CH_2OH \left(ethanol\right) + 2CO_2 \left(carbon\ dioxide\right) \tag{1.1}$$

In this kind of production process, bioethanol is derived from a variety of sugar and starch-rich crops, which includes grain, corn, sugarcane, and sugar beet. The process of traditional production of this kind of substitute fuel is a well-known and easy process that only consists of the fermentation of the sugar, similar to the process used to prepare beverages like whisky or vodka. The scale of production is in hundreds of thousands of liters and one can get a good view of these traveling through the Napa Valley in California.

There is another process of making bioethanol wherein bioethanol can be derived from materials that have lignocellulose, which is primarily a strengthening substance found in the tissues of woody plant such as straw, cornstalks, wood chippings, or other organic materials that are often considered waste. Once fully developed, this method will reduce the cost of bioethanol while preserving the use of crops for food purpose as well as reduce the carbon dioxide footprint. In this process, the biomass goes through a step that reduces the size of the material so that it is easier to handle and to make the production process more efficient. It is much like the grinding process that the agricultural residues go through so that the particles have uniform size.

The next step is to treat the biomass in which the hemicellulose fraction of the biomass is broken down into simple sugars. It happens with the help of a simple chemical reaction called hydrolysis, which occurs when dilute sulfuric acid is mixed with the biomass feedstock. In this reaction, the complex chains of sugars in the hemicellulose are broken and that results in the releasing of simple sugars. The complex hemicellulose sugars are transformed into a mix of soluble five-carbon sugars, xylose and arabinose, and soluble six-carbon sugars, mannose and galactose. Small portion of the cellulose is also transformed into glucose. There are few enzymes that are used like the cellulase enzymes, which hydrolyze the cellulose part of the biomass. These enzymes are either produced in the last-mentioned step or are to be bought.

After the hydrolysis of cellulose, the glucose and pentose are fermented which gives "ethanol broth" as an output. A final step of dehydration removes the excess water from ethanol, and this step is therefore called *ethanol recovery*. Then, the other by-products that include products like lignin are used to produce electricity that is required for the production of ethanol. It is anticipated that within the next 5–10 years, this process will be widely used and the future bioprocess engineering needs will rise sharply in this field.

1.5.3 Metabolic Manufacturing of Chemicals and Drugs

A good example of how the metabolites in a bioprocess end up yielding a product of use is the production of alcohol wherein carbohydrates are consumed to produce alcohol and carbon dioxide. One of the earliest exploitation of metabolic pathways was the manufacture of antibiotics like penicillin wherein a fungus produces this antibiotic in its natural growth cycle. Since then, thousands of combinations of living organisms and chemicals added to the nutrition resulted in fine chemicals and drugs. The manufacturing process is a typical upstream reaction where the biomass is grown under optimal conditions and the secreted product or the product contained within the body of the living organisms is removed and purified. The scale of production for most of these systems is into thousands of liters, and since the end product is generally stable, these systems provide many low-cost opportunity of purifying them.

1.5.4 Recombinant Manufacturing of Drugs

With the production of insulin using genetically modified bacteria, the science of recombinant manufacturing has become the most significant discovery. The manufacturing process of this technique is similar to all other upstream and downstream processes except that the living organisms have been genetically modified to include human genes. The bioprocess engineer is not likely to be part of the team constructing the organism but from this point forward, it is a standard manufacturing process, with one significant caveat—the disposition of the living organisms at the end of the process. Contrary to a popular belief, the genetically modified organisms are generally not harmful to man or the environment as they are unable to survive in nature. A good example is that of the CHO cells—they are pretty innocuous, modified, or unmodified and there are no specific requirements of decontaminating the culture. The same holds true of some non-pathogenic bacteria if they are unable to survive. The National Institute of Health provides a list of organisms that need specific decontamination and also the level of manufacturing that makes it optional or mandatory. These details are provided in Chapter 11.

The manufacturing systems are scaled to thousands of liters, the largest being around 100,000 L used by a firm in Korea. However, with improved yields from better-designed organisms, the trend is shifting toward smaller vats for fermentation. The fact that the yields from several batches can be combined makes it easier to utilize smaller apparatus. The developments in the downstream processing, more particularly the purification of the products, have also improved the finished yields, provided higher purity products and thus reduced the cost of manufacturing. Generally, the cost of manufacturing of a monoclonal antibody using 5,000 L or higher volumes is about \$300–\$400/g; this compares to \$3,000–\$5,000 for cytokines in bacterial cultures and even \$50–\$100,000/g for some molecules in mammalian cells. However, the cost of manufacturing should be reviewed in a proper perspective of their dosing. A monoclonal antibody may require a dose of 25–50 mg, whereas a cytokine produced in a mammalian cell may have a dose in micrograms. Insulin is one good example where the large patient dose makes it a very large manufacturing operation and as a result only a handful (no more than 3–4) companies around the world produce commercial, grade insulin.

1.6 ECONOMIC PREDICTIONS AND CAREERS IN BIOPROCESS ENGINEERING

Trained, qualified bioprocess engineers are always in big demand; the roles they play include the following:

- Develop a process for newly discovered technology for proof of principle and commercial production
- Optimize the process for cost-effectiveness as well as regulatory compliance
- Scale up process to desired commercial level
- Manufacture products in upstream and downstream systems
- Provide products ready for use on a repeated batch uniformity

One can see clearly the commercial importance of the profession. However, to be an efficient engineer, the qualifications must be periodically reviewed for compliance with the changing needs, even when in a continuing job situation. New methods, equipment, instruments, and trends arise almost every day. A company will not generally change a process; once it has been established, there is always a need to be ready for changes. This field of business is called *benchmarking*; we need to be fully aware of what others are doing. An interesting example comes from the use of CHO cells in a roller bottle wherein they adhere to the wall of the bottle to express recombinant proteins; developed about 30 years ago, the process yielded such blockbuster drugs as erythropoietin with sales into billions of dollars; the inventor of the drug, Amgen (Thousand Oaks, CA), used this tedious and regulatory-unfriendly process that required roller bottles in hundreds of thousands running simultaneously to provide the large worldwide need. Whereas Amgen developed a bioreactor process for its newer molecules, the archaic process of using the roller bottles continued because the cost of changing the regulatory filings will be prohibitive. There being no other option, the company instead chose to shut down the manufacturing of erythropoietin and instead began promoting the newer generation drugs used for the same purpose. Nevertheless, erythropoietin remains one of the most desired drugs and now the biosimilar manufacturers have taken it over but they are using much more efficient bioreactor systems that do not require large capital investment and also allow use of CHO cells that do not require animal components.

One of newer advances in the field of manufacturing is the use of disposable systems. Whereas most of the larger companies are still using fixed stainless steel systems, the newer companies are more likely to use a disposable system; it is for this reason that we have included a detailed chapter on the use of disposable systems (Chapter 11).

1.7 SKILLS NEEDED FOR FUTURE BIOPROCESS ENGINEERS

The best way to assess the marketable skills in any field is to review what the market is requiring today. The broad spectrum of fields of biotechnology that feeds the needs of the future bioprocess engineers teaches us that this is indeed a dynamic field. Many disciplines of biotechnology were not even discovered just a couple of decades ago, for example, the science of recombinant manufacturing of proteins, one of the most promising field of new job opportunities did not exist 20 years ago. There is always a lag between what the market needs and how we are training the manpower; it is when we keep a close tab on the changing dynamics of the technical fields that we are able to provide the manpower of the future.

A survey toward the end of 2012 showed that there were over a thousand jobs available for senior bioprocess engineers. Given below would be a typical description of the position and the qualifications required.

A successful candidate should have a PhD degree or master's degree with >3 years academic and/or industrial laboratory experience in multiple areas related to chemical engineering, fermentation, heat/mass transport, bioprocessing, and automated process development. An incumbent should be entrepreneurial minded with experience/understanding of one or more of the following areas: fermentation, microbial cell banking, medium development and optimization, metabolic network analysis, continuous culture operation, high-throughput screening and Department of Energy techniques, biostatistics, formulation, purification, analytical chemistry, molecular biology techniques, microbiology, and automated process development. He or she should have deep technical experience and a track record of success in previous endeavors within relevant areas. Additionally, the bioprocess engineer should have significant interest in team-based innovation, have strategic collaboration experience, have a strong technical and industrial network, and be well respected by his or her peers. A successful candidate will be driven by the ability of solving complex multidisciplinary problems with an evolving data set and solution space.

A bioprocess engineer should possess excellent leadership and interpersonal skills and have demonstrated a successful track record delivering against challenging commitments. He or she should have deep scientific grounding and aptitude and have a high degree of scientific integrity. The bioprocess engineer should be confident, be execution focused, be team oriented, and have the ability to motivate others.

The qualifications described above are for a mid-level recruitment; however, for a starting position as well as even a higher-level position, there will be little difference in the technical skills required; the main difference is the years of experience and the management capabilities.

We have tried to design this book for the current and future bioprocess engineers (with 10 years horizon); many techniques and technologies that were considered primary for bioprocess engineers of the yore have been reduced in emphasis or deleted; these have been replaced by the future skill sets needed.

Briefly, a prospective bioprocess engineer should, at a minimum, be able to

- Fully understand the biological systems that drive the industry, from metabolite focus to genetically modified systems.
- Collect, present, and analyze data from all types of experiments required for scale up and optimization of processes.
- Suggest technological means to convert a laboratory-scale process into an industrial-scale system.
- Appreciate and understand the need for regulatory compliance in the manufacture of biological products intended for humans.
- Apply and understand various common unit operations and the mathematics involved in applying them to an industrial process.
- Scale up an upstream and downstream process.
- Provide validation documentation for all processes.
- Use computers fluently, from data collection, analysis, and interpretation to operating various engineering drawing software and flowchart presentation.
- Prepare and maintain records and communication paperwork methodically and for presentation to the regulatory authorities during audits.

APPENDIX 1A: TIME LINE OF BIOTECHNOLOGY DEVELOPMENT

8000 BC

Humans domesticated crops and livestock.
Potatoes first cultivated for food.

4000–2000 BC

Biotechnology was first used to leaven bread and ferment beer, using yeasts (Egypt).
Production of cheese and fermentation of wine (Sumeria, China, and Egypt).
Babylonians controlled date palm breeding by selectively pollinating female trees with pollen from certain male trees.

2500–2000 BC

The ancient Egyptians made wine using fermentation techniques based on an understanding of the microbiological processes that occur in the absence of oxygen.

Egyptians also applied fermentation technologies to make dough rise during bread making. Due in part to this application, there were more than 50 varieties of bread in Egypt more than 4,000 years ago.

In wetter parts of the Nile valley, Egyptians also bred geese and cattle to meet their society's nutritional and dietary needs.

1750 BC

The Sumerians brew beer.

500 BC

The Chinese used moldy soybean curds (first recorded antibiotic usage) as an antibiotic to treat boils.

AD 100

First insecticide: powdered chrysanthemums (China).

1322

An Arab chieftain first used artificial insemination to produce superior horses.

1492

Beginning with his first visit to the Americas in 1492, Christopher Columbus and other explorers introduced corn, native to the Americas, to the rest of the world, and European growers adapted the plant to their unique growing conditions. Spanish navigators also returned with potatoes, which are native to the Andes in South America. Two centuries after their European introduction, potatoes were a staple in Ireland, Germany, and other European countries.

1590

Janssen invented the microscope.

1663

Hooke discovered the existence of the cell.

1675

Leeuwenhoek discovered bacteria.

1761

Koelreuter reported successful crossbreeding of crop plants in different species.

1797

Jenner inoculated a child with a viral vaccine to protect him from smallpox.

1830

Proteins discovered.

1833

First enzyme discovered and isolated.

1835–1855

Schleiden and Schwann proposed that all organisms are composed of cells, and Virchow declared, "Every cell arises from a cell."

1857

Pasteur proposed that microbes cause fermentation.

1859

Charles Darwin published a book on the theory of evolution by natural selection. The concept of carefully selecting parents and culling the variable progeny greatly influenced plant and animal breeders in the late 1800s despite their ignorance of genetics.

1864

In 1864, French chemist Louis Pasteur developed the process named after him and known today as pasteurization, which uses heat to destroy harmful microorganisms in products. The products are then sealed airtight for safety. Pasteur's scientific breakthrough enhanced quality of life, allowing products such as milk to be transported without spoiling.

1865

Science of genetics began: Austrian monk Gregor Mendel studied garden peas and discovered that genetic traits are passed from parents to offspring in a predictable way—the laws of heredity.

1870–1890

Using Darwin's theory, plant breeders crossbreed cotton, developing hundreds of
varieties with superior qualities.
Farmers first inoculated fields with nitrogen-fixing bacteria to improve yields.
William James Beal produced the first experimental corn hybrid in the laboratory.

1877

A technique for staining and identifying bacteria was developed by Koch in 1878.
The first centrifuge was developed by Laval in 1879.
Fleming discovered chromatin, the rod-like structures inside the cell nucleus that
later came to be called *chromosomes*.

1900

Drosophila (fruit flies) was used in the early studies of genes.
Mendel's work rediscovered.

1902

The term *immunology* first appeared.

1906

The term *genetics* was introduced.

1911

The first cancer-causing virus was discovered by Rous.
Alfred Sturtevant created the first *Drosophila* gene map in 1911.

1914

Bacteria were used to treat sewage for the first time in Manchester, England.

1915

Phages, or bacterial viruses, were discovered.

1919

First use of the word *biotechnology* in print.

1920

The human growth hormone was discovered by Evans and Long.

1926

In the early twentieth century, agricultural expert Henry Wallace applied the principles of hybridization to develop new, higher-yielding seeds. Wallace went on to apply his scientific innovation to a business model as one of the early leaders of Pioneer Hi-Bred International, Inc., today a DuPont business. A precursor to more advanced cross-breeding and eventually biotechnology, hybridization is the process of crossing plant varieties to produce crops with more favorable traits—or combining genes from two or more varieties of a plant species to produce improved seed. For example, a breeder might eliminate a plant's thorns by cross-breeding with a thornless variety. The often imprecise process of traditional plant breeding took years to control for desired traits.

1928

Penicillin was discovered as an antibiotic by Alexander Fleming.
A small-scale test of formulated *Bacillus thuringiensis* (Bt) for corn borer control began in Europe. Commercial production of this biopesticide began in France in 1938.
Karpechenko crossed radishes and cabbages, creating fertile offspring between plants of different genera.
Laibach first used embryo rescue to obtain hybrids from wide crosses in crop plants—known today as *hybridization*.

1930

U.S. Congress passed the Plant Patent Act, enabling the products of plant breeding to be patented.

1933

Hybrid corn, developed by Henry Wallace in the 1920s, was commercialized. Growing hybrid corn eliminated the option of saving seeds. The remarkable yields outweighed the increased costs of annual seed purchases, and by 1945, hybrid corn accounted for 78% of U.S.-grown corn.

1938

The term *molecular biology* was coined.

1940

American Oswald Avery demonstrated that DNA is the *transforming factor* and is the material of genes.

1941

The term *genetic engineering* was first used by Danish microbiologist A. Jost in a lecture on reproduction in yeast at the technical institute in Lwow, Poland.

1942

The electron microscope was used to identify and characterize a bacteriophage—a virus that infects bacteria.
Penicillin was mass-produced in microbes.

1944

DNA was proven to carry genetic information—Avery et al.
Waksman isolated streptomycin, an effective antibiotic for tuberculosis.
First successful IVF of an immature egg.
Large-scale manufacture of penicillin was achieved.

1946

Discovery that genetic material from different viruses can be combined to form a new type of virus, an example of genetic recombination.
Recognizing the threat posed by loss of genetic diversity, the U.S. Congress provided funds for systematic and extensive plant collection, preservation, and introduction.

1947

McClintock discovered transposable elements, or *jumping genes*, in corn.

1949

Pauling showed that sickle-cell anemia is a *molecular disease* resulting from a mutation in the protein molecule hemoglobin.

1950–1952

Artificial insemination of livestock using frozen semen (a longtime dream of farmers) was successfully accomplished.

1952

Cloning of frog embryonic cells by nuclear transfer resulted in the birth of tadpoles. Enzymes used in manufacturing of detergents.

1953

The scientific journal *Nature* published James Watson and Francis Crick's manuscript describing the double helical structure of DNA, which marked the beginning of the modern era of genetics. People did not know where genes lived until DNA was *discovered* or understood in the early 1950s. British scientist Rosalind Franklin's DNA research formed the foundation for James Watson and Francis Crick's 1953 discovery of the structure of DNA, the ladder-like double helix. Watson and Crick perfected the DNA's structural model that Franklin explored earlier.

Understanding DNA was essential to the exploration of biotechnology, cells are the basic unit of living matter in all organisms, and DNA carries the information determining what traits a cell will have. With biotechnology, scientists could express favorable traits by lending DNA from one organism to another. From the beginning, scientists saw the potential for new drugs designed to help the body do what it could not do on its own, or crops able to protect themselves from disease. For example, through biotechnology-developed built-in protection, researchers have developed corn plants resistant to rootworm, beetle-like pests that, in early larval stages, feed on the plant's roots. Every year, corn rootworm costs around $1 billion to farmers.

1955

An enzyme involved in the synthesis of a nucleic acid was isolated for the first time.

1956

Kornberg discovered the enzyme DNA polymerase I, leading to an understanding of how DNA is replicated.

The fermentation process was perfected in Japan.

1958

Sickle-cell anemia was shown to occur due to a change of a single amino acid.

DNA was made in a test tube for the first time.

1959

Systemic fungicides were developed.

The steps in protein biosynthesis were delineated.

Also in the 1950s

Discovery of interferons.
First synthetic antibiotic.

1960

Exploiting base pairing, hybrid DNA–RNA molecules were created.
Messenger RNA was discovered.

1961

USDA registered first biopesticide: *Bacillus thuringiensis* or Bt.

1963

New wheat varieties developed by Norman Borlaug increased yields by 70%.

1964

The International Rice Research Institute in the Philippines started the Green Revolution with new strains of rice that double the yield of previous strains if given sufficient fertilizer.

1965

Harris and Watkins successfully fuse mouse and human cells.

1966

The genetic code was cracked, demonstrating that a sequence of three nucleotide bases (a codon) determines each of the 20 amino acids. (Two more amino acids have since been discovered.)

1967

The first automatic protein sequencer was perfected.

1969

An enzyme was synthesized in vitro for the first time.

1970

Norman Borlaug received the Nobel Peace Prize (see 1963).

Discovery of restriction enzymes that cut and splice genetic material, opening the way for gene cloning.

1971

First complete synthesis of a gene.

1972

The DNA composition of humans was discovered to be 99% similar to that of chimpanzees and gorillas.

Recombinant DNA molecules were first produced.

Genentech, the first commercial biotech company was founded.

Initial work with embryo transfer.

1973

Stanley Cohen and Herbert Boyer perfected techniques to cut and paste DNA (using restriction enzymes and ligases) and reproduced the new DNA in bacteria.

The National Institutes of Health formed a Recombinant DNA Advisory Committee to oversee recombinant genetic research.

In 1973, researchers Stanley Cohen and Herbert Boyer were the first to apply this technique. Working to help people living with diabetes, they lifted genetic materials from one organism's DNA and copied them into another organism's genetic material. This is the story of insulin.

The human body produced insulin to regulate blood sugar levels. Diabetes occurred when the body does not produce insulin or cannot produce enough insulin. People with diabetes often need injections of insulin, which the doctors first provided the patients through supplies taken from pigs and cows.

However, scientists did not know the long-term effects of having animal insulin in your body. In 1978, Boyer was able to take pieces of human DNA and isolate a gene for insulin using biotechnology. He then inserted it into bacteria, which allowed the gene to reproduce a larger quantity of insulin for diabetics. This scientific advancement vastly improved the quality of life for many people living with diabetes and guaranteed their safety.

1975

Government first urged to develop guidelines for regulating experiments in recombinant DNA: Asilomar Conference, California.

The first monoclonal antibodies were produced.

1976

The tools of recombinant DNA were first applied to a human inherited disorder.
Molecular hybridization was used for the prenatal diagnosis of alpha thalassemia.
Yeast genes were expressed in *E. coli* bacteria.
The sequence of base pairs for a specific gene was determined (A, C, T, G).
First guidelines for recombinant DNA experiments released: National Institutes of
    Health–Recombinant DNA Advisory Committee.

1976–1977

DNA sequencing methods developed.

1977

First expression of human gene in bacteria.
Procedures developed for rapidly sequencing long sections of DNA using
    electrophoresis.

1978

High-level structure of virus first identified.
Recombinant human insulin first produced.
North Carolina scientists showed that it is possible to introduce specific mutations at
    specific sites in a DNA molecule.
Thirumalachar issued patent for a process for the production of insulin by geneti-
    cally transformed fungal cells.

1979

Human growth hormone first synthesized.

Also in the 1970s

Discovery of polymerases.
Techniques for rapid sequencing of nucleotides perfected.
Gene targeting.
RNA splicing.

1980

The U.S. Supreme Court, in the landmark case *Diamond v. Chakrabarty*, approved the
    principle of patenting recombinant life forms, which allowed the Exxon oil com-
    pany to patent an oil-eating microorganism.
The U.S. patent for gene cloning was awarded to Cohen and Boyer.

The first gene-synthesizing machines were developed.

Researchers successfully introduced a human gene—one that codes for the protein interferon—into a bacterium.

Cohen got a patent for a process for producing biologically functional chimeras.

Nobel Prize in chemistry was awarded for creation of the first recombinant molecule to Berg, Gilbert, and Sanger.

1981

Scientists at Ohio University produced the first transgenic animals by transferring genes from other animals into mice.

Chinese scientist became the first to clone a fish—a golden carp.

1982

Applied Biosystems, Inc., introduced the first commercial gas phase protein sequencer, dramatically reducing the amount of protein sample needed for sequencing.

First recombinant DNA vaccine for livestock developed.

First biotech drug approved by FDA: human insulin produced in genetically modified bacteria.

First genetic transformation of a plant cell: petunia.

1983

The polymerase chain reaction (PCR) technique was conceived. PCR, which uses heat and enzymes to make unlimited copies of genes and gene fragments, later became a major tool in biotech research and product development worldwide.

The first genetic transformation of plant cells by TI plasmids was performed.

The first artificial chromosome was synthesized.

The first genetic markers for specific inherited diseases were found.

First whole plant grown from biotechnology: petunia.

First proof that modified plants passed their new traits to offspring: petunia.

Axel got a patent for a process of inserting DNA into eukaryotic cells and for producing proteinaceous materials.

1984

The DNA fingerprinting technique was developed.

A sheep was cloned from early embryos—first verified cloning of a mammal by the process of nuclear transfer.

The first genetically engineered vaccine was developed.

The entire genome of the human immunodeficiency virus was cloned and sequenced.

1985

Genetic markers found for kidney disease and cystic fibrosis.

Genetic fingerprinting entered as evidence in a courtroom.

Transgenic plants resistant to insects, viruses, and bacteria were field-tested for the first time.

The NIH approved guidelines for performing gene-therapy experiments in humans.

The polymerase chain reaction (PCR) was invented.

1986

First recombinant vaccine for humans: hepatitis B.

First anticancer drug produced through biotech: interferon.

The U.S. government published the *Coordinated Framework for Regulation of Biotechnology*, establishing more stringent regulations for rDNA organisms than for those produced with traditional genetic modification techniques.

A University of California–Berkeley chemist described how to combine antibodies and enzymes (abzymes) to create pharmaceuticals.

The first field tests of transgenic plants (tobacco) were conducted.

The Environmental Protection Agency approved the release of the first transgenic crop—gene-altered tobacco plants.

The Organization of Economic Cooperation and Development (OECD) Group of National Experts on Safety in Biotechnology stated: "Genetic changes from rDNA techniques will often have inherently greater predictability compared to traditional techniques" and "risks associated with rDNA organisms may be assessed in generally the same way as those associated with non-rDNA organisms."

First automated DNA sequencing instrument was developed.

1987

First approval for field test of modified food plants: virus-resistant tomatoes.

Frostban, a genetically altered bacterium that inhibits frost formation on crop plants, was field tested on strawberry and potato plants in California, the first authorized outdoor tests of a recombinant bacterium.

1988

Harvard molecular geneticists were awarded the first U.S. patent for a genetically altered animal—a transgenic mouse.

A patent for a process to make bleach-resistant protease enzymes to use in detergents was awarded.

Congress funded the Human Genome Project, a massive effort to map and sequence the human genetic code as well as the genomes of other species.

1989

First approval for field test of modified cotton: insect-protected (Bt) cotton.
Plant Genome Project began.
Pre-implantation genetic diagnosis (PGD) was performed for the first time to identify X-linked diseases.

Also in the 1980s

Studies of DNA used to determine evolutionary history.
Recombinant DNA animal vaccine approved for use in Europe.
Use of microbes in oil spill cleanup: bioremediation technology.
Ribozymes and retinoblastomas identified.

1990

Chy-Max™, an artificially produced form of the chymosin enzyme for cheese making, was introduced. It was the first product of recombinant DNA technology in the U.S. food supply.
The Human Genome Project—an international effort to map all the genes in the human body—was launched.
The first experimental gene therapy treatment was performed successfully on a 4-year-old girl suffering from an immune disorder.
The first transgenic dairy cow—used to produce human milk proteins for infant formula—was created.
First insect-protected corn: Bt corn.
First food product of biotechnology approved in the United Kingdom: modified yeast.
First field test of a genetically modified vertebrate: trout.

1992

American and British scientists unveiled a technique for testing embryos in vitro for genetic abnormalities such as cystic fibrosis and hemophilia.
The FDA declared that transgenic foods are *not inherently dangerous* and do not require special regulation.
American and British scientists unveiled a technique for testing embryos in vitro for genetic abnormalities such as cystic fibrosis and hemophilia.
Intracytoplasmic sperm injection (ICSI) was developed to assist in cases of severe male infertility.

1993

Merging two smaller trade associations created the Biotechnology Industry Organization (BIO).

1994

First FDA approval for a whole food produced through biotechnology: Flavr Savr tomato.

The first breast cancer gene was discovered.

Approval of recombinant version of human DNase, which broke down protein accumulation in the lungs of CF patients.

BST commercialized as POSILAC bovine somatotropin. The Flavr Savr tomato—the first genetically engineered whole food approved by the FDA was on the market.

1995

The first baboon-to-human bone marrow transplant was performed on an auto-immune deficiency syndrome patient.

The first full gene sequence of a living organism other than a virus was completed, for the bacterium *Haemophilus influenzae.*

Gene therapy, immune system modulation, and recombinantly produced antibodies entered the clinic in the war against cancer.

1996

The discovery of a gene associated with Parkinson's disease provided an important new avenue of research into the cause and potential treatment of the debilitating neurological ailment.

Monsanto's first plant biotechnology products (Roundup Ready Soy and anola and Bollgard Cotton) planted commercially.

"Dolly" the sheep was the first successful clone from an adult mammalian cell conceived through the process of nuclear transfer.

1997

First animal cloned from an adult cell: a sheep named Dolly in Scotland.

First weed- and insect-resistant biotech crops commercialized: Roundup Ready® soybeans and Bollgard® insect protected cotton.

Biotech crops grown commercially on nearly 5 million acres worldwide: Argentina, Australia, Canada, China, Mexico, and the United States.

A group of Oregon researchers claimed to have cloned two Rhesus monkeys.

A new DNA technique combined PCR, DNA chips, and a computer program providing a new tool in the search for disease causing genes.

1998

University of Hawaii scientists cloned three generations of mice from nuclei of adult ovarian cumulus cells.

Human embryonic stem cell lines were established.

Scientists at Japan's Kinki University cloned eight identical calves using cells taken from a single adult cow.

The first complete animal genome, for the *C. elegans* worm, was sequenced.

A rough draft of the human genome map was produced, showing the locations of more than 30,000 genes.

Five Southeast Asian countries formed a consortium to develop disease-resistant papayas.

Also in the 1990s

First conviction using genetic fingerprinting in the United Kingdom.

Discovery that hereditary colon cancer is caused by defective DNA repair gene.

Recombinant rabies vaccine tested in raccoons.

Biotechnology-based biopesticide approved for sale in the United States.

Patents issued for mice with specific transplanted genes.

First European patent on a transgenic animal issued for transgenic mouse sensitive to carcinogens.

Isolation of gene that clearly participates in the normal process of regulating weight.

Breast cancer susceptibility genes cloned.

Biotechnology Industry Organization formed.

One-step fermentation production process for riboflavin engineered.

2000

First complete map of a plant genome developed: *Arabidopsis thaliana.*

Biotech crops grown on 108.9 million acres in 13 countries.

Golden rice announcement allowed the technology to be available to developing countries in hopes of improving the health of undernourished people and preventing some forms of blindness.

First biotech crop field-tested in Kenya: virus-resistant sweet potato.

Rough draft of the human genome sequence was announced.

First complete map of the genome of a food plant completed: rice.

Chinese National Hybrid Rice Research and Development Center researchers reported developing a *super rice* that could produce double the yield of normal rice.

Complete DNA sequencing of the agriculturally important bacteria, *Sinorhizobium meliloti*, a nitrogen-fixing species, and *Agrobacterium tumefaciens*, a plant pest.

A single gene from *Arabidopsis* inserted into tomato plants to create the first crop able to grow in salty water and soil.

RNA interference (RNAi) identified.

First report of human embryos cloned from a body cell (developed to early six-cell stage).

Targeted gene-based therapeutic Gleevec approved by FDA for leukemia treatment.

Biometric identification systems for airport security and border controls.

2002

The first draft of a functional map of the yeast proteome, an entire network of protein complexes and their interactions, was completed. A map of the yeast genome was published in 1996.

International consortia sequenced the genomes of the parasite that causes malaria and the species of mosquito that transmits the parasite.

The draft version of the complete map of the human genome was published, and the first part of the Human Genome Project came to an end ahead of schedule and under budget.

Scientists made great progress in elucidating the factors that control the differentiation of stem cells, identifying over 200 genes that are involved in the process.

Biotech crops grown on 145 million acres in 16 countries, a 12% increase in acreage grown in 2001. More than one-quarter (27%) of the global acreage was grown in nine developing countries.

Researchers announced successful results for a vaccine against cervical cancer, the first demonstration of a preventative vaccine for a type of cancer.

Scientists completed the draft sequence of the most important pathogen of rice, a fungus that destroys enough rice to feed 60 million people annually. By combining an understanding of the genomes of the fungus and rice, scientists will elucidate the molecular basis of the interactions between the plant and the pathogen.

Scientists were forced to rethink their view of RNA when they discovered how important small pieces of RNA are in controlling many cell functions.

Cattle cloned for commercial purpose.

Cargill Dow introduced 100% renewable bioplastic onto the market, produced in prototype biorefinery.

2003

First synthetic bacteriophage. Hamilton Smith et al. of the Institute of Biological Energy Alternatives (Rockville, MD) published their paper on the creation of first bacteriophage from synthetic oligonucleotides. This research revolutionized the field of biotechnology, raising serious concerns about biological warfare hazards.

FDA reorganized its biological division taking all recombinant drugs from Center for Biologics Research and Evaluation (CBER) to CDER; FDA also issued guidelines on comparability protocols for biologicals starting a system that will eventually result in the approval of biogeneric products in the United States.

Completed version of the human genome published.

Virus genome synthesized from scratch

2004

FDA refused to accept biogeneric application for somatropin by Sandoz.

FDA holded its first public hearing and opened forum for discussion of *follow-on* biologic products. BioPartners filed biogeneric application for interferon in Europe; it was accepted for review as *biosimilar* product.

2010

Biologics Price Competition and Innovation Act of 2009 (BPCI Act).

The BPCI Act of 2009 was originally sponsored and introduced on June 26, 2007, by Senator Edward Kennedy (D-MA). It was formally passed under the Patient Protection and Affordable Care Act (PPAC Act), signed into law by President Barack Obama on March 23, 2010. The BPCI Act was an amendment to the Public Health Service Act (PHS Act) to create an abbreviated approval pathway for biological products that are demonstrated to be highly similar (biosimilar) to a Food and Drug Administration (FDA) approved biological product. The BPCI Act was similar, conceptually, to the Drug Price Competition and Patent Term Restoration Act of 1984 (also referred to as the *Hatch–Waxman Act*), which created biological drug approval through the Federal Food, Drug, and Cosmetic Act (FFD&C Act). The BPCI Act aligned with the FDA's longstanding policy of permitting appropriate reliance on what is already known about a drug, thereby saving time and resources and avoiding unnecessary duplication of human or animal testing.

FDA approved the first generic enoxaparin injection without requiring clinical trials on July 23, 2010; the Sanofi application was based on carbohydrate characterization technology developed by Momenta.

2011

First successful artificially grown organ implanted in humans.

2012

FDA issued draft guidelines for biosimilar biological products.

Therapeutic Proteins International received the first U.S. patent for combined processing of upstream and downstream engineering together in a flexible plastic bag.

Therapeutic Proteins International produced the first bacterial proteins, GCSF, in a flexible disposable plastic bag.

2

Introduction to Molecular Biology

LEARNING OBJECTIVES

1. Understand the fundamental mechanisms governing genetic information transfer.
2. Utilize the fundamentals of transcription and translation to *decode* the amino acid sequence carried within the genetic information.
3. Recognize how mechanisms of genetic information transfer can be altered or exploited for development of biological assays and therapies.

2.1 INTRODUCTION

Molecular biology examines the transfer of information within a cell, which is the basic functional unit of life. Cells exist as single cellular organisms up to the basic functional and structural units of tissues and organs within the body. The challenges associated with multiple tasks required for cells from movement to metabolism need unique proteins at unique moments in time. Much as you or I would rely on instructions when we carry out a task or our computer relies on code when we request it to carry out a calculation, cells carry with them the genetic code to produce all required proteins. This genetic code and how the information contained within it is transferred and translated to produce proteins is the primary focus of molecular biology.

2.2 BUILDING BLOCKS OF LIFE: DNA, RNA, AND PROTEINS

DNA (deoxyribonucleic acid), RNA (ribonucleic acid), and proteins are the three fundamental biopolymers of life. DNA is the message; it is a long polymer chain composed of four nucleotides. A nucleotide is a nucleobase, adenine, cytosine, guanine, or thymine (A, C, G, and T), linked to deoxyribose phosphate. These four nucleotides pair with each other, A with T and C with G. Ultimately, the pairs of these four unique nucleotides store genetic information in much the same way that a computer stores information through binary with a series of 1's and 0's. RNA is the translator; it carries the message and also translates the message into a protein with a few exceptions, such as ribosomal RNA that acts in a similar way to a protein. RNA is similar in structure to DNA, composed of a nucleobase with uracil (U) used in place of thymine and the sugar ribose phosphate in place of deoxyribose phosphate. Similar to DNA, the nucleotides in RNA pair with each other, C with G and A with U. Proteins are the end result of this information transfer and are capable of carrying out unique functions. Proteins have a high degree of structural diversity relative to DNA and RNA; the organization of 21 unique amino acids provides the wide array diversity required of proteins. The organization of these amino acids ultimately dictates the structure and function of the proteins. The principle governing the flow of genetic information to structural and functional proteins within a cell was first postulated by Francis Crick and is termed the *central dogma of molecular biology*. Crick discussed the central dogma of molecular biology in an article titled "Central Dogma of Molecular Biology" published in *Nature* in 1970. Crick identified that there are 9 possible mechanisms for information transfer between these three biopolymers. He deemed the first 3 mechanisms general, commonly observed within a cell; the second 3 were deemed special; and the final 3 were deemed to never occur. Examining the general case, we find the typical flow of information within a cell.

$$\text{DNA} \leftrightarrow \text{DNA} \rightarrow \text{RNA} \rightarrow \text{Protein} \tag{2.1}$$

Here we see first that DNA is capable of transferring information back to itself, which would be DNA replication. Second, we note that DNA is capable of transferring information to RNA, which would be transcription. Finally, we note that RNA is capable of transferring information to proteins, which would be translation. These three transfers underpin the frequent moment-to-moment activities within a cell. DNA replication is a key component of cell division. DNA transcription to RNA allows a single gene (instruction set) to be transferred out of the nucleus. Finally, RNA translation converts the genetic message carried by RNA to a useable protein. The coding of a protein sequence within messenger RNA (mRNA) is accomplished through usage of the genetic code that identifies each amino acid in the protein with a three-nucleotide sequence (a codon). Marshall Nirenberg and his colleagues deciphered the genetic code in the early 1960s. Figure 2.1 provides the breakdown between codons and amino acids.

Examining the special case of information transfer within cells, we find the following relationships:

$$\text{RNA} \leftrightarrow \text{RNA} \rightarrow \text{DNA} \rightarrow \text{Protein} \tag{2.2}$$

Here we see first that RNA is capable of transferring information back to itself. This could be through RNA replication, which is fundamental to many viruses that do not contain DNA. It is also found in RNA editing and silencing processes that occur in eukaryotic cells, essentially a posttranscriptional modification of RNA leading to either loss of function (silencing) or a modification/repair of function (editing). Next it is possible that RNA transfers information back to DNA. This is most often found in viruses. Retroviruses use reverse transcription to convert RNA to DNA in the infected host cell. Reverse transcription is also found in quantitative molecular biology techniques such as RT-PCR

Second letter

First letter		U	C	A	G	Third letter
U	U	UUU ⎤ Phe	UCU ⎤	UAU ⎤ Tyr	UGU ⎤ Cys	U
	C	UUC ⎦	UCC	UAC ⎦	UGC ⎦	C
	A	UUA ⎤	UCA ⎥ Ser	UAA Stop	UGA Stop	A
	G	UUG ⎦ Leu	UCG ⎦	UAG Stop	UGG Trp	G
C	U	CUU ⎤	CCU ⎤	CAU ⎤ His	CGU ⎤	U
	C	CUC ⎥ Leu	CCC ⎥ Pro	CAC ⎦	CGC ⎥ Arg	C
	A	CUA	CCA	CAA ⎤ Gin	CGA	A
	G	CUG ⎦	CCG ⎦	CAG ⎦	CGG ⎦	G
A	U	AUU ⎤	ACU ⎤	AAU ⎤ Asn	AGU ⎤ Ser	U
	C	AUC ⎥ Ile	ACC ⎥	AAC ⎦	AGC ⎦	C
	A	AUA ⎦	ACA Thr	AAA ⎤ Lys	AGA ⎤ Arg	A
	G	AUG Met	ACG ⎦	AAG ⎦	AGG ⎦	G
G	U	GUU ⎤	GCU ⎤	GAU ⎤ Asp	GGU ⎤	U
	C	GUC ⎥ Val	GCC ⎥ Ala	GAC ⎦	GGC ⎥ Gly	C
	A	GUA	GCA	GAA ⎤ Glu	GGA	A
	G	GUG ⎦	GCG ⎦	GAG ⎦	GGG ⎦	G

Figure 2.1 The genetic code converts information stored in DNA to function proteins through mRNA. Above is a table detailing the amino acids corresponding to the nucleotide sequences present in mRNA.

(reverse transcription polymerase chain reaction), which uses the enzymes necessary for reverse transcription to convert RNA back to cDNA prior to amplification. RT-PCR is an excellent tool that enables the expansion of intracellular RNA to identify expression levels of particular genes. The third type of special information transfer, DNA to protein, has yet to be identified occurring naturally, but has been demonstrated experimentally. In 1965, McCarthy and Holland were the first to demonstrate that denatured eukaryotic DNA combined with protein extract from *Escherichia coli* was capable of directly serving as a template for protein translation in the absence of any RNA intermediate.

Examining the case of information transfer thought to never occur, we find the following relationships:

$$\text{DNA} \leftarrow \text{Protein} \leftrightarrow \text{Protein} \rightarrow \text{RNA} \qquad (2.3)$$

To date, there has been no true demonstration of the types of information transfer thought to never occur; however, there have been several *near misses*. In regard to protein transferring information to DNA, the field of epigenetics has demonstrated information transfer in

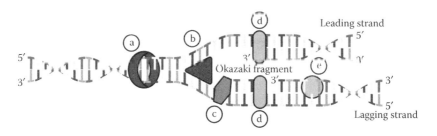

Figure 2.2 DNA replication begins with topoisomerase unwinding the double helix (a), followed by helicase splitting the DNA into single strands (b), then DNA primase generates a single RNA primer (c), and DNA polymerase binds to the RNA primer and generates complementary strands (termed Okazaki fragments) (d), finally, the Okazaki fragments are joined together by DNA ligase (e).

terms of proteins capable of acetylating and methylating DNA. This results in alterations in DNA conformation resulting in increases and decreases in the binding of transcription factors and subsequent regulation of the corresponding genes (Figure 2.2).

2.3 DNA REPLICATION

The process of DNA replication occurs through several key steps all using specialized proteins referred to as *enzymes*:

1. Topoisomerases facilitate the unknotting of DNA, converting the double helix into an unwound double strand of DNA. This is accomplished through generating a series of transient breaks in the DNA structure.
2. The double-stranded DNA is separated into two single strands. The process of separating the DNA is accomplished by helicase enzymes and results in two single strands of DNA that will serve as templates for the leading and lagging strands of the daughter DNA.
3. The two single strands of DNA are *primed* for replication. This occurs via DNA primase (which is a type of RNA polymerase) adding short RNA primers to the template strands. DNA primase only creates a single RNA primer on the template for the leading strand; however, multiple primers are added to the lagging strand template.
4. The base pairs in the two template strands are matched to their complement. DNA polymerase travels along and reads the template strands from the 3′ to 5′ direction. As the DNA polymerase reads the template strand, it attaches the corresponding complementary nucleotide to the template strand, thus generating the daughter strand of DNA in the 5′ to 3′ direction. The formation of the leading strand proceeds unimpeded trailing just behind the unwinding of uncopied DNA by helicase. However, the formation of the lagging strand occurs in spurts as DNA polymerase *runs into* existing segments of double strand of DNA. This discontinuous formation of the lagging strand necessitated DNA primase generating multiple primers

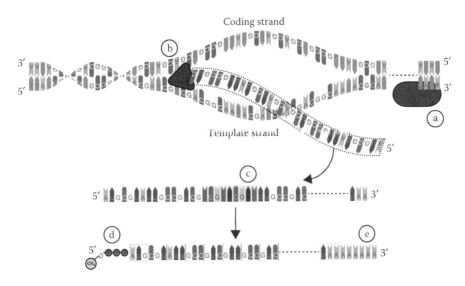

Coding strand

Template strand

Figure 2.3 The process of DNA transcription begins with transcription factor binding (a), then RNA polymerase generates a complementary RNA sequence (b), and finally concludes with posttranslational modifications (c–e).

on the lagging strand template to complete replication. Finally, DNA polymerase is not capable of connecting these segments leading to the formation of Okazaki fragments.

5. The Okazaki fragments are joined together. DNA ligase repairs the *nicks* leftover by DNA polymerase. There will be a single nick at the beginning of replication on the leading strand and multiple nicks on the lagging strand at each Okazaki fragment. DNA ligase repairs these nicks by inserting the appropriate complementary nucleotide (Figure 2.3).

2.4 TRANSCRIPTION

The first step in decoding the DNA to produce functional proteins is through the process of transcription. Eukaryotes and prokaryotes undergo a similar process for the transcription of DNA. In eukaryotes, the process is as follows:

1. Transcription factors bind segments of the DNA to coordinate the transcription of genes. A common transcription factor binding region is referred to as the *TATA box*. The TATA box is found in nearly a quarter of all human genes and contains the nucleotide sequence, 5'-TATAAA-3', and is approximately 25 base pairs upstream of the appropriate gene. Transcription factor binding to the TATA box facilitates the unwinding of the DNA in the preparation of RNA polymerase binding and transcribing the appropriate gene. The binding of transcription factors to the gene of interest is referred to as the *pre-initiation step* of transcription.

2. RNA polymerase binding to the DNA is facilitated by transcription factors and is the initiation step of transcription. As RNA polymerase begins to travel down the template strand of the gene moving toward the 5′ end, it generates the complementary RNA sequence to the template strand, which matches the original coding strand. The process of generating a complementary RNA sequence is similar to that for DNA except RNA contains the nucleotide uracil in lieu of thymine. The process of RNA polymerase generating RNA is referred to as the *elongation step* of transcription.

3. After the generation of the RNA, it is processed through several posttranslational modifications. The combination of these posttranslational modifications is referred to as the *termination step* of transcription. The first posttranslational modification addresses regions in the RNA that interrupt the coding sequence for the desired protein. These interrupting sequences in the RNA are referred to as *introns*. Likewise, the coding sequences on either side of the introns are referred to as *exons*. Once an RNA transcript has been generated, the introns are spliced out and the exons are joined together. The resulting RNA sequence will have a start codon composed of the nucleotide sequence, AUG, and a stop codon composed of either UAA, UGA, or UAG. The sequence between the start and stop codon is referred to as the *open reading frame* (ORF).

4. The second posttranslational modification that most eukaryotic mRNA undergoes is capping of the 5′ end with a *reversed* methylated guanine nucleotide by linking the 5′ end of the guanine nucleotide with the 5′ end of the mRNA through a triphosphate linkage. The capping allows the mRNA to cross the nuclear membrane, prevents degradation, and aids mRNA translation by ribosomes.

5. The final posttranslational modification is polyadenylation of the 3′ end, generating a poly(A) tail. Polyadenylation is the addition of multiple adenosines to the 3′ end of the mRNA. The poly(A) tail facilitates the transport of the mRNA out of the nucleus. It also serves as an mRNA lifetime marker. As the mRNA is translated, the poly(A) tail is shortened through a separate enzymatic mechanism. The ability of the mRNA transcript to block its degradation is reduced, the shorter the poly(A) tail becomes until eventually the mRNA transcript is degraded in the cytoplasm (Figure 2.4).

2.5 TRANSLATION

Translation is the final step in converting the genetic message into a functional protein. Similar to transcription, both eukaryotes and prokaryotes undergo translation through similar mechanisms with the eukaryotes being slightly more complex. In eukaryotes, the process is as follows:

1. The first step in translation is initiation. The initiation step involves the binding of cap-binding proteins and the 40S ribosome: methionine aminoacyl-tRNA complex, which together bind the 5′ cap of the mRNA transcript. The cap-binding proteins facilitate the binding of the 40S ribosome:methionine aminoacyl-tRNA complex and also facilitate the binding to the poly(A) tail to generate an mRNA loop. Once the cap-binding proteins, ribosome, and aminoacyl-tRNA are bound to the mRNA, the complex travels toward the 3′ end until it reaches the start codon, AUG.

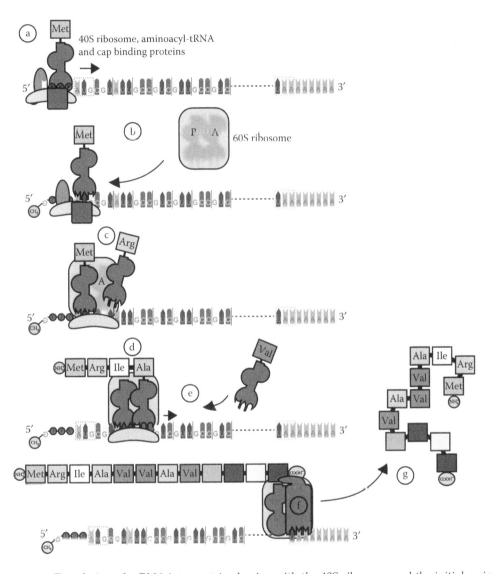

Figure 2.4 Translation of mRNA into proteins begins with the 40S ribosome and the initial amino acid tRNA (methionine aminoacyl-tRNA) binding the mRNA (a), then the 60S ribosome binds the 40S ribosome (b), and together they facilitate the binding of appropriate tRNAs based on the mRNA sequence (c), and promote the cleavage of the amino acid from the tRNA while forming a peptide bond to the nascent peptide chain (d), this process repeats down the mRNA (e), until a stop codon terminates the peptide chain formation releasing the protein (f), and the protein undergoes posttranslational modification (g).

2. Once the 40S ribosome. methionine aminoacyl-tRNA complex is at the start codon, the larger 60S ribosome binds. The 60S:40S ribosome combination (80S) serves as the machinery that organizes and orchestrates the formation of an amino acid sequence corresponding to the codons contained in the mRNA. A codon is a series of three nucleotides that codes for a specific amino acid. The 80S ribosome has two aminoacyl-tRNA binding sites. The 5′ side is referred to as the *peptide (P) site* and contains the aminoacyl-tRNA that is tethered to the growing peptide chain. The 3′ side is referred to as the *aminoacyl (A) site* and contains aminoacyl-tRNA conjugated to the amino acid that will be added to the growing peptide chain. After the ribosome complex is assembled, the process of elongation begins.

3. The first step in elongation is the binding of the aminoacyl-tRNA that corresponds to the codon in the A site of the 80S ribosome. The enzyme aminoacyl-tRNA synthetase has previously catalyzed the formation of an ester bond between the aminoacyl-tRNA and corresponding amino acid. The ester bond is formed on the carboxylic end of the amino acid and will eventually be displaced by the peptide bond linking the amino acid to the growing peptide chain. The process whereby the corresponding aminoacyl-tRNA binds the A site of the 80S ribosome is simply a function of having many unique aminoacyl-tRNAs present in the cytoplasm and relying on diffusion to ultimately provide the correct one to the A site of the ribosome.

4. The second step in elongation is the formation of a peptide bond between the amino acids occupying the A and P sites on the ribosome complex. Prior to peptide bond formation, there is a free amine group on the P site amino acid. The 80S ribosome contains a peptidyltransferase, which catalyzes the reaction between the amine on the A site amino acid and the ester linking the P site amino acid to the tRNA. Once complete, the P site tRNA is no longer linked to the peptide chain.

5. The third step in elongation is to move the mRNA relative to the ribosome and allow the next codon to occupy the A site of 80S ribosome; proteins called *elongation factors* in both eukaryotes and prokaryotes facilitate the movement of the mRNA allowing the positioning of the next codon and corresponding aminoacyl-tRNA in the A site of the 80S ribosome.

6. The final step in generating the amino acid sequence, but not the final step in generating a functional protein, is termination. Once the A site of the 80S ribosome is a stop codon, proteins called *release factors* bind. In eukaryotes, there is one release factor that recognizes all three stop codons, whereas in prokaryotes there are three unique release factors. The release factor catalyzes the cleavage of the P site amino acid from the aminoacyl-tRNA without forming a new peptide bond. The result is a COOH functional group at the end of the peptide chain.

7. The final step in generating a functional protein is posttranslational modification. Posttranslational modification involves folding of the protein, cutting between amino acids, forming disulfide bonds, and the addition of functional groups. These functional groups can allow proteins to operate as on/off switches, which is a key feature in intracellular signaling.

2.6 GENES

By definition, a *gene* includes the entire nucleic acid sequence necessary for the expression of its product (peptide or RNA). Such a sequence may be divided into a *regulatory region* and a *transcriptional region*. The regulatory region could be near or far from the transcriptional region. The transcriptional region consists of *exons* and *introns*. Exons encode a peptide or functional RNA. Introns will be removed after transcription.

As shown in Figure 2.5, a typical DNA molecule consists of *genes, pseudogenes,* and *extragenic region*. Pseudogenes are nonfunctional genes. They often originate from mutation of duplicated genes. Because duplicated genes have many copies, the organism can still survive even if a couple of them become nonfunctional.

Gene family refers to a set of genes with homologous sequences. For example, *H2A, H2B, H3,* and *H4* are in the same histone gene family. Their products have similar structures and functions.

Most proteins do not need duplicated genes, because the mRNA molecule transcribed from one gene can be translated into many copies of its protein product. However, rRNA and tRNA are the final gene products. In order to accelerate the production process, all species contain an array of tandemly repeated RNA genes. The number of repeats ranges from tens to 24,000. There are four types of rRNA in mammalian cells: 28S, 5.8S, 5S, and 18S. In the human genome, 28S, 5.8S, and 18S are clustered together. They form a single transcription unit, which will be separated by specific enzymes after transcription. *Pre-rRNA* refers to their precursor. In humans, a repeat unit for the pre-rRNA has about 40 kb in length, including a 13-kb transcription unit and a 27-kb untranscribed spacer region. The transcription unit contains three spacers: ETS, ITS1, and ITS2. They will be removed during RNA processing.

A stretch of DNA sequence often repeats several times in the total DNA of a cell. For example, the following DNA sequence is just a small part of a *telomere* located at the ends of each human chromosome (Figure 2.6):

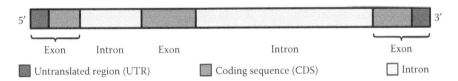

| Exon | Intron | Exon | Intron | Exon |

▮ Untranslated region (UTR)   ▮ Coding sequence (CDS)   ☐ Intron

Figure 2.5   General organization of the DNA sequence. Only the exons encode a functional peptide or RNA. The coding region accounts for about 3% of the total DNA in a human cell.

```
. . . GGTTAGGGTTAGGGTTAGGGTTAGGGTTAGGGTTA
GGGTTAGGGTTAGGGTTAGGGTTAGGGTTAGGGTTAGG
GTTAGGGTTAGGGTTAGGGTTAGGGTTAGGGTTAG . . .
```

Figure 2.6   An entire telomere, about 15 kb, is constituted by thousands of the repeated sequence *GGGTTA*.

Experimentally, the number of repeated copies can be classified on the basis of *DNA reassociation kinetics*. The total DNA is first randomly cleaved into fragments with an average size of about 1000 bp. Then, they are heated to separate the complementary strands of each fragment. Subsequently, temperature is reduced to allow strand reassociation. If a fragment contains a sequence which is repeated many times in the total DNA, it will have greater chance to find a complementary strand and reassociate more quickly than other fragments with less repetitive sequences.

Based on the reassociation rate, DNA sequences are divided into three classes:

- *Highly repetitive*: About 10%–15% of mammalian DNA reassociates very rapidly. This class includes *tandem repeats*.
- *Moderately repetitive*: Roughly 25%–40% of mammalian DNA reassociates at an intermediate rate. This class includes *interspersed repeats*.
- *Single copy (or very low copy number)*: This class accounts for 50%–60% of mammalian DNA.

Tandem repeats are an array of consecutive repeats. They include three subclasses: satellites, minisatellites, and microsatellites. The name *satellites* comes from their optical spectra.

Interspersed repeats are repeated DNA sequences located at dispersed regions in a genome. They are also known as *mobile elements* or *transposable elements*. A stretch of DNA sequence may be copied to a different location through *DNA recombination*. After many generations, such sequence (the repeat unit) could spread over various regions. Mobile elements were first discovered by Barbara McClintock in the 1940s from her studies of corn (http://www.geneticorigins.org/geneticorigins/pv92/media1.html). Subsequently, mobile elements were found in all kinds of organisms. In mammals, the most common mobile elements are *LINEs* and *SINEs*.

Genome is the total genetic information of an organism. For most organisms, it is the complete DNA sequence. For RNA viruses, the genome is the complete RNA sequence, since their genetic information is encoded in RNA.

2.7 MUTATIONS

As with all aspects of life, genetic information transfer is not flawless. Mutations within the DNA occur often. These mutations can be repaired without altering the translation of the genetic message; however, they can also propagate permanently into the genetic message with either positive or negative outcomes. It is natural to think that mutations in DNA would be a rare occurrence; however, an examination of the frequency behind the number of mutations yields some surprising results.

For example, in humans there are approximately

$$2.5*10^{-8} \frac{\text{mutations}}{\text{base}*\text{generation}} \tag{2.4}$$

This appears to be a very small mutation rate until we take into account that there are approximately $3.2*10^{10}$ base pairs in human DNA, which results in around 800 mutations/generation.

The most common mutation is the point mutation. A point mutation occurs when cytosine is swapped for a thymine or an adenine is swapped for a guanine. Due to the redundancy in codons for amino acids, often-times a point mutation in part of the protein coding sequence that is not repaired may not affect anything at all. A point mutation that results in the same amino acid or a very similar amino acid that does not affect the resulting protein is referred to as a *silent mutation*. If the point mutation results in a different amino acid that does affect protein function, it is referred to as a *missense mutation*. Finally, a point mutation that results in a stop codon, which has a deleterious effect on the protein, is referred to as a *nonsense mutation*.

Next, there are insertion mutations. Insertion mutations significantly alter the gene function because they shift the ORF altering every downstream codon. Similar to insertions, there can be deletions where a single nucleotide is removed which result in an altered reading frame.

Small-scale mutations are often repaired. One of the most common point mutations is the spontaneous deamination of cytosine or methylated cytosine. Methylation is a key for epigenetic regulation of gene expression and will be discussed later in the text. The result of deamination of a methylated cytosine is uracil, which is not normally a nucleotide found in DNA and is repaired by the enzyme endonuclease. The result of deamination of an unmethylated cytosine is thymine, which creates a G/T mismatch in the DNA and is repaired by thymine-DNA-glycosylase. The deamination of cytosine to thymine is the most common mutation.

Not all mutations are small scale, large-scale mutations also occur. These can be amplifications where large copies of chromosomal regions are repeated. These types of mutations result in an upregulation of the genes on the regions that are repeated. Finally, there can also be large-scale deletions, which result in loss of large amounts of chromosomal regions. Large-scale mutations are not nearly as common as small-scale mutations; however, they are often fatal during fetal development so identifying the prevalence of large-scale mutations is challenging.

Examining the effect mutations have on function, we find several possible outcomes. The first is a loss of function mutation that results in a diminished effect of the targeted gene. Loss of function mutations are typically recessive, a good example would be cystic fibrosis. Cystic fibrosis is caused by a mutation in the gene coding for cystic fibrosis transmembrane conductance regulator (CFTR) on both of the two matching chromosomes. CFTR is an ion channel that operates in epithelial membranes. Lacking functional CFTR results in an ion imbalance leading to altered osmotic pressure that decreases the fluid present in mucous secretions, making these secretions viscous.

The next possible effect a mutation can have on function would be a gain of function. These are often dominant mutations and result in one copy of the gene gaining new or abnormal function. An example of a gain of function mutation would be sickle cell disease. The red blood cells coded by the mutated gene demonstrate a sickle cell morphology and clump together.

The next type of mutation would a dominant negative mutation. This mutation results in a mutant protein antagonizing the wild type, or natural, protein. An example of a dominant negative mutation would be Marfan syndrome where the expression of the mutant fibrillin protein blocks the wild type fibrillin protein. Fibrillin is an extracellular matrix protein and its misfolding in Marfan syndrome affects the connective tissues.

Any mutation, either dominant or recessive, can result in developmental challenges that do not permit an embryo to proceed to birth. These are referred to as *lethal mutations*. Finally, it is possible for a mutation to fix a previous mutation. This is referred to as a *back mutation or reversion*.

2.8 CHROMOSOME

The organization of genes depends on special structures referred to as *chromosomes*. Since chromosomes play a very large role in the processing of living systems, a separate discussion of them is warranted.

A chromosome is an organized structure of DNA and protein found in cells. It is a single piece of coiled DNA containing many genes, regulatory elements, and other nucleotide sequences. Chromosomes also contain DNA-bound proteins, which serve to package the DNA and control its functions. Chromosomal DNA encodes most or all of an organism's genetic information; some species also contain plasmids or other extra chromosomal genetic elements.

Chromosomes vary widely between different organisms. The DNA molecule may be circular or linear and can be composed of 100,000 to over 3,750,000,000 nucleotides in a long chain. Typically, eukaryotic cells (cells with nuclei) have large linear chromosomes and prokaryotic cells (cells without defined nuclei) have smaller circular chromosomes, although there are many exceptions to this rule. Also, cells may contain more than one type of chromosome; for example, mitochondria in most eukaryotes and chloroplasts in plants both have their own small chromosomes.

In eukaryotes, proteins and DNA associate in a condensed structure called *chromatin* that packages nuclear chromosomes. This allows the very long DNA molecules to fit into the cell's nucleus. The structure of chromosomes and chromatin varies through the cell cycle. Chromosomes are the essential unit for cellular division and must be replicated, divided, and passed successfully to daughter cells to ensure the genetic diversity and survival of progeny. Chromosomes may exist as either duplicated or unduplicated. Unduplicated chromosomes are single linear strands, whereas duplicated chromosomes contain two identical copies (called *chromatids*) joined by a centromere.

In practice, *chromosome* is a rather loosely defined term. In prokaryotes and viruses, the term *genophore* is more appropriate when no chromatin is present, although historically the term *chromosome* has been used regardless of chromatin content. In prokaryotes, DNA is usually arranged as a loop, which is tightly coiled in on itself, sometimes accompanied by one or more smaller, circular DNA molecules called *plasmids*. These small circular genomes are also found in mitochondria and chloroplasts, reflecting their bacterial origins. The simplest genophores are found in viruses: these DNA or RNA molecules are either short and linear or circular genophores that often lack structural proteins.

Prokaryotes—bacteria and archaea—typically have a single circular chromosome, but many variations exist. Most bacteria's chromosome can range in size from only 160,000 base pairs in the endosymbiotic bacterium *Candidatus Carsonella ruddii*, to 12,200,000 base pairs in the soil-dwelling bacterium *Sorangium cellulosum*. Spirochaetes of the genus *Borrelia* are a notable exception to this arrangement, with bacteria such as *Borrelia burgdorferi*, the cause of lyme disease, containing a single linear chromosome.

Prokaryotic chromosomes have less sequence-based structure than eukaryotes. Bacteria typically have a single point (the origin of replication) from which replication starts, whereas some archaea contain multiple replication origins. The genes in prokaryotes are often organized in operons and do not usually contain introns, unlike eukaryotes.

Prokaryotes do not possess nuclei. Instead, their DNA is organized into a structure called the *nucleoid*. The nucleoid is a distinct structure and occupies a defined region of the bacterial cell. This structure is, however, dynamic and is maintained and remodeled by the actions of a range of histone-like proteins, which associate with the bacterial chromosome. In archaea, the DNA in chromosomes is even more organized, with the DNA packaged within structures similar to eukaryotic nucleosomes.

Bacterial chromosomes tend to be tethered to the plasma membrane of the bacteria. In molecular biology applications, this allows for its isolation from the plasmid DNA by centrifugation of lysed bacteria and pelleting of the membranes (and the attached DNA).

Prokaryotic chromosomes and plasmids are, like eukaryotic DNA, generally supercoiled. The DNA must first be released into its relaxed state to allow access for transcription, regulation, and replication to take place.

Eukaryotes possess multiple large linear chromosomes contained in the cell's nucleus. Each chromosome has one centromere, with one or two arms projecting from the centromere, although, under most circumstances, these arms are not visible as such. In addition, most eukaryotes have a small circular mitochondrial genome, and some eukaryotes may have additional small circular or linear cytoplasmic chromosomes.

In the nuclear chromosomes of eukaryotes, the uncondensed DNA exists in a semi-ordered structure, where it is wrapped around histones (structural proteins), forming a composite material called *chromatin*.

Chromosomes in humans can be divided into two types: autosomes and sex chromosomes. Certain genetic traits are linked to a person's sex and are passed on through the sex chromosomes. The autosomes contain the rest of the genetic hereditary information. Both autosomes and sex chromosomes act in the same way during cell division. Human cells have 23 pairs of chromosomes (22 pairs of autosomes and one pair of sex chromosomes), giving a total of 46 per cell. In addition to these, human cells have many hundreds of copies of the mitochondrial genome. Sequencing of the human genome has provided a great deal of information about each of the chromosomes.

In a nondividing cell, chromosomes are not visible by light microscopy, because chromatin is spread throughout the nucleus. During the metaphase of cell division, the chromatin condenses and becomes visible as chromosomes. At this time, each chromosome has been duplicated. A chromosome becomes two sister chromatids attached at the centromere.

Chromosomes are normally viewed under microscope after treated with chemical dyes, such as *Giemsa*. The chromosome will appear as a series of alternate dark and light bands. If Giemsa is used, the dark band is called *G-band* or G-positive band, and the light band is named G-negative band. Similar banding patterns can be observed by using another dye, quinacrine. However, if chromosomes were treated in a hot alkaline solution before staining with Giemsa, a reverse pattern would be observed, namely, the original dark band would become a light band, and vice versa. For this reason, the G-negative band is also known as the *R-band*. Each chromosome consists of two arms separated by the centromere. The long arm and short arm are labeled *q* (for queue) and *p* (for petit), respectively. At the lowest resolution, only a few major bands can be distinguished, which are labeled q1, q2, q3; p1, p2, p3; and so on, counting from the centromere. Higher resolution reveals sub-bands, labeled q11, q12, q13, and so on. Sub-sub-bands identified by even higher resolution are labeled q11.1, q11.2, q11.3, and so on. Traditionally, the short arm (p) is displayed on top of the long arm (q).

A germ cell (sperm or egg) contains only one set of chromosomes. This germ cell with only one set of chromosomes is referred to as *haploid* and is represented as 1n. Somatic cells (cells other than germ cells) of sexually reproducing organisms are diploid, denoted by 2n because they contain two sets of chromosomes. In humans, the haploid chromosome number is 23, but the diploid chromosome number is 46.

Sex chromosomes determine the sex of an organism. A human somatic cell has two sex chromosomes: X and Y in male and two X in female. A human germ cell has one sex chromosome: X or Y in a sperm and X in an egg. When an X-sperm is combined with an egg, the resulting *zygote* (fertilized egg) will contain two X chromosomes. A person developed from the XX-zygote will have the characteristics of a female. Combination of a Y-sperm and an egg will produce a male. The gene that plays an important role in sex determination is sex-determining region Y, located on chromosome Y. This gene is critical for testis formation (Figure 2.7).

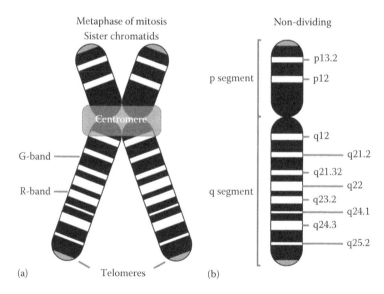

Figure 2.7 Schematic drawing of chromosomes. (a) During the metaphase of cell division, a chromosome becomes two sister chromatids attached at the centromere. (b) Notations about the chromosome bands. This figure uses human chromosome 17 as an example.

2.9 DNA CLONING

The understanding about the living forms and their structure described above should provide sufficient background to understand one of the most significant techniques utilized in many bioprocessing industries—DNA cloning.

DNA cloning is a technique for reproducing DNA fragments by a cell-based approach or using a PCR. The cell-based approach involves a vector, a foreign strand of nucleic acid, to carry the DNA fragment of interest into the host cell. The DNA fragment to be cloned is inserted into a vector, which also contains an antibiotic-resistance gene. The recombinant DNA enters into the host cell and proliferates. This stage is called *transformation* because the function of the host cell is altered. An example of the cells infected by this process includes *E. coli*, which are generally resistant to uptake of the plasmid DNA from the medium and require prior treatment such as exposure to $CaCl_2$. Even then, only one *E. coli* cell in about 10,000 cells may take up a plasmid DNA molecule. To weed out the *E. coli* cells that did not take up the plasmid DNA, the culture is treated with the antibiotic for which a resistant gene has been inserted. Finally, the desired DNA clones are isolated. Chapter 9 goes into greater detail about recombinant protein manufacturing involving DNA clones.

The PCR method relies on thermal cycling, consisting of cycles of repeated heating and cooling of the process for DNA melting and enzymatic replication of the DNA. Primers (short DNA fragments) containing sequences complementary to the target region along with a DNA polymerase (after which the method is named) are key components that enable selective and repeated amplification. As PCR progresses, the DNA generated is used as a template for further replication, setting in motion a chain reaction in which the DNA template is exponentially amplified. PCR can be extensively modified to perform a wide array of genetic manipulations. In 1993, Kary Mullis was awarded the Nobel Prize in chemistry along with Michael Smith for their work on PCR.

Almost all PCR applications employ a heat-stable DNA polymerase, such as Taq polymerase, an enzyme originally isolated from the bacterium *Thermus aquaticus*. This DNA polymerase enzymatically assembles a new DNA strand from DNA building blocks, nucleotides, by using single-stranded DNA as a template and DNA oligonucleotides (also called *DNA primers*), which are required for the initiation of DNA synthesis. The vast majority of PCR methods use thermal cycling, that is, alternately heating and cooling the PCR sample to a defined series of temperature steps. These thermal cycling steps are necessary first to physically separate the two strands of a DNA double helix. Thermal cycling heats the DNA to a high temperature in a process called *DNA melting*. At a lower temperature, the DNA polymerase acts to selectively amplify the target DNA and then uses each strand as the template in DNA synthesis. The selectivity of PCR results from the use of primers that are complementary to the DNA region targeted for amplification under specific thermal cycling conditions.

Questions

1. What is the purpose of DNA?
2. What is the purpose of RNA?

3. If only around 1% of all DNA in eukaryotes encodes for proteins but approximately 80% of DNA is transcribed, is there any function for the remaining ~79% of transcripts?

   Answer: Yes, it encodes for regulatory RNA, like miRNA and also functional RNA such as tRNA and ribosomal RNA.

4. Describe the *special* cases of information transfer possible in biology and detail examples when they occur?

5. A single transcription factor is often capable of reading and transcribing DNA coding for very diverse proteins necessary for multiple types of mature cells. Assuming the same transcription factor is key in mature muscle and bone cells, what prevents the expression of myogenic (muscle) proteins in the osteoblast (bone cell)?

   Answer: There are existing modifications to either the DNA directly, through methylation, or to the underlying histone proteins, through both methylation and acetylation, that increases or decreases the affinity of the transcription factor for a given gene set. Often, genes that are downregulated will have methylated DNA and genes that are upregulated will have acetylated histone proteins.

6. Sociologists often explain that a person is a combination of nature (the genes they are born with) and nurture (the environment they are exposed to). Is there a way for nurture to alter the nature?

7. For the following sequences, identify the template strand, coding strand, and RNA strand:

$$3' - ATCGTTGGCATA - 5'$$
$$5' - TAGCAACCGTAT - 3'$$
$$3' - AUCGUUGGCAUA - 5'$$

8. Justify your response to question 7 by detailing what specifically led to the determination of the RNA strand.

9. Single-stranded DNA weighs approximately 304 Da/nucleotide, single-stranded RNA weighs approximately 321 Da/nucleotide, and the average amino acid in a protein weighs 110 Da. For a protein that is 20 amino acids long created from mRNA with no introns, which portion of the genetic message had the most mass in the cell?

10. A simple way to determine the concentration of DNA in a sample is to measure the absorbance of the sample at 260 nm. The Beer–Lambert law relates absorbance to concentration. $A = \varepsilon * b * c$, where A is the absorbance, ε is the extinction coefficient, b is the path length of the cuvette, and c is the concentration. For an unknown sample of DNA, the absorbance was measured to be 0.2 at 260 nm. The extinction coefficient for double-stranded DNA, ε_{260} nm, is 0.02 $(\mu g/ml)^{-1}$ cm^{-1}. A common laboratory device for measuring DNA, the NanoDrop, operates with a 1-mm path length. What is the concentration measured?

    Answer: By rearranging the Beer–Lambert law and converting the units to be consistent, we see that $c = A/\varepsilon b = 0.2/0.02$ (mL/µg) cm*1 mm*(1 cm/10 mm) = 100 µg/mL.

11. The typical mass of DNA in a mammalian cell is around 6 pg. Approximately how many base pairs are contained in the average mammalian cell?

12. What is the amino acid sequence that the following mRNA transcript codes for?

$$3' - AGUUUUAUCCCCGAUGUGCCGAAGUGGAGAGGAGUA - 5'$$

13. Eukaryotic mRNA typically contains a single ORF; however, prokaryotic mRNA often contains multiple ORFs. For the following mRNA sequence, how many ORFs are there?

$$5' - AUGUUAUGUUGAUCGAUGUCUAAAGGAUAA - 3'$$

Answer: We can identify the ORFs by looking for AUG:

$$5' - AUGUUAUGUUGAUCGAUGUCUAAAGGAUAA - 3'$$

There are 3 ORFs in this prokaryotic mRNA.

14. For the following DNA/RNA sequence identify the mutation in the template strand and comment on what the expected effect of this mutation would be:

$$3' - TACAGGGTACCACCTCAGATT - 5'$$
$$5' - ATGTCCCATGGTGGAGTTTAA - 3'$$
$$5' - AUGUCCCAUGGUGGAGUCUAA - 3'$$

15. Researchers have recently began to use DNA and RNA sequences to generate functional conformations by relying on complementary sequences to bind and non-complementary sequences to permit bending and folding, like a protein or ribosomal RNA, as opposed to solely carrying genetic information. For the following RNA-based aptamer sequence identify what shape would be generated:

$$5' - AUUACGAUCAUGGAAAUCGUAAU - 3'$$

16. The genome size for the typical RNA virus, like HIV, is approximately 10,000 nucleotides. The mutation rate for these viruses can approach 10^{-3} mutations/base * generation and they can progress from one generation to the next in approximately 50 h. How many mutations would you expect over the course of a week?
    Answer:

$$\frac{10^{-3}\,\text{mutations}}{\text{base} * \text{generation}} * 10,000\,\text{bases} * 1\,\text{week} * \frac{7\,\text{days}}{\text{week}} * \frac{24\,\text{h}}{\text{day}} * \frac{1\,\text{generation}}{50\,\text{h}} = 336\,\text{mutations}$$

17. Based on the number of mutations found in question 16, how does this complicate treatment strategies for RNA viruses?

18. In the context of the chromosome, what is the region called that codes for the production of a protein?

19. Alleles are genes present on the two matched chromosomes, are they always the same and if not, what determines the eventual protein expression pattern?

20. How are chromosomes important in the regulation of cell function?

3

Introduction to Biochemistry

LEARNING OBJECTIVES

1. Recognize the differences in the structure and how they correlate to function between DNA and RNA.
2. Understand the three levels of organization demonstrated by a protein   primary, secondary, and tertiary—and how each level regulates protein function.
3. Utilize the fundamentals of basic chemistry to appreciate energy transfer in cells through the metabolism of multiple components.

3.1 INTRODUCTION

Biochemistry is the study of the biological processes that occur in organisms. In the scope of biochemistry and molecular biology, biochemistry examines the structure–function relationships in biomolecules, whereas molecular biology examines information transfer between biomolecules. More specifically, biochemistry seeks to generate an understanding of how biomolecules contribute to the processes that drive all functions in prokaryotes, archaea, and eukaryotes. This chapter will begin with an examination of the structure of DNA and RNA and then proceed through an overview of other biomolecules, specifically proteins, carbohydrates, and lipids, and will conclude with an introduction and overview of several basic metabolic pathways.

3.2 DNA STRUCTURE

A nucleotide is composed of three parts: pentose, base, and phosphate group. In DNA or RNA, a pentose is associated with only one phosphate group, but a cellular free nucleotide (such as adenosine triphosphate [ATP]) may contain more than one phosphate group. If all phosphate groups are removed, a nucleotide becomes a nucleoside.

In cells, a free nucleotide may contain one, two, or three phosphate groups. The energy carrier ATP has three phosphate groups; ADP (adenosine diphosphate) has two phosphate groups; and AMP (adenosine monophosphate) has one phosphate group. If all phosphate groups are removed, a nucleotide becomes a nucleoside such as adenosine. Table 3.1 lists various nucleosides and nucleotides.

In a nucleic acid chain, two nucleotides are linked by a phosphodiester bond, which may be formed by the condensation reaction similar to the formation of the peptide bond. In cells, such a process has been found in the ligation between two nucleic acid fragments. However, RNA polymerase or DNA polymerase usually synthesizes the whole nucleic acid chain. Like peptide chains, a nucleic acid chain also has orientation: its 5' end contains a free phosphate group and 3' end contains a free hydroxyl group. Synthesis of a nucleic acid chain always proceeds from 5' to 3'. Therefore, unless specified otherwise, the sequence of a nucleic acid chain is written from 5' to 3' (left to right).

In DNA or RNA, a nucleic acid chain is also called a *strand*. A DNA molecule typically contains two strands, whereas most RNA molecules contain a single strand. The length of a nucleic acid chain is represented by the number of *bases*. In the case of a double-stranded nucleic acid, bases are paired between two strands. Therefore, its length is given by the number of *base pairs* (bp), 1 kb = 1,000 bases or bp; 1 Mb = 1 million bases or bp. *Oligonucleotides* refer to short nucleic acid chains (<50 bases or bp) and *polynucleotides* have longer chains. The chemical

Table 3.1 Cellular Nucleosides and Nucleotides

Base	Nucleoside (= Base + Pentose)		Nucleotide (= Nucleoside + Phosphate)		
	Ribonucleoside	Deoxyribo-nucleoside	NMP dNMP	NDP dNDP	NTP dNTP
Purines					
Adenine	Adenosine	Deoxyadenosine	AMP dAMP	ADP dADP	ATP dATP
Guanine	Guanosine	Deoxyguanosine	GMP dGMP	GDP dGDP	GTP dGTP
Pyrimidines					
Cytosine	Cytidine	Deoxycytidine	CMP dCMP	CDP dCDP	CTP dCTP
Thymine	Thymidine	Deoxythymidine	TMP dTMP	TDP dTDP	TTP dTTP
Uracil	Uridine	Deoxyuridine	UMP dUMP	UDP dUDP	UTP dUTP

Note: dNMP, deoxynucleoside monophosphate; dNDP, deoxynucleoside diphosphate; dNTP, deoxynucleoside; triphosphate; NDP, nucleoside diphosphate; NMP, nucleoside monophosphate; NTP, nucleoside triphosphate; (nucleoside = ribonucleoside; deoxynucleoside = deoxyribonucleoside).

structure of pentose, which contains five carbon atoms, is labeled as C1′ to C5′. The pentose is called *ribose* in RNA and *deoxyribose* in DNA, because the DNA's pentose lacks an oxygen atom at C2′. Recall that RNA stands for *ribonucleic acid* and DNA stands for *deoxyribonucleic acid*. There are five different bases, each denoted by a single letter as given in the parenthesis. They are as follows:

- Adenine (A)
- Cytosine (C)
- Guanine (G)
- Thymine (T)
- Uracil (U)

Among them, A, C, G, and T exist in DNA and A, C, G, and U exist in RNA.

A and G contain a pair of fused rings, classified as *purines*. C, T, and U contain only one ring, classified as *pyrimidines*. The chemical structure of uracil is simpler than thymine, and thus why RNA uses uracil, instead of thymine. The reason why DNA uses thymine is because it pairs well with uracil but so does adenine.

A DNA molecule has two strands, held together by the hydrogen bonding between their bases. Adenine can form *two* hydrogen bonds with thymine; cytosine can form *three* hydrogen bonds with guanine. Although other base pairs (e.g., [G:T] and [C:T]) may also form hydrogen bonds, their strengths are not as strong as (C:G) and (A:T) found in natural DNA molecules. Figure 3.1 shows an example of base pairing between two strands of DNA.

Due to the specific base pairing, the two strands of DNA are *complementary* to each other. Hence, the nucleotide sequence of one strand determines the sequence of another strand. For example, in Figure 3.1, the sequence of the two strands can be written as 5′-Act-3′ and 3′-Tga-5′.

Note that they obey the (A:T) and (C:G) pairing rule. If we know the sequence of one strand, we can deduce the sequence of another strand. For this reason, a DNA database needs to store only the sequence of one strand. By convention, the sequence in a DNA database refers to the sequence of the 5′ to 3′ strand (left to right). In a DNA molecule, the two strands are not parallel, but intertwined with each other. Each strand looks like a helix. The two strands form a *double helix* structure, which was first discovered by James D. Watson and Francis Crick in 1953. In this structure, also known as the *B form*, the helix makes a turn every 3.4 nm, and the distance between two neighboring base pairs is 0.34 nm. Hence, there are about 10 pairs/turn. The intertwined strands make two grooves of different widths, referred to as the *major groove* and the *minor groove*, which may facilitate binding with specific proteins.

In a solution with higher salt concentrations or with alcohol added, the DNA structure may change to an *A form*, which is still right handed, but every 2.3 nm makes a turn and there are 11 base pairs/turn. Furthermore, a DNA molecule with alternating G–C sequences in alcohol or high concentrations of salt in solution will exhibit a structure called the *Z form*, because its bases seem to zigzag. Z DNA is left-handed. One turn spans 4.6 nm, comprising 12 base pairs/turn.

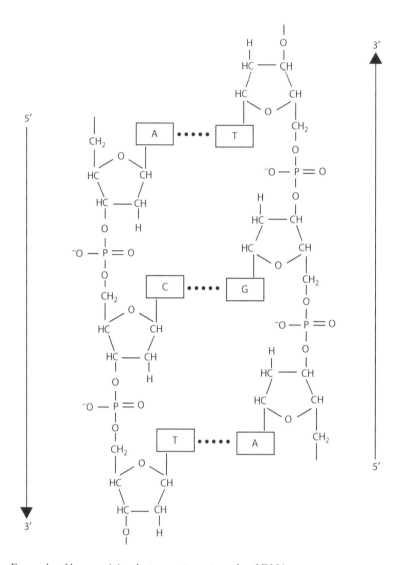

Figure 3.1 Example of base pairing between two strands of DNA.

3.3 RNA STRUCTURE

Most cellular RNA molecules are single stranded. They may form secondary structures such as stem-loop and hairpin. The major role of RNA is to participate in protein synthesis. This requires three classes of RNA, which are listed as follows:

1. *Messenger RNA (mRNA)*: mRNA is transcribed from DNA, carrying information for protein synthesis. Three consecutive nucleotides in mRNA encode an amino acid or a stop signal for protein synthesis. The trinucleotide is known as a *codon*.

2. *Transfer RNA (tRNA)*: The major role of tRNA is to *translate* mRNA sequences into amino acid sequences. A tRNA molecule consists of 70–80 nucleotides. Some nucleotides in tRNA have been modified, such as *dihydrouridine (D)*, *pseudouridine* (Ψ), and *inosine (I)*. In dihydrouridine, a hydrogen atom is added to each C5 and C6 of uracil. In pseudouridine, the ribose is attached to C5, instead of the normal N1. Inosine plays an important role in codon recognition. In addition to these modifications, a few nucleosides are methylated.

3. *Ribosomal RNA (rRNA)*: In prokaryotes, the rRNA has three types—23S, 5S, and 16S. In mammals, four types of rRNA have been found—28S, 5.8S, 5S, and 18S. The unit *S* stands for Svedberg, which is a measure of the sedimentation rate. After rRNA molecules are produced in the nucleus, they are transported to the cytoplasm, where they combine with tens of specific proteins to form a ribosome. In prokaryotes, the size of a ribosome is 70S, consisting of two subunits—50S and 30S. The size of a mammalian ribosome is 80S, comprising a 60S and a 40S subunit. Proteins in the larger subunit are designated as L1, L2, L3, and so on (L = large). In the smaller subunit, proteins are denoted by S1, S2, S3, and so on (S = small).

3.4 PROTEIN STRUCTURE AND FUNCTION

Proteins are made of amino acids that are composed of an amino group (NH_2), a carboxyl group (COOH), and an R (alklyl) group and have the general formula: $R–CH(NH_2)–COOH$. The R group, called a *side chain in proteins*, differs among various amino acids.

3.4.1 Amino Acids

There are over 300 naturally occurring amino acids on earth, but the genetic code is based on only 20 amino acids, which are classified based on their physicochemical properties. Acidic amino acids include aspartic acid (aspartate) and glutamatic acid (glutamate). Basic amino acids include lysine, arginine, and histidine. The neutral amino acids when placed in a neutral solution, the R group of a basic amino acid, may gain a proton and become positively charged. Interaction between positive and negative R groups may form a *salt bridge*, which is an important stabilizing force in proteins. The aromatic amino acids include tyrosine, tryptophan, and phenylalanine. The amino acids that include sulfur atoms in their R groups are cysteine and methionine; a disulfide bond between two cysteine residues provides for stabilization of the globular structure; methionine is where the synthesis of all peptide chains starts. The uncharged hydrophilic amino acids include serine, threonine, asparagine, and glutamine, and these are capable of forming hydrogen bonds. The inactive hydrophobic amino acids include glycine, alanine, valine, leucine, and isoleucine. There are also amino acids with special structure like proline, which is an exception in that the R group is not directly connected to the amino group. Table 3.2 lists the 20 amino acids.

Amino acids are optically active. Optical activity is assessed by the rotation of a plane of light as it passes through a sample. Optical activity was measured prior to advanced techniques that are capable of determining the three-dimensional structure. The assignment of optical activity was demarcated with the letter D or the + sign for clockwise rotation of the

Table 3.2 Twenty Amino Acids

Name	Symbol		R group	Terminal group	Hydro-phobicity
	3 Lett.	1 Lett.			
Aspartate	Asp	D			−3.5
Glutamate	Glu	E			−3.5
Lysine	Lys	K	$H_3\overset{+}{N}-CH_2-CH_2-CH_2-CH_2$		−3.9
Arginine	Arg	R	$H_2N-C-NH-CH_2-CH_2-CH_2$ $\overset{\|\|}{\underset{+}{NH_2}}$		−4.5
Histidine	His	H			−4.2
Tyrosine	Tyr	Y			−1.3
Tryptophan	Trp	W			−0.9

(*Continued*)

Table 3.2 (*Continued*) Twenty Amino Acids

Name	Symbol		R group	Terminal group	Hydro-phobicity
	3 Lett.	1 Lett.			
Phenylalanine	Phe	F	$\bigcirc - CH_2 -$ (benzene ring)	$\begin{array}{c} H \\ | \\ -C-COO^- \\ | \\ NH_3 \\ + \end{array}$	2.8
Cysteine	Cys	C	$HS-CH_2-$	$\begin{array}{c} H \\ | \\ -C-COO^- \\ | \\ NH_3 \\ + \end{array}$	2.5
Methionine	Met	M	$CH_3-S-CH_2-CH_2-$	$\begin{array}{c} H \\ | \\ -C-COO^- \\ | \\ NH_3 \\ + \end{array}$	1.9
Serine	Ser	S	$HO-CH_2-$	$\begin{array}{c} H \\ | \\ -C-COO^- \\ | \\ NH_3 \\ + \end{array}$	−0.8
Threonine	Thr	T	$\begin{array}{c} CH_3-CH- \\ | \\ OH \end{array}$	$\begin{array}{c} H \\ | \\ -C-COO^- \\ | \\ NH_3 \\ + \end{array}$	−0.7
Asparagine	Asn	N	$\begin{array}{c} NH_2 \\ \backslash \\ C-CH_2- \\ // \\ O \end{array}$	$\begin{array}{c} H \\ | \\ -C-COO^- \\ | \\ NH_3 \\ + \end{array}$	−3.5
Glutamine	Gln	Q	$\begin{array}{c} NH_2 \\ \backslash \\ C-CH_2-CH_2- \\ // \\ O \end{array}$	$\begin{array}{c} H \\ | \\ -C-COO^- \\ | \\ NH_3 \\ + \end{array}$	−3.5

(Continued)

69

Table 3.2 (*Continued*) Twenty Amino Acids

Name	Symbol		R group	Terminal group	Hydro-phobicity
	3 Lett.	1 Lett.			
Glycine	Gly	G		$H-\overset{\overset{\displaystyle H}{|}}{\underset{\underset{\displaystyle NH_3^+}{|}}{C}}-COO^-$	−0.4
Alanine	Ala	A		$CH_3-\overset{\overset{\displaystyle H}{|}}{\underset{\underset{\displaystyle NH_3^+}{|}}{C}}-COO^-$	1.8
Valine	Val	V	$\overset{CH_3}{\underset{CH_3}{>}}CH$	$\overset{\overset{\displaystyle H}{|}}{\underset{\underset{\displaystyle NH_3^+}{|}}{C}}-COO^-$	4.2
Leucine	Leu	L	$\overset{CH_3}{\underset{CH_3}{>}}CH-CH_2$	$\overset{\overset{\displaystyle H}{|}}{\underset{\underset{\displaystyle NH_3^+}{|}}{C}}-COO^-$	3.8
Isoleucine	Ile	I	$CH_3-CH_2-\underset{\underset{\displaystyle CH_3}{|}}{CH}$	$\overset{\overset{\displaystyle H}{|}}{\underset{\underset{\displaystyle NH_3^+}{|}}{C}}-COO^-$	4.5
Proline	Pro	P	$\overset{CH_2}{\underset{CH_2}{}}\underset{CH_2}{>}$	$\overset{\overset{\displaystyle H}{|}}{\underset{\underset{\displaystyle N\;H}{|}}{C}}-COO^-$	−1.6

Note: Hydrophilic amino acids have negative values.

light and L or − sign for counterclockwise rotation of the light. Figure 3.2 demonstrates the D and L forms of glyceraldehyde.

A second configuration notation uses the symbols R and S and was developed by Cahn, Ingold, and Prelog. Configuration is assigned by *looking* down the bond to the lowest priority substituent and assigning R to the configuration where the remaining substituents are

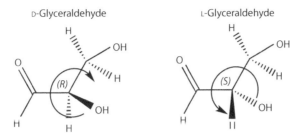

Figure 3.2 Representation of the stereochemistry of glyceraldehyde.

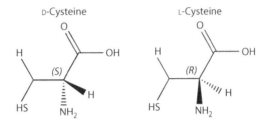

Figure 3.3 Representation of the stereochemistry of L-cysteine, which, unlike the other amino acids, demonstrates an *R* conformation. An additional outlier is glycine, which has no stereochemistry.

arranged clockwise with decreasing polarity; similarly, S is assigned to the form where the substituents are arranged counterclockwise.

General priorities with R/S notation demonstrate the following for the substituents attached to the carbon: **SH > OH > NH$_2$ > COOH > CHO > CH$_2$OH > C$_6$H$_5$ > CH$_3$ > H.**

Groups that contain an additional carbon chain are ranked based on points of divergence, that is, a CH$_2$CH$_2$OH is greater than a CH$_2$CH$_2$NH$_2$.

The configuration of amino acids has historically used the D/L notation with reference to the absolute configuration of glyceraldehyde rather than the more modern R/S designation. All of the amino acids used in proteins are of L configuration. However, because of the differences in determining stereochemistry, in the R/S notation L-cysteine is R where the other amino acids are all S. Figure 3.3 shows the stereochemistry of cysteine.

Finally, a few amino acids demonstrate multiple stereocenters. The amino acids with multiple stereocenters are threonine and isoleucine. Figure 3.4 demonstrates the stereochemistry of L-threonine and L-isoleucine.

3.4.2 Peptide

A peptide is a chain of amino acids held together by peptide bonds formed by a condensation reaction (Figure 3.5). Polypeptides are long peptides and oligopeptides are short with less than 10 amino acids. One or more peptides with a total of more than 50 amino acids are called *proteins*. The primary structure of a protein refers to its amino acid sequence.

The amino acid in a peptide is also called a *residue*. Figure 3.6 shows the amino acid sequence of hemoglobin.

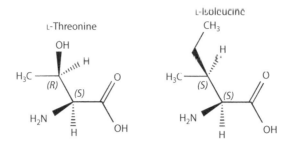

Figure 3.4 Representation of the stereochemistry of L-threonine and L-isoleucine.

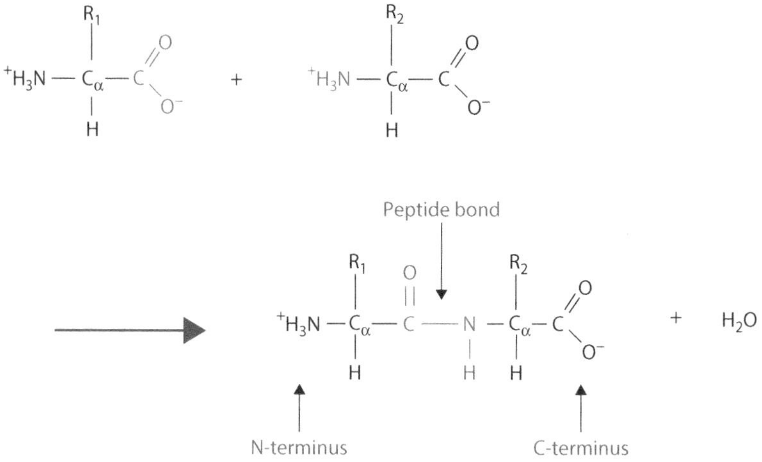

$$^+H_3N - \underset{\underset{H}{|}}{\overset{\overset{R_1}{|}}{C_\alpha}} - C \overset{O}{\underset{O^-}{\diagup}} \quad + \quad ^+H_3N - \underset{\underset{H}{|}}{\overset{\overset{R_2}{|}}{C_\alpha}} - C \overset{O}{\underset{O^-}{\diagup}}$$

Peptide bond

$$^+H_3N - \underset{\underset{H}{|}}{\overset{\overset{R_1}{|}}{C_\alpha}} - \overset{\overset{O}{\parallel}}{C} - \underset{H}{\overset{}{N}} - \underset{\underset{H}{|}}{\overset{\overset{R_2}{|}}{C_\alpha}} - C \overset{O}{\underset{O^-}{\diagup}} \quad + \quad H_2O$$

N-terminus   C-terminus

Figure 3.5 Formation of the peptide bond by condensation reaction.

```
 1   2   3   4   5   6     7    8   9   10
val–his–leu–thr–pro– glu – glu –lys–ser–ala
                     lys–C  gly–G
                     val–S

11  12  13  14  15  16  17  18  19  20  21
–val–thr–ala–leu–try–gly–lys–val–asp–val–asp

22  23  24  25  26   27  28  29  30  31
–glu–val–gly–gly– glu –ala–leu–gly–arg–leu–
ala–A₂              lys–E
```

Figure 3.6 Amino acid sequence of hemoglobin.

3.4.3 Helix Structure

In a protein, certain domains may form specific structures such as alpha helix (α helix) and beta strand (β strand), which constitute the secondary structure of the protein. The α helix is a common secondary structure of proteins and is a right-handed coiled or spiral conformation (helix), in which every backbone N–H group donates a hydrogen bond to the backbone C=O group of the amino acid four residues earlier (hydrogen bonding). Among types of local structure in proteins, the α helix is the most regular and the most predictable from sequence, as well as the most prevalent. Figure 3.7 shows an α helix.

In an α helix, every 3.6 residues make one turn, the distance between two turns is 0.54 nm, and the C=O (or N–H) of one turn is hydrogen bonded to N–H (or C=O) of the neighboring turn. The α helix conformation is stabilized by hydrogen bonds, and the sizes and charges of side chains are important. For example, alanine has a greater tendency to form α helices than proline.

An α helix can be either right-handed or left-handed. In an amphipathic α helix, one side of the helix contains mainly hydrophilic amino acids, and the other side contains mainly hydrophobic amino acids. The amino acid sequence of amphipathic α helix alternates between hydrophilic and hydrophobic residues every 3 to 4 residues, since the α helix makes a turn for every 3.6 residues.

Beta strand is a structural unit of protein β sheets. This is an extended stretch of polypeptide chains typically 3 to 10 amino acids long that forms hydrogen bonds with other β strands in the same β sheet. The β sheet (also β-pleated sheet) is the second form of regular secondary structure in proteins, only somewhat less common than the α helix. Beta sheets consist of β strands connected laterally by at least two or three backbone hydrogen bonds, forming a generally twisted, pleated sheet. A β strand is a stretch of polypeptide chain typically 3 to 10 amino acids long with the backbone in an almost fully extended

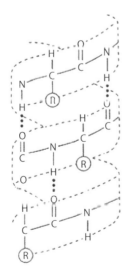

••• Hydrogen bond

(R) = Amino acid side chain

Figure 3.7 An alpha helix.

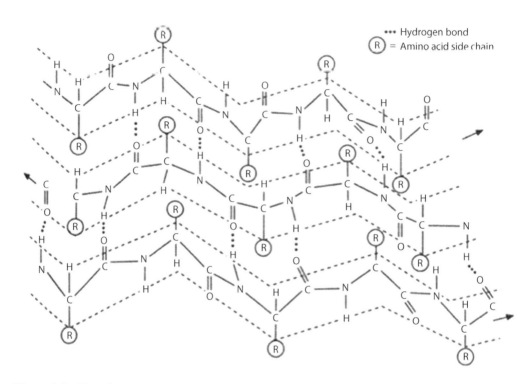

Figure 3.8 Beta sheet.

conformation. The higher-level association of β sheets has been implicated in formation of the protein aggregates and fibrils observed in many human diseases, notably the amyloidoses such as Alzheimer's disease. Figure 3.8 shows a β sheet.

In a β strand, the torsion angle of N–Ca–C–N in the backbone is about 120°. A β sheet consists of two or more hydrogen bonded β strands. The two neighboring β strands may be parallel if they are aligned in the same direction from one terminus (N or C) to the other, or antiparallel if they are aligned in the opposite direction. A β barrel is a closed β sheet.

3.4.4 Motif

The motif is a characteristic domain structure consisting of two or more α helices or β strands. Common examples include coiled coil, helix-loop-helix, zinc finger, and leucine zipper. Many proteins also contain specific domains such as the SH2 domain. Figure 3.9 shows various types of motifs.

The three-dimensional structure is also called the *tertiary structure* Figure 3.10 shows an example of tertiary structure. If a protein molecule consists of more than one polypeptide, it also has the *quaternary structure*, which specifies the relative positions among the polypeptides (subunits) in a protein (Figure 3.11).

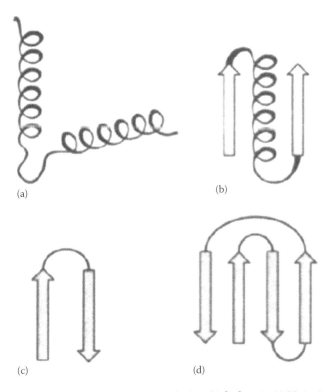

Figure 3.9 Various types of motifs. (a) Helix-loop-helix, (b) βαβ unit, (c) Hairpin, (d) Greek key.

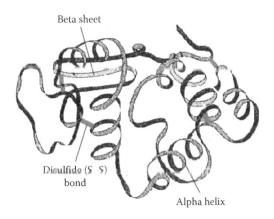

Figure 3.10 Tertiary structure of proteins.

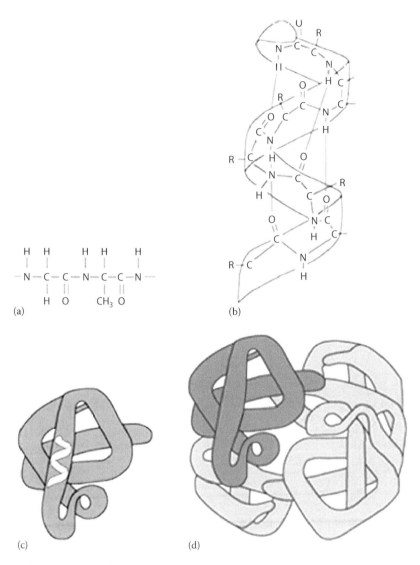

Figure 3.11 Primary, secondary, tertiary, and quaternary structures. (a) The primary structure is composed of a linear sequence of amino acid residues of proteins. (b) The secondary structure indicates the local spatial arrangement of the polypeptide backbone yielding an extended α-helical or β-pleated sheet structure as depicted by the ribbon. (c) The tertiary structure illustrates the three-dimensional conformation of a subunit of the protein, while the quaternary structure (d) indicates the assembly of multiple polypeptide chains into an intact, tetrameric protein. (Data from Baynes, J.W. and Dominiczak, M.H. *Medicinal Biochemistry*, 2nd Edition, Elsevier, 2005, p. 18.)

3.4.5 Other Proteins

Enzymes are large biological molecules responsible for a large number of chemical conversions in life reactions. They are highly selective catalysts, greatly accelerating both the rate and specificity of metabolic reactions, from the digestion of food to the synthesis of DNA. Most enzymes are proteins, although some catalytic RNA molecules have been identified. Enzymes adopt a specific three-dimensional structure and may employ organic (e.g., biotin) and inorganic (e.g., magnesium ion) cofactors to assist in catalysis. Since enzymes are of great importance in bioprocessing, a Chapter 6 deals with their description.

In addition to enzymes and membrane proteins, there are many other proteins with various cellular functions. This page is not intended to be comprehensive, but lists only a few important examples.

1. *Chaperones*: Involved in protein folding.
2. *Conjugated proteins*: Covalently bonded to prosthetic groups such as glycoproteins and metalloproteins.
3. *Cytokines*: Regulate immunity, inflammation, apoptosis, and hematopoiesis.
   a. *Interleukins*: Cytokines that act specifically as mediators between leukocytes. Presently there has been 36 Interleukins identified. These interleukins typically serve to stimulate proliferation, activation and differentiation of leukocytes.
   b. *Interferons (IFNs)*: Cytokines that can *interfere* with viral growth. They also have the ability to inhibit proliferation and modulate immune responses. Four types of IFNs have been identified: IFN-α, IFN-β, IFN-ω, and IFN-γ. The first three are type I IFNs that have relatively high antiviral potency. IFN-γ is the type II IFN, also called *immune IFN*. Type I IFNs are produced by macrophages, neutrophils, and other somatic cells in response to infection by viruses or bacteria. After they are released, they may bind to their receptors that are expressed on most cell types, resulting in the production of over 30 different proteins in the target cell. Among them, two enzymes play a critical role in the inhibition of viral replication: RNA-dependent protein kinase and 2'–5' oligoadenylate synthetase (2–5A synthetase). Both enzymes can be activated by double-stranded RNA, which may be present in some viruses. The activated RNA-dependent protein kinase can phosphorylate protein eIF2 to inhibit protein synthesis. The 2–5A synthetase produces oligoadenylate that can bind and activate a cellular endonuclease to degrade mRNA. IFN-γ is produced in activated T-helper cell 1 (and natural killer cells, particularly in response to IL-2 and IL-12). Its production is suppressed by IL-4, IL-10, and transforming growth factor-β. Binding of IFN-γ to its receptor increases the expression of class I major histocompatibility complex on all somatic cells. It also enhances the expression of class II major histocompatibility complex on antigen-presenting cells. IFN-γ may also activate macrophages, neutrophils, and natural killer cell cells.

   c. *Tumor necrosis factors (TNF)*: Cytokines produced mainly by macrophages and
      T lymphocytes that help regulate the immune response and hematopoiesis
      (blood cell formation). There are two types of TNF, which are as follows:
      i. *TNFα*—also called *cachectin*, produced by macrophages
      ii. *TNFβ*—also called *lymphotoxin*, produced by activated CD4+ T cells
   d. *Chemokines*: Cytokines that may activate or chemoattract leukocytes. Each
      chemokine contains 65 ~ 120 amino acids, with molecular weight of 8 ~ 10 kD.
      Their receptors belong to G-protein-coupled receptors. Since the entry of human
      immunodeficiency virus into host cells requires chemokine receptors, their antag-
      onists are being developed to treat acquired immune deficiency syndrome.
4. *Hormones*: Examples are insulin, growth hormone, and prolactin.
5. *Prions*
6. *Structural proteins*: Collagen, myosin.
7. *Transcription factors*: Regulate gene transcription.
8. *Ubiquitin*: Marker for protein degradation. If a protein binds to ubiquitin, it will
   be degraded by proteasome.

3.5 CARBOHYDRATES

Carbohydrates are organic compounds that consist only of carbon, hydrogen, and oxygen,
usually with a hydrogen:oxygen atom ratio of 2:1 (as in water); in other words, with the
empirical formula $C_m(H_2O)_n$. (Some exceptions exist; for example, deoxyribose, a component of DNA, has the empirical formula $C_5H_{10}O_4$.) Carbohydrates are not technically
hydrates of carbon. Structurally it is more accurate to view them as polyhydroxy aldehydes and ketones. The term is most common in biochemistry, where it is a synonym of
saccharide.

   The carbohydrates (saccharides) are divided into four chemical groupings: monosaccharides, disaccharides, oligosaccharides, and polysaccharides. In general, the monosaccharides and disaccharides, which are smaller (lower molecular weight) than carbohydrates,
are commonly referred to as *sugars*. The word *saccharide* comes from the Greek word
σάκχαρον (sákkharon), meaning *sugar*. While the scientific nomenclature of carbohydrates is complex, the names of the monosaccharides and disaccharides vary, often ending
in the suffix -ose. For example, blood sugar is the monosaccharide glucose, table sugar
is the disaccharide sucrose, and milk sugar is the disaccharide lactose (see Figures 3.12
through 3.15).

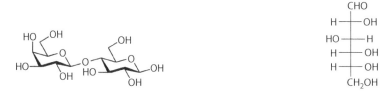

Figure 3.12 Lactose.   **Figure 3.13** Glucose.

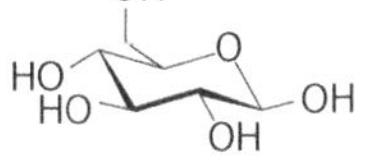

Figure 3.14   Glucose: Three-dimensional structure. 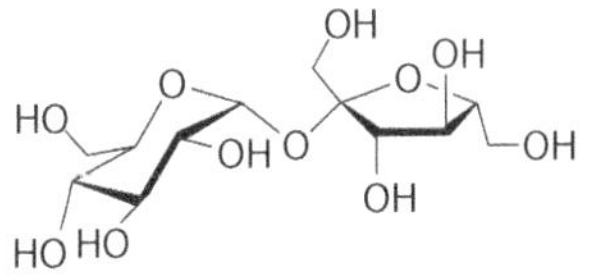   **Figure 3.15**   Sucrose.

Carbohydrates perform numerous roles in living organisms. Polysaccharides serve for the storage of energy (e.g., starch and glycogen) and as structural components (e.g., cellulose in plants and chitin in arthropods). The 5-carbon monosaccharide ribose is an important component of coenzymes (e.g., ATP, flavin adenine dinucleotide [FAD], and nicotinimide adenine dinucleotide [NAD]) and the backbone of the genetic molecule known as *RNA*. The related deoxyribose is a component of DNA. Saccharides and their derivatives include many other important biomolecules that play key roles in the immune system, fertilization, preventing pathogenesis, blood clotting, and development.

Natural saccharides are generally built of simple carbohydrates called *monosaccharides* with general formula $(CH_2O)_n$ where n is three or more. A typical monosaccharide has the structure $H-(CHOH)_x(C=O)-(CHOH)_y-H$, that is, an aldehyde or ketone with many hydroxyl groups added, usually one on each carbon atom that is not part of the aldehyde or ketone functional group. Examples of monosaccharides are glucose, fructose, and glyceraldehydes. However, some biological substances commonly called *monosaccharides* do not conform to this formula (e.g., uronic acids and deoxy-sugars such as fucose), and there are many chemicals that do conform to this formula but are not considered to be monosaccharides (e.g., formaldehyde CH_2O and inositol $[CH_2O]_6$) (Figures 3.12–3.15).

The open-chain form of a monosaccharide often coexists with a closed ring form where the aldehyde/ketone carbonyl group carbon (C=O) and hydroxyl group (−OH) react forming a hemiacetal with a new C–O–C bridge.

Monosaccharides can be linked together into what are called *polysaccharides* (or oligosaccharides) in a large variety of ways. Many carbohydrates contain one or more modified monosaccharide units that have had one or more groups replaced or removed. For example, deoxyribose, a component of DNA, is a modified version of ribose; chitin is composed of repeating units of *N*-acetyl glucosamine, a nitrogen-containing form of glucose.

Monosaccharides are the simplest carbohydrates in that they cannot be hydrolyzed to smaller carbohydrates. They are aldehydes or ketones with two or more hydroxyl groups. The general chemical formula of an unmodified monosaccharide is $(C \cdot H_2O)_n$, literally a *carbon hydrate*. Monosaccharides are important fuel molecules as well as building blocks for nucleic acids. The smallest monosaccharides, for which $n = 3$, are dihydroxyacetone and D- and L-glyceraldehydes.

The α and β are anomers of glucose. Note the position of the hydroxyl group (red or green) on the anomeric carbon relative to the CH_2OH group bound to carbon 5: they are either on the opposite sides (α) or on the same side (β) (Figures 3.16 and 3.17).

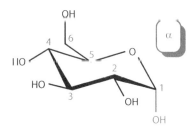

Figure 3.16   The α anomer of glucose.

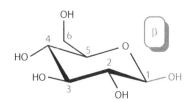

Figure 3.17   The β anomer of glucose.

Monosaccharides are classified according to three different characteristics: the placement of its carbonyl group, the number of carbon atoms it contains, and its chiral handedness. If the carbonyl group is an aldehyde, the monosaccharide is an aldose; if the carbonyl group is a ketone, the monosaccharide is a ketose. Monosaccharides with three carbon atoms are called *trioses*, those with four are called *tetroses*, five are called *pentoses*, six are called *hexoses*, and so on. These two systems of classification are often combined. For example, glucose is an aldohexose (a six-carbon aldehyde), ribose is an aldopentose (a five-carbon aldehyde), and fructose is a ketohexose (a six-carbon ketone).

Each carbon atom bearing a hydroxyl group (−OH), with the exception of the first and last carbons, is asymmetric, making them stereo centers with two possible configurations each (R or S). Because of this asymmetry, a number of isomers may exist for any given monosaccharide formula. The aldohexose D-glucose, for example, has the formula $(C \cdot H_2O)_6$, of which all but two of its six carbon atoms are stereogenic, making D-glucose one of 24 = 16 possible stereoisomers. In the case of glyceraldehydes, an aldotriose, there is one pair of possible stereoisomers, which are enantiomers and epimers. 1, 3-dihydroxyacetone, the ketose corresponding to the aldose glyceraldehydes, is a symmetric molecule with no stereocenters. The assignment of D or L is made according to the orientation of the asymmetric carbon furthest from the carbonyl group: in a standard Fischer projection if the hydroxyl group is on the right the molecule is a D sugar, otherwise it is an L sugar. The D- and L- prefixes should not be confused with d- or l-, which indicate the direction that the sugar rotates plane polarized light. This usage of d- and l- is no longer followed in carbohydrate chemistry.

Glucose can exist in both a straight-chain and ring form. The aldehyde or ketone group of a straight-chain monosaccharide will react reversibly with a hydroxyl group on a different carbon atom to form a hemiacetal or hemiketal, forming a heterocyclic ring with an oxygen bridge between two carbon atoms. Rings with five and six atoms are called *furanose* and *pyranose forms*, respectively, and exist in equilibrium with the straight-chain form.

During the conversion from straight-chain form to the cyclic form, the carbon atom containing the carbonyl oxygen, called the *anomeric carbon*, becomes a stereogenic center with two possible configurations: The oxygen atom may take a position either above or below the plane of the ring. The resulting possible pair of stereoisomers is called *anomers*. In the α anomer, the –OH substituent on the anomeric carbon rests on the opposite side (*trans*) of the ring from the CH_2OH side branch. The alternative form, in which the CH_2OH substituent and the anomeric hydroxyl are on the same side (*cis*) of the plane of the ring, is called the β *anomer*.

Monosaccharides are the major source of fuel for metabolism, being used both as an energy source (glucose being the most important in nature) and in biosynthesis. When monosaccharides are not immediately needed by many cells, they are often converted to more space-efficient forms, such as polysaccharides. In many animals, including humans, this storage form is glycogen, especially in liver and muscle cells. In plants, starch is used for the same purpose.

Particular types of monosaccharides are D-ribose and deoxyribose, the five carbon ring-structured sugar molecules that are essential components of DNA and RNA (Figure 3.18).

Disaccharides are formed by the condensation of two monosaccharides. For example, maltose forms when two molecules of glucose condense. Sucrose, also known as *table sugar*, is a common disaccharide. It is composed of two monosaccharides: D-glucose (left) and D-fructose (right). Two joined monosaccharides are called a *disaccharide*, and these are the simplest polysaccharides. Examples include sucrose and lactose. They are composed of two monosaccharide units bound together by a covalent bond known as a *glycosidic linkage* formed via a dehydration reaction, resulting in the loss of a hydrogen atom from one monosaccharide and a hydroxyl group from the other. The formula of unmodified disaccharides is $C_{12}H_{22}O_{11}$. Although there are numerous kinds of disaccharides, a handful of disaccharides are particularly notable.

Lactose, a disaccharide composed of one D-galactose molecule and one D-glucose molecule, occurs naturally in mammalian milk. The systematic name for lactose is O-β-D-galactopyranosyl-(1→4)-D-glucopyranose. Other notable disaccharides include maltose (two D-glucoses linked α-1,4) and cellulobiose (two D-glucoses linked β-1,4).

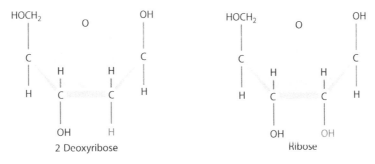

Figure 3.18 The structures of 2-deoxyribose and ribose, which are the monosaccharides that comprise the backbone of DNA and RNA, respectively.

Disaccharides can be classified into two types: reducing and non-reducing disaccharides; if the functional group is present in bonding with another sugar unit it is called a *reducing disaccharide* or *biose*.

Amylose is a straight chain of glucose molecules linked by an α-1,4 glycosidic linkage; the molecular weight of amylose ranges between thousands to half a million daltons (Figure 3.19).

Amylopectin is a branched chain D-glucose where branching occurs between the glycosidic hydroxyl group and one chain and the −6 carbon of another glucose—α-1,6 glycosidic linkage (Figure 3.20).

Glycogen is a branched chain of glucose molecules that resemble amylopectin; it is highly branched and contains about 12 glucose units in straight chain with molecular weight of 5 million daltons (Figure 3.21).

Cellulose is a long unbranched chain of D-glucose with molecular weight between 50,000 and one million daltons; the linkage between glucose monomers in cellulose is a β-1,4 glycosidic linkage, which is resistant to enzymatic hydrolysis making this one of the

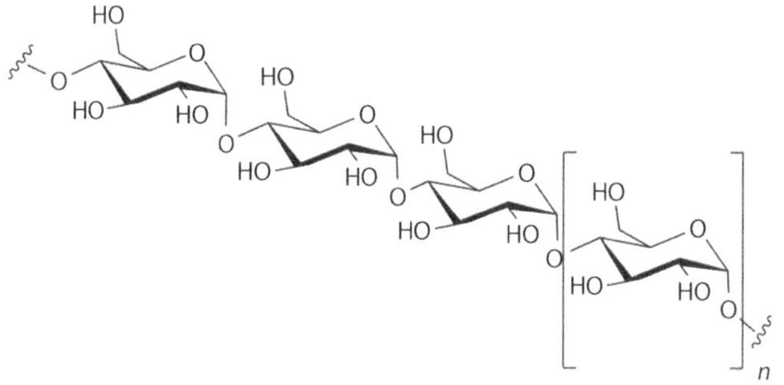

Figure 3.19   Depiction of the straight chain polysaccharide, amylose.

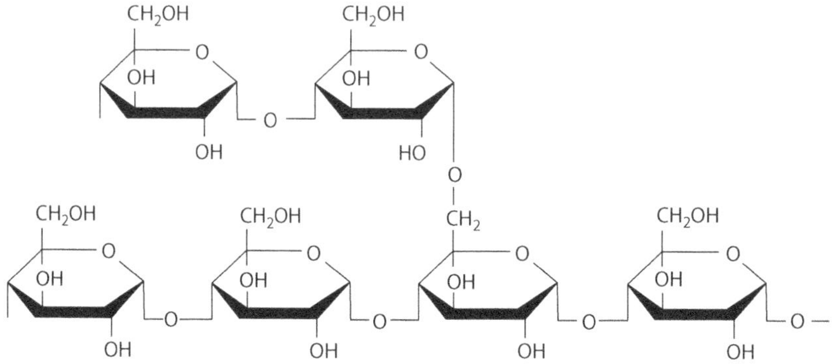

Figure 3.20   Depiction of the branched chain polysaccharide, amylopectin.

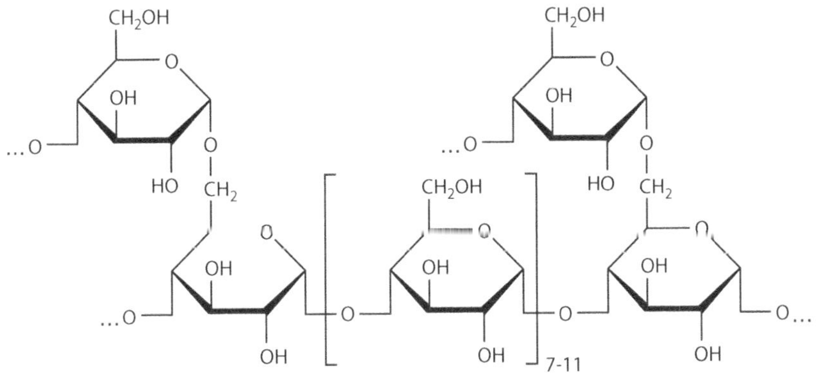

Figure 3.21 Depiction of the structure of the branched polysaccharide glycogen, which is composed of glucose subunits and looks similar to amylopectin; however, it contains increased branching.

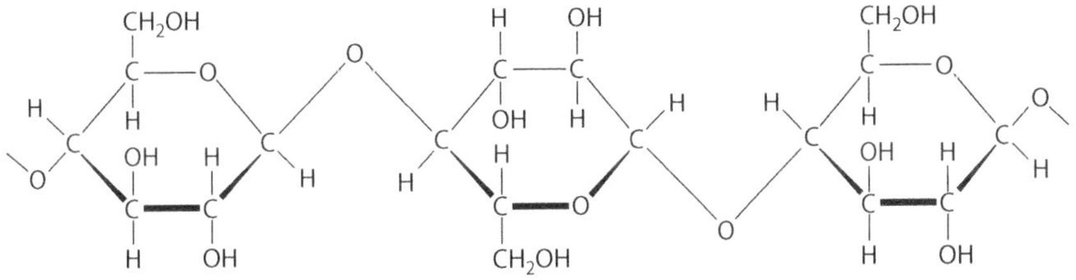

Figure 3.22 Depiction of the unbranched polysaccharide cellulose, which is composed of glucose subunits.

challenging aspects of bioprocessing, for a successful breakage would provide extensive source of energy (Figure 3.22).

Carbohydrates are not necessary building blocks of other molecules, and the body can obtain all its energy from protein and fats. The brain and neurons generally cannot burn fat for energy, but instead use glucose or ketones. Humans can synthesize some glucose (in a set of processes known as *gluconeogenesis*) from specific amino acids, which originate from the glycerol backbone in triglycerides and in some cases from fatty acids. Carbohydrate and protein contain 4 cal/g, while fats contain 9 cal/g. In the case of protein, this is somewhat misleading, as only some amino acids are usable for fuel.

Organisms typically cannot metabolize all types of carbohydrate to yield energy. Glucose is a nearly universal and an accessible source of calories. Many organisms also have the ability to metabolize other monosaccharides and disaccharides, though glucose is preferred. In *Escherichia coli*, for example, the lac operon will express enzymes for the digestion of lactose when it is present, but if both lactose and glucose are present the lac operon is repressed, resulting in the glucose being used first. Polysaccharides are also common sources of energy. Many organisms can easily breakdown starches into glucose; however, most organisms cannot metabolize cellulose or other polysaccharides like chitin and arabinoxylans. Some bacteria and protists can metabolize these types of carbohydrates.

83

Ruminants and termites, for example, use microorganisms to process cellulose. Even though these complex carbohydrates are not very digestible, they may comprise important dietary elements for humans called *dietary fiber*, and these carbohydrates enhance digestion among other benefits.

3.6 LIPIDS, FATS, AND STEROIDS

Lipids constitute a group of naturally occurring molecules that include fats, waxes, sterols, fat-soluble vitamins (such as vitamins A, D, E, and K), monoglycerides, diglycerides, triglycerides, phospholipids, and others. The main biological functions of lipids include energy storage, signaling, and acting as structural components of cell membranes. More broadly they are defined as hydrophobic (water hating) or amphiphilic (water and oil loving) small molecules. The amphiphilic nature of some lipids allows them to form structures such as vesicles, liposomes, or membranes in an aqueous environment. Biological lipids originate entirely or in part from two distinct types of biochemical subunits or *building blocks*: ketoacyl and isoprene groups. Using this approach, lipids may be divided into eight categories: fatty acids, glycerolipids, glycerophospholipids, sphingolipids, saccharolipids, and polyketides (derived from condensation of ketoacyl subunits), and sterol lipids and prenol lipids (derived from condensation of isoprene subunits).

Although the term *lipid* is sometimes used as a synonym for fats, fats are a subgroup of lipids called *triglycerides*. Lipids also encompass molecules such as fatty acids and their derivatives (including tri-, di-, and monoglycerides and phospholipids), as well as other sterol-containing metabolites such as cholesterol. Although humans and other mammals use various biosynthetic pathways to both break down and synthesize lipids, some essential lipids cannot be made this way and must be obtained from the diet.

Fatty acids, or fatty acid residues when they form part of a lipid, are a diverse group of molecules synthesized by chain elongation of an acetyl-CoA primer with malonyl-CoA or methylmalonyl-CoA groups in a process called *fatty acid synthesis*. They are made of a hydrocarbon chain that terminates with a carboxylic acid group; this arrangement confers the molecule with a polar, hydrophilic end, and a nonpolar, hydrophobic end that is insoluble in water.

A typical structure of fatty acids is $CH_3-(CH_2)_n-COOH$; these are one of the most fundamental categories of biological lipids and are commonly used as building blocks of more structurally complex lipids. The carbon chain, typically 4–24 carbons long, may be saturated or unsaturated and may be attached to functional groups containing oxygen, halogens, nitrogen, and sulfur. Where a double bond exists, there is the possibility of either a *cis* or *trans* geometric isomerism, which significantly affects the molecule's configuration. *Cis*-double bonds cause the fatty acid chain to bend, an effect that is compounded with more double bonds in the chain. This in turn plays an important role in the structure and function of cell membranes. Most naturally occurring fatty acids are of the *cis* configuration, although the *trans* form does exist in some natural and partially hydrogenated fats and oils.

Fatty acid chains differ by length, often categorized as short to very long.

- Short-chain fatty acids are fatty acids with aliphatic tails of fewer than six carbons (i.e., butyric acid).
- Medium-chain fatty acids are fatty acids with aliphatic tails of 6–12 carbons, which can form medium-chain triglycerides.
- Long-chain fatty acids are fatty acids with aliphatic tails 13–21 carbons.
- Very long chain fatty acids are fatty acids with aliphatic tails longer than 22 carbons.

Table 3.3 shows the structure of unsaturated fatty acids, and Table 3.4 shows the structure of saturated fatty acids.

Examples of biologically important fatty acids are the eicosanoids, derived primarily from arachidonic acid and eicosapentaenoic acid, that include prostaglandins, leukotrienes, and thromboxanes. Docosahexaenoic acid is also important in biological systems, particularly with respect to sight. Other major lipid classes in the fatty acid category are the fatty esters and fatty amides. Fatty esters include important biochemical intermediates such as wax esters, fatty acid thioester coenzyme A derivatives, fatty acid thioester acyl carrier protein derivatives, and fatty acid carnitines. The fatty amides include *N*-acyl ethanolamines, such as the cannabinoid neurotransmitter anandamide. Figure 3.23 shows common lipid forms.

Table 3.3 Unsaturated Fatty Acids

Common Name	Chemical Structure	Δx	*C:D	$n-x$
Myristoleic acid	$CH_3(CH_2)_3CH=CH(CH_2)_7COOH$	cis-$\Delta 9$	14:1	$n-5$
Palmitoleic acid	$CH_3(CH_2)_5CH=CH(CH_2)_7COOH$	cis-$\Delta 9$	16:1	$n-7$
Sapienic acid	$CH_3(CH_2)_8CH=CH(CH_2)_4COOH$	cis-$\Delta 6$	16:1	$n-10$
Oleic acid	$CH_3(CH_2)_7CH=CH(CH_2)_7COOH$	cis-$\Delta 9$	18:1	$n-9$
Elaidic acid	$CH_3(CH_2)_7CH=CH(CH_2)_7COOH$	trans-$\Delta 9$	18:1	$n-9$
Vaccenic acid	$CH_3(CH_2)_5CH=CH(CH_2)_9COOH$	trans-$\Delta 11$	18:1	$n-7$
Linoleic acid	$CH_3(CH_2)_4CH=CHCH_2CH=CH(CH_2)_7$ COOH	cis,cis-$\Delta 9,\Delta 12$	18:2	$n-6$
Linoelaidic acid	$CH_3(CH_2)_4CH=CHCH_2CH=CH(CH_2)_7$ COOH	trans,trans-$\Delta 9,\Delta 12$	18:2	$n-6$
α-Linolenic acid	$CH_3CH_2CH=CHCH_2CH=CHCH_2$ $CH=CH(CH_2)_7COOH$	cis,cis,cis-$\Delta 9,\Delta 12,\Delta 15$	18:3	$n-3$
Arachidonic acid	$CH_3(CH_2)_4CH=CHCH_2CH=CHCH_2$ $CH=CHCH_2CH=CH(CH_2)_3COOHNIST$	cis,cis,cis,cis-$\Delta 5,\Delta 8,\Delta 11,\Delta 14$	20:4	$n-6$
Eicosapentaenoic acid	$CH_3CH_2CH=CHCH_2CH=CHCH_2$ $CH=CHCH_2CH=CHCH_2CH=CH(CH_2)_3$ COOH	cis,cis,cis,cis,cis-$\Delta 5,\Delta 8,\Delta 11,$ $\Delta 14,\Delta 17$	20:5	$n-3$
Erucic acid	$CH_3(CH_2)_7CH=CH(CH_2)_{11}COOH$	cis-$\Delta 13$	22:1	$n-9$
Docosahexaenoic acid	$CH_3CH_2CH=CHCH_2CH=CHCH_2$ $CH=CHCH_2CH=CHCH_2CH=CHCH_2$ $CH=CH(CH_2)_2COOH$	cis,cis,cis,cis,cis, cis-$\Delta 4,\Delta 7,\Delta 10,$ $\Delta 13,\Delta 16,\Delta 19$	22:6	$n-3$

*C: Number of carbons and D: number of double bonds.

Note: $n-x$: a double bond is at xth carbon counting from the terminal methyl carbon designated as or omega. For example, omega-C fatty acids ($n-3$).

Table 3.4 Saturated Fatty Acids

Common Name	Chemical Structure	C:D
Caprylic acid	$CH_3(CH_2)_6COOH$	8:0
Capric acid	$CH_3(CH_2)_8COOH$	10:0
Lauric acid	$CH_3(CH_2)_{10}COOH$	12:0
Myristic acid	$CH_3(CH_2)_{12}COOH$	14:0
Palmitic acid	$CH_3(CH_2)_{14}COOH$	16:0
Stearic acid	$CH_3(CH_2)_{16}COOH$	18:0
Arachidic acid	$CH_3(CH_2)_{18}COOH$	20:0
Behenic acid	$CH_3(CH_2)_{20}COOH$	22:0
Lignoceric acid	$CH_3(CH_2)_{22}COOH$	24:0
Cerotic acid	$CH_3(CH_2)_{24}COOH$	26:0

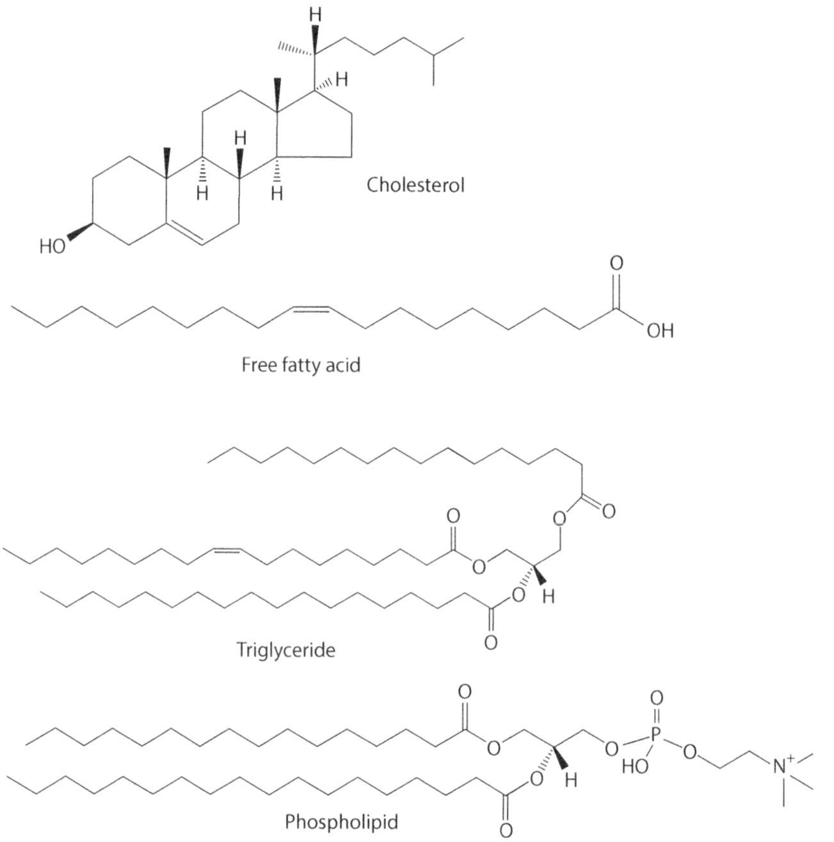

Figure 3.23 Structures of some common lipids. At the top are cholesterol and oleic acid. The middle structure is a triglyceride composed of oleoyl, stearoyl, and palmitoyl chains attached to a glycerol backbone. At the bottom is the common phospholipid, phosphatidylcholine.

Glycerolipids are composed mainly of mono-, di-, and tri-substituted glycerols, the most well known being the fatty acid triesters of glycerol, called *triglycerides*. The word *triacylglycerol* is sometimes used synonymously with *triglyceride*, though the latter lipids contain no hydroxyl group. In these compounds, the three hydroxyl groups of glycerol are each esterified, typically by different fatty acids. Because they function as an energy store, these lipids comprise the bulk of storage fat in animal tissues. The hydrolysis of the ester bonds of triglycerides and the release of glycerol and fatty acids from adipose tissue are the initial steps in metabolizing fat.

Additional subclasses of glycerolipids are represented by glycosylglycerols, which are characterized by the presence of one or more sugar residues attached to glycerol via a glycosidic linkage. Examples of structures in this category are the digalactosyldiacylglycerols found in plant membranes and seminolipid from mammalian sperm cells.

Glycerophospholipids, usually referred to as *phospholipids*, are key components of the lipid bilayer of cells, as well as being involved in metabolism and cell signaling. Neural tissue, including the brain, contains relatively high amounts of glycerophospholipids, and alterations in their composition have been implicated in various neurological disorders. Glycerophospholipids may be subdivided into distinct classes, based on the nature of the polar headgroup at the sn-3 position of the glycerol backbone in eukaryotes and eubacteria, or the sn-1 position in the case of archaebacteria. Examples of glycerophospholipids found in biological membranes are phosphatidylcholine (also known as PC, GPCho, or lecithin), phosphatidylethanolamine (PE or GPEtn), and phosphatidylserine (PS or GPSer). In addition to serving as a primary component of cellular membranes and binding sites for intra- and intercellular proteins, some glycerophospholipids in eukaryotic cells, such as phosphatidylinositols and phosphatidic acids, are either precursors of or, themselves, membrane-derived second messengers. Typically, one or both of these hydroxyl groups are acylated with long-chain fatty acids, but there are also alkyl-linked and 1Z-alkenyl-linked (plasmalogen) glycerophospholipids, as well as dialkylether variants in archaebacteria. Figure 3.24 shows the structure of a phosphatidyl ethanolamine.

Sphingolipids are a complicated family of compounds that share a common structural feature, a sphingoid base backbone that is synthesized *de novo* from the amino acid serine and a long-chain fatty acyl CoA, then converted into ceramides, phosphosphingolipids, glycosphingolipids, and other compounds. The major sphingoid base of mammals

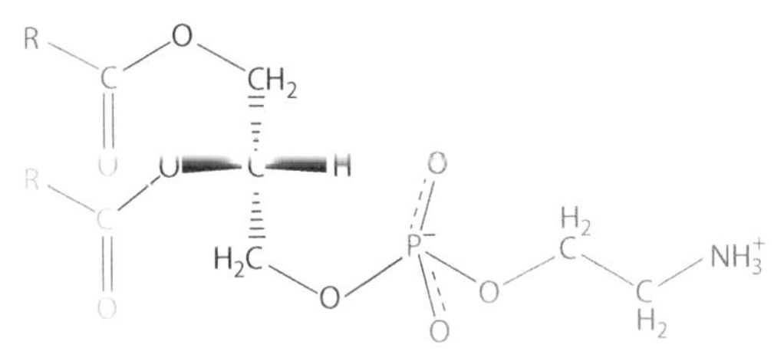

Figure 3.24   Structure of phosphatidyl ethanolamine.

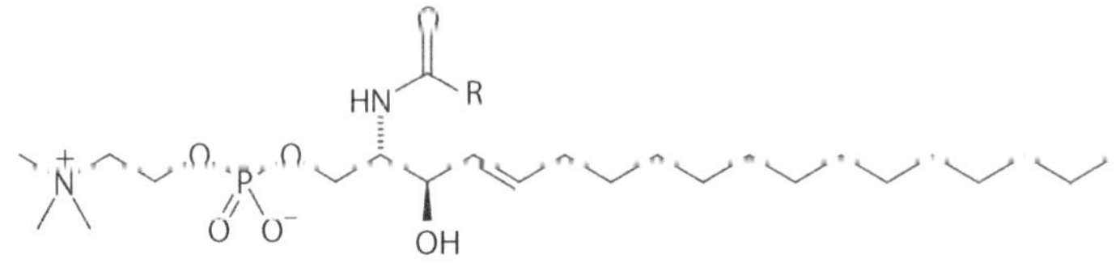

Figure 3.25 Structure of sphingomyelin.

is commonly referred to as *sphingosine*. Ceramides (*N*-acyl-sphingoid bases) are a major subclass of sphingoid base derivatives with an amide-linked fatty acid. The fatty acids are typically saturated or monounsaturated with chain lengths from 16 to 26 carbon atoms. Figure 3.25 shows the structure of sphingomyelin.

The major phosphosphingolipids of mammals are sphingomyelins (ceramide phosphocholines), whereas insects contain mainly ceramide phosphoethanolamines, and fungi have phytoceramide phosphoinositols and mannose-containing headgroups. The glycosphingolipids are a diverse family of molecules composed of one or more sugar residues linked via a glycosidic bond to the sphingoid base. Examples of these are the simple and complex glycosphingolipids such as cerebrosides and gangliosides.

Sterol lipids, such as cholesterol and its derivatives, are an important component of membrane lipids, along with the glycerophospholipids and sphingomyelins. The steroids, all derived from the same fused four-ring core structure, have different biological roles as hormones and signaling molecules. The 18-carbon (C18) steroids include the estrogen family, whereas the C19 steroids comprise the androgens such as testosterone and androsterone. The C21 subclass includes the progestogens as well as the glucocorticoids and mineralocorticoids. The secosteroids, comprising various forms of vitamin D, are characterized by cleavage of the B ring of the core structure. Other examples of sterols are the bile acids and their conjugates, which in mammals are oxidized derivatives of cholesterol and are synthesized in the liver. The plant equivalents are the phytosterols, such as β-sitosterol, stigmasterol, and brassicasterol; the latter compound is also used as a biomarker for algal growth. The predominant sterol in fungal cell membranes is ergosterol.

Prenol lipids are synthesized from the five-carbon-unit precursors isopentenyl diphosphate and dimethylallyl diphosphate that are produced mainly via the mevalonic acid pathway. The simple isoprenoids (linear alcohols, diphosphates, etc.) are formed by the successive addition of C5 units and are classified according to the number of terpene units. Structures containing greater than 40 carbons are known as *polyterpenes*. Carotenoids are important simple isoprenoids that function as antioxidants and as precursors of vitamin A. Another biologically important class of molecules is exemplified by the quinones and hydroquinones, which contain an isoprenoid tail attached to a quinonoid core of non-isoprenoid origin. Vitamin E and vitamin K, as well as the ubiquinones, are examples of this class. Prokaryotes synthesize polyprenols (called *bactoprenols*) in which the terminal isoprenoid unit attached to oxygen remains unsaturated, whereas in animal polyprenols (dolichols) the terminal isoprenoid is reduced.

Saccharolipids describe compounds in which fatty acids are linked directly to a sugar backbone, forming structures that are compatible with membrane bilayers. In the saccharolipids, a monosaccharide substitutes for the glycerol backbone present in glycerolipids and glycerophospholipids. The most familiar saccharolipids are the acylated glucosamine precursors of the lipid A component of the lipopolysaccharides in Gram-negative bacteria. Typical lipid A molecules are disaccharides of glucosamine, which are derived with as many as seven fatty-acyl chains. The minimal lipopolysaccharide required for growth in *E. coli* is Kdo2-Lipid A, a hexa acylated disaccharide of glucosamine that is glycosylated with two 3-deoxy-D-manno-octulosonic acid (Kdo) residues.

Polyketides are synthesized by polymerization of acetyl and propionyl subunits by classic enzymes as well as by iterative and multimodular enzymes that share mechanistic features with the fatty acid synthases. They comprise a large number of secondary metabolites and natural products from animal, plant, bacterial, fungal, and marine sources and have great structural diversity. Many polyketides are cyclic molecules whose backbones are often further modified by glycosylation, methylation, hydroxylation, oxidation, and/or other processes. Many commonly used antimicrobial, antiparasitic, and anticancer agents are polyketides or polyketide derivatives, such as erythromycins, tetracyclines, avermectins, and antitumor epothilones.

Eukaryotic cells are compartmentalized into membrane-bound organelles that carry out different biological functions. The glycerophospholipids are the main structural component of biological membranes, such as the cellular plasma membrane and the intracellular membranes of organelles; in animal cells, the plasma membrane physically separates the intracellular components from the extracellular environment. The glycerophospholipids are amphipathic molecules (containing both hydrophobic and hydrophilic regions) that contain a glycerol core linked to two fatty acid-derived *tails* by ester linkages and to one *head* group by a phosphate ester linkage. While glycerophospholipids are the major component of biological membranes, other non-glyceride lipid components such as sphingomyelin and sterols (mainly cholesterol in animal cell membranes) are also found in biological membranes.

In plants and algae, the galactosyldiacylglycerols and sulfoquinovosyldiacylglycerol, which lack a phosphate group, are important components of membranes of chloroplasts and related organelles and are the most abundant lipids in photosynthetic tissues, including those of higher plants, algae, and certain bacteria.

Bilayers have been found to exhibit high levels of birefringence (an optical property of a material having a refractive index that depends on the polarization and propagation direction of light), which can be used to probe the degree of order (or disruption) within the bilayer using techniques such as dual polarization interferometry and circular dichroism (often abbreviated as CD).

Figure 3.26 shows the self-organization of phospholipids, a spherical liposome, a micelle, and a lipid bilayer. A biological membrane is a form of lipid bilayer. The formation of lipid bilayers is an energetically preferred process when the glycerophospholipids described above are in an aqueous environment. This is known as the *hydrophobic effect*. In an aqueous system, the polar heads of lipids align toward the polar, aqueous environment, while the hydrophobic tails minimize their contact with water and tend to cluster

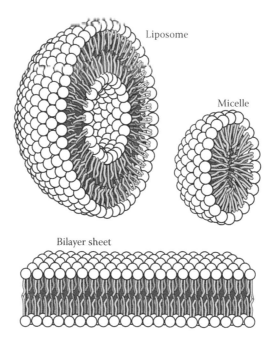

Figure 3.26 Self-organization of phospholipids.

together, forming a vesicle. Depending on the concentration of the lipid, this biophysical interaction may result in the formation of micelles, liposomes, or lipid bilayers. Other aggregations are also observed and form part of the polymorphism of amphiphile (lipid) behavior. Phase behavior is an area of study within biophysics and is the subject of current academic research.

Micelles and bilayers form in the polar medium by a process known as the *hydrophobic effect*. When dissolving a lipophilic or amphiphilic substance in a polar environment, the polar molecules (i.e., water in an aqueous solution) become more ordered around the dissolved lipophilic substance, since the polar molecules cannot form hydrogen bonds to the lipophilic areas of the amphiphile. So in an aqueous environment, the water molecules form an ordered *clathrate* cage around the dissolved lipophilic molecule.

Beta-oxidation is the metabolic process by which fatty acids are broken down in the mitochondria and/or in peroxisomes to generate acetyl-CoA. For the most part, fatty acids are oxidized by a mechanism that is similar to, but not identical to, a reversal of the process of fatty acid synthesis. That is, two-carbon fragments are removed sequentially from the carboxyl end of the acid after steps of dehydrogenation, hydration, and oxidation to form a β-keto acid, which is split by thiolysis. The acetyl-CoA is then ultimately converted into ATP, CO_2, and H_2O using the citric acid cycle and the electron transport chain. Hence, the Krebs cycle can start at acetyl-CoA when fat is being broken down for energy if there is little or no glucose available.

3.7 BASIC METABOLIC PATHWAYS

The main source of energy for cells comes in the form of ATP. All cell types use a number of metabolic pathways to ultimately produce ATP. Metabolic pathways in eukaryotic cells are relatively straightforward, photosynthesis in plant cells and metabolism of glucose in mammalian cells. Prokaryotic cells are capable of wide range of metabolic pathways including photosynthesis; glucose metabolism; metabolism of nitrogen, phosphorous, and sulfur containing compounds; metabolism of hydrocarbons; and metabolism of CO_2.

3.7.1 Glycolysis and the Citric Acid Cycle

Glucose metabolism is a metabolic pathway that is shared between eukaryotic and prokaryotic cells. The metabolism of glucose can occur both in the presence, aerobic, and absence, anaerobic, of oxygen. Regardless of oxygen, the first step in each is the conversion of glucose to pyruvate through the process of glycolysis (Figure 3.27). The overall reaction for glycolysis is

$$\text{Glucose} + 2\text{ADP} + 2\text{NAD}^+ + 2\text{P}_i \rightarrow 2\text{pyruvate} + 2\text{ATP} + 2\left(\text{NADH} + \text{H}^+\right) \tag{3.1}$$

The most straightforward way to proceed from glycolysis would be the single step enzymatic conversion of pyruvate to lactate by lactate dehydrogenase:

$$\text{Pyruvate} + \text{NADH} + \text{H}^+ \rightarrow \text{lactate} + \text{NAD}^+ \tag{3.2}$$

This process, while straightforward, fails to make the most out of pyruvate and only occurs in eukaryotes and prokaryotes when there is not sufficient oxygen. Instead, in the presence of oxygen, both eukaryotes and prokaryotes will use the citric acid cycle and electron transport chain to covert pyruvate into additional energy. Figure 3.28 provides an overview of the citric acid, or Krebs, cycle. The conversion of one pyruvate through the citric acid cycle has the following overall reaction:

$$\text{Pyruvate} + 4\text{NAD}^+ + \text{FAD} + \text{CoA-SH} + \text{GDP} + \text{P}_i + 2\text{H}_2\text{O}$$
$$\rightarrow \text{CoA} + 4\left(\text{NADH} + \text{H}^+\right) + \text{FADH}_2 + \text{GTP} + 3\text{CO}_2 \tag{3.3}$$

Likewise, the net conversion of glucose by glycolysis and the citric acid cycle proceeds through the following reaction:

$$\text{Glucose} + 10\text{NAD}^+ + 2\text{FAD} + 2\text{CoA-SH} + 2\text{ADP} + 2\text{GDP} + 4\text{P}_i + 4\text{H}_2\text{O}$$
$$\rightarrow 2\text{CoA} + 10\left(\text{NADH} + \text{H}^+\right) + 2\text{FADH}_2 + 2\text{ATP} + 2\text{GTP} + 6\text{CO}_2 \tag{3.4}$$

Examining the overall equation, the key energy providing components are NADH, FADH$_2$, guanosine triphosphate (GTP), and ATP. GTP is directly converted to ATP. NADH and FADH$_2$ are converted to ATP through the electron transport chain. In the cytoplasm of prokaryotes and the mitochondria of eukaryotes, the electron transport chain pulls electrons off NADH and FADH$_2$ and uses those electrons to transfer 6H$^+$ for NADH and 4H$^+$ for FADH$_2$ across the

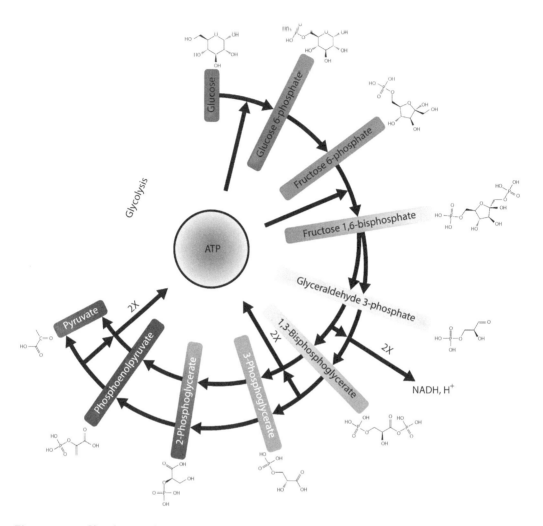

Figure 3.27 Glycolysis is the breakdown of glucose to pyruvate. This process initially requires two moles of ATP per glucose in the breakdown of glucose to glyceraldehyde 3-phosphate; however, the second half of glycolysis results in the production of 4 mol of ATP per glucose resulting in a net 2 mol of ATP per glucose.

mitochondrial membrane. These protons flow back into the mitochondria due to a potential gradient through ATP synthase, which uses the transport of $2H^+$ across the membrane to drive the conversion of $ADP + P_i \rightarrow ATP$. Thus, the $68H^+$ pumped across the mitochondrial membrane by the oxidation of NADH to NAD^+ and $FADH_2$ to FAD have the potential to generate 34 ATPs, which when added to the 4 ATPs produced directly (2 from the direct conversion of GTP to ATP) by glycolysis and the citric acid cycle nets a total of 38 potential ATPs. In reality, some ATPs are used in the transport of pyruvate and ADP and some protons leak back across the mitochondrial membrane leading to a typical net of 29–30ATP per glucose.

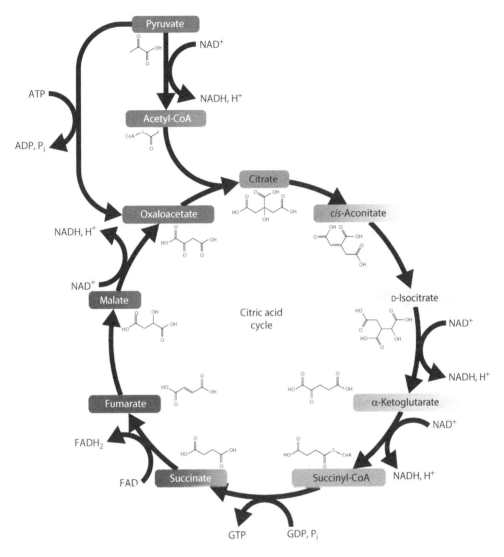

Figure 3.28 Demonstration of the major components in the citric acid cycle, which converts pyruvate to citric acid (citrate) and then onto oxaloacetate while generating GTP that is readily exchanged to ATP in a 1:1 relationship and the coenzymes NADH and FADH$_2$, which are converted to ATP through the electron transport chain.

3.7.2 Photosynthesis

It is widely recognized that plants and some prokaryotes undergo photosynthesis; however, contrary to popular belief, photosynthesis does not produce ATP. Instead photosynthesis is a precursor to glycolysis and the citric acid cycle. Photosynthesis occurs in specialized organelles called *chloroplasts* and is divided into both light-dependent reactions and light independent reactions. The light-dependent reactions use water and light to produce ATP and oxygen and proceed as follows:

$$2H_2O + 2NADP^+ + 3ADP + 3P_i \xrightarrow{h\nu} 2NADPH + 2H^+ + 3ATP + O_2 \tag{3.5}$$

Next, the light-independent reactions proceed through a process referred to as the *Calvin cycle*. The Calvin cycle does not require it to be dark; it simply proceeds without any energy provided by light. The Calvin cycle will consume ATP and produce sugars. Three turns around the Calvin cycle yields the following net reaction:

$$3CO_2 + 6NADPH + 5H_2O + 9ATP$$
$$\rightarrow \text{glyceraldehyde-3-phosphate} + 2H^+ + 6NADP^+ + 9ADP + 8P_i \tag{3.6}$$

Two glyceraldehyde-3-phosphates are readily combined to form glucose, as well as other carbohydrates. A quick inspection of the light-dependent reactions that produce energy and the reducing coenzyme NADPH reveals all the ATP and NADPH produced with light are consumed without light to produce ever more complex sugars from CO_2. The net photosynthesis reaction for the production of glucose (from two glyceraldehyde-3-phosphates) is

$$6CO_2 + 6H_2O \xrightarrow{h\nu} C_6H_{12}O_6 + 6O_2 \tag{3.7}$$

To produce energy in the form of ATP, plants simply use the glucose generated by photosynthesis in the respiration processes, glycolysis and the citric acid cycle.

3.7.3 Nitrogen Cycle

The final mechanism of metabolism covered in this chapter deals with the sequestration and conversion of nitrogen to ammonia, nitrite, and nitrate. Nitrogen is a key compound in many biomolecules, for example, amino acids, and is attained either by the breakdown of existing biomolecules or sequestration of nitrogen present in the atmosphere. Atmospheric nitrogen, N_2, is very stable. The first step of converting N_2 into useful intermediates is referred to as *nitrogen fixation*. Nitrogen fixation occurs in prokaryotes (both bacteria and archaea) called *diazotrophs* and proceeds as follows:

$$N_2 + 8H^+ + 8e^- + 16ATP \rightarrow 2NH_3 + H_2 + 16ADP + P_i \tag{3.8}$$

Diazotrophs are unique in their ability to sequester nitrogen from the atmosphere allows for independence from any external fixed nitrogen source, which is required of all other prokaryotes and eukaryotes. Examination of the nitrogen fixation equation reveals that it requires an enormous amount of cellular energy to proceed. This is due to high activation energy of N_2, EA = 420 kJ/mol (approximately 10× the energy required to vaporize water during boiling). Once nitrogen is fixed as ammonia, it is readily consumed through downstream reactions leading to the production of biomolecules such as glutamate, which is instrumental in the formation of amino acids.

The next step in the nitrogen cycle is the conversion of ammonia to either nitrite or nitrate. This process is referred to as *nitrification*. Nitrification occurs through the following reactions:

$$NH_3 + O_2 \rightarrow NO_2^- + 3H^+ + 2e^-$$ (3.9)

$$NO_2^- + H_2O \rightarrow NO_3^- + 2H^+ + 2e^-$$ (3.10)

Unlike nitrogen fixation, both nitrification steps are energy producing thanks to the protons generated. The first nitrification step is carried out by prokaryotes, both ammonia-oxidizing bacteria and ammonia-oxidizing archaea. The second nitrification step is less well understood, but it is known to be carried out by *Nitrospina* and *Nitrobacter* in marine environments.

Questions

1. What is the difference between a nucleotide and a nucleoside?
   Answer: A nucleotide includes the sugar (either deoxyribose or ribose), the base (adenine, thymine, etc.), and at least one phosphate. A nucleoside also contains the sugar and the base, but no phosphate.
2. Draw the nucleosides for the four nucleotides in DNA.
3. Double-stranded DNA demonstrates a helical structure because of the bonding between two complementary strands. What type of bond is formed between complementary strands of DNA and how does the bond vary depending on the nucleotides present?
4. High concentrations of salt are known to mediate the transformation of DNA from the typical B form to either the A or Z form. From the standpoint of chemistry, what could the addition of salt do to the DNA structure that would lead to a conformation change?
5. A mutation that occurs more often than any other specific mutation in a mammalian cell results in the deamination of 5-methylcytosine. Once 5-methylcytosine is deaminated, what is the resulting nucleotide? If this occurs in DNA, what downstream effects could it have and how can it be addressed?
   Answer: Deamination of 5-methylcytosine results in thymine, which can be corrected by thymine-DNA glycosylase. If uncorrected, since thymine is a nucleotide found in DNA, the mutation produces the typical by-products of a point mutation.
6. The deamination of cytosine in DNA results in a separate nucleotide. Is this nucleotide normally found in DNA? If it is normally found in DNA, what challenge would the repair of this mutation present?
7. What type of DNA mutation would be the most difficult to detect and repair?
8. What are the key structural differences between DNA and RNA?
9. The three key polymers of biology are DNA, RNA and proteins; however, carbohydrates and lipids are also important. What are the key differences between carbohydrates and lipids?

10. Phospholipids are capable of self-organizing into membranes, what underlying principle of chemistry allows for the phenomenon?
    Answer: Intermolecular forces—Van der Waals forces promote the packing of the fatty acid tails. Hydrogen bonding and ionic interactions link the hydrophilic heads together.
11. Amino acids exist in either a D or an L conformation, which conformation is found exclusively in proteins?
12. In proteins, an α helix and a β sheet are examples of what?
13. In proteins, combinations of multiple α helices and β sheets comprise supersecondary structures that are not to the level of complexity of a tertiary structure, what name is given to these combinations of α helices and β sheets?
14. The potassium ion channel is composed of four identical proteins that integrate with one another to form a functional ion channel. What level of protein organization corresponds to functional units composed of multiple proteins?
15. The Krebs cycle relies on the oxidation of multiple components. Oxidation results in the liberation of an electron, what is the most common electron acceptor in the Krebs cycle?
16. The Krebs cycle takes citrate and through a number of reactions converts it to oxaloacetate. The process can be restarted by the conversion of oxaloacetate back to citrate, what is required for this conversion?
    Answer: A single acetyl-CoA is required to convert oxaloacetate back to citrate.
17. If the oxidation of NADH allows for the transport of 6H+ across the membrane, which ultimately contribute to the formation of ATP?
    a. How much ATP is generated per NADH oxidized?
    b. How much ATP is generated per $FADH_2$ oxidized?
18. Into what form is glucose converted for entry into the Krebs cycle?
19. Where in a eukaryotic cell does the Krebs cycle take place?
20. The math for the Krebs cycle indicates a gain of 38 ATPs per glucose, why is the net gain typically only around 30 ATPs?

4

Introduction to Cellular Biology and Microbiology

LEARNING OBJECTIVES

1. Understand the fundamental constituents required of a cell.
2. Recognize the shift in complexity and key differences between eukaryotic and prokaryotic cells.
3. Understand the necessity for organelles in eukaryotic cells and how they assist in maintaining cell function.
4. Grasp the necessity of intracellular signal transduction to overcome limitations in intracellular transport.

4.1 INTRODUCTION

Living entities are characterized by their ability to multiply, grow, or otherwise sustain their existence and are made of chains of carbon atoms, with a few other atoms, such as nitrogen or phosphorous. How a living entity, such as an organism, uses these elemental sources and energy to multiply is a vast subject that requires a clear understanding of cell biology. It is fascinating how, given the same elements and energy, the organisms behave differently and survive under a broad range of environments, from −20°C to +120°C, from very acidic to very basic pH, in the presence or absence of water or oxygen, and so on. These living organisms are classified based on whether they contain a nucleus, an internal membrane surrounding genetic material. Those with a nucleus are classified as *eukaryotes* and those without a nucleus are *prokaryotes*.

4.2 GENERAL CELL STRUCTURE

For the traditional scope of bioprocessing, the living entities of importance are of microbial nature and have a few things in common: they all contain cytoplasm, a viscous material that holds proteins, ribosomes, metabolites, and ions; they all have a plasma membrane,

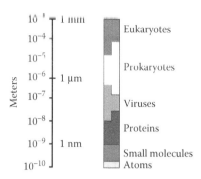

Figure 4.1 Relative sizes of life domains compared to chemical molecules.

which is a cell membrane that surrounds the cytoplasm and is composed of a phospholipid bilayer, associated proteins and carbohydrates; and finally, the generic material DNA (deoxyribonucleic acid) that stores the code for the entire characteristics of the organism.

The DNA material in a eukaryotic cell resides inside the nucleus and mitochondria (a part of nucleus and is in turn a membrane-bound organelle). A prokaryotic cell contains a single DNA molecule, which has no specific boundary within the cytoplasm. Both are capable of forming spores; the spores of prokaryotes have high heat resistance.

The size of these forms of life is also differentiated and scales with the complexity of the life form (Figure 4.1). A broad description of shapes, habitat, and general properties is listed in Table 4.1. Figures 4.2 and 4.3 provide outline structures of these domain organisms.

Table 4.1 Types of Organisms

Characteristic	Label
Grow below 20°C	Psychrophiles
Grow between 20°C and 50°C	Mesophiles (these can be infectious to humans because of the body temperature of 37.5°C)
Grow above 50°C	Thermophiles (geysers of Yellow stone National Park)
Require oxygen	Aerobic
Inhibited by oxygen	Anaerobic
Adaptable to different conditions	Facultative
Need little nutrients	Cyanobacteria (called because blue-green algae)
Spherical or elliptical	Cocci (coccus)
Cylindrical or rod	Bacilli (bacillus)
Spiral-shaped	Spirilli (spirillum)
Producing methane, intolerant of oxygen (live in swamps)	Methanogen

(Continued)

Table 4.1 (*Continued*)   Types of Organisms

Characteristic	Label
Live in high concentration of salt (Salt Lake City, Dead Sea)	Halophiles
Living in extreme environment conditions and lack peptidoglycan in the cell wall	Archaea (e.g., thermophiles and halophiles)
Living in extreme conditions and contain pseudoglycans (composed of N-acetyltalosaminuronic acid, instead of N-acetylmuramic in peptidoglycan)	Often archaea
Cell walls composed of three layers: periplastic, thin layer of peptoglycan, and an outer membrane and no periplasmic space—sensitive to lysozyme and penicillin; they also develop stain to Gram reagent	Gram positive
Small, often unicellular, reproductive unit of plants, algae, fungi, protozoa, and bacteria	Spores; bacterial spores have thick walls, which can withstand varying temperatures, humidity, and other unfavorable conditions

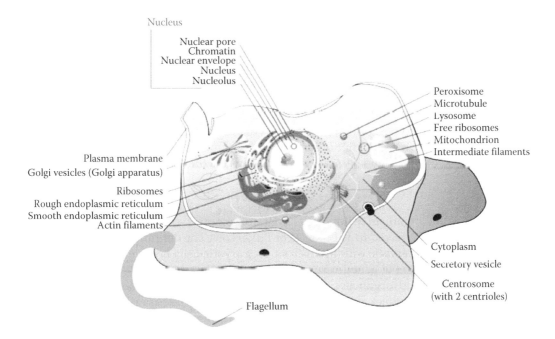

Figure 4.2   Structure of a eukaryotic cell.

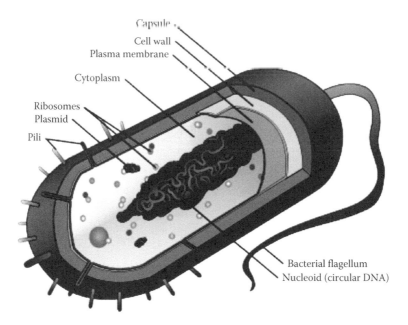

Figure 4.3   Structure of a prokaryotic cell.

4.3 EUKARYOTES, PROKARYOTES, ARCHAEA, AND VIRUSES

From this collection of structures, a division takes place—either with the presence or absence of a nucleus. The divisions with nuclei are called *eukaryotic* (e.g., Chinese hamster ovary cell; see Figure 4.2; remember the *eu* of nucleus for *eu*karyotic), and those without a nucleus are categorized as *prokaryotic* (e.g., bacteria; see Figure 4.3). A third type, Archaea, includes organisms that survive in extreme conditions, such as thermophiles (very hot environments) and acidophiles (acidic conditions). Thus, the living domains are divided into three types: prokaryotic, eukaryotic, and archaea. A fourth group of biological entities, the viruses, are not organisms in the same sense that eukaryotes, archaeans, and bacteria are classified. However, they are of considerable biological importance.

4.3.1 Eukaryotes

A eukaryote is an organism whose cells contain complex structures enclosed within membranes; they are referred to as Eukarya or Eukaryota. The defining membrane-bound structure that sets eukaryotic cells apart from prokaryotic cells is the nucleus, or nuclear envelope, within which the genetic material is carried. Most eukaryotic cells also contain other membrane-bound organelles such as mitochondria, chloroplasts, and the Golgi apparatus. All large complex organisms are eukaryotes, including animals, plants, and fungi. The group also includes many unicellular organisms.

Cell division in eukaryotes is different from that in prokaryotes. It involves separating the duplicated chromosomes, through movements directed by microtubules. There are two types of division processes, mitosis and meiosis. In mitosis, one cell divides to produce two genetically identical cells. In meiosis, which is required in sexual reproduction, one diploid cell (having two instances of each chromosome, one from each parent) undergoes recombination of each pair of parental chromosomes, and then two stages of cell division, resulting in four haploid cells (gametes). Each gamete has just one complement of chromosomes, each a unique mix of the corresponding pair of parental chromosomes.

Eukaryotes represent a tiny minority of all living things; even in a human body there are 10 times more prokaryotes than human eukaryotic cells. However, due to their much larger size, their collective worldwide biomass is estimated at about equal to that of prokaryotes.

Eukaryotic DNA is divided into several linear bundles called *chromosomes*, which are separated by a microtubular spindle during nuclear division. The nucleus is surrounded by a double membrane (commonly referred to as a *nuclear envelope*) with pores that allow material to move in and out. Various tube- and sheet-like extensions of the nuclear membrane form the endoplasmic reticulum or ER, which is involved in protein transport and maturation. It includes the rough ER where ribosomes are attached to synthesize proteins, which enter the interior space or lumen. Subsequently, they generally enter vesicles, which bud off from the smooth ER. In most eukaryotes, these protein-carrying vesicles are released and further modified in stacks of flattened vesicles, called *Golgi bodies* or *dictyosomes*.

Vesicles may be specialized for various purposes. For instance, lysosomes contain enzymes that break down the contents of food vacuoles, and peroxisomes are used to break down peroxide, which is toxic otherwise. Many protozoa have contractile vacuoles, which collect and expel excess water, and extrusomes, which expel material used to deflect predators or capture prey. In higher plants, most of a cell's volume is taken up by a central vacuole, which primarily maintains its osmotic pressure.

Plants and various groups of algae also have plastids. Again, these have their own DNA and developed from endosymbiotes, in this case cyanobacteria. They usually take the form of chloroplasts, which like cyanobacteria contain chlorophyll and produce organic compounds (such as glucose) through photosynthesis. Others are involved in storing food. Although plastids likely had a single origin, not all plastid-containing groups are closely related. Instead, some eukaryotes have obtained them from others through secondary endosymbiosis or ingestion.

An animal cell is a form of eukaryotic cell that makes up many tissues in animals. The animal cell is distinct from other eukaryotes, most notably plant cells, as they lack cell walls and chloroplasts, but they have smaller vacuoles. Due to the lack of a rigid cell wall, animal cells can adopt a variety of shapes, and a phagocytic cell can even engulf other structures. There are many different cell types. For instance, there are approximately 210 distinct cell types in the adult human body.

Plant cells are quite different from the cells of the other eukaryotic organisms. Their distinctive features are as follows:

- A large central vacuole (enclosed by a membrane, the *tonoplast*), which maintains the cell's turgor and controls movement of molecules between the cytosol and sap.
- A primary cell wall contains cellulose, hemicellulose, and pectin, deposited by the protoplast on the outside of the cell membrane; this contrasts with the cell walls

of fungi, which contain chitin, and the cell envelopes of prokaryotes, in which peptidoglycans are the main structural molecules.

- The plasmodesmata, linking pores in the cell wall that allow each plant cell to communicate with other adjacent cells; this is different from the functionally analogous system of gap junctions between animal cells.
- Plastids, especially chloroplasts that contain chlorophyll, the pigment that gives plants their green color and allows them to perform photosynthesis.
- Higher plants, including conifers and flowering plants (Angiospermae), lack the flagellae and centrioles that are present in animal cells.

Fungal cells are most similar to animal cells, with the following exceptions:

- A cell wall that contains chitin.
- Less definition between cells; the hyphae of higher fungi have porous partitions called *septa*, which allow the passage of cytoplasm, organelles, and, sometimes, nuclei. Primitive fungi have few or no septa, so each organism is essentially a giant multinucleate supercell; these fungi are described as coenocytic.
- Only the most primitive fungi, chytrids, have flagella.

Nuclear division is often coordinated with cell division. This generally takes place by mitosis, a process that allows each daughter nucleus to receive one copy of each chromosome. In most eukaryotes, there is also a process of sexual reproduction, typically involving an alternation between haploid generations, wherein only one copy of each chromosome is present, and diploid generations, wherein two are present, occurring through nuclear fusion (syngamy) and meiosis. There is considerable variation in this pattern, however.

Eukaryotes have a smaller surface area to volume ratio than prokaryotes and thus have lower metabolic rates and longer generation times. In some multicellular organisms, cells specialized for metabolism will have enlarged surface areas, such as intestinal villi.

Eukaryotes are generally classified as follows:

- Kingdom Protista
- Kingdom Plantae
- Kingdom Fungi
- Kingdom Animalia

4.3.2 Prokaryotes

Prokaryotes lack the internal substructures of eukaryotes, which limits the degree to which a prokaryote can specialize. For example, a single eukaryotic cell in the human body contains the necessary DNA to specialize into anything from an osteoblast capable of depositing dense extracellular matrix that promotes mineralization necessary for bone formation to a hepatocyte capable of internalizing and metabolizing carbohydrates and toxins in addition to synthesizing proteins and other key biomolecules such as cholesterols, bile salts, and phospholipids. Prokaryotes do not possess the extensive specialization of eukaryotes, which allows for a smaller overall size and allocation of nutrients primarily toward replication. This small size permits an increased metabolic rate because prokaryotes have more membrane area relative to cytoplasmic volume, allowing for rapid transport in and out of the cell interior. Likewise, the small size, lack of specialization capacity, and increased metabolic rate lead to a very high rate of replication and result in a cell well suited for the singular focus of many bioprocessing applications.

4.3.2.1 Bacteria

The bacteria naming process is complex; the science of taxonomy deals with it, and as an example, shown below is a scientific classification of the most common bacteria *Escherichia coli*

Scientific classification
Domain: Bacteria
Kingdom: Eubacteria
Phylum: Proteobacteria
Class: Gammaproteobacteria
Order: Enterobacteriales
Family: Enterobacteriaceae
Genus: *Escherichia*
Species: *E. coli*
Binomial name: *Escherichia coli* (Migula 1895), Castellani and Chalmers 1919
Synonyms: *Bacillus coli communis* Escherich (1885)

Given below is a description of how bacterial species are identified and classified:

1. Bacterial species
   a. *Similar individuals*: A bacterial species is a population of cells with similar characteristics. This definition is very different from how plant and animal species are often defined, which usually involves something to do with sex.
   b. *Resemble fossil species*:
      i. *Bacterial species* resemble the way fossil species are distinguished (i.e., phylogenetic species concept).
      ii. Normally plant and especially animal species are defined as populations of interbreeding or potentially interbreeding individuals that do not breed with individuals of other, like-defined populations.
      iii. For fossils, on the other hand, it cannot be determined who interbred, or could have, with whom. Consequently, fossil species are defined only in terms of character resemblance, just as are bacteria.
2. *Bergey's Manual*
   a. *Bergey's Manual* is a guide to distinguishing bacterial species based on phenotypic differences between isolates.
3. Strain
   a. A *strain* is a subset of a bacterial species differing from other bacteria of the same species by some minor but identifiable difference.
   b. A *strain* is "a population of organisms that descends from a single organism or pure culture isolate. Strains within a species may differ slightly from one another in many ways." (Prescott et al., 1996, p. 392)
   c. *Strains* are often created in the laboratory by mutagenizing existing *strains* or *wild-type* examples of bacterial species.

103

  d. The term *strain* is also applicable to eucaryotic microorganisms, as well as to viruses.
4. Type strain
  a. A type strain is the nomenclatural type of the species or the reference point to which all other strains will be compared, and is consequently thoroughly characterized. The type strain thus determines whether future strains belong within that species.
5. Serovar (serotype)
  a. A *serovar* is a strain differentiated by serological means.
  b. Individual strains of *Salmonella* spp. are often distinguished and distinguishable by serological means.
6. Biovar (biotype)
  a. *Biovars* are strains that are differentiated by biochemical or other non-serological means.
7. Morphovar (morphotype)
  a. A *morphovar* is a strain that is differentiated on the basis of morphological distinctions.
8. Isolate (i-so-lit)
  a. An *isolate* is a pure culture derived from a heterogeneous, wild population of microorganisms.
  b. The term *isolate* is also applicable to eucaryotic microorganisms as well as to viruses.
9. Classification
  a. Placement of an organism within a scheme relating different types of organisms, such as that presented in Woese's universal tree, is known as *classification*.
  b. Organisms are classified for scientific purposes.
10. Identification
  a. *Identification* is the determination of whether an organism (or isolate in the case of microorganisms) should be placed within a group of organisms known to fit within some classification scheme.
  b. Organisms are identified for practical purposes, such as diagnosis of disease.
  c. A number of identification techniques are available.
    i. Many different criteria may be employed for identification, though it is often desirable to employ the easiest techniques possible.
    ii. What techniques and tests may be necessary, however, depend on what organism is being identified and how much detail into the organism's classification you are interested.
    iii. Techniques include the following:
       A. Morphological identification
       B. Differential staining
       C. Use of differential media
       D. Serological methods
       E. Flow cytometry

    F.   Phage typing
    G.   Protein analysis
    H.   Comparisons of nucleotide sequences

11. Morphological identification
   a. A number of morphological characteristics are useful in bacterial identification. These include the presence or absence of the following structures:
      i.   Endospores
      ii. Flagella
     iii. Glycocalyx
   b. Additional considerations include the following:
      i.   Colony morphology
      ii. Cell shape
     iii. Cell size

12. Serological methods (agglutination test, ELISA, Western blot)
   a. *Antibodies*
      i.   *Serological methods* employ antibodies and include the following methods:
         A.   Agglutination tests
         B.   ELISAs
         C.   Western blots
      ii. It is antibody binding that all *serological tests* ultimately detect.
   b. The basic premise behind all of these tests is that antibodies are highly selective in terms of the proteins (or other cell structures) to which they bind, to the point that they are able to distinguish the proteins coming from one bacterial species among many species, or even one strain among many strains.

13. Flow cytometry
   a. *Flow cytometry* is a technique that can employ serological methods (but does not necessarily) that analyze cells suspended in a liquid medium by light, electrical conductivity, or fluorescence as the cells individually pass through a small orifice.

14. Phage typing
   a. Bacteriophages (or phages) are viruses that infect bacteria.
   b. Phages can be very specific in what bacteria they infect and the pattern of infection by many phages may be employed in *phage typing* to distinguish bacterial species and strains.

15. Protein analysis (gel electrophoresis, sodium dodecyl sulfate-polyacrylamide gel electrophoresis (SDS-PAGE), establishment of clonality)
   a. The size and other differences between proteins among different organisms may be determined very easily employing methods of protein separation using methods collectively known as *gel electrophoresis.*
   b. SDS-PAGE
      i.   One popular technique goes by the name *SDS-PAGE.*
      ii. Note that another name for *SDS* is *sodium lauryl sulfate,* a detergent you will find in many shampoos.
   c. Such methods are very good at detecting small differences between isolates and are especially good at *establishing clonality.*

16. Comparison of nucleotide sequences [Southern blot, nucleic acid hybridization, restriction fragment length polymorphism, DNA fingerprinting]

   a. The actual sequence of bases (nucleotides) in the genome of organisms may be inferred or actually determined (nucleotide sequencing) by a variety of methods.
   b. Various methods of inference are as follows:
      i.   Southern blotting
      ii. Nucleic acid hybridization
      iii. Restriction fragment length polymorphism comparison (DNA fingerprinting)
   c. Another technique that is worth knowing about is PCR, which stands for polymerase chain reaction, a method of amplifying specific regions of DNA found in an organism's genome by selectively catalyzing the replication of those regions.

4.3.2.2 Gram Staining

One of the most common method of identification is Gram staining. A typical example would be *E. coli*, which is gram negative when fixed in Gram's reagent (Hans Christian Gram used it first in 1884). The method involves use of a crystal violet dye; all bacteria will be stained purple; next, iodine is added and then ethanol. The gram-positive cells would remain purple and the gram-negative cells will become colorless. If the organic dye is added, it will turn gram-negative cells red leaving gram-positive cells purple. Figure 4.4 shows the structure of a gram-negative *E. coli*; gram positive structure will be the same except without the outer membrane. Instead, it will have a thick cell wall with multiple layers of peptidoglycan. Gram-positive cells also contain teichoic acids covalently bonded to peptidoglycans. The absence of an outer membrane and presence of only the cytoplasmic membrane make gram positive cells excellent choice as engines to produce proteins, because the proteins are excreted. In most gram-negative organisms, proteins expressed as inclusion bodies need to be excised from the organism first (Figure 4.4).

Some bacteria are neither gram-positive nor gram-negative such as Mycoplasma with no cell walls. These organisms produce a variety of infections including contaminating culture media and manufacturing facilities; later in Chapter 16, we will dwell more on the nuisance of mycoplasma contamination and how to test recombinant cells for mycoplasma contamination.

4.3.3 Archaea

The Archaea constitute a domain of single-celled microorganisms. These microbes have no cell nucleus or any other membrane-bound organelles within their cells. In the past, Archaea had been classified with bacteria as prokaryotes (or Kingdom Monera) and named archaebacteria, but this classification is regarded as outdated. In fact, the Archaea have an independent evolutionary history and show many differences in their biochemistry from other forms of life, and so they are now classified as a separate domain in the three-domain system (Figure 4.5). In this system, the phylogenetically distinct branches of evolutionary descent are the Archaea, Bacteria, and Eukaryota. Archaea are further divided into four recognized phyla, but many more phyla may exist. Of these groups, the

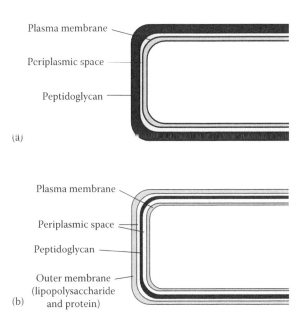

(a)

(b)

Plasma membrane

Periplasmic space

Peptidoglycan

Plasma membrane

Periplasmic space

Peptidoglycan

Outer membrane
(lipopolysaccharide
and protein)

Figure 4.4 Schematic descriptions of (a) gram-positive and (b) gram-negative bacteria.

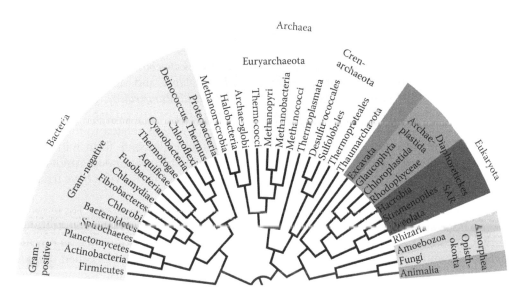

Figure 4.5 Three domains of life.

Crenarchaeota and the Euryarchaeota are the most intensively studied. Classification is still difficult, because the vast majority have never been studied in the laboratory and have only been detected by analysis of their nucleic acids in samples from the environment.

Archaea and bacteria are quite similar in size and shape, although a few archaea have very strange or unusual shapes, such as the flat and square-shaped cells of *Haloquadratum walsbyi*. Despite this visual similarity to bacteria, archaea possess genes and several metabolic pathways that are more closely related to those of eukaryotes, notably the enzymes involved in transcription and translation. Other aspects of archaean biochemistry are unique, such as their reliance on ether lipids in their cell membranes. Archaea use a much greater variety of sources of energy than eukaryotes: ranging from familiar organic compounds such as sugars, to ammonia, metal ions, or even hydrogen gas. Salt-tolerant archaea (the Haloarchaea) use sunlight as an energy source, and other species of archaea fix carbon; however, unlike plants and cyanobacteria, no species of archaea is known to do both. Archaea reproduce asexually by binary fission, fragmentation, or budding; unlike bacteria and eukaryotes, no known species form spores.

Initially, archaea were seen as extremophiles that lived in harsh environments, such as hot springs and salt lakes, but they have since been found in a broad range of habitats, including soils, oceans, marshlands, and the human colon and navel. Archaea are particularly numerous in the oceans, and the archaea in plankton may be one of the most abundant groups of organisms on the planet. Archaea are now recognized as a major part of Earth's life and may play roles in both the carbon cycle and the nitrogen cycle. No clear examples of archaeal pathogens or parasites are known, but they are often mutualists or commensals. One example is the methanogens that inhabit the gut of humans and ruminants, where their vast numbers aid digestion. Methanogens are used in biogas production and sewage treatment, and enzymes from extremophile archaea that can endure high temperatures and organic solvents are exploited in biotechnology.

Individual archaea range from 0.1 to over 15 μm in diameter and occur in various shapes, commonly as spheres, rods, spirals, or plates. Other morphologies in the Crenarchaeota include irregularly shaped lobed cells in *Sulfolobus*, needle-like filaments that are less than half a micrometer in diameter in *Thermofilum*, and almost perfectly rectangular rods in *Thermoproteus* and *Pyrobaculum*. *Haloquadratum walsbyi* are flat, square archaea that live in hypersaline pools. These unusual shapes are probably maintained both by their cell walls and a prokaryotic cytoskeleton. Proteins related to the cytoskeleton components of other organisms exist in archaea, and filaments form within their cells, but in contrast to other organisms, these cellular structures are poorly understood. In *Thermoplasma* and *Ferroplasma*, the lack of a cell wall means that the cells have irregular shapes and can resemble amoebae.

Some species form aggregates or filaments of cells up to 200 μm long. These organisms can be prominent in biofilms. Notably, aggregates of *Thermococcus coalescens* cells fuse together in culture, forming single giant cells. Archaea in the genus *Pyrodictium* produce an elaborate multicell colony involving arrays of long, thin hollow tubes called *cannulae* that stick out from the cells' surfaces and connect them into a dense bush-like agglomeration. The function of these cannulae is not settled, but they may allow communication or nutrient exchange with neighbors.

Archaea and bacteria have generally similar cell structure, but cell composition and organization set the archaea apart. Like bacteria, archaea lack interior membranes and organelles. Like bacteria, archaea cell membranes are usually bounded by a cell wall and they swim using one or more flagella. Structurally, archaea are most similar to gram-positive bacteria. Most have a single plasma membrane and cell wall and lack a periplasmic space; the exception to this general rule is *Ignicoccus*, which possess a particularly large periplasm that contains membrane-bound vesicles and is enclosed by an outer membrane.

Archaea recycle elements such as carbon, nitrogen, and sulfur through their various habitats. Although these activities are vital for normal ecosystem function, archaea can also contribute to human-made changes and even cause pollution.

Extremophile archaea, particularly those resistant either to heat or to extremes of acidity and alkalinity, are a source of enzymes that function under these harsh conditions. These enzymes have found many uses. For example, thermostable DNA polymerases, such as the Pfu DNA polymerase from *Pyrococcus furiosus*, revolutionized molecular biology by allowing the PCR to be used in research as a simple and rapid technique for cloning DNA. In industry, amylases, galactosidases, and pullulanases in other species of *Pyrococcus* that function at over 100°C (212°F) allow food processing at high temperatures, such as the production of low lactose milk and whey. Enzymes from these thermophilic archaea also tend to be very stable in organic solvents, allowing their use in environmentally friendly processes in green chemistry that synthesize organic compounds. This stability makes them easier to use in structural biology. Consequently, the counterparts of bacterial or eukaryotic enzymes from extremophile archaea are often used in structural studies.

In contrast to the range of applications of archaean enzymes, the use of the organisms themselves in biotechnology is less developed. Methanogenic archaea are a vital part of sewage treatment, since they are part of the community of microorganisms that carry out anaerobic digestion and produce biogas. In mineral processing, acidophilic archaea display promise for the extraction of metals from ores, including gold, cobalt, and copper. Archaea host a new class of potentially useful antibiotics. A few of these archaeocins have been characterized, but hundreds more are believed to exist, especially within Haloarchaea and *Sulfolobus*. These compounds differ in structure from bacterial antibiotics, so they may have novel modes of action. In addition, they may allow the creation of new selectable markers for use in archaeal molecular biology.

4.3.4 Viruses

Often classified as the fourth domain, viruses are non-living entities and thus form their own classification.

Viruses are the smallest organisms, with diameters ranging from 20 to 300 nm ($1 \text{ nm} - 10^{-9} \text{ m}$) comprising a capsid (having a helical or icosahedral shape) that contains the genetic materials and enzymes. Some viruses also contain an envelope surrounding the capsid. The viruses are classified into the following seven categories according to the Baltimore Classification based on genetic contents and replication strategies of viruses.

1. dsDNA viruses
2. ssDNA viruses

3. dsRNA viruses
4. (+)-Sense ssRNA viruses
5. (−)-Sense ssRNA viruses
6. RNA reverse transcribing viruses
7. DNA reverse transcribing viruses

where *ds* represents *double strand* and *ss* denotes *single strand*. The genetic material in all types of cells is dsDNA, but some viruses use RNA or ssDNA to carry genetic information. Table 4.2 lists examples of common viruses.

The life cycle of viruses starts with attachment, that is, a specific binding between viral surface proteins and their receptors on the host cellular surface. This specificity determines the host range of a virus. For instance, the human immunodeficiency virus (HIV) attacks only human's immune cells (mainly T cells), because its surface protein, gp120, can interact with CD4 and chemokine receptors on the T cell's surface. The attachment phase is followed by uncoating wherein the viral capsid is degraded by viral enzymes or host enzymes; then comes replication that involves assembly of viral proteins and genetic materials produced in the host cell; and the final phase of release wherein viruses escape from the host cell by causing cell rupture (lysis). Enveloped viruses (e.g., HIV) typically *bud* from the host cell. During the budding process, a virus acquires the

Table 4.2   Examples of Common Viruses

Class	Nucleic Acid	Examples	Envelope	Genome Size (kb)
I	dsDNA	Herpes virus	Yes	120–220
		Poxvirus	Yes	130–375
		Adenovirus	No	3.0–4.2
		Papillomavirus	No	5.3–8.0
II	ssDNA	Adeno-associated virus	No	5.0
III	dsRNA	Reovirus	No	18–311[a]
IV	(+) ssRNA	Togavirus	Yes	9.7–11.8
		Poliovirus	No	7.4
		Foot-and-mouth disease virus	No	7.5
				10.5
		Hepatitis A virus	No	
		Hepatitis C virus	Yes	
V	(−) ssRNA	Influenza virus	Yes	12–15[a]
VI	(reverse) RNA	HIV	Yes	9.7
VII	(reverse) DNA	Hepatitis B virus	Yes	3.1

Notes: ss = single strand; ds = double strand.

   (+) RNA is the one that can function as mRNA for the synthesis of proteins and (−) RNA cannot function as mRNA.

[a] Reovirus and influenza virus have segmented RNA genomes; the total length is shown here.

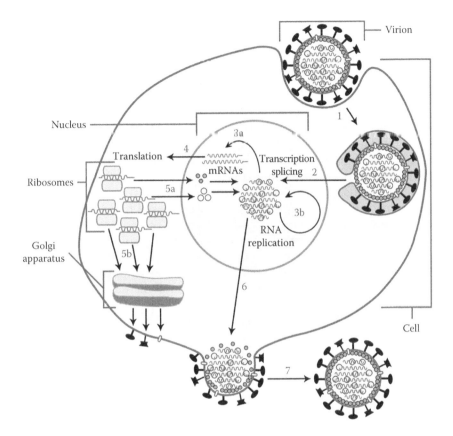

Figure 4.6 Typical virus life cycle.

phospholipid envelope containing the embedded viral glycoproteins. Figure 4.6 shows a typical virus life cycle.

4.3.4.1 Bacteriophages

A good example of viruses is that of bacteriophages, which are frequently encountered in bioprocessing and these include dsDNA phages with contractile tails, such as T4; ssDNA phages with long flexible tails, such as λ; dsDNA phages with stubby tails, such as p22; ssDNA phages, such as ΦX174; and ssRNA phages, such as MS2. Bacteriophages have two life cycles: lytic and lysogenic. In the lytic cycle, λ phages replicate rapidly and eventually cause lysis of the host cell. In the lysogenic cycle, the viral DNA circularizes and integrates into the host DNA. Then, λ phages may replicate with the host cell. Under certain conditions (e.g., ultraviolet irradiation of cells), the λ phages may transform from the lysogenic cycle to the lytic cycle. This transformation is mainly controlled by two proteins: cI (also known as λ *repressor*) and Cro; an increase in cI proteins promotes the lysogenic cycle, whereas an increase in Cro proteins promotes the lytic cycle.

4.4 INTRACELLULAR ORGANELLES

Due to the comparatively large size of a eukaryotic cell in addition to possessing the capacity for specialization, there is a need for increased intracellular organization. Eukaryotes demonstrate this through a series of membrane-bound structures referred to as *organelles*.

The largest organelle in a eukaryote is the nucleus. The nucleus is separated from the interior of the cell by two lipid bilayers. The nucleus contains the chromosomal DNA of the cells. The DNA exists as multiple long chains. Each of these chains is associated with DNA-binding proteins, histones, which organize the DNA into unique chromosomes. In addition to chromosomal DNA, the nucleus contains within it a separate organelle, the nucleolus. The nucleolus is where ribosomes, an amalgamation of RNA and proteins capable of carrying out a function as opposed to transferring information like mRNA, are assembled.

The outer lipid bilayer of the nucleus extends into the cytoplasm to form the ER. These nuclear membrane projections form thin interconnected sacs, referred to as *cisternae*. The ER is further classified by the presence of ribosomes on the cytoplasmic side of the cisternae membranes. The ER presenting ribosomes is termed the *rough endoplasmic reticulum* (rough ER). The ER with no ribosomes is termed the *smooth endoplasmic reticulum* (smooth ER). The ribosomes present on the rough ER hint toward the core function, which is the production of proteins. Specifically, the rough ER plays a key role in the production of proteins to be secreted. The smooth ER facilitates the production of lipids, phospholipids, and steroids. Additionally, the smooth ER metabolizes carbohydrates and steroids in addition to detoxification of drugs and other compounds. Hepatocytes in the liver contain a large amount of smooth ER relative to other human eukaryotic cells.

Another eukaryotic organelle with two lipid bilayers is the mitochondrion. The primary function of mitochondria is the generation of energy in the form of adenosine triphosphate (ATP). Most of the ATP and GTP generation in mitochondria is through the Krebs, or citric acid, cycle. The Krebs cycle begins with acetyl coenzyme A (acetyl-CoA), which is generated by the metabolism of proteins, lipids, and carbohydrates. The Krebs cycle was previously detailed in Chapter 3. Additionally, mitochondria store intracellular Ca^{2+} ions and are involved in the regulation of cell fate. Finally, one curious aspect of mitochondria is they present their own unique DNA. Mitochondrial DNA is circular and double stranded. The presence of the circular mitochondrial DNA in addition to the fact that mitochondria divide through binary fission, similar to prokaryotic division, supports the endosymbiotic theory which states that several eukaryotic organelles began as symbioses between single-celled organisms.

The Golgi apparatus is separated from the cytosol by a single lipid bilayer. Similar to the ER, the membrane of the Golgi apparatus is organized into thin sacs, or cisternae. The Golgi apparatus is key in organizing, transporting, and posttranslational modifying of proteins and lipids within the cell. The Golgi apparatus synthesizes an additional organelle, the lysosome. Lysosomes are small membrane-bound vesicles containing hydrolytic enzymes and internal pH of ~4. The enzymes and low pH are necessary for the primary function of the lysosome, which is the degradation of intracellular debris and waste products.

Similar to lysosomes, peroxisomes are small membrane-bound intracellular vesicles. However, peroxisomes demonstrate a neutral pH and contain enzymes capable of generating hydrogen peroxide. The enzymes and hydrogen peroxide in peroxisomes promote the catabolism of fats and amino acids in addition to detoxification, for example, some ingested ethanol is converted to acetaldehyde in peroxisomes through hydrogen peroxide-mediated oxidation. The remaining ethanol is metabolized to acetaldehyde in the cytoplasm through the enzyme alcohol dehydrogenase.

There are several plant cell-specific organelles, vacuoles and chloroplasts, that serve to store water and generate energy through photosynthesis, respectively.

Organelles are not the only key features within a cell. The cytoskeleton is key to cell shape and function. The cytoskeleton is composed of biopolymers that organize into fibers and are capable of generating and withstanding mechanical forces. These biopolymers are microfilaments, intermediate filaments, and microtubules. Microfilaments are linear chains composed of the protein actin. Bundles of microfilaments, called stress fibers, are capable of generating force through the following two unique mechanisms: First, the polymerization of the actin filaments exerts an outward force stretching the cell membrane. Second, small molecular motors, myosins, are capable of ratcheting adjacent actin filaments together resulting in an inward force. These two mechanisms of force generation are key in cell motility. In an anchorage-dependent eukaryotic cell, the outward stretching of the cell membrane allows for the formation of anchorage points to the underlying surface, a complex formation of multiple proteins referred to as *focal adhesions*. The actin stress fibers are linked to the focal adhesions, and the ability of the stress fiber to contract while tethered to an adhesion ultimately pulls the cell body forward. Actin is not only important for stress fiber formations, but also for providing the cell membrane with structure. Actin filaments arrange on the cytoplasmic side of the cell membrane to form the cortical actin shell. Actin filaments in general help withstand tensile forces applied to the cell. Next, intermediate filaments are so named because they demonstrate a larger diameter than actin, but a smaller diameter than the microtubules, approximately 10 nm. Intermediate filaments are elastic and durable. They are found in the cytoplasm, primarily in cells under mechanical strain, where they transmit mechanical forces. Intermediate filaments also stabilize the nuclear membrane. Finally, the microtubules are hollow tubes, 25 nm in diameter, composed of the protein tubulin. Microtubules are the stiffest of the cytoskeletal filaments and serve several purposes. First, microtubules serve as a transit system in the cell, coordinating the movement of vesicles through microtubule-binding motor proteins that can travel both ways along the microtubule in a motor protein-specific manner. Second, microtubules are a major structural component of the cytoskeleton. Due to the increased stiffness relative to actin, microtubules provide support under compression.

Much like the cytoskeleton, the cytosol is an integral part of the cell that is not a classical organelle. The cytosol is a key element of the cell and is the intracellular fluid that fills the space between the nuclear and organelle membranes and the cell membrane. The combination of the cytosol, cytoskeleton, and organelles comprises the cytoplasm. Stating that cytosol is simply fluid does not provide the whole story. Approximately 70% of the cytosol is water with many dissolved ions. The remaining 30% is dissolved macromolecules, such as proteins. Thirty percent may not initially sound very high; however, it translates to approximately 300 mg/ml, which is an incredibly viscous solution. Researchers have only recently recognized the importance of accounting for the viscous nature of the cytosol in addition to the compartmentalization of the cytosol by the lattice network, that is, the cytoplasm in examining the interactions between proteins expected to take place in the cytosol. By generating systems that mimic the crowded nature of the cytosol, future molecular biologists and biochemists will be able to examine protein interactions in a biologically relevant manner. Already research into macromolecular crowding had demonstrated decreased enzymatic reaction rates and increased sensitivity of the resulting reaction rate to the physicochemical properties of the substrate. Early studies indicate that this macromolecular crowding ultimately reduces the Michaelis constant K_m for the respective enzymatic reactions. As will be discussed in Chapter 6, Michaelis–Menten kinetics and the modeling thereof are key areas of current and future bioprocess engineering; thus, developing an experimental system that mimics native biology is of paramount importance to ensure the accuracy of mathematical models.

4.5 CELLULAR TRANSPORT

A simple examination of transport processes reveals that diffusion is not sufficient for intracellular transport of large macromolecules. Examining the idealized case that negates the crowded nature of the cytosol, diffusion coefficients, D, for small molecules and proteins in water are 1×10^{-5} and 1×10^{-7} cm^2/s, respectively. One-dimensional diffusion can be approximated with the relationship for random walk: $\langle x \rangle = q \cdot D \cdot t$, where $\langle x^2 \rangle$ is the mean squared displacement; q adjusts for the number of dimensions diffusion is in and is 2, 4, or 6 for one, two, or three dimensions; D is the diffusion coefficient; and t is time. Figure 4.7 demonstrates a random walk in two dimensions. Notice that despite the time increasing an equal amount between each frame, the max distance any one of the three molecules reaches remains nearly constant.

If we assume small molecule and protein transport across a bacterium of ~5 μm, we find times on the order of 0.01–1 s. In contrast, those same molecules diffusing across a ~50 μm eukaryotic cell would take 1–100 s, a significantly larger time. Taking into account

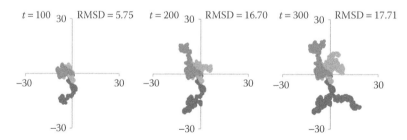

Figure 4.7 A simple model of diffusion based on a random walk model demonstrating that the max distance traveled by any of the three molecules remains nearly constant across the time points which is substantiated by the small shift in root mean squared displacement (RMSD) from a time of 200 to 300s.

that the cytosol and the diffusion coefficient for proteins decreases at least an additional order of magnitude leading to times approaching hours for a single protein to diffuse the distance of a cell. This introduces an interesting question, is a timescale of hours reasonable for protein transport in a cell? First, we define reasonable as the ability for a cell to maintain normal function. Perhaps the secretion of extracellular matrix proteins would be appropriate on the order of hours; however, the production and secretion of insulin would be severely hampered if hours were required for transport out of a cell. To compensate for the relatively long times required for transport to the extracellular space by diffusions, cells have developed active mechanisms that package and transport proteins in intracellular vesicles, membrane-bound mobile compartments. These vesicles are transported along microtubules by several proteins. Kinesins and dyneins are two families of proteins involved in this vesicle transport. Kinesins tether to vesicles and travel toward the (+) end of the microtubule through an ATP-dependent mechanism, whereas dyneins tether to vesicles and travel toward the (−) end of the microtubule also through an ATP-dependent mechanism. Microtubule polymerization often begins at the microtubule organizing center, which contains a ring of γ-tubulin that serves as a nucleation site for the outward, in the (+) direction, growth of the microtubules. The maximum velocity for kinesin-mediated transport is 3.8 µm/s, which rapidly outpaces diffusion, taking only 13 s to travel the distance of our 50 µm cell. Typically, kinesins travel around slightly less than 1 µm/s, which still provides transport much quicker than diffusion. Vesicle-mediated active transport has an additional benefit in that once the proteins are packaged in a vesicle it is easy for that vesicle to directly fuse to the cell membrane and deliver the contents into the extracellular space. This brings up another key issue of intracellular transport, crossing membranes.

In the cytoplasm, proteins are not freely permitted to cross plasma membranes; however, often proteins are synthesized in areas where they are not needed, which necessitates some mechanism to transport the protein across a membrane. The cell membrane permits protein transfer to the extracellular space through exocytosis, which occurs through vesicle fusion as mentioned in Section 4.5 in either a Ca^{2+}-dependent or -independent mechanism. The Ca^{2+}-dependent exocytosis is often found in neurons where the neurotransmitter is released in response to cell Ca^{2+}-mediated depolarization of the cell. Ca^{2+}-independent exocytosis is a constitutive, or continuous, process. Likewise, endocytosis governs the transport of extracellular proteins to the intracellular space. Endocytosis occurs through receptor-dependent and -independent mechanisms. Receptor-dependent endocytosis is assisted by the proteins clathrin and caveolin that mediate the formation of invaginations into the cell in response to an extracellular protein binding a cell membrane receptor, which then pinches off in the intracellular space forming small 50–100 nm diameter vesicles. Receptor-independent endocytosis is through a process referred to as *pinocytosis* and results in large 500 nm–5 µm diameter intracellular vesicles filled with extracellular fluid. Finally, a specialized type of receptor-mediated endocytosis is the process of *phagocytosis*. Phagocytosis occurs when an unwanted particle, for example, debris and bacteria, binds the surface ligands and results in the formation of an intracellular phagolysosome that digests the material contained within. Not all protein transport across membranes is governed by vesicle budding and fusion. Special pores permit transport of proteins into

115

the nucleus. These pores span the nuclear membrane and open to allow proteins that are labeled for nuclear importation. Ion transport across membranes also occurs through both active and passive mechanisms. Passive ion channels permit bidirectional selective ion transport in a gated or ungated manner without energy consumption. Gated ion channels are either closed or open and respond to electrical, chemical, and physical stimuli. Active ion transport occurs through ion pumps. Ion pumps use chemical energy, typically ATP, to transport ions against an electrochemical gradient. The most common ion pump is the Na^+/K^+ ion pump, which transports three Na^+ out of the cell in exchange for two K^+ transported into the cell. The Na^+/K^+ ion pump helps polarize the cell by decreasing positively charged intracellular ions. Intracellular transport of ions typically occurs through diffusion since the small size of an ion is not affected by the viscosity and complexity of the cytoplasm.

4.6 INTRACELLULAR SIGNAL TRANSDUCTION

Cell behavior is governed by the proteins actively being synthesized at any given moment in time, which is referred to as the cell's *phenotype*. Likewise, changes and maintenance in this cell behavior is governed by gene expression, which is referred to as *genotype*, and is dictated by proteins binding and reading the DNA. These DNA reading proteins are referred to as *transcription factors* and the difference between a neuron and osteoblast (bone forming cell) is a function of which transcription factors are being expressed and are in an *on* state. The ability of a cell to shift its genotype and subsequently its phenotype depends on an ability to respond to extracellular signals. These extracellular signals could result in a depolarization of the cell through ion fluxes; however, ion transport alone is not near complex enough to govern all possible fate outcomes of a single cell. Instead there are numerous unique intracellular signaling proteins. These signaling proteins often have *on* and *off* states determined by whether a preceding reaction has resulted in the phosphorylation of one of the amino acids on the signaling protein. Once phosphorylated, the signaling protein's affinity for its substrate, often another signaling protein, increases allowing binding and phosphorylation. Typically, the final protein activated is a transcription factor that then goes on to affect changes in gene expression. While at first this concept may seem complex, it is actually both elegant and functional. Consider that we have already established diffusion as ineffective at transporting proteins quickly, now if we also account for a diffusing protein that is only in an *on* state for a very brief period of time before a secondary reaction reduces it back to an *off* state, it is clear that we need some help to transfer a signal. Numerous second messengers that exist throughout the cytosol allow the first receptor at the membrane to be activated and then pass that signal downstream through reactions and small amounts of diffusion with each second messenger. Additionally, since the *on* state and *off* state of proteins are often governed by independent reactions, a single *on* protein can react with numerous second messengers. A simple analogy would be a relay race where each runner could then hand a baton off to five additional runners, allowing for both amplification and transmission of a signal. Inside the cell, the combination of diffusion and reaction kinetics results in a series of waves where the first is sharp and tall

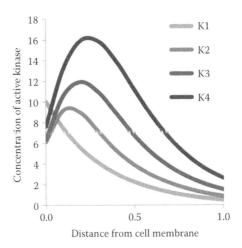

Figure 4.8 Simplified representation of steady-state signal transduction through a series of four kinases (K1–K4). Notice the peak activity for each subsequent kinase moves toward 1 in addition to increasing in amplitude.

and each subsequent second messenger presents progressively wider waves eventually generating an effective concentration of the terminal second messenger capable of affecting changes in gene expression. Figure 4.8 demonstrates this amplification and transmission for a steady-state signal originating at the cell membrane and propagating through second messenger signaling.

Signal transduction will be examined in much greater detail including the modeling of both the transport and underlying reactions in Chapter 6.

Questions

1. Define in your own words what a cell is.
2. Detail the key differences between eukaryotic and prokaryotic cells.
3. If you are concerned that eukaryotic cells in culture may have become contaminated by prokaryotic cells, a typical first step would be to use a Gram stain to identify which cell wall the bacteria demonstrate and then select an appropriate antibiotic. However, if your culture is contaminated with mycoplasma, a very small prokaryote that is ubiquitous in cell cultures, it would not stain either Gram positive or negative due to lacking a cell wall altogether. Propose a method to identify whether mycoplasma may be present.
   Answer: There are numerous correct answers. For example, staining for DNA will identify small extracellular particles. Likewise, gene analysis techniques such as PCR can be used to identify mycoplasma-specific genes.
4. Detail the organelles involved in protein synthesis through the eventual secretion to the extracellular space by beginning with gene expression.

5. Cells express structural proteins that ultimately constitute the cytoskeleton and help to both maintain shape and apply forces. Actin filaments in the cytoskeleton are capable of applying both tensile and compressive forces. Describe how each of these forces is generated.

   Answer: Tensile forces are applied to the cell by polymerization of actin—pushing the cell membrane out. Compressive forces are applied through the intermediate protein, myosin, which ratchets adjacent actin filaments together—pulling the cell membrane in.

6. Muscle tissue is comprised of specialized cells termed *myoblasts* that fuse into multinucleated tubes termed *myotubules*. The formation of these myotubules is associated with an increase in a particular organelle due to the high energy needs of muscle tissue. Which organelle is upregulated in myotubules?

7. Why is it necessary for the specialized function of eukaryotic cells to have multiple organelles?

8. If we assume the diffusion coefficient for glucose, a primary energy source in the cell, is 300 μm^2/s; justify the need for organelles in eukaryotic cells.

9. The protein tubulin assembles into microtubules in the cytoplasm. What purpose do these microtubules have?

   Answer: They serve as *highways* for transport of intracellular vesicles and are capable of resisting compressive forces applied to the cell.

10. Based on intracellular diffusion, why did evolution generate complex signal transduction pathways?

    Answer: Diffusion is slow, and thus, the reactions driving the signaling molecule back to the *off* state would dominate the system. Signal transduction allows the amplification of the signal through multiple reactions with secondary signaling molecules that overcomes diffusion limitations.

11. Compare and contrast the replication mechanisms used by both eukaryotes and prokaryotes.

12. Does the ability of one signaling molecule to activate multiple downstream signaling molecules benefit the signal propagation?

13. What types of mechanisms does a cell use to modify the intracellular potential gradient? (Hint: Ions have a charge that affects intracellular potential.)

14. What is the net effect of the sodium/potassium pump in cells relative to the potential gradient in the cell?

15. Often in propagating a signal from one cell to the next, the cell membrane resting potential is dramatically shifted. How does the cell return back to the baseline resting potential?

    Answer: The cell depolarizes to propagate a signal. The original potential of the cell is around −40 to −80 mV. Depolarization increases this voltage and sodium/potassium pumps serve to decrease the potential back down to the resting state.

16. What are the steps involved with viral infection and propagation of a virus?

17. You are developing a genetic engineering strategy that will use a virus to insert a foreign, but beneficial, genetic fragment. This fragment is about 10,000 bp, what virus (and by proxy the associated viral packaging proteins) is appropriate for this size of nucleic acid?

18. Virus usually refers to an organism that uses a eukaryotic cell as a host. Is there a synonymous microorganism that uses a prokaryotic cell as a host and what is it?
19. How are viruses classified?
20. Based on the information presented so far, considering the genetic complexity of microorganisms, which is the most appropriate choice for efficient production of a therapeutic protein?

5

Reaction Stoichiometry, Thermodynamics, and Kinetics

LEARNING OBJECTIVES

1. Understand the fundamentals of reaction chemistry and determination of stoichiometric coefficients.
2. Recognize that diffusion and convection are the fundamental processes bringing reactants together.
3. Recognize that thermodynamics affect the behavior of a reaction in multiple ways.
4. Implement rate laws and mass balances to solve reactions.

5.1 INTRODUCTION

Chemistry provides the foundation for understanding and analyzing many processes in bioprocess engineering. This chapter will cover the basics of reaction stoichiometry, thermodynamics, and kinetics, including energy and material balances, mass transfer, fluid dynamics, free energy and the Arrhenius equation, and fundamental reaction kinetics, and will include a brief overview of numerical methods for modeling advanced reaction kinetics. In short, it is a chapter that briefly discusses many topics that build the foundation for future topics and is intended to serve as a reference and refresher more so than a detailed educational overview.

5.2 MASS AND ENERGY BALANCES

Physicists are constantly discovering ever-smaller particles; however, in the context of chemistry and reaction kinetics a reasonable starting point is the atom. An atom is a particle of matter that is the smallest unit capable of defining a chemical element. Despite atoms being composed of electrons, neutrons, and protons (which are each composed of smaller particles), neither electrons, neutrons, nor protons can define a chemical element—a chemical element is the specific combination of electrons, neutrons, and protons, or the atom. If we assume that a system is closed to any transfer of material, either matter or energy, then sum of the masses present initially will be equal to the sum of the masses present at any point in the future. This concept is the law of conservation of mass, put simply, mass is neither created nor destroyed by chemical reactions. A second law that aids in the analysis of basic chemical reactions is the law of definite proportions, or Proust's law, which states that any sample of a chemical compound will always contain the exact same proportion of elements by mass. Together, the law of conservation of mass and the law of definite proportions are the foundation for John Dalton's atomic theory, which states the following:

1. All elements are made of matter, and matter is made of atoms.
2. Each element is characterized by the mass and properties of its atoms, which are unique to that element.
3. Chemical compounds are formed by the combination of elements whose atoms are in whole number ratios, that is, atoms are not split.
4. Chemical reactions only rearrange the atoms present.

Dalton's atomic theory explains basic chemical reactions. Obviously, we recognize now that atoms can be destroyed via nuclear reactions and likewise that not all atoms in an element are identical in mass. Atoms of an element that have altered masses are referred to as isotopes and still maintain the same chemical properties of the other atoms present in the element.

Similar to mass, the conservation of energy states that energy is neither created nor destroyed. Thus in an isolated system, the energy present at the beginning is equal to the energy present at any point in the future. The conservation of energy does allow for the changes in the form of energy present, which aids in evaluating numerous chemical systems. For instance, an explosion converts a large amount of chemical energy to kinetic energy. It is also important to note that mass is related to energy through the mass–energy equivalence, which ultimately establishes that the mass of a system is merely a measure of the energy present. The mass–energy equivalence is represented by the very recognizable equation:

$$E = m \cdot c^2 \tag{5.1}$$

where:
  E is the energy
  m is the mass
  c is the speed of light, 299,792,458 m/s in a vacuum

Having established that mass and energy are conserved and related, we can establish mass and energy balances for the total mass/energy that state

$$\text{Input} = \text{output} + \text{accumulation} \tag{5.2}$$

If we consider a single element in a system, which can undergo a chemical reaction, then the mass balance becomes

$$\text{Input} + \text{generation} = \text{output} + \text{accumulation} + \text{consumption} \qquad (5.3)$$

5.3 FUNDAMENTALS OF CHEMICAL REACTIONS

Implementing a mass balance is the most straightforward method to determine the equivalent amounts of elements/compounds involved in a chemical reaction. Take for instance the simple formation of water from hydrogen and oxygen gases:

$$H_2 + O_2 \rightarrow H_2O \qquad (5.4)$$

A simple inspection of the above equation reveals that only one oxygen atom is used for every two hydrogen atom, thus as written the mass balance would not hold up. A simple visual inspection reveals that placing a two in front of the H_2 and H_2O would give us the following:

$$2H_2 + O_2 \rightarrow 2H_2O \qquad (5.5)$$

Now the reaction is balanced, four hydrogen atoms and two oxygen atoms are found on both sides of the equation. The determination of the appropriate coefficients to place in front of each element or compound in a chemical reaction is referred to as *stoichiometry* and is essentially a mass balance with the left side of the equation being the input and the right side of the equation being the output. Keep in mind that to truly treat the system as a mass balance, the quantities of the elements present in the compounds being reacted would have to be converted to mass. This can be accomplished through molecular weights, which provide the mass of an element per mole. A mole is simply a measure of the number of particles present. For a chemical compound, one mole corresponds to 6.022×10^{23} atoms. Thus, 1 mol of H_2 gas, which has a molecular weight of 2.02 g/mol, would weigh 2.02 g. A mass balance on the reaction producing water would be the following based on the molecular weights of hydrogen and oxygen atoms being 1.01 g/mol and 16.00 g/mol, respectively, and assuming we are beginning with 2 mol of H_2 and 1 mol of O_2:

$$2\,\text{mol} \cdot \left(1.01\frac{g}{\text{mol}} + 1.01\frac{g}{\text{mol}} \right) + 1\,\text{mol} \cdot \left(16.00\frac{g}{\text{mol}} + 16.00\frac{g}{\text{mol}} \right) \rightarrow$$

$$2\,\text{mol} \cdot \left(1.01\frac{g}{\text{mol}} + 1.01\frac{g}{\text{mol}} + 16.00\frac{g}{\text{mol}} \right) = 36.04\ g \rightarrow 36.04\ g$$

$$(5.6)$$

Notice that when the stoichiometric coefficients are determined, the mass balance is satisfied regardless of whether we started with 2 mol of H_2 or 200 mol of H_2.

Chemical reactions in bioprocess often involve multiple steps leading to a single end product. For these more complicated multiple reaction systems, solving all the balanced chemical equations can quickly become cumbersome. For these scenarios, a matrix approach is valuable. To analyze stoichiometric relationships with matrices, first we identify the species in the system and the elements that compose these species. Then, a formula matrix, $F = F_{ki}$, which corresponds to element k in species i is formulated. The rows of the formula matrix are the elements and the columns are the species. Similarly, we can establish a matrix based on the stoichiometric coefficients of the species within each reaction in a system, $V = V_{ij}$, which corresponds to species i in reaction j. The rows of the stoichiometric matrix are the species and the columns are the reactions, the products have positive values and the reactants have negative values in the matrix. We know from fundamentals in general chemistry that the mass of every element in a closed system is conserved. We can realize this relationship with the following simple equation:

$$F \cdot V = 0 \tag{5.7}$$

An example of using a matrix approach to deal with the stoichiometry of multiple reactions can be seen in the following example using the watergas shift reaction, which produces hydrogen from hydrocarbons and is useful in generating fuel for fuel cells. First, we have the chemical reactions

$$C_3H_8 + 3H_2O \rightarrow 3CO + 7H_2 \tag{5.8}$$

$$CO + H_2O \rightarrow CO_2 + H_2 \tag{5.9}$$

Both of these reactions are balanced; the elements involved are C, H, and O; and the species are C_3H_8, CO_2, CO, H_2O, and H_2. The formula matrix would be

$$F_{ki} = \begin{bmatrix} 3 & 1 & 1 & 0 & 0 \\ 8 & 0 & 0 & 2 & 2 \\ 0 & 2 & 1 & 1 & 0 \end{bmatrix} \tag{5.10}$$

With the rows corresponding to the elements: C, H, and O, from top to bottom, and the columns corresponding the species: C_3H_8, CO_2, CO, H_2O, and H_2, from left to right. Next, we establish the stoichiometric matrix for the two equations with the rows corresponding to the species: C_3H_8, CO_2, CO, H_2O, and H_2, from top to bottom, and the columns corresponding to reactions 1 and 2, from left to right. The stoichiometric matrix would be

$$V_{ij} = \begin{bmatrix} -1 & 0 \\ 0 & 1 \\ 3 & -1 \\ -3 & -1 \\ 7 & 1 \end{bmatrix} \tag{5.11}$$

Examining the dot product, it is evident that the system is balanced because

$$F \cdot V = \begin{bmatrix} 0 & 0 \\ 0 & 0 \\ 0 & 0 \end{bmatrix} = 0 \tag{5.12}$$

This may seem odd since to balance the overall system would require 3 mol of CO to be used in Equation 5.14. We can correct this by balancing Equation 5.14 to match the products produced in Equation 5.13 as follows:

$$C_3H_8 + 3H_2O \rightarrow 3CO + 7H_2 \tag{5.13}$$

$$3CO + 3H_2O \rightarrow 3CO_2 + 3H_2 \tag{5.14}$$

The new stoichiometric matrix and the dot product of the two are

$$V_{ij} = \begin{bmatrix} -1 & 0 \\ 0 & 3 \\ 3 & -3 \\ -3 & -3 \\ 7 & 3 \end{bmatrix} \text{and } F \cdot V = \begin{bmatrix} 0 & 0 \\ 0 & 0 \\ 0 & 0 \end{bmatrix} \tag{5.15}$$

This demonstrates that as long as the individual reactions in a system are correctly balanced, the dot product between the formula and stoichiometric matrices will always be zero. The use of matrices has more value than simply determining whether the stoichiometry is balanced, the formula matrix can provide information regarding the number of reactions, and the stoichiometric coefficients of those reactions even if they are unknown. To establish the maximum number of equations in an unknown system, we first determine the unit matrix form of our formula matrix. Using the above system, we first rearrange the columns as follows (matrix algebra is not affected by column order and this step simply allows the downstream math to reach the unit matrix more efficiently):

$$\begin{array}{c} \\ C \\ H \\ O \end{array} \begin{array}{ccccc} CO & H_2 & H_2O & CO_2 & C_3H_8 \\ \begin{bmatrix} 1 & 0 & 0 & 1 & 3 \\ 0 & 2 & 2 & 0 & 8 \\ 1 & 0 & 1 & 2 & 0 \end{bmatrix} \end{array} \tag{5.16}$$

First, we subtract row 1 from row 3

$$
\begin{array}{c}
 \\
C \\
H \\
O
\end{array}
\begin{array}{ccccc}
CO & H_2 & H_2O & CO_2 & C_3H_8 \\
\left[\begin{array}{ccccc}
1 & 0 & 0 & 1 & 3 \\
0 & 2 & 2 & 0 & 8 \\
0 & 0 & 1 & 1 & -3
\end{array}\right]
\end{array}
\tag{5.17}
$$

Then, we multiply row 2 by 1/2

$$
\begin{array}{c}
 \\
C \\
H \\
O
\end{array}
\begin{array}{ccccc}
CO & H_2 & H_2O & CO_2 & C_3H_8 \\
\left[\begin{array}{ccccc}
1 & 0 & 0 & 1 & 3 \\
0 & 1 & 1 & 0 & 4 \\
0 & 0 & 1 & 1 & -3
\end{array}\right]
\end{array}
\tag{5.18}
$$

Finally, we subtract row 3 from row 2

$$
\begin{array}{c}
 \\
C \\
H \\
O
\end{array}
\begin{array}{ccccc}
CO & H_2 & H_2O & CO_2 & C_3H_8 \\
\left[\begin{array}{ccccc}
1 & 0 & 0 & 1 & 3 \\
0 & 1 & 0 & -1 & 7 \\
0 & 0 & 1 & 1 & -3
\end{array}\right]
\end{array}
\tag{5.19}
$$

Once the unit matrix is determined, it no longer represents a matrix with species and elements and should be rearranged such that the linearly independent species occupy the rows

$$
\begin{array}{c}
 \\
CO \\
H_2 \\
H_2O
\end{array}
\begin{array}{ccccc}
CO & H_2 & H_2O & CO_2 & C_3H_8 \\
\left[\begin{array}{ccccc}
1 & 0 & 0 & 1 & 3 \\
0 & 1 & 0 & -1 & 7 \\
0 & 0 & 1 & 1 & -3
\end{array}\right]
\end{array}
\tag{5.20}
$$

The number of linearly independent columns in our matrix denotes the rank of the matrix; in this case, the rank of the matrix is 3. The rank of the matrix is equal to the number of component species, CO, H_2, and H_2O. The noncomponent species would then be CO_2 and C_3H_8. Furthermore, the degrees of freedom, which denotes the maximum number of reactions necessary is equal to the total number of species minus the rank of formula matrix. For the above example, 5-rank(F) = 5 − 3 = 2. Based on the degrees of freedom for this example, there are a maximum of two equations needed, which are represented by the vectors in the matrix for the noncomponent species and result in the following equations:

$$
CO_2 = CO - H_2 + H_2O
\tag{5.21}
$$

$$
C_3H_8 = 3CO + 7H_2 - 3H_2O
\tag{5.22}
$$

After rearranging and converting back to a chemical equation, remember that negative values are products and positive values are reactants

$$H_2 + CO_2 - CO - H_2O = 0 \tag{5.23}$$

$$CO + H_2O \rightarrow CO_2 + H_2 \tag{5.24}$$

and

$$3CO + 7H_2 - 3H_2O - C_3H_8 = 0 \tag{5.25}$$

$$C_3H_8 + 3H_2O \rightarrow 3CO + 7H_2 \tag{5.26}$$

Despite making no assumption about the equations in our system, following the method outlined above knowing only the species present results in the same two balanced chemical equations for watergas shift reactions that were used in the beginning.

5.4 BASIC MASS TRANSFER: DIFFUSION AND CONVECTION

Mass transfer is of extreme importance to bioprocess engineering. Mass transfer in most systems for bioprocess engineering proceeds through a combination of diffusion and convection. Diffusion is the net movement of a substance from an area of high concentration to one of low concentration. Eventually, diffusion in a closed system will result in a single uniform concentration of the substance. Advection is the movement of a substance due to the bulk movement of the fluid the substance is contained within. Finally, convection is the combination of diffusion and advection. Thus, the rate of transport of substance i is the sum of the rates of transport of the diffusive velocity and bulk fluid velocity.

$$v_i = v_{i,\text{diffusion}} + v_{\text{bulk fluid}} \tag{5.27}$$

The flux of the substance is the amount of substance that passes through a unit area. This can be determined for both fixed and moving coordinates. A system that has no advection would result in the flux being the same regardless of the coordinates chosen. In fixed coordinates, the mass flux, n_i, is simply

$$n_i = \rho_i v_i \tag{5.28}$$

To convert to a molar flux we can use the molar concentration, C_i, in lieu of the density

$$N_i = C_i v_i \tag{5.29}$$

If we would like to consider just the flux due to diffusion, J, then the bulk fluid velocity is subtracted from the total velocity

$$j_i = \rho_i \left(v_i - v_{\text{bulk fluid}} \right) = \rho_i v_{i,\text{diffusion}} \tag{5.30}$$

$$J_i = C_i \left(v_i \quad v_{\text{bulk fluid}} \right) = C_i v_{i,\text{diffusion}} \tag{5.31}$$

If we assume that the substance i is dissolved in a solvent at a very low concentration, then the above relationships can be simplified to

$$N_i = J_i + C_i v_{\text{solvent}} \tag{5.32}$$

Diffusion can be evaluated in several different ways. First, we can examine the solute in the solvent fluid as a continuum, and second, we can evaluate solute stochastically. The continuum approach is best dealt with by using Fick's laws. Fick's first law establishes a function relating diffusive flux to a concentration gradient under steady-state conditions. In a single dimension, Fick's first law states

$$J_i = -D_{ij} \frac{dC_i}{dx} \tag{5.33}$$

where D_{ij} is the diffusivity or diffusion coefficient of solute i in solvent j and has units of length^2 × time^{-1}. Expanding Fick's first law to multiple dimensions is generalized by the multiplying the diffusion coefficient by the concentration gradient

$$J_i = -D_{ij} \nabla C_i \tag{5.34}$$

Under unsteady-state conditions, Fick's second law introduces time dependence, and for a single and multiple dimensions, respectively, states

$$\frac{\partial C_i}{\partial t} = D_{ij} \frac{\partial^2 C_i}{\partial x^2} \text{ and } \frac{\partial C_i}{\partial t} = D_{ij} \nabla^2 C_i \tag{5.35}$$

As with solving most engineering problems, boundary conditions are key for solving Fick's laws. Some common boundary conditions are as follows: assuming the concentration goes to zero as the distance goes to ∞; if there is a solid impenetrable boundary, the flux at that boundary is zero; and if there is a gas:liquid interface, the flux across the interface is equal to the flux at both the gas and liquid phase on either side of the interface.

The molecular mechanism for evaluating diffusion was briefly discussed in Chapter 4. At the molecular scale, diffusion involves a few molecules moving and transferring energy between each other. To evaluate this, we treat diffusion as a random walk. Consider that a single particle in a one-dimensional system can move either forward or backward and that the selection of either direction is random. Over a long time, the net movement of the particle will generate a mean displacement of zero; however, during that time the particle travels a substantial distance and the maximum distance traveled from the origin at any particular point gradually increases. The derivation of Brownian motion of a particle in one, two, or three dimensions is available from many sources and will not be presented here; however, the net result in one dimension is

$$\langle x^2 \rangle = 2D_{ij}t \tag{5.36}$$

where, $\langle x^2 \rangle$ is the mean squared displacement, $\langle x(t) - x_0 \rangle^2$, at time t. Extending this relationship to multiple dimensions results in the following equation:

$$\langle r^2 \rangle = \alpha D_{ij}t \tag{5.37}$$

where α is equal to 2, 4, and 6 for one-, two-, and three-dimensional diffusions, respectively. For systems where D_{ij} is unknown, it can be found using the Stokes–Einstein equation:

$$D_{ij} = \frac{k_B T}{f} \tag{5.38}$$

where:
   f is the shape factor to determine drag on the particle diffusing
   k_B is the Boltzmann constant, 1.38×10^{-23} J/K
   T is the temperature

For a simple sphere, f is a function of viscosity, μ, and the particle radius, R.

$$f = 6\pi\mu R \tag{5.39}$$

5.5 BASIC FLUID DYNAMICS

Much like the discussion on diffusion, fluid dynamics can easily occupy an entire textbook. This section will briefly cover the two most relevant aspects of fluid dynamics for bioprocess engineering, the Navier–Stokes equation and the Reynolds number. The Navier–Stokes equation is derived by applying Newton's second law, force = mass · accleration, to fluid motion. In the most general form, the Navier–Stokes equation for incompressible fluid flow is stated as follows.

$$\rho\left(\frac{\partial v}{\partial t} + v \cdot \nabla v\right) = -\nabla P + \mu\nabla^2 v + \rho \cdot g \tag{5.40}$$

where:
   ρ is the density
   v is the velocity
   t is the time
   P is the pressure
   μ is the viscosity
   $\rho * g$ accounts for force due to gravity

Examining the above equation, the left-hand side represents the potential inertial forces present, whereas the right-hand side represents the forces due to pressure, viscosity, and gravity. Based on the assumptions made in the system of interest, the Navier–Stokes equation can be simplified. Typically, we consider systems with laminar flow, which would reduce the left-hand side to 0. Additionally, the Navier–Stokes equation is readily expanded to generate solutions for fluid flow in different coordinate systems. For instance, in cylindrical coordinates, the Navier–Stokes equation in r, θ, and z directions would be

$$r: \rho\left(\frac{\partial v_r}{\partial t} + v_r\frac{\partial v_r}{\partial r} + \frac{v_\theta}{r}\frac{\partial v_r}{\partial \theta} - \frac{v_\theta^2}{r} + v_z\frac{\partial v_r}{\partial z}\right) =$$
$$-\frac{\partial P}{\partial r} + \mu\left\{\frac{\partial}{\partial r}\left[\frac{1}{r}\frac{\partial}{\partial r}(rv_r)\right] + \frac{1}{r^2}\frac{\partial^2 v_r}{\partial \theta^2} - \frac{2}{r^2}\frac{\partial v_\theta}{\partial \theta} + \frac{\partial^2 v_r}{\partial z^2}\right\} + \rho g_r$$

(5.41)

$$\theta: \rho\left(\frac{\partial v_\theta}{\partial t} + v_r\frac{\partial v_\theta}{\partial r} + \frac{v_\theta}{r}\frac{\partial v_\theta}{\partial \theta} + \frac{v_r v_\theta}{r} + v_z\frac{\partial v_\theta}{\partial z}\right) =$$
$$-\frac{1}{r}\frac{\partial P}{\partial \theta} + \mu\left\{\frac{\partial}{\partial r}\left[\frac{1}{r}\frac{\partial}{\partial r}(rv_\theta)\right] + \frac{1}{r^2}\frac{\partial^2 v_\theta}{\partial \theta^2} + \frac{2}{r^2}\frac{\partial v_r}{\partial \theta} + \frac{\partial^2 v_\theta}{\partial z^2}\right\} + \rho g_\theta$$

(5.42)

$$z: \rho\left(\frac{\partial v_z}{\partial t} + v_r\frac{\partial v_z}{\partial r} + \frac{v_\theta}{r}\frac{\partial v_z}{\partial \theta} + v_z\frac{\partial v_z}{\partial z}\right) =$$
$$-\frac{\partial P}{\partial z} + \mu\left[\frac{1}{r}\frac{\partial}{\partial r}\left(r\frac{\partial v_z}{\partial r}\right) + \frac{1}{r^2}\frac{\partial^2 v_z}{\partial \theta^2} + \frac{\partial^2 v_z}{\partial z^2}\right] + \rho g_z$$

(5.43)

If we examine these equations under the assumptions that fluid flows in a tube of length L at steady state and under laminar and incompressible flow conditions, then the left side of the equations, which describe inertial effects, would be zero. Likewise, if there are no inertial effects and it is steady state, velocity in the r- and θ-directions is also zero. These assumptions reduce the system of three equations to just the right side of the equation describing velocity in the z-direction. Thus, the resulting equation describing fluid flow in a tube is

$$z: 0 = -\frac{\partial P}{\partial z} + \mu\left[\frac{1}{r}\frac{\partial}{\partial r}\left(r\frac{\partial v_z}{\partial r}\right) + \frac{1}{r^2}\frac{\partial^2 v_z}{\partial \theta^2} + \frac{\partial^2 v_z}{\partial z^2}\right] + \rho g_z$$

(5.44)

Which if we neglect the effect of gravity, and account for laminar and steady-state flow and rearrange yields

$$z: \frac{\partial P}{\partial z} = \mu\left[\frac{1}{r}\frac{\partial}{\partial r}\left(r\frac{\partial v_z}{\partial r}\right)\right]$$

(5.45)

Solving the above is straightforward, first we examine the left-hand side by setting each of the left and the right sides equal to some constant C_1. Then, we see

$$\frac{\partial P}{\partial z} = C_1, \quad \int_{P_1}^{P_2} \partial P = C_1 \int_0^L \partial z, \quad P_2 - P_1 = C_1 L, \quad C_1 = \frac{P_2 - P_1}{L} \tag{5.46}$$

Similarly, we can now integrate the right side of the equation

$$C_1 = \mu \left[\frac{1}{r} \frac{\partial}{\partial r} \left(r \frac{\partial v_z}{\partial r} \right) \right], \quad \int \frac{C_1 r}{\mu} \partial r = \left(r \frac{\partial v_z}{\partial r} \right), \quad \int \frac{C_1 r}{2\mu} + \frac{C_2}{r} \partial r = \int \partial v_z \tag{5.47}$$

$$\frac{C_1 r^2}{4\mu} + C_2 \ln(r) + C_3 = v_z, \quad \frac{(P_2 - P_1) r^2}{4\mu L} + C_2 \ln(r) + C_3 \tag{5.48}$$

To solve for the two unknown constants, first we know that the velocity is finite at all possible values of r, including $r = 0$. Because the $\ln(r)$ has a discontinuity at 0, $C_2 = 0$. To solve C_3, we evaluate at the boundaries, which we assume are no-slip: $v_z = 0$ at $r = R$ where R is the radius of the tube

$$\frac{(P_2 - P_1) R^2}{4\mu L} + C_3 = 0, \quad \frac{(P_2 - P_1) R^2}{4\mu L} = -C_3 \tag{5.49}$$

Finally, we recognize the pressure at the end of the pipe is lower than that at the beginning and rewrite the solved equation for velocity in a pipe as

$$\frac{(P_1 - P_2) R^2}{4\mu L} - \frac{(P_1 - P_2) r^2}{4\mu L} = v_z \tag{5.50}$$

The above was derived for a very specific case where there was pressure driven, steady state, incompressible, and laminar flow without any external forces. Often it is useful to determine what the expected behavior of a solution will be before making such assumptions. A simple dimensionless number, the Reynolds number, can provide a quick determination of the fluid profile present. The Reynolds number is determined as follows:

$$\mathrm{Re} = \frac{\rho v L}{\mu} \text{ or } \mathrm{Re} = \frac{v L}{\nu} \tag{5.51}$$

where L is a characteristic dimension of the system, the diameter for a tube, or the height between two parallel plates. The top portion of the Reynolds number represents the inertial forces in a system, whereas the bottom represents the viscous forces. It follows then that if Re is high, inertia dominates, and if Re is low, viscous forces dominate. The threshold for making a laminar flow assumption would be Re < 2,300.

5.6 BASIC THERMODYNAMICS

Two major thermodynamic characteristics are important for the description of bio-chemical reactors in process modeling, that is, heats of reaction and thermodynamic equilibrium. The heat of reaction determines the amount of heat to be removed by appropriate cooling since most biological reactions are run isothermally. Heat changes are determined by reaction enthalpies, ΔH. The heat of reaction, ΔH, can be calculated from the heats of formation or heats of combustion:

$$\sum_{i=1}^{n} v_i \Delta HFi = \sum_{i=1}^{n} v_i \Delta HCi \tag{5.52}$$

where:
ΔHFi is the heat of formation of component i
ΔHCi is the heat of combustion of component i having stoichiometric coefficients v_i

If heats of formation are not available, heats of combustion can be determined experimentally from calorimetric measurement. The resulting heat of reaction, ΔH, is negative for exothermic reactions and positive for endothermic reactions by convention. Whole-cell growth and product formation is a more complex process, and we have available only empirical data, ideally from relevant experiments or by empirical correlation, for example, typical energy yield coefficients, to calculate the total heat production as described earlier. Chemical equilibrium is defined by the equilibrium constant, for example, for the reaction specified in Equation 5.53:

$$K = \frac{CvC}{AvA \, BvB} \tag{5.53}$$

Gibbs free energy of a reaction, ΔG, is related to reaction enthalpy, ΔH, and reaction entropy, ΔS. At standard conditions indicated by superscript 0:

$$\Delta G^0 = \Delta H^0 - T\Delta S^0 \tag{5.54}$$

where T is the absolute temperature. The equilibrium constant is related to Gibbs free energy of a reaction by

$$\Delta G^0 = -RT\ln K \tag{5.55}$$

where R is the universal gas constant. An example of an enzymatic equilibrium reaction is the isomerization of glucose to fructose used to produce fructose corn syrup. This is an endothermic reaction with $\Delta H = 2{,}670$ J/mol, $\Delta G = 349$ J/mol, and specific heat (C_p) = 76 J/mol K at 25°C. From this, the calculated equilibrium constants at 30°C and 60°C are 0.886 and 1.034, respectively, as calculated by the van't Hoff equation. For this reaction, the equilibrium conversion, xe, is defined as

$$xe = 1/(1+K) \tag{5.56}$$

A temperature increase from 30°C to 60°C therefore allows an increase in the equilibrium conversion of about 8%. High temperature is thus desirable but may be limited by decreased enzyme stability at elevated temperature. While variation of temperature is feasible for simple enzyme-catalyzed reactions, it is less often used for cell-based processes since the temperature-range optimal performance is quite narrow, not usually more than a few degrees Celsius. Furthermore, growth and fermentation processes are irreversible processes. Therefore, thermodynamically possible conversion is not influenced by the usual temperature changes allowed.

5.7 BASIC REACTION KINETICS

Reaction kinetics describes the way that a group of reactants area consumed leading to the formation of products. The two key concepts for solving and understanding most reaction systems are mass balances and rate laws. The mass balance we have covered above. Developing a rate law for a particular reaction is straightforward; take the following reaction with rate constant k and stoichiometric coefficients V_i.

$$V_A A + V_B B \xrightarrow{k} V_C C + V_D D \tag{5.57}$$

The general rate law for the above reaction would then be

$$\text{Rate} = k[A]^x [B]^y \tag{5.58}$$

The overall order of the reaction is the sum of the exponents for each reactant in the rate law and would be $x + y$. The order of the reaction with respect to $[A]$ is x and with respect to $[B]$ is y. The overall order of the reaction, and the order with respect to the individual reactants, can be any positive number and is not limited to an integer. It is possible for the order to be negative with respect to one of the reactants; however, the overall order is still positive but is classified as undefined. If the reactants, $[A]$ and $[B]$, collide and react in one singular event, which is rare for reactions involving more than two molecules, then the reaction can be said to be elementary. For an elementary reaction, the general rate law for the previous reaction would be

$$\text{Rate} = k[A]^{V_A} [B]^{V_B} \tag{5.59}$$

If we want to examine the loss of $[A]$ for the above reaction and assuming it is elementary then the rate law for the loss of $[A]$ would be

$$\frac{-d[A]}{dt} = V_A k[A]^{V_A} [B]^{V_B} \tag{5.60}$$

Likewise for the other reactants and products the rate laws would be

$$\frac{-d[B]}{dt} = V_B k [A]^{V_a} [B]^{V_R} \tag{5.61}$$

$$\frac{d[C]}{dt} = V_C k [A]^{V_A} [B]^{V_B} \tag{5.62}$$

$$\frac{d[D]}{dt} = V_D k [A]^{V_A} [B]^{V_B} \tag{5.63}$$

Each of these individual rate laws are derived by multiplying the governing rate law by each of the components stoichiometric coefficients. In general the stoichiometry of the reaction can provide information about the rate loss or gain of each species as they relate to each other in the following way, for the equation:

$$V_A A + V_B B \xrightarrow{k} V_C C + V_D D \tag{5.64}$$

$$\frac{-1}{V_A} \cdot \frac{d[A]}{dt} = \frac{-1}{V_B} \cdot \frac{d[B]}{dt} = \frac{1}{V_C} \cdot \frac{d[C]}{dt} = \frac{1}{V_D} \cdot \frac{d[D]}{dt} \tag{5.65}$$

When we consider reaction order, the most common involving a single reactant is the first-order reaction. A first-order reaction with a single reactant is straightforward to solve and analyze and is useful in applications ranging from radioactive decay to eukaryotic cell growth. The analysis of a first-order reaction can be determined by establishing the rate laws and mass balances followed by integration of the rate law and appropriate substitution of the mass balance to determine functions describing the loss and gain of the products and reactants. The following is a simple example of a first-order reaction:

$$A \xrightarrow{k} B \tag{5.66}$$

$$\text{Mass balance: } [A]_0 - [A] = [B] - [B]_0 \tag{5.67}$$

$$\text{Rate law: } -\frac{d[A]}{dt} = k[A] \tag{5.68}$$

$$\text{Integration of the rate law: } \int_{[A]_0}^{[A]} -\frac{d[A]}{[A]} = \int_0^t k \cdot dt, -\left(\ln[A] - \ln[A]_0 \right) \tag{5.69}$$

$$= kt$$

$$\text{Rearranging: } \frac{\ln[A]}{\ln[A]_0} = -kt, \frac{[A]}{[A]_0} = e^{-kt}, [A] = [A]_0 e^{-kt} \tag{5.70}$$

Finally, now that we have developed a solution for $[A]$, we can easily solve for $[B]$ using the mass balance:

$$[B] = [A]_0 \left(1 - e^{-kt}\right) + [B]_0 \tag{5.71}$$

Often times, it is useful to characterize reactions in terms of their half-lives, which is simply the time it takes for the concentration of the product to drop by half. For the previous first-order equation, we can find the half-life as follows:

$$\frac{1}{2}[A]_0 = [A]_0 e^{-kt_{1/2}}, \ \frac{1}{2} = e^{-kt_{1/2}}, \quad \ln\left(\frac{1}{2}\right) = -kt_{1/2}, \ t_{1/2} = \frac{\ln(2)}{k} \tag{5.72}$$

Next to a first-order reaction, zero-order reactions are also common in biological processes in that they are characteristic of enzymatic reactions where the substrate concentration greatly exceeds the enzyme concentration. If the reaction, $A \xrightarrow{k} B$, is zero order, the following solution can be found describing $[A] = f(t)$:

$$-\frac{d[A]}{dt} = k[A]^0, \ \int_{A_0}^{A} -dA = \int_0^t k \cdot dt, \ [A] = [A]_0 - kt \tag{5.73}$$

The half-life for a zero-order reaction can be found similar to that of a first-order reaction and yields, $t_{1/2} = [A]_0/2k$. Finally, it is possible for higher-order reactions to be functions of only a single reactant and a general solution can be found as follows, where n corresponds to the order with respect to $[A]$ for all values other than 1

$$-\frac{d[A]}{dt} = k[A]^n, \ \int_{[A]_0}^{[A]} -\frac{d[A]}{[A]^n}$$

$$= \int_0^t k \cdot dt, \ \frac{1}{[A]^{n-1}} \tag{5.74}$$

$$= (n-1)kt + \frac{1}{[A]_0^{n-1}}$$

Reactions involving more than one reactant, of the same or mixed order, quickly become cumbersome to solve analytically, and it becomes prudent to approximate these reactions in software. The simplest method of analyzing these higher-order reactions is a spreadsheet where the integration can be approximated by

$$f(t+\Delta t) = f(t) + \frac{df(t)}{dt} \cdot \Delta t \qquad (5.75)$$

The only challenge in using this approximation is selecting an appropriate Δt. A good starting point is found with a relationship combining the starting concentrations of the products and the rate constant, where n again corresponds to the reaction order

$$\Delta t = \frac{\sum [\text{Products}]^{n-1}}{4k} \qquad (5.76)$$

Figure 5.1 illustrates a reaction solved by the above approximation versus the same reaction solved analytically with the mean squared error between the two curves being approximately 6%. Halving the Δt brings the mean squared error down to 1.3%, but increases the computational expense. In contrast, doubling the Δt increases the mean squared error to 28%, which is a poor approximation for most scenarios.

Often times with kinetic data, the goal is not to analyze or model the reaction, but instead to determine the rate constants or the order of the reaction. There exist straightforward strategies for determining both the rate constant and order of a reaction. Examining the solutions for the first- and zero-order reactions, we can linearize each by rearranging as follows:

$$\text{First order:} \ \ln[A] = -kt + \ln[A]_0 \qquad (5.77)$$

$$\text{Zero order:} \ [A] = -kt + [A]_0 \qquad (5.78)$$

Each of these fit the typical format of a line, $y = mx + b$. First-order reactions will demonstrate a linear relationship when the ln() of the reactant is plotted against time. The slope of this line is $-k$. Likewise, a zero-order reaction will demonstrate a linear relationship

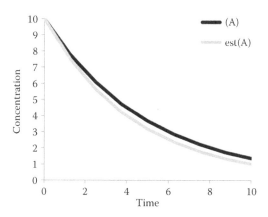

Figure 5.1 Comparison of the change in concentration of [A] for an analytical solution to first-order reaction kinetics and estimated solution.

when the reactant is plotted against time and again, the slope of the line is $-k$. Reactions of nth order, when $n \neq 1$, also produce a linear relationship when $1/[A]^{n-1}$ is plotted versus t, the slope produced is $(n-1)*k$. Additionally, relationships can be established if the rate or the half-life is known for multiple initial conditions by ensuring there is an initial condition (and likewise and equation) for each unknown and solving as appropriate.

The approach of identifying rate laws and mass balances holds for equations involving more than one reactant and also those that are not one direction, take the simple reversible reaction

$$A \underset{k_{-1}}{\overset{k_1}{\rightleftharpoons}} B \tag{5.79}$$

$$\text{Rate laws:} -\frac{d[A]}{dt} = k_1[A] - k_{-1}[B] = \frac{d[B]}{dt} \tag{5.80}$$

$$\text{Mass balance:} [A]_0 - [A] = [B] - [B]_0 \tag{5.81}$$

$$\text{Expansion:} \frac{d[A]}{dt} + [A](k_1 + k_{-1}) = k_{-1}([A]_0 + [B]_0) \tag{5.82}$$

Solving the non-homogenous linear first-order differential equation, we get the following:

$$[A] = \frac{k_{-1}([A]_0 + [B]_0)}{k_1 + k_{-1}}\left[1 - e^{-(k_1+k_{-1})t}\right] + [A]_0 e^{-(k_1+k_{-1})t} \tag{5.83}$$

$$[B] = [B]_0 - \frac{k_{-1}([A]_0 + [B]_0)}{k_1 + k_{-1}}\left[1 - e^{(k_1+k_{-1})t}\right] + [A]_0\left[1 - e^{(k_1+k_{-1})t}\right] \tag{5.84}$$

Reversible reactions eventually reach equilibrium values of $[A]_f$ and $[B]_f$ that are directly related to the ratio between the rate constants, $k_{-1}/k_1 = [A]_f/[B]_f$; Figure 5.2 provides a graphical example of a reversible reaction where $[A]_0 = 10$ [M] and $[B]_0 = 0$ [M] and k_1 is double k_{-1}.

Another common group of reactions are those involving intermediates. Again, the simple approach of identifying the rate laws and mass balances allows for a straightforward solution. Take the following:

$$[A] \overset{k_1}{\rightarrow} [B] \overset{k_2}{\rightarrow} [C] \tag{5.85}$$

$$\text{Rate laws:} -\frac{d[A]}{dt} = k_1[A], \quad \frac{d[B]}{dt} = k_1[A] - k_2[B], \quad \frac{d[C]}{dt} = k_2[B] \tag{5.86}$$

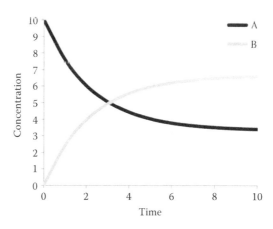

Figure 5.2 Example of first order reversible reaction where [B] is initially 0 [M], [A] is initially 10 [M] and the forward reaction rate constant is double the reverse reaction rate constant.

$$\text{Mass balance}: \left[A\right]_0 - \left[A\right] = \left(\left[B\right] - \left[B\right]_0\right) + \left(\left[C\right] - \left[C\right]_0\right) \tag{5.87}$$

The solution for the loss of [A] follows simple first-order reaction kinetics, $\left[A\right] = \left[A\right]_0 e^{-k_1 t}$, which we can plug into the rate law for the loss of [B] as follows:

$$\frac{d\left[B\right]}{dt} = k_1 \left[A\right]_0 e^{k_1 t} - k_2 \left[B\right] \tag{5.88}$$

Now the integrated rate law for [B] can be determined by solving the first-order non-homogenous linear differential equation to find

$$\left[B\right] = \frac{k_1 \left[A\right]_0}{k_2 - k_1} \left(e^{-k_1 t} \quad e^{-k_2 t}\right) + \left[B\right]_0 e^{-k_2 t} \tag{5.89}$$

This is true for all values of k_1 and k_2 except when $k_1 = k_2$, in which case following the same process of identifying the rate law and substituting k_1 for k_2 yields

$$\left[B\right] = k_1 \left[A\right]_0 t e^{-k_1 t} + \left[B\right]_0 e^{-2k_1 t} \tag{5.90}$$

Finally, once [A] and [B] are determined, the integrated rate law for [C] can be found by substitution into the mass balance:

$$\left[C\right] = \left[A\right]_0 + \left[B\right]_0 + \left[C\right]_0 - \left[A\right] - \left[B\right] \tag{5.91}$$

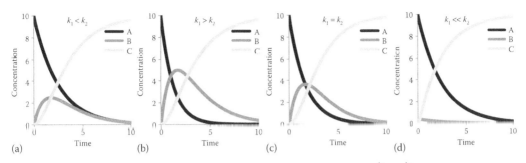

Figure 5.3 Representation of potential intermediate reactions for $[A] \xrightarrow{k_1} [B] \xrightarrow{k_2} [C]$: the typical case, A, where the reaction driving the intermediate formation is slightly slower than the reaction forming the product; the rare case, B, where a stable intermediate emerges; the exceedingly rare case, C, where the rate for the two reactions are identical; and the relatively common case, D, of a reactive intermediate.

Intermediate reactions typically proceed with a $k_1 < k_2$. The first scenario, when $k_1 < k_2$, generates a stable intermediate, or an intermediate that demonstrates a peak concentration higher than the reactant concentration at that time point. The other possibility is when $k_1 \ll k_2$, which describes a highly reactive intermediate that demonstrates a concentration that is near zero throughout the lifetime of the reaction. Figure 5.3 provides a graphical representation of the types of relationships between k_1 and k_2 and the resulting behavior of the concentrations of the reactant [A], intermediate [B], and product [C].

Finally, a discussion on reaction kinetics would be remiss without including the potential for thermodynamics to affect reaction. The effect of temperature on reaction rates can proceed through three different variants. The first demonstrates a gradual increase in rate with temperature. The second demonstrates a rapid increase in rate above a threshold temperature, for example, an explosion. Finally, reactions may increase to a threshold temperature above which the rate decreases, for example, and enzymatic reaction where the decrease is due to the denaturation of the enzyme. The relationship between temperature and the reaction rate constant, k, is described by the Arrhenius equation.

$$k = Ae^{-E_a/RT} \tag{5.92}$$

where:
   A is a pre-exponential factor that has units matching the expected units for k depending on the order of the reaction
   E_a is the activation energy for the reaction
   R is the ideal gas constant, for example, 8.314 J/mol K
   T is the temperature

Figure 5.4 is a representation of these three potential temperature dependence mechanisms.

139

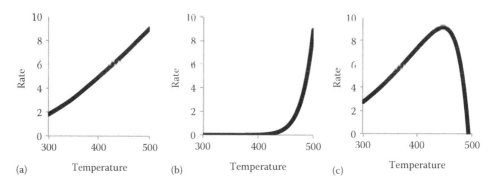

Figure 5.4 Representation of possible temperature dependence for reactions. (a) A typical gradual increase in rate with temperature, *A*; (b) an explosive increase in rate above a threshold temperature, *B*; and (c) competing reactions where the inhibitory reaction dominates the rate above a threshold temperature, *C*.

Questions

1. Four grams of hydrogen peroxide, H_2O_2, decompose into water and oxygen. What mass of each of the products is formed by the decomposition?
   Answer: First, we balance the reaction and determine the molecular weights of the components: $2H_2O_2 \rightarrow 2H_2O + O_2$ with molecular weights for H_2O_2, H_2O, and O_2 equal to 34, 18, and 32 g/mol. Then, we use stoichiometry: $4g \cdot [1/34(g/mol)] \cdot (2\,mol\,H_2O/2\,mol\,H_2O_2) \cdot 18(g/mol) = 2.12\,g\,H_2O$ and $4g \cdot [1/34(g/mol)] \cdot (1\,mol\,O_2/2\,mol\,H_2O_2) * 32(g/mol) = 1.88\,g\,O_2$. As expected, the total mass in the system remains 4 g.

2. Using the solution obtained for question 1, the amount of water formed underwent electrolysis to further separate the water into hydrogen and oxygen. If the bond energies for H–O, H–H, and O–O are 467, 432, and 204 kJ/mol, what quantity of energy is consumed or produced to drive the electrolysis?

3. The molecular weight of ethanol is 46.07 g/mol, the density of ethanol is 0.789 g/cm^3. How many molecules of ethanol are present in 1 mL, assuming a 100% solution of ethanol?
   Answer: 0.789 g/cm^3 * 1 cm^3/mL * 1 mL = 0.789 g, 0.789 g/46.07 g/mol = 0.01713 mol, 0.01713 mol * 6.022 × 10^{23} molec/mol = 1.03 × 10^{22} molecules.

4. Use the matrix approach to identify the number of reactions, and what those reactions are, and balance the fictional overall reaction: $AB + BC_2 + A_3D_2 \rightarrow AC_2 + B_3D_2$

5. A drug delivery strategy was designed to treat a tumor of approximately 1 cm in diameter. The drug has a half-life of 2 h and is implanted into the middle of the tumor. Assuming a diffusion coefficient for the drug of 1.0×10^{-5} cm^2/s, will the treatment strategy be effective?

6. For the scenario presented in question 5, what if the drug was a protein-based therapeutic with a half-life of 2 h and a diffusion coefficient of 5×10^{-7} cm^2/s?

7. For the scenario detailed in question 6, what is the maximal distance the drug can reasonably treat if it is delivered at a concentration equal to 10× the effective dose? *Answer*: Based on the half-life, the time required for the drug to fall to the effective concentration is 6.6 h because [Concentration] = [Concentration]$_0 e^{-t[\ln(2)/\text{half-life}]}$. Then, if we approximate the tumor based on one-dimensional diffusion, the maximum diffusion distance would be about 26 μm.

8. What is the rate law and overall reaction order for the reaction of glucose, $C_6H_{12}O_6$, with oxygen to form carbon dioxide and water?

9. For the elementary reaction: $2A + B \rightarrow P$:
   a. Solve for $[A] = f(t)$
   b. Solve for $[A] = f(t)$ if $B_0 \gg A_0$

10. The irreversible hydrolysis of alanine ethyl ester to alanine and ethanol occurs in an ice water bath and has an activation energy of 10 kJ/mol and a pre-exponential factor of 1.5×10^{-2} M/s. The density of water is 1,000 g/L and the molecular weight of water is 18.02 g/mol. Assume the reaction is elementary. Below is the chemical structure for alanine ethyl ester

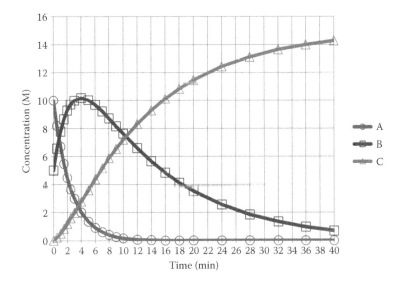

   a. Write and balance the equation for the hydrolysis of alanine ethyl ester to alanine.
   b. Find the integrated rate law for the production of alanine.
   c. What is the concentration of alanine after 2 min if the original concentration was 10 M?

11. For the following graph:

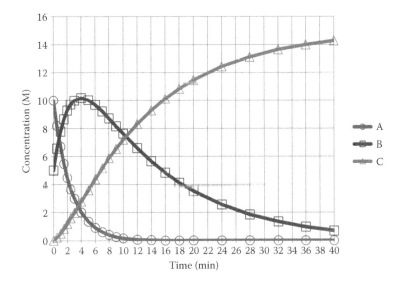

a. What is the type of reaction occurring? (e.g., parallel and reversible)
   Answer: The reaction depicted is a series reaction with the intermediate, *B*. The stoichiometric relationship is 1:1:1 for *A*:*B*:*C* based on the mass balance that $(A_0 - A) = (B - B_0) + (C - C_0)$.

b. What can be determined regarding the initial concentrations?
   Answer: *A* is 10 M, *B* is 5 M, and *C* is 0 M.

c. What can be determined regarding the rate constants?
   Answer: The reaction forming the intermediate is faster than the reaction consuming the intermediate, hence a stable intermediate is formed.

12. For the following graph:

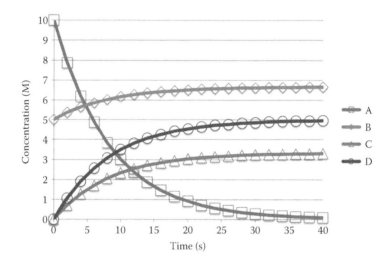

a. What is the type of reaction occurring? (e.g., parallel and reversible)
b. What can be determined regarding the initial concentrations?
c. What can be determined regarding the rate constants?

13. For the following data:

$(dA/dt)_i$ **M/s**	$[A]_0$ **M**	$[B]_0$ **M**
1.000	1	1
5.657	2	2
12.728	2	3

a. What is the overall order of the reaction?
b. What is the order of the reaction with respect to *A*?
c. What is the order of the reaction with respect to *B*?

14. The reversible hydrolysis of ethyl acetate to ethanol and acetic acid has an activation energy of 1 kJ/mol and a pre-exponential factor of 1.5×10^{-2} M^{x}s^y. The reaction

is proceeding at 98.6°F. The density of water is 1,000 g/L and the molecular weight of water is 18.02 g/mol. Assume the reaction is elementary and that reversible reaction is negligible when carried out at 98.6°F. Below is the chemical structure for ethyl acetate:

a. Write and balance the equation for the hydrolysis of ethyl acetate to ethanol and acetic acid.
b. Find the integrated rate law for the loss of ethyl acetate.
c. What is the concentration of ethyl acetate after 2 min if the original concentration was 10 mM?

15. For the simple reversible reaction, $A \leftrightarrow B$, with $k_1 = 1/2 * k_{-1}$, what are the equilibrium concentrations if
   a. $[A]_0 = 10$ M, $[B]_0 = 0$ M
   b. $[A]_0 = 10$ M, $[B]_0 = 5$ M

16. The concentration of the enzyme alkaline phosphatase can be determined because it catalyzes the conversion of 4-nitrophenylphosphate to p-nitrophenol. The product, p-nitrophenol is yellow and can be quantified by measuring the absorbance at 405 nm, absorbance is proportional to concentration. The following absorbances were obtained

Time	0	1	2	3	4	5	6	7	8
Absorbance	0.5	1.5	1.83	2	2.1	2.17	2.21	2.25	2.28

To correct for the absorbance caused by the assay plate, you took a reading at 600 nm and recorded the following:

Time	0	1	2	3	4	5	6	7	8
Absorbance	0.52	0.48	0.5	0.49	0.47	0.5	0.53	0.5	0.51

What is the overall order of the conversion of 4-nitrophenylphosphate to p-nitrophenol? (15pts) Absorbance $= \varepsilon * b * [C]$, $\varepsilon * b = 0.2/M$

17. The reaction, $A \xrightarrow{k} B + 2C$, can be monitored by measuring the concentration of C, from the following values calculate the overall order of the reaction if $A_0 - 10$ M: (15pts)

T (s)	C (M)
0	0.000
1	10.000
2	13.333
3	15.000
4	16.000
5	16.667
6	17.143
7	17.500
8	17.778
9	18.000
10	18.182

Answer: First determine the concentration of the reactant A, $2(A_0 - A) = C - C_0$, $A = A_0 - C/2$, then examine the $\ln[A]$ and $1/[A]$ to determine if the reaction is first or second order.

T (s)	A (M)	Ln (A)	1/A
0	10.000	2.303	0.1
1	5.000	1.609	0.2
2	3.333	1.204	0.3
3	2.5	0.916	0.4
4	2.0	0.693	0.5

The relationship is linear with $1/A$, thus second order.

6

Kinetics of Enzymes and Cell Growth

LEARNING OBJECTIVES

1. Understand the fundamentals of enzymatic reactions from the perspective of basic reaction kinetics.
2. Derive the Michaelis–Menten equation based on either rapid equilibrium or quasi-steady-state assumptions.
3. Determine the type of enzymatic reaction present when presented with experimental data.
4. Recognize how enzyme kinetics are key to the regulation of eukaryotic and prokaryotic cell growth.
5. Model the growth of eukaryotic and prokaryotic cells in culture.

6.1 INTRODUCTION

Enzymes are typically proteins capable of increasing the rate of a reaction. They demonstrate remarkable specificity for their substrate and their activity can be modulated. Biological process, whether it is immediately apparent or not, relies almost entirely on enzymes. Take the rather simple example of a hormone regulating the differentiation of stem cells. Examining this process, enzymes are the receptors that the hormone binds, enzymes propagate the signal through the cytoplasm, enzymes modify the methylation pattern of the DNA and regulate the transcription pattern of genes, and finally enzymes mediate the formation of proteins that will ultimately define the lineage of the stem cell. This chapter will explore enzyme kinetics, both directly and indirectly through cell growth models.

6.2 BASIC MICHAELIS–MENTEN KINETICS

Michaelis–Menten kinetics relies on the law of mass action, which is derived from the assumptions of free diffusion and thermodynamically driven random collision. However, many biochemical or cellular processes deviate significantly from these conditions, because of macromolecular crowding, phase separation of the enzyme/substrate/product, or one- or two-dimensional molecular movement. In these situations, a fractal Michaelis–Menten kinetics may be applied.

Some enzymes operate with kinetics, which are faster than diffusion rates, which would seem to be impossible. Several mechanisms have been invoked to explain this phenomenon. Some proteins are believed to accelerate catalysis by drawing their substrate in and pre-orienting them by using dipolar electric fields. Other models invoke a quantum-mechanical tunneling explanation, whereby a proton or an electron can tunnel through activation barriers, although for proton tunneling this model remains somewhat controversial. Quantum tunneling for protons has been observed in tryptamine. This suggests that enzyme catalysis may be more accurately characterized as *through the barrier* rather than the traditional model, which requires substrates to go *over* a lowered energy barrier.

In biochemistry, Michaelis–Menten kinetics is one of the simplest and best-known models of enzyme kinetics. It is named after German biochemist Leonor Michaelis and Canadian physician Maud Menten. The model takes the form of an equation describing the rate of enzymatic reactions, by relating reaction rate v to [S], the concentration of a substrate S. Its formula is given by

$$v = \frac{d[P]}{dt} = \frac{V_{max}[S]}{K_m + [S]} \tag{6.1}$$

Here, V_{max} represents the maximum rate achieved by the system, at maximum (saturating) substrate concentrations. The Michaelis constant K_m is the substrate concentration at which the reaction rate is half of V_{max}. Biochemical reactions involving a single substrate are often assumed to follow Michaelis–Menten kinetics, without regard to the model's underlying assumptions (Figure 6.1).

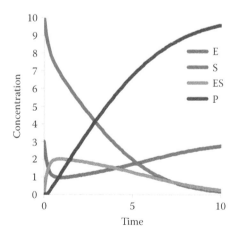

Figure 6.1   Change in concentrations over time for enzyme E, substrate S, complex ES, and product P.

In 1903, French physical chemist Victor Henri found that enzyme reactions were initiated by a bond between the enzyme and the substrate. His work was taken up by German biochemist Leonor Michaelis and Canadian physician Maud Menten who investigated the kinetics of an enzymatic reaction mechanism, invertase, that catalyzes the hydrolysis of sucrose into glucose and fructose. In 1913, they proposed a mathematical model of the reaction. It involves an enzyme E binding to a substrate S to form a complex ES, which in turn is converted into a product P and the enzyme. This may be represented schematically as

$$E + S \underset{k_r}{\overset{k_f}{\rightleftharpoons}} ES \xrightarrow{k_{cat}} E + P \tag{6.2}$$

where:

k_f, k_r, and k_{cat} denote the rate constants

The double arrows between S and ES represent the fact that enzyme–substrate binding is a reversible process

Under certain assumptions—such as the enzyme concentration being much less than the substrate concentration—the rate of product formation is given by

$$v = \frac{d[P]}{dt} = V_{max} \frac{[S]}{K_m + [S]} = k_{cat}[E]_0 \frac{[S]}{K_m + [S]} \tag{6.3}$$

The reaction rate increases with increasing substrate concentration, asymptotically approaching its maximum rate V_{max}, attained when all enzyme is bound to substrate. It also follows that $V_{max} = k_{cat}[E]_0$, where $[E]_0$ is the enzyme concentration. k_{cat}, the turnover number, is maximum number of substrate molecules converted to product per enzyme molecule per second.

The Michaelis constant K_m is the substrate concentration at which the reaction rate is at half-maximum and is an inverse measure of the substrate's affinity for the enzyme—as a small K_m indicates high affinity, meaning that the rate will approach V_{max} more quickly. The value of K_m is dependent on both the enzyme and the substrate, as well as conditions such as temperature and pH.

The model is used in a variety of biochemical situations other than enzyme–substrate interaction, including antigen–antibody binding, DNA–DNA hybridization, and protein–protein interaction. It can be used to characterize a generic biochemical reaction, in the same way that the Langmuir equation can be used to model generic adsorption of biomolecular species. When an empirical equation of this form is applied to microbial growth, it is referred to as the *Monod equation*.

Parameter values vary wildly between enzymes (Table 6.1). The constant k_{cat}/K_m is a measure of how efficiently an enzyme converts a substrate into product. It has a theoretical upper limit of 108–1,010/M s, enzymes working close to this, such as fumarase, are termed superefficient.

Michaelis–Menten kinetics have also been applied to a variety of spheres outside of biochemical reactions, including alveolar clearance of dusts, the richness of species pools, clearance of blood alcohol, the photosynthesis–irradiance relationship, and bacterial phage infection.

147

Table 6.1 Michaelis–Menten parameters for several common enzymes.

Enzyme	K_m (M)	K_{cat} (1/s)	K_{cat}/K_m (1/M s)
Chymotrypsin	1.5×10^{-2}	0.14	9.3
Pepsin	3.0×10^{-4}	0.50	1.7×10^3
Tyrosyl-tRNA synthetase	9.0×10^{-4}	7.6	8.4×10^3
Ribonuclease	7.9×10^{-3}	7.9×10^2	1.0×10^5
Carbonic anhydrase	2.6×10^{-2}	4.0×10^5	1.5×10^7
Fumarase	5.0×10^{-6}	8.0×10^2	1.6×10^8

Applying the law of mass action, which states that the rate of a reaction is proportional to the product of the concentrations of the reactants, gives a system of four nonlinear ordinary differential equations that define the rate of change of reactants with time t:

$$\frac{d[S]}{dt} = -k_f[E][S] + k_r[ES] \tag{6.4}$$

$$\frac{d[E]}{dt} = -k_f[E][S] + k_r[ES] + k_{cat}[ES] \tag{6.5}$$

$$\frac{d[ES]}{dt} = +k_f[E][S] - k_r[ES] - k_{cat}[ES] \tag{6.6}$$

$$\frac{d[P]}{dt} = +k_{cat}[ES] \tag{6.7}$$

In this mechanism, the enzyme E is a catalyst, which only facilitates the reaction, so its total concentration, free plus combined, $[E] + [ES] = [E]_0$ is a constant. This conservation law can also be obtained by adding Equations 6.5 and 6.6 leading to

$$\frac{d[E]}{dt} + \frac{d[ES]}{dt} = 0$$

indicating that all the enzyme present in the system is either free or bound to substrate.

In their original analysis, Michaelis and Menten assumed that the substrate is in instantaneous chemical equilibrium with the complex, and thus, $k_f[E][S] = k_r[ES]$. Combining this relationship with the enzyme conservation law, the concentration of complex is

$$[ES] = \frac{[E]_0[S]}{K_d + [S]} \tag{6.8}$$

where $K_d = k_r/k_f$ is the dissociation constant for the enzyme–substrate complex. Hence, the velocity of the reaction—the rate at which P is formed—is

$$v = \frac{d[P]}{dt} = \frac{V_{max}[S]}{K_d + [S]}$$

(6.9)

where $V_{max} = k_{cat}[E]_0$ is the maximum reaction velocity.

6.2.1 Quasi-Steady-State Approximation

An alternative analysis of the system was undertaken by British botanist G.E. Briggs and British geneticist J.B.S. Haldane in 1925. They assumed that the concentration of the intermediate complex does not change on the timescale of product formation—known as the *quasi-steady-state assumption* or *pseudo-steady-state hypothesis*. Mathematically, this assumption means $k_f[E][S] = k_r[ES] + k_{cat}[ES]$. Combining this relationship with the enzyme conservation law, the concentration of complex is

$$[ES] = \frac{[E]_0[S]}{K_m + [S]}$$

(6.10)

where:

$$K_m = \frac{k_r + k_{cat}}{k_f}$$

(6.11)

is known as the Michaelis constant. k_r, k_{cat}, and k_f are, respectively, the constants for substrate unbinding, conversion to product, and binding to the enzyme. Hence, the velocity of the reaction is

$$v = \frac{d[P]}{dt} = \frac{V_{max}[S]}{K_m + [S]}$$

(6.12)

6.2.1.1 Assumptions and Limitations

The first step in the derivation applies the law of mass action, which is reliant on free diffusion. However, in the environment of a living cell where there is a high concentration of proteins, the cytoplasm often behaves more like a gel than a liquid, limiting molecular movements and altering reaction rates. While the law of mass action can be valid in heterogeneous environments, it is more appropriate to model the cytoplasm as a fractal, in order to capture its limited-mobility kinetics.

The resulting reaction rates predicted by the two approaches are similar, with the only difference being that the equilibrium approximation defines the constant as K_d, while the quasi-steady-state approximation uses K_m. However, each approach is founded upon a different assumption. The Michaelis–Menten equilibrium analysis is valid if the substrate reaches equilibrium on a much faster timescale than the product is formed or, more precisely, that

$$\epsilon_d = \frac{k_{cat}}{k_r} \ll 1 \tag{6.13}$$

By contrast, the Briggs–Haldane quasi-steady-state analysis is valid if

$$\epsilon_m = \frac{[E]_0}{[S]_0 + K_m} \ll 1 \tag{6.14}$$

Thus, it holds if the enzyme concentration is much less than the substrate concentration. Even if this is not satisfied, the approximation is valid if K_m is large.

In both the Michaelis–Menten and Briggs–Haldane analyses, the quality of the approximation improves as decreases. However, in model building, Michaelis–Menten kinetics are often invoked without regard to the underlying assumptions.

It is also important to remember that, while irreversibility is a necessary simplification in order to yield a tractable analytic solution, in the general case product formation is not in fact irreversible. The enzyme reaction is more correctly described as

$$E + S \underset{k_{r1}}{\overset{k_{f1}}{\rightleftarrows}} ES \underset{k_{r2}}{\overset{k_{f2}}{\rightleftarrows}} E + P \tag{6.15}$$

In general, the assumption of irreversibility is a good one in situations where one of the below is true:

1. The concentration of substrate(s) is very much larger than the concentration of products:

$$[S] \gg [P]$$

   This is true under standard in vitro assay conditions and is true for many in vivo biological reactions, particularly where the product is continually removed by a subsequent reaction.
2. The energy released in the reaction is very large, that is,

$$\Delta G \ll 0$$

In situations where neither of these two conditions hold (i.e., the reaction is low energy and a substantial pool of product[s] exists), the Michaelis–Menten equation breaks down, and more complex modeling approaches explicitly taking the forward and reverse reactions into account must be taken to understand the enzyme biology.

6.2.2 Determination of Constants

The typical method for determining the constants V_{max} and K_m involves running a series of enzyme assays at varying substrate concentrations [S] and measuring the initial reaction rate. *Initial* here is taken to mean that the reaction rate is measured after a relatively short time period, during which it is assumed that the enzyme–substrate complex has formed, but that the substrate concentration held approximately constant, and so the equilibrium or quasi-steady-state approximation remains valid. By plotting reaction rate against concentration, and using nonlinear regression of the Michaelis–Menten equation, the parameters may be obtained.

Before computing facilities to perform nonlinear regression became available, graphical methods involving linearization of the equation were used. A number of these were proposed, including the Eadie–Hofstee diagram, Hanes–Woolf plot, and Lineweaver–Burk plot; of these, the Hanes–Woolf plot is the most accurate. However, while useful for visualization, all three methods distort the error structure of the data and are inferior to nonlinear regression. Nonetheless, their use can still be found in modern literature, and a thorough evaluation of the three techniques to linearize the Michaelis–Menten equation is detailed in Section 6.3.

In 1997, Santiago Schnell and Claudio Mendoza derived a closed form solution for the time course kinetics analysis of the Michaelis–Menten kinetics. The solution, known as the *Schnell–Mendoza equation*, has the form

$$\frac{[S]}{K_m} = W\left[\frac{[S]_0}{K_m} \cdot \exp\left(\frac{[S]_0}{K_m} - \frac{V_{max}}{K_m}t\right)\right] \tag{6.16}$$

where W is the Lambert-W function. It has been used to estimate V_{max} and K_m from time course data.

6.3 MICHAELIS–MENTEN KINETICS WITH INHIBITION

Several mechanisms can lead to inhibition of enzyme function, resulting in alteration of V_m, K_m, or both. Competitive inhibition is a form of enzyme inhibition where binding of the inhibitor to the active site on the enzyme prevents binding of the substrate and vice versa.

Figure 6.2 provides a diagram of the three common types of inhibition. The enzyme is depicted in green, the substrate in blue, the product in purple, and the various possible inhibitors in red. In competitive inhibition, the inhibitor competes with the substrate to bind the enzyme. In uncompetitive inhibition, the enzyme binding the substrate allows the inhibitor to bind and the inhibitor blocks the conversion of the substrate to products. Finally, in noncompetitive inhibition the inhibitor does not depend in any way on substrate binding, but blocks conversion to products when the inhibitor is bound to the enzyme.

Most competitive inhibitors function by binding reversibly to the active site of the enzyme. As a result, many sources state that it is the defining feature of competitive

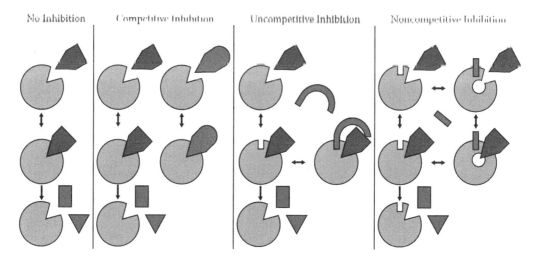

No Inhibition   Competitive Inhibition   Uncompetitive Inhibition   Noncompetitive Inhibition

Figure 6.2 Diagram of the three common types of inhibition.

inhibitors. This, however, is a misleading oversimplification, as there are many possible mechanisms by which an enzyme may bind either the inhibitor or the substrate but never both at the same time. For example, allosteric inhibitors may display competitive, non-competitive, or competitive inhibition.

In competitive inhibition, at any given moment, the enzyme may be bound to the inhibitor, the substrate, or neither, but it cannot bind both at the same time. In virtually every case, competitive inhibitors bind in the same binding site as the substrate, but same-site binding is not a requirement. A competitive inhibitor could bind to an allosteric site of the free enzyme and prevent substrate binding, as long as it does not bind to the allosteric site when the substrate is bound. In competitive inhibition, the maximum velocity (V_{max}) of the reaction is unchanged, while the apparent affinity of the substrate to the binding site is decreased (the K_d dissociation constant is apparently increased). The change in K_{m} (Michaelis–Menten constant) is parallel to the alteration in K_d. Any given competitive inhibitor concentration can be overcome by increasing the substrate concentration in which case the substrate will outcompete the inhibitor in binding to the enzyme. Competitive inhibition increases the apparent value of the Michaelis–Menten constant, $K_{\mathrm{m}}^{\mathrm{app}}$, such that rate of reaction, v, is given by

$$v = \frac{V_{\mathrm{max}}[S]}{K_{\mathrm{m}}^{\mathrm{app}} + [S]} \qquad (6.17)$$

where:
$K_{\mathrm{m}}^{\mathrm{app}} = K_{\mathrm{m}}\left[1 + ([I]/K_i)\right]$
K_i is the inhibitor's dissociation constant
$[I]$ is the inhibitor concentration

V_{max} remains the same because the presence of the inhibitor can be overcome by higher substrate concentrations. K_m^{app}, the substrate concentration that is needed to reach $V_{max}/2$, increases with the presence of a competitive inhibitor. This is because the concentration of substrate needed to reach V_{max} with an inhibitor is greater than the concentration of substrate needed to reach V_{max} without an inhibitor.

In the simplest case of a single-substrate enzyme obeying Michaelis–Menten kinetics, the typical scheme

$$E + S \underset{k_{-1}}{\overset{k_1}{\rightleftarrows}} ES \overset{k_2}{\longrightarrow} E + P \tag{6.18}$$

is modified to include binding of the inhibitor to the free enzyme:

$$EI + S \underset{k_3}{\overset{k_{-3}}{\rightleftarrows}} E + S + I \underset{k_{-1}}{\overset{k_1}{\rightleftarrows}} ES + I \overset{k_2}{\longrightarrow} E + P + I \tag{6.19}$$

Note that the inhibitor does not bind to the ES complex and the substrate does not bind to the EI complex. It is generally assumed that this behavior is indicative of both compounds binding at the same site, but that is not strictly necessary. As with the derivation of the Michaelis–Menten equation, assume that the system is at steady state, that is, the concentration of each of the enzyme species is not changing.

$$\frac{d[E]}{dt} = \frac{d[ES]}{dt} = \frac{d[EI]}{dt} = 0 \tag{6.20}$$

Furthermore, the known total enzyme concentration is $[E]_0 = [E] + [ES] + [EI]$, and the velocity is measured under conditions in which the substrate and inhibitor concentrations do not change substantially and an insignificant amount of product has accumulated.

We can therefore set up a system of equations.

$$[E]_0 = [E] + [ES] + [EI] \tag{6.21}$$

$$\frac{d[E]}{dt} = 0 = -k_1[E][S] + k_{-1}[ES] + k_2[ES] - k_3[E][I] + k_{-3}[EI] \tag{6.22}$$

$$\frac{d[ES]}{dt} = 0 = k_1[E][S] - k_{-1}[ES] - k_2[ES] \tag{6.23}$$

$$\frac{d[EI]}{dt} = 0 = k_3[E][I] - k_{-3}[EI] \tag{6.24}$$

where $[S]$, $[I]$, and $[E]_0$ are known. The initial velocity is defined as $V_0 = d[P]/dt = k_2[ES]$, so we need to define the unknown $[ES]$ in terms of the knowns $[S]$, $[I]$, and $[E]_0$.

153

From Equation 6.23, we can define E in terms of ES by rearranging to

$$k_1[E][S] = (k_{-1} + k_2)[ES] \tag{6.25}$$

Dividing by $k_1[S]$ gives

$$[E] = \frac{(k_{-1} + k_2)[ES]}{k_1[S]} \tag{6.26}$$

As in the derivation of the Michaelis–Menten equation, the term $(k_{-1} + k_2)/k_1$ can be replaced by the macroscopic rate constant K_m:

$$[E] = \frac{K_m[ES]}{[S]} \tag{6.27}$$

Substituting Equation 6.27 into Equation 6.24, we have

$$0 = \frac{k_3[I]K_m[ES]}{[S]} - k_{-3}[EI] \tag{6.28}$$

Rearranging, we find that

$$[EI] = \frac{K_m k_3[I][ES]}{k_{-3}[S]} \tag{6.29}$$

At this point, we can define the dissociation constant for the inhibitor as $K_i = k_{-3}/k_3$, giving

$$[EI] = \frac{K_m[I][ES]}{K_i[S]} \tag{6.30}$$

At this point, substitute Equations 6.27 and 6.30 into Equation 6.21:

$$[E]_0 = \frac{K_m[ES]}{[S]} + [ES] + \frac{K_m[I][ES]}{K_i[S]} \tag{6.31}$$

Rearranging to solve for ES, we find

$$[E]_0 = [ES]\left(\frac{K_m}{[S]} + 1 + \frac{K_m[I]}{K_i[S]} \right) = [ES]\frac{K_m K_i + K_i[S] + K_m[I]}{K_i[S]} \tag{6.32}$$

$$[ES] = \frac{K_i [S][E]_0}{K_m K_i + K_i [S] + K_m [I]} \tag{6.33}$$

Returning to our expression for v, we now have

$$v = k_2 [S] = \frac{k_2 K_i [S][E]_0}{K_m K_i + K_i [S] + K_m [I]} = \frac{k_2 [S][E]_0}{K_m + [S] + K_m ([I]/K_i)} \tag{6.34}$$

Since the velocity is maximal when all the enzyme is bound as the enzyme–substrate complex, $V_{max} = k_2[E]_0$. Replacing and combining terms finally yields the conventional form:

$$v = \frac{V_{max} [S]}{K_m \left[1 + ([I]/K_i) \right] + [S]} \tag{6.35}$$

Analysis of the solution for competitive inhibition reveals that there is a net decrease on the reaction rate due to an increase in K_m, which indicates more substrate is required to reach the half-maximal velocity of the reaction.

Other common types of inhibition are the confusingly named, uncompetitive inhibition and non-competitive inhibition. With uncompetitive inhibition, the inhibitor binds [ES] preventing the conversion of the substrate to product. The reaction scheme for uncompetitive inhibition is

$$E + S \xrightleftharpoons[k_{-1}]{k_1} \quad ES \xrightarrow{k_2} \quad E + P$$
$$+$$
$$I \tag{6.36}$$
$$k_3 \updownarrow k_{-3}$$
$$ESI$$

This scheme can be solved following a similar process detailed for competitive inhibition. The resulting expression for the velocity, v, with uncompetitive inhibition is

$$v = \frac{\left\{ V_{max} / \left[1 + ([I]/K_i) \right] \right\}[S]}{\left\{ K_m / \left[1 + ([I]/K_i) \right] \right\} + [S]} \quad \text{or} \quad v = \frac{V_{max}^{app} [S]}{K_m^{app} + [S]} \tag{6.37}$$

Where both V_{max} and K_m are corrected to apparent forms by dividing each by $\left(1 + [I]/K_i \right)$, thus $V_{max}^{app} = V_{max} / \left(1 + [I]/K_i \right)$ and $K_m^{app} = K_m / \left(1 + [I]/K_i \right)$. If one analyzes the resulting equation a curious observation arises. Intuitively, inhibition would suggest that the overall reaction slows down; however, dividing K_m by a number larger than 1 would result in a decreased K_m and a net increase in the velocity—this decrease indicates the formation of the intermediate [ES] is more favorable than the uninhibited case. Examination of the reaction makes clear that since there is an equilibrium relationship between [ES] and [ESI] and since the total amount of enzyme bound to substrate is the sum of [ES] and [ESI], then because of Le Chatelier's principle there can be more substrate bound to enzyme than the uninhibited case. However, ultimately, the velocity does go down since V_{max} in the numerator is decreased by the same factor. Since the inhibition present in the denominator is added to the [S] and the inhibition in the numerator is multiplied by [S], the result is the decrease in V_{max} dominates the overall reaction slowing the velocity.

Noncompetitive inhibition prevents the conversion of the [S] to product, but does not prevent the binding of the enzyme with the substrate. The reaction scheme for noncompetitive inhibition is

$$
\begin{array}{ccccc}
E + S & \xleftrightarrow[k_{-1}]{k_1} & ES & \xrightarrow{k_2} & E + P \\
+ & & + & & \\
I & & 1 & & \\
k_3 \updownarrow k_{-3} & & k_3 \updownarrow k_{-3} & & \\
EI + S & & ESI & &
\end{array}
\tag{6.38}
$$

Again, solving in a method similar to that detailed for competitive inhibition results in

$$
v = \frac{\left[V_{max}/\left(1+[I]/K\right)\right][S]}{K_m + [S]} \quad \text{or} \quad v = \frac{V_{max}^{app}[S]}{K_m + [S]}
\tag{6.39}
$$

Now only V_{max} is corrected to an apparent form by dividing by $1+[I]/K_i$, thus $V_{max}^{app} = V_{max}/\left(1+[I]/K_i\right)$. It is clear that the net result of the reaction is a decrease in rate to a decrease in the maximal velocity. Le Chatelier's principle does not provide the same benefit as in an uncompetitive reaction because both the free and bound enzyme exist in a similar equilibrium balance with the inhibitor.

Today, computers are more than capable of identifying the key rate parameters for an enzymatic reaction following Michaelis–Menten kinetics; however, that was not always the case. Previously, the easiest method to both find V_{max} and K_m was to linearize the Michaelis–Menten equation. There are three techniques for linearizing; the first is by taking the reciprocal of both the left and right side of the equation:

$$
\frac{1}{v} = \frac{K_m + [S]}{V_{max}[S]} = \frac{K_m}{V_{max}} \cdot \frac{1}{[S]} + \frac{1}{V_{max}}
\tag{6.40}
$$

Plotting $(1/v)$ versus $(1/[S])$ results in a line with slope, K_m/V_{max}, a y-intercept of $1/V_{max}$ and a x-intercept of $-1/K_m$. Hans Lineweaver and Dean Burk first detailed this linearization strategy in 1934. The resulting plot is referred to as a *Lineweaver–Burk plot*. It is not the best method for determining rate constants from experimental data, but was certainly one of the first. It is also a nice graphical representation of the different types of inhibition. Figure 6.3 demonstrates a traditional *V* versus [S] plot and Lineweaver–Burk plots for each of the three inhibition types discussed.

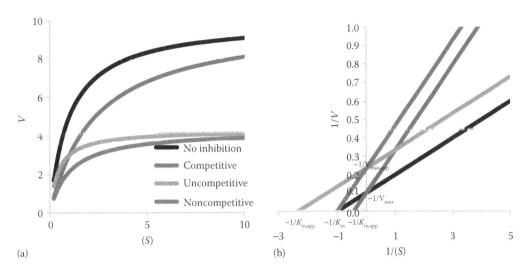

Figure 6.3 *V* versus [*S*] plot for the three types of inhibition (a) and a Lineweaver–Burk plot of the same three types of inhibition (b).

The Lineweaver–Burk plots provide a rapid visual identification of whether the inhibition occurring is competitive, uncompetitive, or non-competitive. Competitive inhibition increases the slope of the line and increases the *x*-intercept. Uncompetitive inhibition maintains the same slope, decreases the *x*-intercept, and increases the *y*-intercept. Finally, non-competitive inhibition increases the slope and increases the *y*-intercept. The problem with the Lineweaver–Burk linearization is that because it is a double reciprocal, low concentrations of [*S*] affect the resulting slope more than high concentrations. Accurate measurements of initial velocities at low [*S*] concentrations are more prone to error, which readily propagate to the kinetic constants determined for the reaction being investigated. A solution is through altered linearization strategies. The first of which, attributed to both Barnet Woolf and Charles Samuel Hanes, independent of one another, is the Hanes–Woolf linearization. The Hanes–Woolf linearization is accomplished as follows:

$$v = \frac{V_{\max}[S]}{K_{\mathrm{m}} + [S]}$$

(6.41)

is both inverted and multiplied through by [*S*] to yield

$$\frac{[S]}{v} = \frac{K_{\mathrm{m}} + [S]}{V_{\max}} \quad \text{or} \quad \frac{[S]}{v} = \frac{1}{V_{\max}}[S] + \frac{K_{\mathrm{m}}}{V_{\max}}$$

(6.42)

Plotting [*S*]/*v* versus [*S*], this linearization demonstrates a *x*-intercept equal to $-K_{\mathrm{m}}$ and a slope of $1/V_{\max}$. Because it does not depend on the inverse of [*S*], it produces much more accurate results than the Lineweaver–Burk linearization. The key challenge with Hanes–Woolf linearization is that both sides are dependent on [*S*]. The final linearization technique

157

of the Michaelis–Menten is the Eadie–Hofstee linearization and it is quite similar to the Hanes–Woolf linearization. The Eadie–Hofstee linearization is accomplished as follows:

$$v = \frac{V_{max}[S]}{K_m + [S]} \tag{6.43}$$

is both inverted and multiplied through by V_{max} to yield

$$\frac{V_{max}}{v} = \frac{K_m + [S]}{[S]} = \frac{K_m}{[S]} + 1 \tag{6.44}$$

then multiplied through by v and rearranged to yield

$$V_{max} = \frac{v K_m}{[S]} + v \quad \text{or} \quad v = -K_m \frac{v}{[S]} + V_{max} \tag{6.45}$$

Plotting v versus $v/[S]$, this linearization demonstrates a y-intercept of V_{max} and a slope of $-K_m$. Similar to the Hanes–Woolf linearization, the Eadie–Hofstee linearization again results in both y and x being dependent on the same variable, v; however, the Eadie–Hofstee linearization proves to be the most robust approach when there is noise present in v and $[S]$. In summary, the best method with reasonable data is the Hanes–Woolf linearization. The best when the data are noisy is Eadie–Hofstee, and the Lineweaver–Burk linearization is worse than either of the other two under nearly every scenario.

A fourth type of inhibition can occur in when additional substrate binds the enzyme–substrate complex and slows the conversion of the bound substrate to product. A reaction scheme depicting substrate inhibition is

$$
E + S \underset{k_{-1}}{\overset{k_1}{\longleftrightarrow}} \quad ES \quad \overset{k_2}{\longrightarrow} \quad E + P
$$
$$
+
$$
$$
S \tag{6.46}
$$
$$
k_3 \updownarrow k_{-3}
$$
$$
SES
$$

While the reaction scheme for substrate inhibition may look similar to that of uncompetitive inhibition, the resulting solution is quite different owing to the presence of $[S]$ at multiple points in the reaction. We can solve for the enzymatic reaction velocity under the influence of substrate inhibition as follows:

$$v = k_2[ES] \tag{6.47}$$

$$[E]_0 = [E] + [ES] + [SES] \tag{6.48}$$

Assuming equilibrium for each of the reversible reactions:

$$k_1[E][S] = k_{-1}[ES] \text{ and } k_3[ES][S] = k_{-3}[SES] \tag{6.49}$$

$$[ES] = \frac{[E][S]}{k_{-1}/k_1} = \frac{[E][S]}{K_m} \text{ and } [SES] = \frac{[ES][S]}{k_{-3}/k_3} = \frac{[ES][S]}{K_{si}} \tag{6.50}$$

Plugging back into the mass balance and velocity equations results in the following solution for substrate inhibition:

$$v = \frac{V_{max}[S]}{K_m + [S] + \left([S]^2/K_{si}\right)} \tag{6.51}$$

Examining the above we can see that when the concentration of the substrate is low relative to K_{si}, the solution simplifies to the typical Michaelis–Menten equation. The $[S]^2$ term creates challenges for linearizing a reaction undergoing substrate inhibition. Not surprisingly, neither a v versus $[S]$ nor Lineweaver–Burk plot looks familiar as presented by Figure 6.4. A further examination of the solution for v in the presence of substrate inhibition reveals that there is a maximal reaction velocity at some concentrate, $[S]$, which we can find by solving for the case when $dv/d[S] = 0$:

$$\frac{dv}{d[S]} = -\frac{K_{si}V_{max}\left([S]^2 - K_{si}K_m\right)}{\left([S]^2 + K_{si}[S] + K_{si}K_m\right)^2} = 0 \tag{6.52}$$

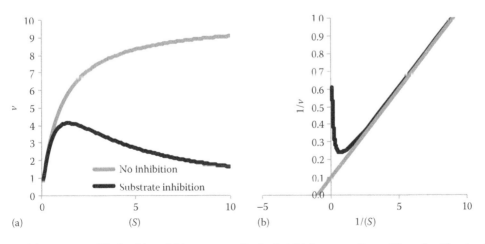

Figure 6.4 v versus $[S]$ plot (a) and Lineweaver–Burk plot (b) for a reaction with and without substrate inhibition.

By inspection it is clear there is a solution when the numerator is equal to 0, which indicates that

$$\left([S]^2 - K_{si}K_m\right) = 0 \text{ or } [S] = \sqrt{K_{si}K_m} \tag{6.53}$$

6.4 pH AND TRANSPORT LIMITATIONS

One final modifier of enzymatic reaction velocities that will be discussed in this chapter is the influence of pH. The general scheme for a reaction in the presence or absence of additional protons can be represented as

$$
\begin{array}{l}
E^- + H^+ \\[4pt]
\updownarrow K_b \\[4pt]
E + S \quad \xleftrightarrow[k_{-1}]{k_1} \quad ES \quad \xrightarrow{k_2} \quad E + P \\[4pt]
+ \\[4pt]
H^+ \\[4pt]
\updownarrow K_a \\[4pt]
EH^+
\end{array}
\tag{6.54}
$$

The above can be solved similar to previous analyses to yield

$$v = \frac{V_{max}[S]}{K_m\left[1 + \left(K_b/[H^+]\right) + \left([H^+]/K_a\right)\right] + [S]} \tag{6.55}$$

We can then establish an apparent K_m and set the derivative of the apparent K_m to 0 to find the optimal pH for the reaction:

$$K_m^{app} = K_m\left(1 + \frac{K_b}{[H^+]} + \frac{[H^+]}{K_a}\right) \text{ and } \frac{dK_m^{app}}{d[H^+]} = \frac{K_m}{K_a} - \frac{K_mK_b}{[H^+]^2} = 0 \tag{6.56}$$

Solving for $[H^+]$ yields

$$[H^+] = K_aK_b \tag{6.57}$$

Thus, the reaction proceeds at a maximal velocity when the pH is between the pK_a and pK_b.

Inhibition is not the only influence that can affect the resulting rate of a reaction. Often enzymes are immobilized onto a surface, for example, a receptor on a cell membrane. In these cases, the reaction is a balance between mass transport and the enzyme reaction kinetics. A simple analysis for mass transfer is to examine the two velocities in the system, the reaction velocity and transport velocity. Since the reaction is occurring on a plane, these velocities, v^*, are represented as [M]*length*s^{-1} where the length for reaction, δ, is the distance from the surface that the immobilized enzymes can bind substrate. The v^* for the reaction and mass transport would then be

$$\text{Reaction velocity}: \quad v^* = \frac{V_{max}^* [S_{surface}]}{K_m + [S_{surface}]} \tag{6.58}$$

$$\text{Transport velocity (flux)}: \quad J = k_L \left([S_{bulk}] - [S_{surface}] \right) \tag{6.59}$$

where:
   k_L is the liquid mass transfer coefficient
   $[S_{bulk}]$ is the bulk fluid [S] concentration
   $[S_{surface}]$ is the [S] concentration at the surface that can bind the tethered or bound
       enzyme

Under steady-state conditions, the reaction velocity is equal to the transport velocity. Often times, either the reaction or the transport limits the overall system. We can use a Damkhöler number, a dimensionless number, to compare the reaction rate to the transport rate and quickly identify whether either are limiting.

$$Da = \frac{\text{maximum reaction rate}}{\text{maximum transport rate}} = \frac{V_{max}^*}{k_L [S_{bulk}]} \tag{6.60}$$

If Da >> 1, then the diffusive transport limits the reaction; likewise, if Da << 1, then the reaction limits. Under reaction limiting conditions, the velocity, v^*, is simply $V_{max}^* [S_{bulk}]/K_m^{app} + [S_{bulk}]$, where

$$K_m^{app} = K_m \left[1 + \frac{V_{max}^*}{k_L \left([S_{bulk}] + K_m \right)} \right] \tag{6.61}$$

Under transport-limiting conditions, the reaction velocity, v^*, is simply $k_L [S_{bulk}]$.

6.5 OTHER ENZYME KINETICS

Many regulatory enzymes do not follow typical Michaelis–Menten kinetics. These enzymes undergo a process referred to as *allosteric regulation*. Allosteric regulation demonstrates a property referred to as *cooperativity*. Cooperativity can be either positive or negative. Positive cooperativity results in the substrate binding the enzyme more rapidly when the enzyme is already bound to substrate. Negative cooperativity results in the substrate binding the enzyme less rapidly when the enzyme is already bound to substrate. Take the following reaction:

$$E + nS \quad \underset{k_{-1}}{\overset{k_1}{\longleftrightarrow}} \quad ES \quad \overset{k_2}{\longrightarrow} \quad E + P \tag{6.62}$$

We can then solve the above similar to the process used in deriving the Michaelis–Menten equations and find that

$$v = \frac{V_{max}[S]^n}{K_d + [S]^n} \tag{6.63}$$

This equation is referred to as the *Hill equation* because it was initially described by Archibald Hill in 1910 in reference to the sigmoidal nature that O_2 bound hemoglobin. n is the Hill coefficient and K_d describes the dissociation of the substrate from the complex; however, since more than one substrate can bind, K_d should not be mistaken for K_m—or a substrate concentration that produces 1/2 the maximal velocity. To identify an equivalent term to K_m, K_h, in the Hill equation, we can solve for [S] at the 1/2 maximal velocity:

$$\frac{V_{max}}{2} = \frac{V_{max}[S]^n}{K_d + [S]^n} \quad \text{rearranging } [S] = K_d^{1/n} = K_h \quad \text{thus} \quad K_d = K_h^n \tag{6.64}$$

Inserting this term into the original equation provides a model of how velocity is affected by cooperativity.

$$v = \frac{V_{max}[S]^n}{K_h{}^n + [S]^n} \tag{6.65}$$

Hill coefficients higher than 1 result in positive cooperativity, whereas Hill coefficients less than 1 result in negative cooperativity, and there is a theoretical lower limit of 0 for the Hill coefficient. When the Hill coefficient is equal to 1, the kinetics of the system are equivalent to Michaelis–Menten kinetics and K_h is equivalent to K_m. Figure 6.5 provides a graphical representation of positive and negative cooperativity. Positive cooperativity results in a sigmoidal curve and negative cooperativity results in a hyperbolic curve.

6.6 PROKARYOTIC AND EUKARYOTIC GROWTH MODELS

Cell growth is as important, or nearly as important, to many applications of bioprocess engineering as is identifying the enzymatic reactions that ultimately govern that cell growth. Cell growth occurs through the process of mitosis. To begin, let us examine a simple example of unrestricted cell growth. With unrestricted cell growth, a single mother cell divides to form two daughter cells and the general reaction is

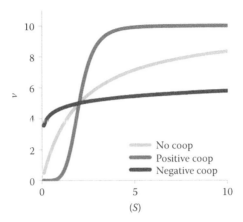

Figure 6.5 Graphical depiction of positive, negative, and no cooperativity as described by the Hill equation. Positive cooperativity yields an S shaped or sigmoidal curve, whereas negative and no cooperativity yield hyperbolic relationships. The case with no cooperativity is the same as would be determined by the Michaelis–Menten equation.

$$\text{Cell} \xrightarrow{\mu} \text{cell} + \text{cell}$$

where μ corresponds to the growth rate. This reaction can be solved similar to the first-order reactions detailed in Chapter 5. First, we will establish a quantity N_{cell} corresponding to the number of cells present. Next, we determine the rate law and integrate:

$$\frac{dN_{cell}}{dt} = \mu N_{cell} \text{ integrated to yield } N_{cell} = N_{cell0}e^{\mu t} \tag{6.66}$$

Similar to the determination of half-life with rate equations in Chapter 5, the doubling time is a useful quantity when describing cell growth and can be found by solving for the time required for the population to double in size:

$$2N_{cell0} = N_{cell0}e^{\mu t_d} \text{ rearranging } t_d = \frac{\ln(2)}{\mu} \tag{6.67}$$

The doubling time for a population of cells varies in a significant amount. Small prokaryotes can double in less than an hour, whereas eukaryotic cells undergoing rapid cell growth rarely have population doubling times faster than 24 h. Examining the cell growth equation derived is disconcerting in that it does not have any control over that cell growth. Instead the population will seemingly grow unrestricted forever. In reality, this is not the case. Prokaryotic, and to an extent eukaryotic, cell growth typically demonstrates four phases:

1. *Lag phase*: When first placed in a new environment, the prokaryotic cells initially adapt to the new environment prior to beginning replication. The lag phase is poorly understood, but it is thought that during this time the prokaryotes

163

begin to upregulate the necessary genes to process the nutrients present in the environment and cell division proteins if they were previously in a stationary phase.

2. *Exponential phase*: This phase corresponds to the growth equation derived above. The cells have transcribed the necessary proteins to convert the nutrients in the system into energy and likewise the necessary proteins for replication. In this phase, there are no limitations on growth. It is often referred to as the *log phase*, because if plotted on a logarithmic axis the growth demonstrates a line with a slope equal to the specific growth rate μ.

3. *Stationary phase*: Eventually unrestricted cell growth results in the presence of some growth restricting factor. This could be due to exhaustion or near exhaustion of key nutrients or the production of a growth arresting molecule, which is key to quorum sensing and often results in a concerted shift in behavior of the bacteria away from proliferation to activities such as producing a biofilm. If the stationary phase is due only to the lack of nutrients, death will begin to occur and the surviving cells will continue to grow by feeding on the newly freed nutrients from the dead cells. The process is referred to as *cryptic growth*.

4. *Death phase*: Either the lack of nutrients or the generation of a hostile environment, which could occur if the metabolism of the bacteria results in a decrease in the pH, both lead to death of the prokaryotes.

The simple model for cell growth did not account for the majority of prokaryotic growth phases. To begin to address the shortcomings in the earlier model, we first examine death. Similar to unrestricted cell growth, cell death is also a first-order reaction of the form:

$$\frac{dN_{cell}}{dt} = -k_D N_{cell} \tag{6.68}$$

Combining the equations for growth and death yields

$$\frac{dN_{cell}}{dt} = \mu N_{cell} - k_D N_{cell} \tag{6.69}$$

which is easily integrated to yield

$$N_{cell} = N_{cell0} e^{(\mu - k_D)t} \tag{6.70}$$

However, as before, we have an equation that describes unrestricted cell growth. The only difference is the growth rate is now decreased by the death rate. To fully understand prokaryotic growth, we need to find a function that determines the growth rate, μ, as a function of the environment. The most straightforward environmental factor affecting growth is food. If we make the assumption that there is essentially one key limiting nutrient, [S], that is processed by enzyme, [E], then we can establish a simple relationship for the growth rate, μ, as a function of substrate concentration:

$$\mu = \frac{\mu_{max}[S]}{K_s + [S]} \qquad (6.71)$$

This equation is the Monod equation, which is named after Jacques Monod who derived it as a method to describe microbial growth. Unlike the Michaelis–Menten equation, which looks quite similar, the Monod equation is empirical—derived because it fits the data, whereas Michaelis–Menten equation was based on enzyme theory μ_{max} in the Monod equation refers to the unrestricted growth rate of the cells and K_s is the half-velocity constant. Combining the Monod equation with the growth equation that includes death and a linear relationship between the substrate consumption and cell number ($[S] = [S]_0 - k_c N_{cell} t$, where k_c is the substrate consumption rate constant) results in the relationship demonstrating a peak cell number at which point the lack of nutrients leads to the death of the cell population (Figure 6.6).

Despite the inclusion of the Monod equation, the resulting relationship does not provide the plateau expected. This is because the plateau, stationary phase, requires some information about the population to serve as feedback. In prokaryotes and eukaryotes, this can be termed *quorum sensing*. Often with eukaryotes in culture, the term *confluency* is used in lieu of quorum sensing. Confluency simply indicates what percent of the available surface area, if the cells are growing in a dish, or volume, if the cells are growing in 3D space, if occupied with cells. To account for the ability of cells to perceive other cells as the space between them diminishes, we need to include a term in our growth equation to account for the population relative to the max population. The most straightforward manner of doing this is to modify the maximum growth rate, μ_{max}, to

$$\mu_{max}^{app} = \mu_{max}\left(1 - \frac{N}{N_{max}}\right) \qquad (6.72)$$

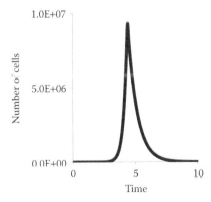

Figure 6.6 Using the simple cell growth equation and incorporating the Monod equation to describe the growth rate with the inclusion of a finite amount of substrate results in a relationship that demonstrates a peak in the number of cells followed by the gradual decline in the population.

where N_{max} represents the total number of cells possible in the space provided. The relationship between N and N_{max} can be substituted for volume, area, or mass as appropriate. By correcting the cell growth equation derived previously with a term for quorum sensing/confluency, we derive the following:

$$N_{cell} = N_{cell0}e^{\left(\{\mu_{max}[1-(N_{cell}/N_{cell,max})][S]\}/K_s+[S]-k_D\right)t}$$ (6.73)

At this point, the cell growth equation has become cumbersome and the easiest method of analysis is to approximate the derivative such that

$$N_{cell,t+\Delta t} = N_{cell,t} + \frac{dN_{cell,t}}{dt} \cdot \Delta t$$ (6.74)

$$\frac{dN_{cell}}{dt} = \mu_{max}N_{cell}\frac{\left[1-\left(N_{cell}/N_{cell,\ max}\right)\right][S]}{K_s+[S]} - k_DN_{cell}$$ (6.75)

Similar to before, approximating this equation and including a consumption term for the substrate results in Figure 6.7.

With a few simple approximations and insertion of appropriate equations for the growth rate and substrate consumption, we have derived a model that represents quite accurately the growth behavior of prokaryotic and eukaryotic cells in culture. The model demonstrates an exponential growth phase, a stationary phase, and a death phase. The model appears to include a lag phase; however, this is simply an artifact from beginning with only a single cell. The model projected in Figure 6.7 was generated with an N_{max} of 1.0×10^7; however, the max that the cells reached was only 9.0×10^6. This is due to the incorporation of the death term with quorum sensing. If we neglect the substrate consumption and focus only on the growth rate, death rate, and quorum sensing terms, we see that at steady state

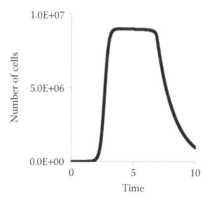

Figure 6.7 Simple cell growth model accounting for growth as a function of substrate, death, quorum sensing, and substrate consumption.

$$\frac{dN_{cell}}{dt} = \mu_{max}N_{cell}\left(1 - \frac{N_{cell}}{N_{cell,max}}\right) - k_D N_{cell} = 0 \tag{6.76}$$

$$\mu_{max}\left(1 - \frac{N_{cell}}{N_{cell,max}}\right) = k_D \tag{6.77}$$

Solving for the cell number at steady state yields

$$\frac{N_{cell}}{N_{cell,max}} = 1 - \frac{k_D}{\mu_{max}} \tag{6.78}$$

The example presented above in Figure 6.7 had a death rate that was 10% the growth rate, which generates a steady-state value equal to 90% $N_{cell,max}$ or 9.0×10^6.

6.7 ADVANCED PROKARYOTIC AND EUKARYOTIC GROWTH MODELS

Returning the equation relating the growth rate with quorum sensing that was included in Section 6.6, we evaluate the relationship between the growth rate and cell number. To simplify, we will make each parameters dimensionless by dividing by their respective maximum values such that

$$\frac{\mu}{\mu_{max}} = 1 - \frac{N_{cell}}{N_{cell,max}} \tag{6.79}$$

Inspection of the above equation reveals a linear relationship. Logically, this does not make sense for most scenarios. Take for instance a large volume of cell growth media that contains two prokaryotic cells. The vast volume and distance between the prokaryotic cells removes the ability for each cell to *perceive* the other through quorum sensing, and as such, the growth rate should remain μ_{max}. A similar problem arises in cell culture dishes, where low values of confluency do not generate the cell-to-cell contacts required to slow the growth rate, but the simple model above would slow the growth rate as soon as a single cell occupied a non-zero area of the culture dish. Kelly Frame and Wei-Shou Hu tackled this issue of confluency in a 1987 article titled "A model for density-dependent growth of anchorage-dependent mammalian cells," which was published in *Biotechnology and Bioengineering*. In their analysis, Frame and Hu determined the following model for controlling growth rate dependent on the confluency in the dish:

$$\mu = \mu_{max}\left\{1 - e^{\left[-C\left(N_{cell,max} - N_{cell}\right)/N_{cell}\right]}\right\} \tag{6.80}$$

The model derived by Frame and Hu provides a constant, C, that can be altered to fit the response of the data to the growth characteristic of multiple populations of cells. Figure 6.8 presents the dimensionless relationship detailing the confluency (N/N_{max}) in a dish and

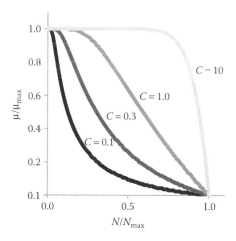

Figure 6.8   Revised model derived by Frame and Hu, relating growth rate to the confluency for anchorage-dependent mammalian cells.

the growth rate for a variety of values for the constant, C. Frame and Hu went on to determine the value for the constant, C, for several cell lines in culture. Their findings demonstrated that mammalian cells in culture are wildly divergent in how the growth rate varies with confluency. Values obtained spanned from just 0.19, indicating a very rapid drop in growth rate with cell growth, for bovine vascular endothelial cells grown in the presence of HDL-transferrin-FGF; to 22, indicating little change in growth rate with cell growth, for the same bovine vascular endothelial cells grown on extracellular matrix-coated dishes without HDL-transferrin-FGF supplementation.

Similar to our approximation of the growth rate in the presence of quorum sensing and confluency, the Monod equation often proves insufficient in detailing the regulation of cell growth rate by the presence of a single substrate. There are multiple other equations similar to the Monod that attempt to model substrate limited growth. The two more common variants that typically outperform the Monod equation are the Moser and Tessier equations. They are stated as follows:

$$\text{Moser}: \ \mu = \mu_{max}\left(\frac{[S]^n}{K_s^{\ n}} + [S]^n\right) \tag{6.81}$$

$$\text{Teissier}: \ \mu = \mu_{max}\left(1 - e^{-[S]/K_s}\right) \tag{6.82}$$

Despite the very dissimilar looking appearance of the Monod, Moser, and Teissier equations, all three follow the same general form if the derivative of (μ/μ_{max}) is found with respect to $[S]$, the following relationship emerges:

$$\frac{d(\mu/\mu_{max})}{d[S]} = K\left(\frac{\mu}{\mu_{max}}\right)^a\left(1 - \frac{\mu}{\mu_{max}}\right)^b \tag{6.83}$$

For the Monod equation: $K = 1/K_s$, $a = 0$, $b = 2$; the Teissier: $K = 1/K_s$, $a = 0$, $b = 1$; and the Moser: $K = n/K_s^{1/n}$, $a = 1 - 1/n$, and $b = 1 + 1/n$. One final variant that is very straightforward but discontinuous is the Blackman relationship. The Blackman relationship states that

$$\text{Blackman}: \quad \mu = \mu_{max} \quad \text{if} [S] \geq 2K_s \quad \text{and} \quad \mu = \left(\frac{\mu_{max}}{2K_s}\right)[S] \text{ if} [S] < 2K_s \tag{6.84}$$

Thus far, substrate limited cell growth has been approximated as the single limiting enzymatic reaction. If that is indeed the case, then it is possible for inhibitors to play a role in substrate limited growth. In principle, there are two mechanisms of inhibition that are possible with substrate limited growth. One is inhibition due to the presence of the substrate, similar to that discussed with general Michaelis–Menten kinetics, and the other is inhibition to the product. When thinking about the product in relation to an enzymatic reaction driving cell growth, it is best to consider that as a negative component in the system—lactic acid for instance is a product of cell growth. Keehyun Han and Octave Levenspiel derived a generalized model for the substrate and product inhibition that can take place in Monod kinetics. Their model states

$$\mu = \frac{\mu_{max}\left[1 - \left([I]/[I]_{max}\right)\right]^n [S]}{K_s\left[1 - \left([I]/[I]_{max}\right)\right]^m + [S]} \tag{6.85}$$

where $[I]$ is the concentration of the inhibitor present, which could be substrate $[S]$ or product $[P]$. The concentration $[I]_{max}$ is the inhibitor concentration that completely stops the reaction. The Han Levenspiel model has coefficients, n and m. These coefficients both determine the type of inhibition and also help fit the data to a model.

1. *Noncompetitive inhibition*: $n > 0$ and $m = 0$
2. *Competitive inhibition*: $n = 0$ and $m < 0$
3. *Uncompetitive inhibition*: n and $m > 0$

The Han Levenspiel model can be analyzed with a Lineweaver–Burk plot similar to general enzyme inhibition. This is accomplished by taking the double reciprocal, thus

$$\mu = \frac{\mu_{max}\left[1 - \left([I]/[I]_{max}\right)\right]^n [S]}{K_s\left[1 - \left([I]/[I]_{max}\right)\right]^m + [S]} \tag{6.86}$$

$$\frac{1}{\mu} = \frac{K_s\left[1 - \left([I]/[I]_{max}\right)\right]^m}{\mu_{max}\left[1 - \left([I]/[I]_{max}\right)\right]^n} \cdot \frac{1}{[S]} + \frac{1}{\mu_{max}\left[1 - \left([I]/[I]\right)\right]^n} \tag{6.87}$$

Thus, a double reciprocal plot of the observed growth rate μ, versus substrate, $[S]$, can be obtained. The substrate will produce similar results for the various types of inhibition as detailed previously. As before, the y-intercept and x-intercept are equal to $-1/K_s^{app}$ and $1/\mu_{max}$, respectively.

Questions

1. There were two approaches to derive the Michaelis–Menten equation. Demonstrate whether or not the rapid equilibrium assumption would also meet the quasi-steady-state assumption.

2. For the following equation $v = V_{m,app} \cdot [S]/K_{m,app} + [S]$ where $V_{m,app} = V_m/1+\left([I]/K_i\right)$ and $K_{m,app} = K_m/1+\left([I]/K_i\right)$ describe what each term means. Draw a graph of the expected curve from the relationship with axes of v versus $[S]$. Label V_m, $V_{m,app}$, K_m, and $K_{m,app}$ on the graph for two unique curves corresponding to an initial concentration of inhibitor, $[I]$, equal to K_i and $[I] = 0$.

3. The enzyme trypsin has the following kinetic constants at an initial concentration of 10^{-6} M acting on a substrate at a concentration of 10^{-3} M:

$$E + S \leftrightarrow ES \rightarrow E + P$$

$$k_1 = 6 \times 10^8 / \text{M s}$$

$$k_{-1} = 5 \times 10^4 / \text{s}$$

$$k_2 = 1 \times 10^3 / \text{s}$$

   a. What is the value of the Michaelis–Menten constant for this enzyme?
      Answer: $k_2/k_{-1} \ll 1$, so assume rapid equation $K_m = 8.5 \times 10^{-5}$ M.
   b. What is the initial rate of product formation?
      Answer: $v = k2[E_0][S_0]/(K_m + [S_0]) = 922 \ \mu$M/s.

4. An enzyme reaction is pH sensitive and can be explained by the following equations and equilibrium/Michaelis–Menten constants:

$$EH \leftrightarrow E^- + H^+, K_2$$

$$EH + H^+ \leftrightarrow EH_2^+, K_1$$

$$EH + S \leftrightarrow EHS \rightarrow EH + P, K_m, k_2$$

Given the following:

$$K_2 = 10^{-5} \ \text{M} \qquad E_0 = 1 \ \mu\text{M}$$

$$K_1 = 10^{-3} \ \text{M} \qquad S = 2 \ \mu\text{M}$$

$$K_m = 5 \times 10^{-6} \ \text{M}$$

$$k_2 = 8 \times 10^{-2} / \text{s}$$

a. At what pH would the reaction proceed at a maximal rate?
b. What is the efficiency of this reaction relative to a case with no pH dependence?
c. Where would you expect to find this enzyme in the body?

5. For the following kinetic data:

No Inhibitor		With Inhibitor	
v (M/min)	S (M)	v (M/min)	S (M)
1.43	0.33	0.95	0.33
2.00	0.50	1.33	0.50
3.33	1.00	2.22	1.00

a. What type of inhibition is occurring?
   Answer: Linearizing and plotting $1/v$ versus $1/S$, a Lineweaver–Burk plot, yields a line for the uninhibited case of $1/v = 0.2 \times \left(1/[S]\right) + 0.1$, which gives a $V_m = 10$ M/min based on the y-int and a $K_m = 2$ M based on the x-int. Following a similar process for the inhibited case yields a line of $1/v = 0.3 \times \left(1/[S]\right) + 0.15$, which gives a $V_m = 6.67$ M/min and a $K_m = 2$ M. Thus, only V_m changed, which indicates noncompetitive inhibition.
b. What is $K_i = f([I])$?
   Answer: From part a, we know that $V_{m,app} = V_m/(1 + [I]/K_i)$, rearranging and solving for $K_i = f([I])$ yields $K_i = 2[I]$.

6. For the following kinetic data:

No Inhibitor		With Inhibitor	
v (M/min)	S (M)	v (M/min)	S (M)
1.43	0.33	1.00	0.33
2.00	0.50	1.43	0.50
3.33	1.00	2.50	1.00

a. What type of inhibition is occurring?
b. What is $K_i = f([I])$?

7. For the following kinetic data:

No Inhibitor		With Inhibitor	
v (M/min)	S (M)	v (M/min)	S (M)
1.43	0.33	1.25	0.33
2.00	0.50	1.67	0.50
3.33	1.00	2.50	1.00

a. What type of inhibition is occurring?

b. At an inhibitor concentration of 0.2 M, what are the values of $K_{m,app}$ and $V_{m,app}$ if applicable?

8. The initial velocities of a reaction were obtained with varying concentration of substrate. The data are suspected to be quite noisy. Use the three linearization strategies to find the error in the obtained K_m and V_m values if the original reaction had values of $K_m = 30\ \mu M$ and $V_m = 80\ \mu M/s$ for the following data:

$[S]_0$ (μM)	V_0 ($\mu M/s$)
1.03	2.35
5.05	10.40
10.3	19.20
21	33.28
30	38.80
53	49.00
92	58.46
470	75.47

9. Using the reaction data in question 8, apply nonlinear regression to find the values for K_m and V_m and compare them to those obtained with the three linearization strategies.

Answer: Using the nonlinear regression solver in Excel to minimize the sum of differences squared between the actual data obtained and a velocity guessed based on varying K_m and V_m values yields:

K_m	32.07661111
V_m	79.98678183

$[S]_0$ (μM)	V_0 ($\mu M/s$)	Calculated V	Square of Difference
1.03	2.35	2.49	0.02
5.05	10.40	10.88	0.23
10.30	19.20	19.44	0.06
21.00	33.28	31.65	2.67
30.00	38.80	38.66	0.02
53.00	49.00	49.83	0.69
92.00	58.46	59.31	0.72
470.00	75.47	74.88	0.35
		Sum of Squares	4.754250696

(Continued)

Lineweaver–Burke		% Error
K_m	36.89	22.96%
V_m	86.48	8.10%
Hanes–Wolff		
K_m	33.32	11.08%
V_m	80.78	0.97%
Eadie–Hofstee		
K_m	33.56	11.86%
V_m	81.18	1.48%
Nonlinear regression		
K_m	32.08	6.92%
V_m	79.99	0.02%

10. Derive an expression for the velocity of an enzymatic reaction with two intermediates:

$$E + S \leftrightarrow ES_1 \leftrightarrow ES_2 \rightarrow E + P$$

11. You are investigating a regulatory enzyme that presents the following data:

$[S]_0$ (µM)	V_0 (µM/s)
1	0.00
5	0.37
10	2.86
20	18.29
30	40.00
50	65.79
100	77.90
500	79.98

    a. Does the enzyme demonstrate Michaelis–Menten kinetics?
    b. Assuming the data fits the Hill equation, what is the value of n?

12. A tethered enzyme demonstrates $V_m - 10$ µM cm/s and $K_m = 1$ µM. The substrate concentration in the bulk liquid is 10 µM and the liquid mass transfer coefficient for the substrate present is 1 cm/s.
    a. What is the steady-state value of the reaction?
    b. What is the limiting factor in the reaction?

13. A population of cells has grown to 10,000,000 in number and reached senescence, a phenomenon characterized by the loss of the ability to duplicate. After 10 h you observe 3.7 million cells remaining in the dish.
    a. What is the death rate?
    b. How long will it take for 90% of the cells to die?
14. It is important to isolate a homogenous population of cells when generating genetically altered clones. You isolate 9 genetically altered cells; however, they are contaminated with 1 unaltered cell. Due to the increased load producing the foreign gene inserted, the genetically altered cells have a doubling time of 24 h, whereas the unaltered cells have a doubling time of 18 h. Assuming there is an abundance of space available for cell growth:
    a. How many days will it take for unaltered cells to reach the same number as the genetically altered cells?
    b. How many days will it take for the unaltered cells to be 10 times the population of genetically altered cells?
    c. If your cell population was originally in a dish that could sustain 20 million cells, what does the above suggest about the number of genetically altered cells present when the dish is full?
15. The conversion of sugars to ethanol by yeast results in the following relationship for the quantity of substrate (glucose), product (ethanol), and number of yeast present over time:

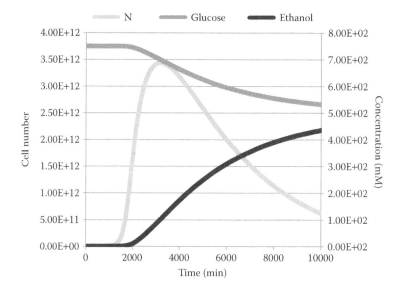

    a. What is occurring?
16. You plate 10,000 cells in a tissue culture dish. The dish has a maximum capacity of 2,000,000 cells. The maximum growth rate of the cells is 0.06/h, and the death

rate of the cells is 0.01/h. The cells consume glucose in the media to grow (weird mutant cells that always consume at a constant rate regardless of the amount present)

$$\frac{-d[\text{Glucose}]}{dt} = k_G \cdot N$$

Where N is the number of cells and $k_G = 5 \times 10^{-10}$ M/h.

The initial concentration of glucose is 25 mM, and the saturation constant, K_s, is equal to 5 mM.

a. Approximately what is the maximum number of cells reached in the dish?
b. If you renew the media after 1 week, what is the maximum number of cells reached?
c. If you renew the media every week, what is the maximum number of cells reached and how long does it take for the cells to reach this maximum?
d. How often must you renew the media for the cells to reach a saturation point (the growth and death rates are equal)?

Answers for all four can be approximations, cells represented in 10,000's and time in days.

17. A population of cells initially at 2,000 is found to have a growth rate of 0.1/h and a death rate of 0.01/h. They also undergo multinucleation, a process where two cells fuse together, at a rate of 0.05/h; however, they will only undergo multinucleation until there are 5 nuclei per cell. The dish holds a maximum of 10,000,000 mononucleated cells.

a. Derive a relationship between the N_{max} and the rate of multinucleation, state all assumptions made.

Answer: Assuming that the total cell area increases directly proportional to the number of nuclei, then N_{max} after all cells have 5 nuclei would be $1/5$ N_{maxo}. The ratio between N_{max} and N_{maxo} tells us how close the popula tion is to being all quintnucleated cells. Using a logistic equation, similar to contact inhibition:

$$\frac{dN_{max}}{dt} = \mu_{multinucleation} \cdot N \cdot \left(\frac{1}{5} - \frac{N_{max}}{10,000,000}\right)$$

b. What is the number of cells present after a long (more than 4 weeks) amount of time?

Answer: After a long time, all the cells have 5 nuclei. $N_{max} = (1/5) \times 10,000,000 = 2,000,000$.

The balance between the growth and death rates at steady state reduces to $N/N_{max} = 1 - (k_d/\mu_g)$. Thus, $N = N_{max} \cdot \left[1 - (k_d/\mu_g)\right] = 2,000,000 \cdot (1 - 0.1) = 1,800,000$.

c. What is the maximum number of cells reached in the dish? An estimate on the order of 100,000's is fine

Answer: This requires a bit of number crunching and taking a $dt = 10$ h and rounding ...

This estimate provides a max of 6,100,000 cells in the dish. A more rigorous approach with a dt of 0.1 provides a max of 5,340,411, which would be unreasonable to do by hand/calculator.

d. Draw a graph approximating the relationship between cell number and time. This does not need to be exact.

Answer:

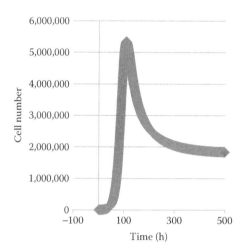

7

Data Management

LEARNING OBJECTIVES

1. Differentiate between a single datum and a set of data and recite the importance of the differentiation.
2. Fully appreciate the need for complying with good laboratory practices.
3. Understand government requirements for electronic data handling.
4. Identify and recognize differences in the sources of error present in data.

7.1 INTRODUCTION

A piece of quantitative or qualitative information is called a *datum* and a set of *datum* is called *data*, a plural form of *datum.* This grammatical observation is frequently ignored. Information is critical to understanding and operating various systems; a datum includes pH value, the flow rate of oxygen, the optical density of a growing culture, or the temperature of a broth. Since the products of bioprocessing are highly dependent on operating conditions, a proper recording, presentation, and analysis of data are critical. Regardless of your hierarchical position in an organization, we will be required to perform all of these data-related functions, and a good basic understanding is absolutely essential to allow decision making and also to comply with the requirements of the regulatory authorities for using data to support a product application.

In this chapter, we will focus on three major aspects of data analysis:

- Data collection, recording, and presentation
- Data types, manipulation, and conclusion drawing
- Automatic data storage and handling and regulatory constraints

A datum is subject to much variability from the inherent variability of the system, the errors of measurement, and the errors of recording. All experiments yield output through instruments that in some way represents the response or the observation about the system under scrutiny, but it is only one surrogate interpretation of the condition of the system.

For example, when using a pH meter to record the pH of a solution, the pH electrode is reading the activity of hydronium ions through a potential generated, which is then processed and fed to a reading device into numbers; even if the pH meter is fully calibrated, the pH value recorded remains subject to myriad of errors. These aspects of error correction fall within the purview of equipment calibration and validation and will not be discussed here. However, once we are able to record a reading, the data analysis begins with its own errors: was it recorded manually or electronically, were there enough decimal points in the reading, if this was a series of reading, were the independent parameters recorded correctly, were the data properly presented, and trend analysis performed and conclusions drawn? If the data were stored electronically, were the hardware and the software validated, and in case of regulatory submission met the critical Code of Federal Regulations (CFR) 21 Part 11 compliant? Were the data retrievable for future audit?

Of great importance is a clear understanding of how to collect and record data; most of these practices are outlined in Section 7.2, a regulation described by the World Health Organization, the Food and Drug Administration (FDA), and the European Commission.

7.2 GOOD LABORATORY PRACTICES

7.2.1 Overview

The scientific measurements (whether they pertain to monitoring contaminants in pharmaceutical products, clinical determinations of blood sugar, characterization of forensic evidence, or testing materials for space missions) are generally recognized as affecting decisions literally concerned with life and death issues. As personal acknowledgment of their responsibility, scientists have traditionally adopted sound laboratory practices directed at assuring the quality of their data. However, until recently these practices were not consistently adopted, enforced, or audited. Because of some notorious historic examples where erroneous data have lead to tragic consequences, national and international agencies have developed guidelines directed at various industries (food, agriculture, pharmaceutical, clinical, environmental, etc.), which fall in the general category of good laboratory practices (GLPs); this is described in CFR 22 Part 58.

Within the United States, federal agencies such as FDA and Environmental Protection Agency (EPA) have produced documents defining laboratory operational requirements, which must be met so that technical data from laboratory studies may be acceptable by those agencies for any legal or contractual purposes. Laboratories doing business with or for these agencies must therefore comply with the specified GLP regulations. So crucial has the issue of maintaining compliance become that many industries report no less than 10%, and occasionally as much as 50%, of their total effort is expended on internal quality assurance (QA). A typical level of effort is 25%.

Because the issue of GLPs is obviously so crucial to modern laboratory operations, but most importantly because GLP is an essential ingredient for any professional scientist, it is highly recommended that all bioprocess engineers read these guidelines thoroughly as they are available at the websites listed in the bibliography section of this chapter.

7.2.2 Elements of GLP

7.2.2.1 Quality Assurance: Establishing Confidence in Reported Data

The primary products of any laboratory concerned with chemical analysis are the analytical data reported for specimens examined by that laboratory. QA for such a laboratory includes all of the activities associated with insuring that chemical and physical measurements are made properly, interpreted correctly, and reported with appropriate estimates of error and confidence levels. QA activities also include those maintaining appropriate records of specimen/sample origins and history (sample tracking), as well as procedures, raw data, and results associated with each specimen/sample. The various elements of QA are itemized as follows:

- Standard operating procedures (SOPs)
- Statistical procedures for data evaluation
- Instrumentation validation
- Reagent/materials certification
- Analyst certification
- Lab facilities certification
- Specimen/sample tracking

7.2.2.2 Standard Operating Procedures

Many volumes could be written regarding each of the QA elements itemized above. However, we can only discuss each briefly here. *SOPs* are what the name implies … procedures, which have been tested and approved for conducting a particular determination. Often, these procedures will have been evaluated and published by the regulatory agency involved (e.g., EPA or FDA); these agencies may not accept analytical data obtained by other procedures for particular analytes. Within any commercial laboratory, SOPs should either be available or developed to acceptable standards, so that any analytical data collected and reported can be tied to a documented procedure. Presumably, this implies that a given determination can be repeated at any later time, for an identical specimen, using the SOPs indicated.

7.2.2.3 Statistical Procedures

Statistical procedures for data evaluation are briefly provided below and for those students who may have not kept up with the science of statistical evaluation, they are advised to read up on it. It should be pointed out, however, that one may not be able to simply select a statistical procedure from a textbook. Many procedural details are optional and arbitrary. Thus, practitioners in bioprocessing industry may adopt certain standards, which are deemed acceptable within that field (e.g., using 95% or 99% confidence levels for particular tests), or they may adopt specific statistical analysis procedures for defining detection limits, confidence intervals, analyte measurement units, and so on. Regulatory agencies often also describe acceptable statistical procedures. All healthcare products produced by biological methods are subject to full compliance with robust data presentation and advanced statistics.

7.2.2.4 Instrumentation Validation

Instrumentation validation is a process inherently necessary for any analytical laboratory. Data produced by *faulty* instruments may give the appearance of valid data. These events are particularly difficult to detect with modern computer-controlled systems, which remove the analyst from the data collection/instrument control functions. Thus, it is essential that some objective procedures be implemented for continuously assessing the validity of instrumental data. These procedures, when executed on a regular basis, will establish the continuing acceptable operation of laboratory instruments within prescribed specifications. Time-related graphical records of the results of these instrument validation procedures are called *control charts*. The *control limits* assigned as upper and lower ranges around the expected instrumental output are generally related to some accepted measure of the random error expected for the overall procedure. Typically, the control limits will be set at $\pm 2\sigma$ (standard deviation). QA procedures will require that whenever a instrument's performance is outside of the *control limits*, use of that instrument to provide analytical reports must be discontinued; the cause of the problem must be determined and fixed if possible; and the instrument must be certified to be operating again with control limits before returning to service for determinations leading to reported analytical data.

7.2.2.5 Reagent and Materials Certification

Reagent and material certification is an obvious element of QA. However, GLP guidelines emphasize that certification must follow accepted procedures and must be adequately documented. Moreover, some guidelines will specify that each container for laboratory reagents/materials must be labeled with information related to its certification value, date, and expiration time. This policy is meant to assure that reagents used are as specified in the SOPs.

7.2.2.6 Certification of Analysis

A certificate of analysis (COA) is a required part of QA. Some acceptable proof of satisfactory training and/or competence with specific laboratory procedures must be established for each analyst. Because the American Chemical Society does not currently have a policy regarding *certification* of chemists or analysts, the requirements for *certification* vary and are usually prescribed by the laboratory in question. These standards would have to be accepted by any agency or client obtaining results from that laboratory.

7.2.2.7 Certification of Laboratory Facilities

Certification of laboratory facilities is normally done by some external agency. For example, an analytical laboratory might be audited by representatives of a federal agency with which they have a contract. An independent laboratory might file documentation with a responsible state or federal agency. The evaluation is concerned with such issues as space (amount, quality, and relevance), ventilation, equipment, storage, hygiene, and so on.

7.2.2.8 Specimen and Sample Tracking

Tracking specimens and samples is an aspect of QA that has received a great deal of attention with the advent of computer-based laboratory information management systems. However, whether done by hand with paper files, or by computer with modern bar-coding techniques, sample tracking is a crucial part of QA. The terms *specimen* and *sample* are often used interchangeably. However, *specimen* usually refers to an item to be characterized chemically, whereas *sample* usually refers to a finite portion of the specimen, which is taken for analysis. When the specimen is homogeneous (such as a stable solution), the sample represents the overall composition of the specimen. However, for heterogeneous specimens (e.g., metal alloys, rock, soil, textiles, foods, polymer composites, vitamin capsules), a sample may not represent the overall composition. Maintaining the distinction in records of analytical results can be crucial to the interpretation of data.

Procedures for assuring adequate specimen/sample tracking will vary among laboratories. The bottom line, however, is that these procedures must maintain the unmistakable connection between a set of analytical data and the specimen and/or samples from which they were obtained. In addition, the original source of the specimen/sample(s) must be recorded and likewise unmistakably connected with the set of analytical data. Finally, in many cases, the *chain-of-custody* must be specified and validated. This is particularly true for forensic samples (related to criminal prosecution) but can also be essential for many other situations as well. For example, a pharmaceutical company developing a new product may be called upon to defend their interpretation of clinical trial tests. Such defense may require the company to establish that specimens collected during these trials could not have been deliberately tampered. That is, they may have to establish an unbroken chain-of-custody, which would remove all doubt regarding the integrity of specimens submitted for chemical analysis.

7.2.2.9 Documentation and Maintenance of Records

A central feature of GLP guidelines is the maintenance of records of specimen/sample origins, chain-of-custody, raw analytical data, processed analytical data, SOPs, instrument validation results, reagent certification results, and analyst certification documents. Maintenance of instrument and reagent certification records provides for post-evaluation of results, even after the passage of several years. Maintenance of all records specified provides documentation, which may be required in the event of legal challenges due to repercussions of decisions based on the original analytical results.

This record-keeping feature of GLP is so critical that vendors are now providing many of these capabilities as part of computer packages for operating modern instruments. For example, many modern computer-based instruments will provide for the indefinite storage of raw analytical data for specific samples in a protected (tamperproof) environment. They also provide for maintenance of historical records of control chart data establishing the operational quality of instruments during any period during which analytical data have been acquired by that instrument.

The length of time over which laboratory records should be maintained will vary with the situation. However, the general guidelines followed in regulated laboratories are to maintain records for at least five years. In practice, these records are being maintained much longer. The development of higher density storage devices for digitized data is making this kind of record-keeping possible. The increasing frequency of litigation regarding chemistry-related commercial products is making this kind of record-keeping essential. Moreover, establishing the integrity of the stored data is becoming a high level security issue for companies concerned about future litigation.

7.2.2.10 Writing and Correcting Data

Data are recorded in laboratory notebooks and only using indelible ink—never using an erasable media. The data are never overwritten or corrected—the wrong entries are crossed out but only minimally to allow readability of the datum crossed out and a new entry made with the initials of the operator. This guideline is the basic practice required by the GLPs and must be followed regardless of the working environment, even when simple experiments or preparatory experiments are conducted. In those rare instances when you may be required to write down data on a loose piece of paper (napkins are frequently used) and then transcribe the data in your notebook, you may not discard the original writing and this must be appended to the book.

7.2.2.11 Data Significance

How sure are you of the data? How accurate is your observation? What is the reproducibility of the numbers reported? These are some of the first questions asked when we collect a set of data to analyze or operate a process. Some of us not cognizant of the mathematical implications find that a datum reported with the largest number of significant figures is more accurate or relevant. We will see why this is not only absurd but takes away the ability to make appropriate presentation of the data.

A datum value reflects a material property with an element of uncertainty; the datum can be accurate or precise or both, yet the uncertainty associated with a value is expressed in the way it is written, the number of figures indicating the uncertainty potential. It is not uncommon to see an inordinate number of figures after the decimal; but even before decimal, the figures can be written in a manner meaningful for the data represented.

An easy way to understand the need not to be superfluous is to count the number of significant figures. For example, the number 19,490 has six significant figures and so is the number 10.098. How many significant figures are required is dependent on two factors. First, what is the multiplicative value of the number? Take for example, the number π. It is 22/7 and can be provided to an infinite number of significant figures. It is, for example, 3.14285714285714 when calculated in a standard calculator that rounds of the rest of the digits. If we are calculating the area of very large circle, say a few hundred million miles, then the number of digits used to signify should be as large as possible, otherwise in most of routine calculations, 3–4 significant figures are sufficient. Notice that we are talking about significant figures, so there must be insignificant figures. Starting from left, each digit in a number represents one-tenth the figure. So, in a three significant digit number such as 114, the digit 4 represents singular percent portion; in this case, the digit 4 is 3.51% of the total number; however if we were examining a number with six significant figures, the last number will represent one-one hundred thousands of fraction. Let us take the same number 139,114; here the last digit 4 adds to only 0.0029%, an insignificant portion compared to the entire number. Since there is likely to be greater variability in the measurement than 0.0029%, the last digit is insignificant and can be dropped and replaced by 0 without affecting the value of the number. To give you a better physical example, when we speak of the deficit the United States government is running we may say it into trillions of dollars and it may suffice to say

4.8 trillion but expanding it to last dollar value for expression purpose will be ludicrous because it does not add to the significance of the value. An interesting incidence was reported a few years ago, when a con artist working in a bank created an account where all of those *insignificant* pennies will be deposited. Banks will generally round of the number after two digits to the right of the decimal point. The first digit to the right of the decimal place is 10 cents, and the second digit, the number of pennies. However, when a bank transaction is made where interest is calculated, the bank computers compute it to several more significant figures. With just this overflow of insignificant one-hundredths and one-millionth of cents, the con artist was able to accumulate millions of dollars without suspicion because no one had lost any money. Zero is like any other digit a significant number unless it is used to locate the position after a decimal point; 0.012, 0.0012, and 0.00012 all have two significant figures.

One of the most ill understood expressions of significant figures comes when using decimal points. A decimal is merely a point where a figure smaller than the unitary figure is present. $10.10 means ten dollars and ten cents; the decimal does not have any contribution to deciding the significant figures; unfortunately, many consider this to be a dividing line in providing a significant figure. A result reported as 1,987.33498 is absurd taking it to nine significant figures, five of which fall into a category of less than unity, which in turn represents in this case one-hundredth of the value. There is also no need to stick to a fixed *two decimal place* reporting; it can be important when the number on the left of the decimal is small. It is all right to report a value of 2.53 (three significant figures) but it is not necessary to report 2,098.53 (six significant figures). Again, how many significant figures are required depends on the nature of the multiplicative value of the number.

Numbers are therefore rounded off to the nearest value to retain the number of significant value; discard all digits right of the nth digit if the $n + 1$ digit is 5 or less; or increase it to next higher number if the $n + 1$ digit is higher than 5:

1,098,769 = 1,098,770
1,098,743 = 1,098,740

When multiplying and dividing, the results are reported to the least significant figures in which any number was represented, and in the case of addition or subtraction, the smaller number of significant value right of the decimal place in any of the number involved in the operation.

To recap, Table 7.1 shows the claimed accuracy in a dataset based on reported significant figures.

These are general guidelines only; in some instances, reporting to two decimal places is the norm (though unfounded), and in other instances, you may be asked to keep a record to higher significant values, which are then rounded off in the end. Please remember that these recording and reporting habits often develop over decades and you will find absurd significant figures reported even in reputable journals. So, if you are told to report everything to nine significant figures or always write the third digit on the right of the decimal place, just do it; this is not a scientific or engineering issue and since reporting more figures does not reduce the validity of data, this should not be a source of argument with

Table 7.1   Claimed Accuracy and Significant Figures Reported

Number of Significant Figures	Claimed Accuracy (%)	Example
1	10	9.0 or 0.9 or 0.09
2	1	99 or 9.9 or 0.99 or 0.099
3	0.1	999 or 99.9 or 9.99 or 0.999 or 0.0999
4	0.01	9,999 or 999.9 or 9.999 or 0.9999 or 0.09999

your superiors. The long discussion on this topic provided here is to educate scientists as they are starting their career to differentiate between expressed significance and actual significance of the data.

7.2.2.12 Accountability

GLP procedures inherently establish accountability for laboratory results. Analysts, instruments, reagents, and analytical methods cannot (and should not) maintain the anonymity that might be associated with a lack of GLP policy. Responsibility for all aspects of the laboratory processes leading to technical results and conclusions is clearly defined and documented. This situation should place appropriate pressure on analysts to conduct studies with adequate care and concern. Moreover, it allows the possibility of identifying more quickly and succinctly the source(s) of error(s) and taking corrective action(s) to maintain acceptable quality of laboratory data.

7.3 ELECTRONIC DATA HANDLING

7.3.1 Background

It is now more common to enter the data directly into an electronic device, a computer, a tablet, or a handwriting conversion device. However, the use of electronic handling of data poses new challenges and requirements that must be clearly understood by all those handling the data. To give the reader a quick understanding, the U.S. FDA has, in the past five years, issued more citations for noncompliance with electronic data handling than for any other reason, including compliance to good manufacturing practices. The citations were issued to companies ranging from small regional outfits to large multinationals. As a result, facilities generating data that are intended for submission to regulatory authorities continue to use a manual system of recording until such time that they are comfortable in switching over to an electronic system.

Electronic data management requires establishment of an elaborate validation and security system that is not likely to be available to smaller institutions. For example, the U.S. FDA requires that all hardware storing data be validated for the accuracy of entry, security of operator identification, use of multiple levels of passwords, and a system to monitor addressing of data stored and its manipulation. While for nonregulatory research, the institutions may not follow these rigorous requirements; when a regulatory submission is planned, these are critical requirements. These regulatory requirements are described in the CFR 21 Part 11 section of the Federal Register. It is important for the students to familiarize themselves with the requirements, if not the details, of this law to be conversant with the system requirements.

7.3.2 CRF 21 Part 11: Electronic Records

Part 11 of Title 21 of the Code of Federal Regulations provides guidance to persons who, in fulfillment of a requirement in a statute or another part of FDA's regulations to maintain records or submit information to FDA, have chosen to maintain the records or submit designated information electronically and, as a result, have become subject to part 11. Part 11 applies to records in electronic form that are created, modified, maintained, archived, retrieved, or transmitted under any records requirements set forth in Agency regulations. Part 11 also applies to electronic records submitted to the Agency under the Federal Food, Drug, and Cosmetic Act (the Act) and the Public Health Service Act (the PHS Act), even if such records are not specifically identified in Agency regulations (§ 11.1). The underlying requirements set forth in the Act, PHS Act, and FDA regulations (other than part 11) are referred to as *predicate rules.*

The Agency (e.g., FDA) enforces the provisions of part 11 including, but not limited to, certain controls for closed systems in § 11.10. For example, the following controls and requirements:

- Limiting system access to authorized individuals
- Use of operational system checks
- Use of authority checks
- Use of device checks
- Determination that persons who develop, maintain, or use electronic systems have the education, training, and experience to perform their assigned tasks
- Establishment of and adherence to written policies that hold individuals accountable for actions initiated under their electronic signatures
- Appropriate controls over systems documentation
- Controls for open systems corresponding to controls for closed systems bulleted above (§ 11.30)
- Requirements related to electronic signatures (e.g., §§ 11.50, 11.70, 11.100, 11.200, and 11.300)

The persons must comply with applicable predicate rules, and records that are required to be maintained or submitted must remain secure and reliable in accordance with the predicate rules.

When persons choose to use records in electronic format in place of paper format, part 11 would apply. On the other hand, when persons use computers to generate paper printouts of electronic records, and those paper records meet all the requirements of the applicable predicate rules and persons rely on the paper records to perform their regulated activities, FDA would generally not consider persons to be *using electronic records in lieu of paper records* under §§ 11.2(a) and 11.2(b). In these instances, the use of computer systems in the generation of paper records would not trigger part 11.

The FDA considers part 11 to be applicable to the following records or signatures in electronic format (part 11 records or signatures):

- Records that are required to be maintained under predicate rule requirements and that are maintained in electronic format *in place of paper format*. On the other hand, records (and any associated signatures) that are not required to be retained under predicate rules, but that are nonetheless maintained in electronic format, are not part 11 records.
- Records that are required to be maintained under predicate rules, that are maintained in electronic format *in addition to paper format*, and that *are relied on to perform regulated activities*.
- In some cases, actual business practices may dictate whether we are *using* electronic records instead of paper records under § 11.2(a). For example, if a record is required to be maintained under a predicate rule and we use a computer to generate a paper printout of the electronic records, but we nonetheless rely on the electronic record to perform regulated activities, the Agency may consider the *use* of the electronic record instead of the paper record. That is, the Agency may take your business practices into account in determining whether part 11 applies.
- Records submitted to FDA, under predicate rules (even if such records are not specifically identified in Agency regulations) in electronic format (assuming the records have been identified in docket number 92S-0251 as the types of submissions, the Agency accepts in electronic format). However, a record that is not itself submitted, but is used in generating a submission, is not a part 11 record unless it is otherwise required to be maintained under a predicate rule and it is maintained in electronic format.
- Electronic signatures intended to be the equivalent of handwritten signatures, initials, and other general signings required by predicate rules. Part 11 signatures include electronic signatures that are used, for example, to document the fact that certain events or actions occurred in accordance with the predicate rule (e.g., approved, reviewed, and verified).

7.3.2.1 Validation

The Agency requires validation of computerized systems (§ 11.10[a] and corresponding requirements in § 11.30). The decision to validate computerized systems, and the extent of the validation, one should take into account the impact the systems have on your ability to meet predicate rule requirements. One should also consider the impact those systems might have on the accuracy, reliability, integrity, availability, and authenticity of required records and signatures. Even if there is no predicate rule requirement to validate a system, in some instances it may still be important to validate the system.

The Agency recommends that clients base their approach on a justified and documented risk assessment and a determination of the potential of the system to affect product quality and safety, and record integrity. For instance, validation would not be important for a word processor used only to generate SOPs.

Computer systems include both hardware and software; the protocols for validating hardware are well defined but the validation of software creates significant problems, and it is a general knowledge that most of the off-the-shelf software programs do not meet FDA's requirement of validation.

7.3.2.2 Audit Trail

The Agency enforces specific part 11 requirements related to computer-generated, time-stamped audit trails (§ 11.10 [e], [k][2] and any corresponding requirement in §11.30). Persons must still comply with all applicable predicate rule requirements related to documentation of, for example, date (e.g., § 58.130[e]), time, or sequencing of events, as well as any requirements for ensuring that changes to records do not obscure previous entries.

Even if there are no predicate rule requirements to document, for example, date, time, or sequence of events in a particular instance, it may nonetheless be important to have audit trails or other physical, logical, or procedural security measures in place to ensure the trustworthiness and reliability of the records. The Agency recommends that we base our decision on whether to apply audit trails, or other appropriate measures, on the need to comply with predicate rule requirements, a justified and documented risk assessment, and a determination of the potential effect on product quality and safety and record integrity. The Agency suggests that we apply appropriate controls based on such an assessment. Audit trails can be particularly appropriate when users are expected to create, modify, or delete regulated records during normal operation.

The copies of electronic records are provided to the Agency by the following:

- Producing copies of records held in common portable formats when records are maintained in these formats
- Using established automated conversion or export methods, where available, to make copies in a more common format (examples of such formats include, but are not limited to, PDF, XML, or SGML)

7.3.2.3 Record Retention

A decision on how to maintain records should be based on predicate rule requirements, a justified and documented risk assessment, and a determination of the value of the records over time.

The Agency does not object if we decide to archive required records in electronic format to nonelectronic media such as microfilm, microfiche, and paper or to a standard electronic file format (examples of such formats include, but are not limited to, PDF, XML, or SGML). Persons must still comply with all predicate rule requirements, and the records themselves and any copies of the required records should preserve their content and meaning. As long as predicate rule requirements are fully satisfied and the content and meaning of the records are preserved and archived, we can delete the electronic version of the records. In addition, paper and electronic record and signature components can coexist (i.e., a hybrid situation) as long as predicate rule requirements are met and the content and meaning of those records are preserved.

7.4 DATA ERRORS

7.4.1 Absolute and Relative Errors

The significant digits are also decided frequently on the output of the instrument recording the data; for example, if a balance is capable of giving ±1 g, then there is no sense reporting weight even to a single decimal place; the last number should be rounded off, for example, a weigh machine recording 138.7 g (yes the output may be provided to any significant value) then the number should be reported as 139 g. In the example given above, we have introduced another concept of absolute error meaning that within a range of 1 g on each side, the values are not accurate; when the absolute error is compared to the total value, we get relative error; in the example above, 139 g weight recorded on a machine with ±1 g uncertainty represents a relative error of (1/139)*100 = 0.72% relative error.

Since the absolute error is estimation and not an actual measurement, reporting it to more than two significant figures is not necessary. For example, in the calculation above, reporting a relative error of 0.7269% will not make any sense.

Absolute errors and relative errors as reported above pertain to a single set of data; when several data are combined in a mathematical formula, the error can be significant; as a rule of thumb, add relative errors when multiplying or dividing. In the example above, the relative error for weight measurement was 0.72%; if the measurement of volume (e.g., to determine the density) has a relative error of 2%, then the final error for density will be 2.72%. For addition or subtraction, the absolute and not the relative errors are added. However, large numbers are subtracted leaving smaller values, the absolute errors can transform into very large relative errors. Let us say a value of 2,890 is subtracted from 2,900 both with absolute error of 10; then, the final answer of 10 will have absolute error of 10% or 100% relative error.

7.4.2 Systematic and Random Errors

Given above was a description of the significant figures in a number and on handling reliability of data. Errors in measurements can be due to a fixed factor such as lack of calibration or unpredictable human errors. The first type is called a *systematic error*; for example, the user did not tare the sample container, which had a weight of 42 g, then 42 g should adjust all measurements down. Additionally, if a calibration error left all readings 10% higher, these corrections can be made after the data are collected. Know that the results obtained in a systematic error are highly reproducible and are thus precise even though not accurate. The second type is random or accidental error due to causes not understood such as human or machine errors where measurements taken repeatedly give different readings or a scattered distribution. To be accurate, the results should have little systematic and little random error.

And finally there are errors that fall in the category of blunders—needless to say it takes a man to err, a computer to blunder.

The goal of obtaining data remains to obtain accurate data that are recorded to reasonable significant figures and thus obviating the systematic and the random errors.

When absolute and correct figures are reported, there is no limit to the significant figures such as in the case of the value of pi or an exact dollar amount but in a collected data, chances are that more than three significant figures will take you below the sensitivity of the methods used to obtain the numbers; a high significant number reported gives a false impression of higher accuracy and reliability deceptively.

To represent the above discussion in a graphical form, Figure 7.1 shows the relative errors.

On a more graphical base, Figure 7.2 shows the description of precision and accuracy on a dartboard.

Interestingly, next time you look at the advertisement of a high-end manual Swiss watch, notice that they tout their *precision movement* not *accurate movement* because none of the watches, particularly the manual ones, are accurate.

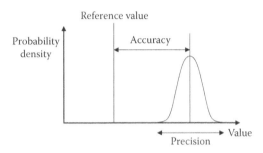

Figure 7.1 Precision–accuracy relationship chart.

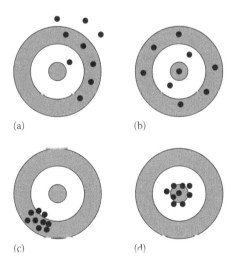

Figure 7.2 Darts thrown representing how precision and accuracy are defined. Key: (a) imprecise and inaccurate; (b) imprecise and accurate (note: the decision to call this observation accurate depends on the range of precision required, e.g., in most circumstances a 5% lack of precision will be readily accepted, in others a much lower range is desired); (c) precise and inaccurate; (d) precise and accurate.

7.5 STATISTICAL ANALYSIS

Randomness in the data was associated above with unpredictable errors; however, there is another aspect of randomness—it is often the data measured. Whereas an electronic instrument might generate an electrical signal with a random range of responses to an impulse, randomness in the values expected to be universal is a common occurrence.

What is the age distribution of the American people? If we plot data on age and the number of people in each group, we will end up with a single distribution curve, it is going to be a bell shaped curve—a Gaussian distribution phenomenon. This bell-shaped curve can be a perfect bell (perfect distribution for a trait that is truly randomized) or skewed to either side depending on the overall general bias. The Japanese show a curve skewed toward the right as more people are living longer and the population is not growing as fast. However, in most developing countries, the curve will be skewed toward the left (lower age) to represent a high rate of birth and a high rate of mortality at an older age.

A coin flipped for enough times will be represented as a flat bar of the two outcomes, not a bell-shaped curve because the outcome is not continuous. The randomness of the two examples given above should not be confused with the randomness in the output of results that form our data. These random errors in measurements can be analyzed using statistical procedures with the aim to find the best estimate of the variable measured and to quantify the extent to which random error affects the data. It is noteworthy that just like the example of age distribution provided above, the random errors also follow a Gaussian (or normal) distribution. Theoretically, if we take an infinite number of readings, then the arithmetic mean of the value will be error free. But we need not go that far. A reasonable number of readings will allow us a clear understanding of the actual value.

We start with an arithmetic mean, which is obtained by adding all values and then dividing the sum by the number of readings taken.

This is a first attempt to define the real value. This value does not give us the precision in measurement, which is measured by how each of the reading deviates from the arithmetic—the residual value. This provides us a statistical parameter called *standard deviation*, σ:

$$\sigma = \sqrt{\frac{\sum^{n}\left(x-\bar{x}\right)^2}{n-1}} \tag{7.1}$$

$$= \sqrt{\frac{\left(x_1-x\right)^2+\left(x_2-\bar{x}\right)^2+\left(x_3-\bar{x}\right)^2+\ldots\left(x_n-\bar{x}\right)^2}{n-1}}$$

Therefore, to report the results of repeated measurements, we quote the mean as the best estimate of the variable, and the standard deviation as a measure of the confidence we place in the result. The units and dimensions of the mean and standard deviation are the same as those of x and the variable is reported as mean $\pm$ standard deviation. It can be readily seen that as the number of observations made increases (n increases), the standard deviation will decrease, but at the same time the arithmetic mean will also become closer to the real value. In those instances where a high value of standard deviation is observed, the goal should be to improve the system rather than try to reduce the standard deviation by repeated measures. Generally, a few dozen readings is about all that one will be able to do to understand the extent of deviation. It is noteworthy at this time to remind that systematic errors, such as those due to poor calibration or validation, are not subject to any statistical analysis since these are constant modulators associated with accuracy and not precision.

7.6 DATA CONCLUSIONS

Data analysis is a collection of methods that help to describe facts, detect patterns, develop explanations, and test hypotheses. The numerical results provided by data analyses are usually simple: It finds the number that describes a typical value and it finds differences among numbers. Data analysis finds averages, like the average pH or the average temperature, and it finds differences like the difference in the optical density of a culture during a fermentation process. Fundamentally, the numerical answers provided by data analyses are that simple. But data analysis is not *about* numbers—it uses them. Data analysis is not about asking, "How does it work?" And that's where data analysis gets tricky. For example, a bacterial culture grown over 8 h showed an increase from the initial optical density of 0.1–12. Mathematically, the culture added an average optical density of 1.49/h. However, without further collection and analysis of data, we will miss out answering the question, "How does it work?" For example, in the example given, the culture doubled in density every 20 min until it reached the value of around 12 and then became stagnant; that time was around 4.5 h. Thus, the end result of data analysis provides the following:

1. Visualization of the general trend of influence of one variable on another
2. Testing of the applicability of a particular model to a process
3. Estimating the value of coefficients in process models
4. Developing new empirical models

Experimental data are either independent variables or dependent variables; the latter is the uncontrolled response. The former can be time, pH, or temperature; the dependent variable can be the optical density and is expressed as a function of the independent variable.

Data are generally represented as tables, graphs, or equations. Tables allow presentation of data of any length and with desired details; however, long tables can become very cumbersome to visualize; as shown above, when the data are presented in a graph form, the results and trends are quickly conveyed—it is this aspect of data analysis that is more important to understand the overall view of the process along with outliers (do not just assume that a reading is an outlier—there is more to it than meets the eye). It also helps additional designs of experiments based on various phases of the experiment. By convention, independent variables are plotted along the *abscissa* (the X-axis), while one or more dependent variables are plotted along the *ordinate* (Y-axis). One of the simplest methods of plotting the data is to use Microsoft Excel; this program has extensive mathematical and statistical tools. It is strongly urged that all those intending to work in any laboratory setting acquire a reasonable expertise in the use of Microsoft Excel. However, know that these data manipulations may not meet the CFR 21 Part 11 compliance, which may or may not be an issue depending on whether the data are submitted for regulatory approval of products or not.

The relationship between the independent and the dependent variables can frequently be presented in equation form where a mathematical relationship can be established. A regression fit may yield a linear relationship such as $y = Ax + B$, where B is the intercept of the straight line on the ordinate; A is the slope; A and B are also called the coefficients, parameters, or adjustable parameters.

A nonlinear regression line will include another mathematical function such as those provided above for an exponential growth model: $X = X_0 e^{-kt}$ is a typical example, where k is the rate constant and t is the time; this is a natural log linear relationship meaning that if the natural log of X is plotting against time, this will yield a straight line with slope equal to $-k$. Plotting the data will allow calculation of k and the data are often fitted to these equations where the output is understood to follow a certain equation.

Earlier discussion of the inherent error in each datum and those errors that can be parsed through statistical analysis must be given consideration when making any conclusions from data analysis. This leads to the use of regression analysis in ascertaining whether a set of data is correctly understood. An easy method is to use Microsoft Excel program to create various regression fits or models that automatically calculate all error terms. However, students must also perform manual calculations of the goodness of fit to impress upon them the role of datum variability; chances are you will rarely perform any manual calculation but statistics is best used when the principles behind the calculations are fully understood or at least fully appreciated. The researcher or technician must always know the difference between a random error, a systematic error, and a blunder and also realize that the largest source of error in any experiment is often caused by human errors. If data are collected incorrectly, very little can be done afterward to make them meaningful. The cliché: garbage in, garbage out is a universal paradigm. And it is for this reason that those working in laboratories must recognize and appreciate all basis statistical methods and their limitations.

When data are plotted (manually or by computer) and a best-fit line is drawn through them, the question always arises as to which points are more important and which ones are not. This is more of a concern when using hand smoothing of data—use of computers takes away that bias as the lines are drawn such that the variance (points predicted by the line and actual point at various intervals) is minimized. However, this also means that the data points with larger value will get more attention; there are, however, models available that place certain weight on data points to make sure this type of error is not forced in automated computations. A popular technique for locating the line or curve, which minimizes the residuals, is *least-squares analysis.* This statistical procedure is based on minimizing the sum of squares of the residuals. There are several variations of the procedure: Legendre's method minimizes the sum-of-squares of residuals of the dependent variable; Gauss's and Laplace's methods minimize the sum of squares of weighted residuals where the weighting factors depend on the scatter of replicate data points. Each method gives different results; it should be remembered that the curve of *best* fit is ultimately a matter of opinion. For example, by minimizing the sum of squares of the residuals, least-squares analysis could produce a curve, which does not pass close to particular data points known beforehand to be more accurate than the rest. Alternatively, we could choose to define the best fit as that which minimizes the absolute values of the residuals, or the sum of the residuals raised to the fourth power. The decision to use the sum of squares is an arbitrary one; many alternative approaches are equally valid mathematically. Points that have large residuals are called *outliers* and thus strongly influence regression; in some instances, these can be thrown out but only after analyzing the data with and without them; statistical models that deal specifically with manipulation of outliers are available and require a much deeper understanding of statistical modeling. GLPs require that you do not throw out any outlier.

In summary, know that the least-squares analysis applies only to data containing random errors and that the variables must be independent; in other words, y cannot be a function of x and allowed to be determined on the nature of the process. For example, if x is time and y is the optical density then regardless of which time of the day the reading is taken, it should not depend on the clock hour; if all readings taken at 2 pm are 10% higher then there is a dependence between x and y. Do not be surprised at the example provided here to illustrate. More sophisticated models are required when there is a suspected dependence between x and y. There is also an assumption made here that the data output is uniform regardless of the life cycle of the experiment; does your equipment heat up and start giving more random error measurements over time? That will require additional corrections. In some instances, it requires applying weighted least-squares analysis.

Plotting data on graph papers was an exercise very common a few years ago, but now as we move on the electronic age, I recommend avoiding this practice because it is not only time wasting, it inevitably results in greater errors and prevents the storage of electronic form of data; the students are again urged to develop as high a level of expertise in Microsoft Excel to begin with. Computer plotting readily provides additional information like error bars, standard deviation bars, and regression coefficients as well the measure of goodness of fit.

7.7 FLOW DIAGRAMS

Flow diagrams are pictorial representations of processes and are used to present relevant process information and data. These can be extremely complex and serve a very useful purpose of summarizing a large volume of data. Figure 8.1 shows a flow diagram of the manufacturing of a recombinant protein. Conditions of experiment as well as outputs recorded can be made part of the flow diagrams. Some flow diagrams are made into decision trees where a certain path is followed if a condition of being true or false arises. Engineering flow diagrams contain extensive details and are routinely used in describing large complex systems.

Questions

1. In statistical analysis, absolute and relative uncertainty exists in the forms of absolute error and relative error. For example, 2.356 ± 0.16 g shows the reading of mass. The uncertainty in this reading is 0.16 g which allows one to judge that this is the actual measuring range by which the reading is uncertain, it is known as the *absolute error*. In the next case, mass is represented by the following expression, $2.356 \pm 1.50\%$ in which the relative error is $\pm 1.50\%$. For the following calculations, follow engineering conventions for significant figures.

   a. Given 2.360 ± 0.56 and 1.420 ± 0.25, find the sum of the two numbers.

   Solution:

   $$(2.360 + 1.420) \pm (0.56 + 0.25) = 3.780 \pm 0.81 = 3.780 \pm 21\%$$

   Answer: $3.780 \pm 21\%$

   b. Given 147 ± 31 gmol/h and 75 ± 13 gmol/h, find the difference between the two numbers.

   Solution:

   $$(147 - 75) \pm (31 + 13) \text{ gmol/h} = 72 \pm 44 \text{ gmol/h} = 72 \text{ gmol/h} \pm 61\%$$

   Answer: 72 gmol/h $\pm 61\%$

   c. Given 0.26 ± 0.012 mol/m^3 and 0.185 ± 0.00756 mol/m^3, find the quotient of the two numbers.

   Solution:

   $$(0.26/0.185) \pm (0.012 + 0.00756) \text{ mol/m}^3 = 1.4 \pm 0.020 \text{ mol/m}^3$$
   $$= 1.4 \text{ mol/m}^3 \pm 1.43\%$$

   Answer: 1.4 mol/m^3 $\pm 1.43\%$

   d. Given 4.56 ± 0.05 g/l and 6.27 ± 0.07 g/l, find the product of the two numbers.

   Solution:

   $$(4.56 \times 6.27) \pm (0.05 + 0.07) \text{ g/l} - 28.59 \pm 0.12 \text{ g/l} = 28.59 \text{ g/l} \pm 0.42\%$$

   Answer: 28.59 g/l $\pm 0.42\%$

2. During fermentation pH is measured at various points of bacterial cells. Six samples are measured with results of 6.17, 6.06, 5.58, 5.45, 6.36, and 6.78.
   a. What is the estimated mean pH of this cycle?
   b. What is the standard deviation of this value?
   c. If 4 more samples were added to the original 6 samples, what would be the mean and standard deviation? Would it change the outcome of the experiment?
   Samples consist of 5.66, 5.97, 6.25, and 6.44.

3. a. During data acquisition, a plot of points is generated on linear graph paper which gives a straight line passing through points (2, 6) and (8, 1.5). Using a plot of y versus x, determine the equation of the line. Use (x_1, y_1) and (x_2, y_2) as a reference coordinate system.

Solution:
The definition of a straight line is represented by the following equation:

$$y = Ax + B$$

A is the slope of the line and is written as

$$A = \frac{(y_2 - y_1)}{(x_2 - x_1)} = \frac{(1.5 - 6)}{(8 - 2)} = \frac{-4.5}{6} = \frac{-3}{4}$$

B is the y-intercept of the line and can be calculated as

$$B = y_1 - Ax_1 = 6 - \left(\frac{-3}{4}\right)(2) = 7.5$$

Therefore, the equation of the straight line is given by $y = -3/4x + 7.5$
Answer: $y = -3/4x + 7.5$

b. A plot of points is generated on linear graph paper which gives a straight line passing through points (2.8, 15.6) and (9.4, 33.5). Use a plot of y versus $x^{1/3}$ to determine the equation of the line.

Solution:
Using the definition of a straight line, the equation is given as

$$y = Ax^{1/3} + B$$

Slope A and y-intercept B are given by

$$A = \frac{y_2 - y_1}{x_2^{1/3} - x_1^{1/3}} = \frac{33.5 - 15.6}{9.4^{1/3} - 2.8^{1/3}} = \frac{17.9}{0.701} = 25.53$$

$$B = y_1 - Ax_1^{1/3} = 15.6 - (25.53)(2.8^{1/3}) = -20.38$$

The equation of the straight line is given by $y = 25.53x^{1/3} - 20.38$
Answer: $y = 25.53x^{1/3} - 20.38$

c. A plot of points is generated on log-log graph paper which gives a straight line passing through points (3, 27) and (525, 2675). Use a plot of y versus x to determine the equation of the line.

Solution:
Using the definition of a straight line, the equation on log log graph paper is given as

$$y = Bx^A$$

or

$$\ln y = \ln B + A\ln x$$

Slope A and y-intercept B are given by

$$A = \frac{(\ln y_2 - \ln y_1)}{(\ln x_2 - \ln x_1)} = \frac{\ln(y_2/y_1)}{\ln(x_2/x_1)} = \frac{\ln 2675 - \ln 27}{\ln 525 - \ln 3} = \frac{\ln(2675/27)}{\ln(525/3)} = \frac{4.596}{5.165} = 0.889$$

$$\ln B = \ln y_1 - A\ln x_1 = \ln(27) - (0.889)\ln(3) = 2.319$$

$$B = e^{2.319} = 10.17$$

The equation of the straight line is given by $y - 10.17x^{0.889}$
Answer: $y = 10.17x^{0.889}$

d. A plot of points is generated on semi-log graph paper which gives a straight line passing through points (1.2, 4.8) and (1.5, 0.065). Use a plot of y versus x to determine the equation of the line.

Solution:
Using the definition of a straight line, the equation on semi-log graph paper is given as

$$y = Be^{Ax}$$

or

$$\ln y = \ln B + Ax$$

Slope A and y-intercept B are given by

$$A = \frac{(\ln y_2 - \ln y_1)}{(\ln x_2 - \ln x_1)} = \frac{\ln(y_2/y_1)}{\ln(x_2 - x_1)} = \frac{\ln 0.065 - \ln 4.8}{1.5 - 1.2} = \frac{\ln(0.065/4.8)}{1.5 - 1.2} = \frac{-4.302}{0.3} = -14.34$$

$$\ln B = \ln y_1 - Ax_1 = \ln(4.8) - (-14.34)(1.2) = 18.77$$

$$B = e^{18.77} = 1.42 \times 10^8$$

The equation of the straight line is given by $y = 1.42 \times 10^8 e^{-14.34x}$
Answer: $y = 1.42 \times 10^8 e^{-14.34x}$

4. Ethanol concentration in a 24-h fermentation broth is measured using a high pressure liquid chromatography. Over the 24-h period, peak areas are measured for five standard ethanol solutions to calibrate the instrument. Each measurement was taken three times for replication purposes. This analysis will help improve the fermentation process to produce the maximum yield of ethanol as a biofuel.

The table below shows the measurements performed during the fermentation process:

Ethanol Concentration (g/l)	Peak Area
4.0	45.55, 52.07, 52.89
13.0	112.65, 113.37, 114.88
19.0	172.05, 174.66, 183.50
25.0	236.48, 236.97, 230.47
33.0	301.80, 303.54, 306.28

a. Determine the mean and standard deviation for the peak areas for each ethanol concentration.
b. Plot the data and show the equation for ethanol concentration as a function of peak area. Show that there is a linear trend with a linear least squares fit of the data.

c. A random sample exhibits a peak area of 125.44. What is the ethanol concentration?

5. Monoclonal antibodies are made by fusing myeloma cells with mouse lymphocytes, thus forming a hybrid cell, *hybridoma*. The concentration of antibodies during continuous culture of hybridoma cells is shown below. Liter per day is used for flow rate and micrograms per milliliter for antibody concentration.

Flow Rate (l/d)	Concentration of Antibodies (µg/ml)
0.12	97.3
0.16	92.1
0.20	86.1
0.22	80.0
0.28	73.8
0.31	65.7
0.39	56.2
0.42	50.3
0.46	47.7
0.51	43.6
0.55	39.9
0.59	31.4
0.62	29.5
0.70	23.3
0.76	19.2
0.79	18.1
0.82	16.2
0.85	15.7
0.93	11.2
1.03	9.6

a. Plot the data points on linear graph paper and determine the *best fit* line using least-squares analysis.

Solution:
The linear least-squares *best fit* line of the data is

$$y = -102.64x + 100.31$$

where:
  y is the concentration of antibodies in µg/ml
  x is the flow rate in l/d

b. Plot the residuals of the antibody concentration versus flow rate after relating the model equation with the actual data. Is there a good fit line for the plotted residuals?

Solution:
Residuals are calculated as the difference between the measured values and the predicted y values obtained from the model equation.

197

Flow Rate (l/d)	Predicted y	Residual
0.12	87.991	9.308
0.16	83.886	8.214
0.2	79.780	6.320
0.22	77.728	2.272
0.28	71.569	2.231
0.31	68.490	−2.790
0.39	60.279	−4.079
0.42	57.120	−6.900
0.46	53.094	−5.394
0.51	47.962	−4.362
0.55	43.857	−3.957
0.59	39.751	−8.351
0.62	36.672	−7.172
0.70	28.461	−5.161
0.76	22.302	−3.102
0.79	19.223	−1.123
0.82	16.144	0.056
0.85	13.065	2.635
0.93	4.854	6.346
1.03	−5.410	15.010

If creating a straight line $y = 0$, the residual values range from being mainly positive, then negative, then positive again while the flow rate increases. Therefore, the residuals are not randomly distributed.

6. Liquid contents in bioreactors are usually mixed by using sparging rods to deliver air into the proprietary disposable bag where the liquid velocity is dependent directly on the gas velocity.

Gas Superficial Velocity, u_G (m/s)	Liquid Superficial Velocity, u_L (m/s)
0.01	0.065
0.02	0.071
0.03	0.078
0.04	0.085
0.05	0.087
0.06	0.088
0.07	0.091
0.08	0.093
0.09	0.097
0.10	0.099

a. Plot the data points on linear graph paper and determine the *best fit* line using least-squares analysis. Is the data fitted well with a linear model?

b. Compare the data on log-log graph paper using the power equation to determine the *best fit* line. Which linear model gives the best results?

7. During a 15-h fermentation period in which sucrose is converted into cellular energy which in turn produces ethanol and carbon dioxide as a by-product, bacterial growth rapidly increases due to yeast under anaerobic conditions. Below are the results of bacterial concentration at each hour of the fermentation process. Plot the data points on linear graph paper and determine the *best fit* line using least-squares analysis. Is the data fitted well with a linear model?

Hours	Cell Concentration (g/l)
0	0
1	0.075
2	0.097
3	0.104
4	0.138
5	0.129
6	0.225
7	0.342
8	0.347
9	0.407
10	0.403
11	0.455
12	0.523
13	0.589
14	0.615
15	0.677

Solution:

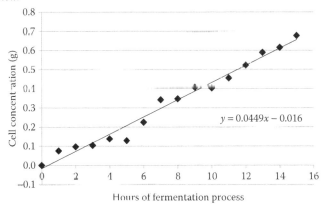

The linear least-squares *best fit* line of the data is

$$y = 0.0449x - 0.016$$

The data are relatively well fitted using the linear model from the measured results.

Section II

Handbook of Bioprocessing

8

Elements of Bioprocessing

LEARNING OBJECTIVES

1. Identify the steps required of a bioprocess.
2. Understand the advantages and disadvantages of possible bioprocessing sterilization procedures.
3. Recognize the different potential bioreactor strategies.
4. Understand the necessary steps required for product concentration and preparation prior to distribution.

8.1 INTRODUCTION

A bioprocess can be divided into the bioreaction section, the upstream processing containing all operations running before the bioreactor step, and the downstream processing with the separation and purification of the product. Figure 8.1 depicts a schematic overview of a general process tree for bioprocesses.

As commonly done in process engineering, we consider unit operations as basic steps in a production process. Typical unit operations in bioprocesses are, for example, sterilization, fermentation, enzymatic reaction, extraction, and filtration or crystallization. A unit procedure we define as a set of operations that take place sequentially in a piece of equipment to adjust pH, and transfer of fermentation broth to another vessel.

8.2 UPSTREAM PROCESSING

Upstream processing includes all unit operations that are necessarily performed before the bioreactor step. Typical upstream steps are the preparation of the medium, the sterilization of the raw materials, and the inoculum preparation.

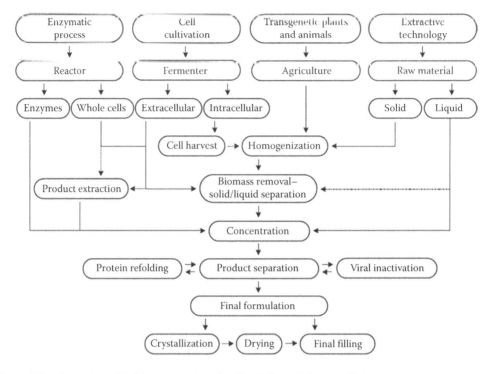

Figure 8.1 General applicable process tree for the different classes of bioprocesses.

8.2.1 Preparation and Storage of Solutions

Mixing and storage operations are used to provide and store solutions that are needed at some point in the process. Examples are the preparation of the medium for the bioreactor or the buffers needed in chromatography. Liquid and solid components are filled in a tank where they are mixed by agitation. After a homogeneous mixture is reached, the solution can be stored in the tank or transferred to a separate storage tank until it is needed in the process. Usually, the material is either sterilized in the tank or in a continuous sterilizer before its use. A decision needs to be made on which materials to store and how much for how long. This decision has a significant impact on the size of the capital investment for storage and the variable cost of materials inventory. It is also an important decision in risk management as it can allow one to absorb process variation in individual unit procedures. If possible, raw material solutions are prepared with high concentrations to keep the volume of the preparation tanks small. The solution then is diluted in the bioreactor by adding sterilized water which might be made continuously and thus is not stored. Usually, carbon and nitrogen sources are prepared in separate tanks to avoid the formation of Maillard or nonenzymatic browning reactions during heat sterilization. The desired volume of the solution has to be defined, for example, 5 m^3 sugar solution, and the composition and the concentration of the components, for example, 400 g/L glucose. The mixing conditions (temperature, agitation, etc.) and the order in which the components are added have to be carefully defined to avoid precipitations. One also identifies the need for automation and process control. The storage conditions might be different from the mixing conditions, particularly with regard to temperature. Especially when using mammalian cell culture, it is necessary to define and validate a maximum storage time for a solution to minimize the risk of contamination or degradation of ingredients.

8.2.2 Sterilization of Input Materials

Input materials are pretreated or sterilized to preclude contamination of the bioreactor. Bacteria and viruses that might be included in the input materials as contaminants are largely destroyed or inactivated. It is important to recognize that inactivation is a probabilistic phenomenon and that one assumes sterile conditions when the possibility of survival of an adventitious agent is less than 10^{-3}. Usually the design is based on the death kinetics of heat-resistant bacterial spores. Sterilization by filtration or by heat is the dominant method used in bioprocesses.

8.2.2.1 Filtration
Gaseous streams are almost exclusively sterilized by filtration. Mostly membrane filters with pore sizes of 0.2–0.3 μm are used. A compressor usually creates the necessary pressure to assure air flow through the membrane filters that retain contaminants. Prefilters are used for dust and other particles. Air filters are also used to remove bioburden from the exhaust gas stream especially to prevent the release of recombinant or pathogenic microorganisms. Product solutions that contain heat-sensitive substances are also filter-sterilized. With the ongoing improvement of membrane filters, the general use of filtration for the sterilization of liquids has increased. In some cases, several consecutive membranes with decreasing pore size are used if there is a high particle load to minimize fouling.

8.2.2.2 Heat Sterilization
Sterilization temperature and exposure time are the key parameters for heat sterilization. The higher the temperature, the lower the sterilization time required to reach the same level of sterilization. Heat sterilization can be done batch-wise or continuously. In batch sterilization, the solution in a tank or the bioreactor is heated most often with steam (in a jacket or sparged directly into the vessel), held at the sterilization temperature for a period of time and then cooling water is used to bring the temperature back to normal operating conditions. Here, often a temperature of 121°C (corresponding to one atmosphere of overpressure) and a holding time of 10 to 20 min are applied. Continuous heat sterilization requires the necessary heat-exchanger network for heating and cooling. However, the time required to sterilize a given volume is much shorter and the energy consumption is up to 80% lower. Although the applied sterilization temperature is higher, usually around 140°C–145°C, heat-sensitive materials are less damaged due to the short exposure time of 120–240 s; this is a consequence of a lower activation energy for thermal degradation than thermal death of bacterial spores. A case, where such sterilization is essential, is the production of riboflavin. In both cases, the heat can be transferred either by direct injection of hot steam into the solution or by indirect heat transfer between the steam and the solution

via a heat exchanger (e.g., the reactor wall or a tube). When the steam is injected directly, the sterilization temperature is reached more quickly. However, this method leads to dilution of the solution resulting from steam condensation. Therefore, the sterilization via a heat exchanger (tubular or plate-and-frame) is more often used, especially in continuous sterilizers. In a bioreactor, steam injection can be useful, if the solution has to be diluted anyway before the inoculation. For injection, the steam has to be appropriately clean. A continuous, countercurrent heat sterilizer typically consists of three heat exchangers. The first heat exchanger heats the cold media using the hot, sterilized media that has been cooled down. The second heat exchanger brings the solution to the sterilization temperature by using steam. The solution then moves through a holding tube. The length of the holding tube is determined by the velocity of the solution and the exposure time necessary for sterilization. Thus, axial dispersion reduces the actual sterilization effect compared to that predicted for plug flow. This axial dispersion has to be considered in the sizing of the heat exchangers. In the following heat exchanger, the hot, already sterilized solution transfers most of its heat to the cold, not yet sterilized, input stream. This step enables the high energy savings compared with batch sterilization to be obtained. The last heat exchanger cools the solution down to the desired exit temperature using cooling water or another cooling agent.

8.2.3 Inoculum Preparation

The inoculum preparation has to provide a sufficient amount of active cells to inoculate the production fermenter. Also called *cell banking system* preserves the strain, for example, in liquid nitrogen, of the cell line that is used in a bioprocess. Each biocatalyst is stored in a large number of vials or ampoules. One vial provides the inoculum for the starter culture of the seed train for each batch. The cells are grown under conditions that enable high cell densities of actively growing cells within a short time. When the cell concentration reaches a certain level, the entire volume is transferred to the second step where it is diluted with fresh medium. This is repeated, sometimes 2–4 more times, until the necessary amount of biomass is available to inoculate the production reactor. The volume factor describes the increase of the volume from one inoculum preparation step to the next. For example, a volume factor of 10 means that the volume of one seed reactor is 10 times larger than that of the preceding seed reactor. Mammalian cell cultures require relatively low volume factors of around 5 to 10, while bacteria and yeast can be prepared with higher volume factors. The volume factor defines the necessary number of inoculum preparation steps. A typical sequence of an animal cell seed train is as follows: (1) T flask, (2) roller bottle, (3) disposable bag bioreactor, (4) first seed reactor, (5) second seed reactor, and finally the production fermenter. The selection of the volume factor will have a significant impact on the size and cost of the seed preparation portion of the plant. The medium's composition and the reaction conditions in the seed train can be different from that of the production stage in order to minimize product formation and to maximize cell growth. For example, mammalian cells can be first grown with serum-containing medium to reach high growth rates. In the last seed reactor, the cells are adapted to serum-free medium that is necessary to minimize the risk of contamination of the final product and to simplify the downstream processing. The modeling of a seed reactor is quite similar to the modeling of the production bioreactor (see Chapter 9).

The carefully planned seed train is important for an optimized scheduling of a process. Especially for processes using mammalian cell culture, the seed train also occupies a considerable amount of the investment and labor costs.

8.2.4 Cleaning-in-Place

After the use of a piece of equipment, cleaning-in-place (CIP) is done to prepare it for the next batch or cycle. The cleaning may be done without removing the equipment or disconnecting it from the process system (in-place). Almost all bioprocess equipment requires CIP operations, often after every batch or cycle. For some consumables such as membranes or chromatographic resins, the harsh cleaning conditions are the main factor that limits their useful life. The empty unit, for example, a reactor, a tank, or a centrifuge, is rinsed with a cleaning agent. The type of cleaning agent, the necessary amount, and the required incubation time have to be defined. A typical CIP sequence is: water—H_3PO_4 (20% w/v)—water—NaOH (5 M)—water. The consumed amount of cleaning agent is either expressed as overall demand, for example, in L or L/m^3, or as a rate such as L/min. The necessary time can be important for the scheduling of the process. The CIP of a unit normally consists of several steps that often run at different temperatures and the whole process can take between a few minutes and a few hours. A typical sequence could be (1) washing with process water, (2) rinsing with a acidic solution, (3) washing with purified water, (4) rinsing with a caustic solution, and (5) washing with purified water.

8.3 BIOREACTOR

8.3.1 Bioreactor Types

8.3.1.1 Stirred Tank Bioreactor

The stirred tank bioreactor is the most commonly used reactor type in bioprocesses. Depending on the complexity of the bioreaction, they range from simple stirred tanks for enzymatic reactions to more sophisticated, aerated fermenters for metabolic bioconversions. The air, usually supplied by a compressor, enters the vessel at the bottom under pressure. The mixing and bubble dispersion are accomplished by mechanical agitation. This requires a relatively high energy input per unit volume. A jacket and/or internal coils allow heating and cooling. The height/diameter quotient varies. The simplest vessels with the smallest surface area per unit volume have a ratio around 1 but in some large-scale fermenters this can exceed 3. For aerated bioreactors, higher ratios are chosen to prolong the contact time between the rising bubbles and the liquid phase.

8.3.1.2 Airlift Bioreactor

In an airlift bioreactor, mixing is achieved without mechanical agitation by the convection caused by the sparged air. Thus, the energy consumption is lower than in a stirred tank reactor. Owing to the low shear levels, airlift bioreactors are used for plant and animal cell culture and for immobilized biocatalysts. The gas is sparged only in one part of the vessel, the so-called riser. The gas holdup and the decreased density of the fluid let the medium move upward in the riser. At the top of the reactor, the bubbles disengage and the now heavier medium moves downward through the nonsparged part of the vessel, the downcomer. The achievable transfer of oxygen is generally lower compared with stirred tank bioreactors.

8.3.1.3 Packed-Bed and Fluidized-Bed Bioreactor

In a packed-bed bioreactor, the immobilized or particulate biocatalyst is filled in a tube-shaped vessel. The medium flows through the column (upward or downward). High velocity of the liquid phase promotes good mass transfer. Compared with a stirred tank reactor, possible particle attrition is small. Often, the medium is recycled and led several times through the column to improve conversion. In this case, an intermediate vessel is needed for storage. The medium flows upward in expanded- or fluidized-bed bioreactors and causes an expansion of the bed at high flow rates. The biocatalyst particles need to have an appropriate size and density. Since the particles are in constant motion, channeling and clogging are avoided.

8.3.2 Unit Procedures

The bioreactor is the core of the flow sheet where the conversion of raw materials to desired product takes place. To run the bioreactor, a number of unit procedures are routinely carried out.

8.3.2.1 Filling and Transfer of Materials in Vessels

These operations are used to bring materials (liquids, solids) into the bioreactor and to transfer parts or the whole reactor volume to the next unit operation at the end of the bioreaction. The parameters that have to be defined for the filling are mass or volume of the input and its composition, or alternatively the concentration of a newly fed substance in the partially filled reactor. For filling and transfer, the duration of the operation should be specified, either by setting the overall filling time or by defining a filling rate, for example, kg/min, to a vessel of known volume. A bioreactor is usually filled up to only 70% or 90% of its overall volume to keep some headspace for foam buildup and the volume increase caused by aeration and subsequent substrate feeding. Additionally, the disengagement of droplets from the exhaust air in the headspace is attempted. The volume that is actually used is called the *working volume of a reactor*.

8.3.2.2 Agitation

A bioreactor is agitated to achieve and maintain homogeneity, to enable efficient heat transfer, and, in the case of an aerated fermentation, for the uniform distribution of the gas phase and gas–liquid mass transfer. An agitator rotates by consuming electrical energy and keeps the fermenter content in motion. Key parameters are the energy demand, expressed either as overall consumption (kW) or as specific consumption (kW/m³), the agitation or mixing time, and sometimes the impeller speed in revolutions per minutes (rpm). Usually, the agitator runs during most of the reaction time of the bioreactor. The energy consumption depends on the rotational speed and the geometry of the agitator, the working volume of the bioreactor, fluid density and viscosity, and baffling of the reactor. Additional equipments

Table 8.1 Average Values of Typical Energy Consumption Steps, Referred to 1 m³ Aqueous Solution

Consumption Step	Energy Demand (MJ)	Energy-Transfer Agent	Average Cost ($)
Heat by 10°C	46.4	Steam (22 kg)	0.10
Cool by 10°C	−46.4	Cooling water (740 kg)	0.06
Agitate for 10 h	32	Electricity (9 kWh)	0.40–0.70
Evaporate	2,510	Steam (1,105 kg)	3.20
Condense	−2,510	Cooling water (40 m³)	3.20
Centrifuge	72	Electricity (20 kWh)	0.90–1.50

Note: For all, an efficiency factor of $\eta = 0.9$ is assumed. Evaporate and condensate consider the energy demand to vaporize water at 100°C to steam at 100°C, and vice versa, respectively. Assumption for cooling water: $\Delta T = 15°C$; assumption for input power agitator: 0.8 kW/m³.

inside the reactor, such as heating coils or thermometer pipes, have a baffling effect and can therefore increase the demand. The specific energy consumption of a bioreactor lies typically between 0.2 and 3.0 kW/m³. At the same stirring rate, aerated fermenters have a lower consumption than do unaerated bioreactors. A good average value is 0.8 kW/m³ (see Table 8.1). The plain mixing of liquids, for example, in the medium's preparation, requires usually around 0.2–0.5 kW/m³.

8.3.2.3 Aeration

The aeration provides oxygen to meet the aerobic demand of the cells during the fermentation and removes gaseous by-product, mainly carbon dioxide. The aeration is specified by the gas used and the aeration rate. Owing to its low cost, air is used in industrial bioprocesses. However, also pure oxygen, pure nitrogen, or air enriched with oxygen or carbon dioxide can be used. The aeration rate typically lies between 0.1 and 2 volume of gas (under atmospheric pressure) per volume of solution per minute (vvm). In large bioreactors, the air utilization is more efficient. Here, a good average aeration rate is 0.5 vvm, while in smaller reactors, the average rate is around 1 vvm. The aeration rate also can vary during the fermentation, for example, when the biomass concentration increases. For citric acid fermentation, a starting rate of 0.1 vvm that is stepwise increased to 0.5–1.0 vvm.

8.3.2.4 Heat Transfer

Heat-transfer operations are necessary to change and control the temperature of the bioreactor, or to keep the temperature constant while exothermic reactions take place in the fermenter. In the case of heating, the heat is transferred from a heat-transfer fluid via a heat-transfer surface to the reactor content or in the case of cooling from the fermenter content to the cooling fluid. Steam is usually used for heating. The heating rate depends on the bioreactor volume, typically at 1.5°C–3.0°C/min for a 10 m³ reactor and at 1°C–2°C/min for a 50 m³ reactor. Commonly used cooling agents are cooling water (around 20°C), chilled water (5°C), or for lower temperatures Freon, glycol, sodium chloride brine, or calcium chloride brine. The final temperature of the cooling agent should be at least 5°C–40°C below the final temperature of the cooled liquid. The heat Q (J) necessary to heat up or cool down a substance i with mass m_i (kg) and specific heat capacity $c_{p,i}$ (J/kg K) from a starting temperature $T0$ to an end temperature $T1$ (temperature change ΔT [K]) is

$$Q = m_i \cdot c_{p,i} \cdot (T0 - T1) = m_i \cdot c_{p,i} \cdot \Delta T \tag{8.1}$$

For a mixture of substances, a good approximation is

$$Q = \sum m_i \cdot c_{p,i} \cdot \Delta T \tag{8.2}$$

In cases where specific heat capacities are not available for all compounds, the heat capacity of water is used as an approximation. In heating operations, steam is the heat-transfer agent. It condenses on the heat-transfer surface without changing its temperature. The heat of condensation is

$$Q = m_S \cdot h_C \tag{8.3}$$

where:
   m_S is the amount of steam (kg)
   h_C is the condensation enthalpy (J/kg)

The condensation enthalpy of steam at 150°C is 2,115 kJ/kg. The necessary amount can be calculated by combining Equations 8.3 and 8.4.

$$Q = \frac{\sum m_i \cdot c_{p,i} \cdot \Delta T}{(\eta - h_C)} \tag{8.4}$$

Thereby the efficiency number η is introduced to the equation to consider heat losses, with $\eta = 0.9$ as a good average. In cooling operations, the heat transported by the cooling agent is

$$Q = m_c \cdot c_{p,c} \left(T_{c,1,av} - T_{c,0} \right) = m_c \cdot c_{p,c} \cdot \Delta T_{c,av} \tag{8.5}$$

where:
   $c_{p,c}$ is the heat capacity of the cooling agent (J/kg K)
   $T_{c,0}$ is the starting temperature of the cooling agent (K)
   $T_{c,1,av}$ is the the average final temperature (K)
   $\Delta T_{c,av}$ is the the average temperature change of the cooling agent (K)

By combining Equations 8.4 and 8.5, the necessary amount of cooling agent can be calculated by:

$$m_c = \frac{\sum m_i \cdot c_{p,i} \cdot \Delta T}{\eta \cdot c_{p,c} \cdot \Delta T_{c,av}} \tag{8.6}$$

Batch cooling, for example, in a jacketed vessel, involves an unsteady heat transfer. That means the temperature difference between the cooling agent and the vessel content varies along the heat-transfer surface and at every point of the surface over time.

However, the heat-transfer rate is proportional to this temperature difference and the heat removed by the cooling agent decreases with a decreasing difference during the cooling operation. Assuming a constant flow rate, the final temperature of the cooling agent decreases during the operation. For a first estimation, it is sufficient to define an average temperature change of the cooling agent. Table 8.1 gives examples for the consumption of heating and cooling steps.

8.3.2.5 Foam Control
The combination of agitation and aeration with the presence of foam-producing and foam-stabilizing substances such as proteins, polysaccharides, and fatty acids can lead to substantial foam formation in the bioreactor. Particularly, aerobic fermentations with complex media tend to have significant foam formation. An overflow of foam can cause blocking of outlet gas lines and filters, a loss of fermenter content, and provide a route for contamination. The foam buildup can be controlled chemically or mechanically. The addition of antifoam agents, usually surface-tension-lowering substances, can deal with even highly foaming cultures. However, they also reduce the oxygen transfer to the cells. Mechanical foam breakers destroy the foam bubbles, for example, by using a disk rotating at high speed at the top of the vessel. Mechanical devices are only efficient for moderately foaming fermentations, and for large bioreactors, they can cause prohibitively high energy consumption. Therefore, the use of chemical antifoam agents often cannot be avoided. The foam problem increases with the fermenter size and cannot be easily predicted. Antifoam agents often have negative impact on oxygen transfer rates and on downstream processes by fouling of membranes.

8.3.2.6 pH Control
Many bioreactions and biocatalysts require a constant pH. In industrial processes, the medium is buffered and pH is adjusted and maintained by adding acids or bases to the bioreactor. If the necessary amounts are not known from experimental data, they can be estimated from the ion-charge balance for the reactor. The sum of the positive charges of the cations is always equal to the sum of the negative charges of the anions. The equation is solved for the ion that is used for pH regulation. For example, if HCl is used, the equation is solved for the chloride concentration. The following equation shows the ion-charge balance of a fermentation producing pyruvic acid where ammonia is used (Ac = acetate, Pyr = pyruvate).

$$\left[NH^{+3} \right] = \left[OH^- \right] + \left[Ac^- \right] + \left[Pyr^- \right] + \left[Cl^- \right] + 2\left[SO_2^{-4} \right] + \left[HSO_2^{-4} \right] + 3\left[PO_3^{-4} \right]$$
$$+2\left[HPO_3^{-4} \right] + \left[H_2PO_3^{-4} \right] - \left[H^+ \right] - \left[Na^+ \right] - \left[K^+ \right] - 2\left[Mg^{2+} \right]$$

(8.7)

The concentrations of the added salts, acids, and bases are usually known. The H^+ and OH^- concentrations at the desired pH are also known. The dissociated and nondissociated parts of an acid, especially weak acids and bases, and the degree of dissociation can be calculated using the following equation:

$$\left[H_{n-L} -_L A^{L-} \right] = \frac{[H^+]^{n-L} \cdot [A]_{tot} \cdot \Pi_{q=0}^L K_{Aq}}{\sum_{m=0}^n \left\{ [H^+]^{n-m} \cdot \Pi_{q=0}^L K_{Aq} \right\}} \text{ with } K_{A0} = 1$$

(8.8)

where:

n is the number of acidic protons

L is the number of dissociated protons

K_{Aq} is the acidity constant of each species

$[A]_{tot}$ is the total concentration of the acid

At pH 7, 99.4% of acetic acid is dissociated ($pK_a = 4.75$).

$$\left[Ac^- \right] = \frac{K_{Ac} \cdot \left[Ac^- \right]_{[tot]}}{\left[H^+ \right] + K_{Ac}} \rightarrow [Ac^-] = \frac{10^{-4.75} \cdot [Ac^-]_{[tot]}}{10^{-7} + 10^{-4.75}} \rightarrow \left[Ac^- \right]$$

$$= 0.99441 \cdot \left[HAc \right]_{[tot]}$$

(8.9)

After the concentrations of all ions are calculated, the necessary amount of acid or base to reach the desired pH can be estimated from the ion-charge balance.

8.3.2.7 Cleaning-in-Place

A bioreactor has to be cleaned after every batch. A typical CIP procedure was presented earlier in Section 8.2.4.

8.4 DOWNSTREAM PROCESSING

In this section, we provide an overview of the downstream unit operations regularly used in bioprocesses. The reader should understand the basic principles and purpose of each unit. This is important for design of the process flow scheme, specification of operating parameters, and subsequent modeling. However, for a deeper understanding of these units and their key parameters the students are referred to textbooks on the subject listed in the bibliography section. All unit operations in downstream processing use one or several differences in the chemical and physical properties of the desired product from other materials in the often complex mixture. Table 8.2 provides an overview of the separation principles of the most regularly used unit operations and the yields that are typically observed. Production methods for bulk chemicals, fine chemicals, and pharmaceuticals differ in the complexity of their downstream processing. This causes differences in overall yield of separation and purification (see Table 8.2). In general, downstream processing is always a tradeoff between yield and purity. High purity is usually paid for with low yield and vice versa. Therefore, one should define early in downstream process design how pure the product needs to be. It is important to realize that downstream processing methods are highly dependent on the bioreaction and upstream steps. High concentrations of the product and low concentrations of by-products and residual substances are always beneficial. The first step of downstream processing is the deliberate selection of the raw materials used in the bioreactor.

Here, a lower product concentration from the bioreaction may be economically favorable if it allows a simplified downstream process. Every additional separation and purification step means additional capital and operating costs and an additional product loss.

Table 8.2 Separation Principles of the Separation Methods Regularly Used in Bioprocesses

Method	Separation Principle	Typical Yield (%)	Separated Product
Centrifugation	Specific density	90–99	Cells and particles
Sedimentation	Specific density	80–99	Cells and particles
Microfiltration	Size/phase	80–99	Cells and particles
Ultrafiltration	Size		Cell debris, proteins, and polymers
Chromatography		60–99	
Gel filtration	Size/phase		Large molecules
Ion exchange	Ionic change		Ions
Hydrophobic interaction	Hydrophobicity		Hydrophilic or hydrophobic molecules
Reversed phase	Hydrophobicity/ diffusivity-specific binding		Hydrophilic or hydrophobic molecules
Affinity	Molecular recognition		Molecules with specific epitopes
Electrodialysis	Ionic charge/diffusivity	70–99	Ions
Extraction	Solubility/phase affinity	70–99	Hydrophilic or hydrophobic molecules
Distillation	Volatility	80–99	Volatiles
Drying/evaporation	Volatility	97–99	High-boiling molecules
Crystallization	Phase change	60–95	Crystallized solids

Therefore, as a general principle the number of downstream steps should be kept to a minimum to meet target purity as well as process robustness. Often, different unit operations can be used to achieve a separation. To select the most appropriate alternative, many characteristics of the unit operations have to be considered such as purity/selectivity, yield, operating cost, necessary investment cost, possible denaturation of product, process robustness, separation conditions, and product concentration after the step

8.4.1 Biomass Removal

In most bioprocesses using cells, the first downstream step is the separation of the biomass from the fermentation broth. There are several unit operations available for this purpose. Widely used are centrifugation, microfiltration, rotary vacuum filtration, and decanting/ sedimentation. These unit operations are described in the Sections 8.4.4.1 through 8.4.4.4. The choice of method for a given process depends on a number of parameters. The concentration, particle size, and density of the biomass and the density and viscosity of the broth determine design, scale of operation, and operating conditions. For small particles such as bacteria or yeast cells, centrifuges or membrane filtration is often the most efficient. The necessary time for the separation, the required yield of removal, the possible

213

degradation or denaturation of the product, and the investment and operating costs of the unit have to be considered as well. In many cases, prior experience with or ownership of a piece of equipment influences the decision.

8.4.2 Homogenization/Cell Disruption

If the product is intracellular, it is necessary to break open the cells to release the product into the solution before further purification. The available techniques include mechanical and nonmechanical methods such as enzymatic digestion of the cell wall, treatment with solvents and detergents, freezing and thawing, and osmotic shock. Most often used are high-pressure homogenization and mechanical bead milling. In the high-pressure homogenization, the slurry is pumped through a narrow valve at a very high pressure (up to 1,200 bar). The large pressure drop behind the valve causes strong shear forces that lead to a disruption of the cells. Often several passes through a homogenizer are necessary to recover the product. The shear forces can lead to denaturation of intracellular proteins. In the mechanical bead mill homogenization, the slurry is fed to a chamber with a rapidly rotating stirrer filled with steel or glass bead, or other abrasives. High shear forces and impact during the grinding cause cell disruption.

8.4.3 Concentration

After the bioreaction, the product concentration is usually relatively low. It may be reasonable to have first a concentration step to reduce the volume of the product stream that has to be processed through the subsequent units and thus reducing equipment size and energy consumption of these units. There are three methods available for this purpose.

8.4.3.1 Partial Evaporation of the Solvent
The solution is heated up to vaporize some of the solvent, usually water. This method requires a heat-stable product with a low vapor pressure to keep the product loss small and causes high energy costs. At reduced pressure, evaporation is possible at lower temperature but vacuum equipment is required.

8.4.3.2 Filtration
A semipermeable membrane retains the product in the retentate but transfers most of the solvent through the membrane. This step can also remove some impurities with a lower molecule size. This is most useful for harvesting large molecules such as proteins. Energy for maintaining the pressure for the mass transfer is necessary.

8.4.3.3 Precipitation
The product is precipitated by adding a precipitation agent or by changing chemical or physical conditions (temperature, pH, etc.) and is subsequently separated by filtration or centrifugation. Costs incurred for the precipitation agent and the separation of the solid product. This method requires a product that can be easily and selectively precipitated without degradation and is especially useful when several impurities can be separated that do not precipitate.

8.4.4 Phase Separation

As a rule, the simplest separation should be applied first. Therefore, many downstream processes start with the separation of the different phases that leave the bioreactor. Furthermore, phase separations are often used later in the process as well. They include centrifugation, filtration, sedimentation, and condensation steps.

8.4.4.1 Centrifugation

Centrifugation is based on density differences between solid particles and a solution or between two immiscible liquids. The sedimentation force is amplified by the particle or drop size in a centrifugal field in the centrifuge. In many bioprocesses, centrifugation is used for biomass removal and solid separation. Disk-stack centrifuges are applied most often, but also basket and tubular bowl centrifuges are used. Sometimes a pretreatment is necessary, for example, heating, pH change, or addition of filter aids (see also Table 8.2), to increase particle size. The maximum throughput of a centrifuge is defined by the sigma factor and the settling velocity. The sigma factor describes the centrifuge in terms of an equivalent area referenced to a settling tank and is the basis for scaling the centrifuge. It is expressed in m^2 and equals the area of a sedimentation tank that would be necessary to realize the same separation work. The settling velocity is specific for the feed that has to be separated. It is determined by the size and density of the particles (e.g., the average cell size lies between 0.5 and 5 µm) and the density and viscosity of the solution. The best separation is realized at low viscosity, for large particles, and large density differences. For most biological materials, the density difference with water is usually small.

8.4.4.2 Filtration

Filtration is used to separate particles or large molecules from a suspension or solution. A semipermeable membrane splits the components according to their size. The permeate includes most of the solvent and small molecules that pass through the membrane. The retentate is a concentrate of the particles and large molecules that are retained by the membrane. Pressure is the driving force for flow through the membrane. Filtration is used for biomass and cell debris removal, concentration of product solutions, and sterile filtration of final product solutions. The different filter types vary in their pore sizes. Microfilters have a pore size of 0.1–10 µm. They are used to retain particles. Ultrafiltration uses pore sizes of 0.001–0.1 µm and keeps back large molecules like proteins, peptides, and other large, dissolved molecules. The molecular weight cutoff of a membrane is the molecular weight of a globular protein that is 90% retained. It determines the retention (or rejection) of a molecule that lies between 0% and 100%. Further unit parameters are the concentration factor (quotient feed/retentate) and the filtrate flux through the membrane. Depending on the particle concentration and viscosity of the feed, the flux typically lies between 20 and 250 L/m^2 h for microfiltration and between 20 and 100 L/m^2 h for ultrafiltration. According to their flow pattern, one distinguishes dead-end and cross-flow filtrations. In dead-end filtration, the particles are retained as a cake through which solvents must pass. Thus, the pressure drop increases with solids' accumulation. In cross-flow filtration, the feed is moved tangentially along the membrane to reduce concentration polarization or filter-cake thickness and associated pressure drop. The particles are obtained as concentrated slurry. Rotary vacuum filtration is used only for large-scale filtration with large particles. Here, the mass transfer through the membrane is caused by the pressure difference between outside ambient pressure and vacuum inside the drum at the permeate side of the membrane. A horizontal drum, covered with the membrane, is partly submerged in a tank that is filled with the feed slurry. During the filtration, the particles accumulate on the surface of the membrane outside the drum. The drum slowly rotates and the cake is mechanically removed when the membrane is outside the feed solution. This approach is taken for biomass removal in large-volume fermentation processes with filamentous fungi. Diafiltration is used to change the buffer solution. The solvent and the components of the old buffer are transported through the membrane, while the desired (larger) product is retained. At the same time, a new buffer is added continuously or stepwise to the feed, resulting in a complete buffer change after a certain time period.

8.4.4.3 Sedimentation and Decanting

Sedimentation and decanting, like centrifugation, utilize the density differences of substances. In contrast to a centrifuge, only gravity is the driving force. Therefore, sedimentation needs a longer settling time and larger density difference and particle size of the substances than does centrifugation. Sedimentation is applied for large-scale biomass removal mostly in wastewater treatment. Flocculating agents can be added to enhance the sedimentation rate by increasing particle size. Decanting is used for the separation of liquid phases, for example, water and organic solvent. Three layers are usually formed: the solid or heavy liquid phase at the bottom, the light liquid phase on top, and a dispersion phase in between. The key parameters are density and viscosity of the two phases. They determine the settling velocity of the heavy phase and thus the necessary settling time and consequently the required tank size. The residence time lies typically between 5 and 10 min.

8.4.4.4 Condensation

In condensation, vapor is condensed into liquid by cooling. Condensation is used to liquefy the distillate in distillation (e.g., in product separation or solvent recycling) and to turn vaporized steam to liquid water after a crystallization or concentration step. A typical condenser is a shell-and-tube surface condenser. Here, the coolant flows in the tube while the condensation of the vapor occurs at the shell side. Heat is transferred from the vapor through the tube wall to the cooling agent, typically cooling water (see also Table 8.1). Heat of vaporization, boiling point, and partition coefficient of the vapor components are the key parameters. The partition coefficient of a condensation describes the mole fraction of a component in the gaseous and the liquid phase. The initial temperature and the temperature change of the cooling agent are also important and can be economically optimized (see, e.g.,). All these parameters, together with the heat-transfer coefficient of the system, determine the necessary heat-transfer area and thus the equipment size. For the system steam and cooling water, a heat-transfer coefficient of 2,000 kcal/h m^2 °C (2,325 J/s m^2 K) is a typical value.

8.4.5 Product Separation and Purification

Following solids removal, the target product is further separated from impurities and purified to meet predetermined specifications. The most often applied unit operations include extraction, adsorption, chromatography, electrodialysis, and distillation.

8.4.5.1 Extraction

In an extraction step, a molecule is separated from a solution by transferring it to another liquid phase. The separation is based on the different solubilities of the product and the impurities in the feed phase, for example, an aqueous solution and an organic extract solvent phase, and thus the selective partitioning of the product and impurities in the two liquid phases. Extraction is applied in the purification of antibiotics and organic acids and even occasionally proteins. It is regularly used when the product concentration is comparably low or when distillation cannot be applied. The simplest extraction equipment is the so-called mixer/settler. Here, the two liquid phases are mixed in a tank to enable the transfer across the phase boundaries of the product and then a sufficient time is allowed until the phases are separated. However, more often used are differential extraction columns that work continuously with countercurrent liquid flows and consist of several stages or a centrifugal extractor. Here, the heavy phase, usually the aqueous solution, is added at the top of the column and the light phase, normally an organic solvent, is added at the bottom and moves upward. Special equipment is used to disperse the solvent into small droplets that flow through the continuous phase to enable a maximum mass transfer. The density differences of the phases determine upward and downward velocities. A centrifugal extractor often used in antibiotic purification works in principle like a centrifuge. The density differences are amplified by the centrifugal force. The key parameter of an extraction is the partition coefficient. It is defined as the equilibrium concentration of a substance in the extract phase divided by its concentration in the feed phase. The partition coefficient finally determines the product loss of the step. It is usually strongly influenced by temperature, ionic strength, and pH. The maximum solubility of the product in the extract phase and the solubility of the solvents in each other are also important parameters. Since the volume of the extract phase is usually smaller, the extraction also leads to an increase of the product concentration.

8.4.5.2 Distillation

Differences in the volatilities of substances are prerequisites for distillation. Typically, the feed is preheated and enters a continuous distillation column that consists of several (theoretical) stages. The volatile compounds evaporate and the vapor moves upward and leaves the column at the top as distillate. The high-boiling compounds remain in the liquid phase, move downward, and leave the column at the bottom. The distillate is liquefied in a condenser. Parts of the distillate can be recycled to the column to improve separation. A sequence of columns that work at different temperatures can be used when more than one volatile fraction has to be separated. Distillation is an alternative to extraction and adsorption. It is extensively used in the chemical, especially the petrochemical, industries. In bioprocesses, it is employed for the purification of large-volume, low-boiling products such as ethanol and other alcohols. Distillation requires heat stability of the product. The boiling point of the substances and the linear velocity of the vapor are the key parameters. At a smaller scale, also batch distillation is applied. For a crude separation, a so-called flash distillation can be used that consists of only one stage. Distillation is frequently applied for the recovery of organic solvents used in downstream processing.

8.4.5.3 Electrodialysis

In electrodialysis, an electromotive force is used to transport ions through a semipermeable, ion-selective membrane by ion diffusion and thus separate them from an aqueous solution. From the feed, the cations move through a cation membrane into the supplied acid stream. Additionally, or alternatively, the anions move through an anion membrane into the supplied base stream. The remaining stream is the diluate. Electrodialysis is applied for the purification of organic acids, for example, lactic acid (see also Chapter 6). Key parameters are the membrane flux and the transport number. The membrane flux is typically between 100 and 300 g/m^2 h. The transport number is the ratio of the flux of the desired ion and the flux of all ions through the membrane. The product concentration in the acid or base stream can be up to 5 molar.

8.4.5.4 Adsorption

Adsorption is used to retain either the product or impurities on a solid matrix. The solution is led through a column where the target molecules bind to the resin. If impurities are retained, they are immediately eluted from the column with a buffer. If the product is retained, usually a washing step is added in between. The column can be operated as a packed-bed or an expanded bed. Several columns are often used to enable a quasi-continuous processing. Key parameters are the binding capacity and selectivity of the resin, the binding yield of the target and nontarget molecules, and the volume of the eluant. The performance is usually influenced by parameters such as pH and temperature. High recovery yield can be realized with adsorption columns (e.g., 70%–90%), even at quite low product concentrations. Adsorption columns are used, for example, in the purification of vitamins and cyclodextrins (see Chapter 9). A special application is the use of activated carbon for decolorization of liquids.

8.4.5.5 Chromatography

Chromatography is used to resolve and fractionate a mixture of compounds based on differential migration, that is, the selective retardation of solutes during the passage through a chromatography column. The basic principles are identical to purification by adsorption. The solvent (mobile phase) flows through a bed of resin particles (stationary phase), and the solutes travel at different speeds depending on their relative affinity for the resin. Thus, they appear at different times at the column outflow, either directly after the load of the column or the product initially remains retained by the resin and is later eluted with an eluant. Before the elution step, a buffer is used to displace the void fraction of the column. After the elution, a buffer is applied for regeneration and equilibration of the column. The elution is carried out either isocratically or by gradient elution. In an isocratic elution, the composition of the elution buffer is kept constant. In a gradient elution, the composition of the eluant, for example, the salt concentration, is changed continuously or stepwise to improve the fractionation of the attached molecules. The portion of the output stream that contains the desired product is separated from the residual that ideally contains most of the impurities. Several forms of chromatography can be specified. They differ in the mechanism by which the desired substances are retarded or retained in the column; thus, the chemical or physical property differences are exploited to fractionate a mixture. In bioprocesses, five types commonly used are as follows:

1. Gel or exclusion chromatography with molecular sieving that separates molecules according to their size. The column is packed with gel particles of a defined porosity. Large molecules cannot enter these pores and are eluted first, while smaller molecules enter the pores at a rate that is inversely proportional to their size, which increases their elution time. Gel filtration is often used as a polishing step at the end of protein purification. Its capacity is typically low but its resolving power is high.

2. In affinity chromatography, the separation is based on the stereoselective binding of the solute to immobilized molecules, the so-called ligand. The target molecules are retained in the column and then eluted by a change of pH, ionic strength, or buffer composition. Affinity chromatography is highly selective. Examples are the purification of monoclonal antibodies using a protein A ligand or the purification of a recombinant therapeutic protein using a monoclonal antibody as ligand.

3. Ion-exchange chromatography uses the electrostatic attraction between the target molecule that is charged at the given pH and the charged resin. The product is first retained and then eluted by changing the pH or the ionic strength, often using a gradient elution.

4. Hydrophobic interaction chromatography is mainly used for the separation of proteins. Differences in their hydrophobicity are caused by the amino acids exposed at the surface of the molecule. Hydrophobic interaction chromatography uses hydrophobic interactions between the solute and the resin to separate the substances. The product is eluted by a reduction of the (hydrophilic) salt concentration of the mobile phase.

5. Separation in reversed-phase chromatography is based on the uneven distribution of the solutes between two immiscible liquid phases. The less polar of the two solvents is fixed on the column and provides the stationary phase. Such stationary phases are hydrophobic alkyl chains, typically C4, C8, and C18. The column is loaded by applying an aqueous solution. The elution is based on an increase in the concentration of hydrophobic, organic solvents in the mobile phase and occurs in the order of hydrophobicity of the substances, with the most hydrophobic substance at the end. Here, methanol and acetonitrile are often used. Chromatography can be operated in a packed-bed or in an expanded bed column. Key parameters are the binding capacity of the resin, the flow rate of the mobile phase through the column, the specific binding of components to the resin, the necessary volume of eluant, and the volume of the product fraction. Chromatography is used, for example, in the purification of pharmaceuticals, mainly proteins. Since it is usually more expensive than extraction, distillation, or filtration methods, it is mainly used for high-price products.

8.4.6 Viral Inactivation

In the production of pharmaceuticals, inactivation of pathogenic bacteria, viruses, and prions that might occur as contaminants or impurities in the product is necessary. Particular attention is paid to viral inactivation when the product is derived from mammalian cell culture, blood plasma, or transgenic animals. An efficient inactivation step must reduce the concentration of active viruses by greater than 10^6 orders of magnitude. To meet the regulatory requirements, usually a combination of methods is necessary because none of the known methods inactivates all possible contaminants. Standard purification steps like extraction, filtration, and chromatography already lead to marked virus reduction. Additional steps, explicitly designed for virus reduction and applied at different points in the flow sheet, include the following:

1. Micro- and ultrafiltration (not sufficient for small viruses).
2. Heat—either continuous (high temperature, short time) or batch (lower temperature, longer time).
3. UV radiation.
4. Chemical substances, for example, with a high acid or base concentration. The methods are very similar to the methods used for the sterilization of raw materials. However, therapeutic proteins are very sensitive to such treatments. The optimal choice for the process is a combination of methods that guarantee a sufficient viral reduction and keep the denaturation of the protein product, and thus the activity loss, at a minimum.

8.4.7 Protein Solubilization and Refolding

Heterologous proteins produced in bacteria and fungi often form inclusion bodies or water-insoluble pellets inside the cell. While their primary structure, the amino acid sequence, and often also secondary structures are correct, their three-dimensional structure is usually incorrect. Therefore, they are biologically inactive. They are precipitated in a relatively pure form as inclusion bodies. It is, however, possible to solubilize and refold the proteins to their active form. At the end of a cultivation process, the cells are inactivated and separated from the broth, for example, by centrifugation. Then, the cells are disrupted to release the intracellular material and inclusion bodies. In the next step, inclusion bodies are isolated, usually by centrifugation. The inclusion bodies are recovered in the heavy phase, while most of the cell debris remains in the light phase. The inclusion body sludge is washed often while applying mild detergent, for example, Triton-X100, to remove lipids, proteins, and other impurities. In the next step, the pellets are dissolved by adding high concentration of chaotropic reagents such as urea or guanidine hydrochloride and detergents such as sodium dodecyl sulfate. Additionally, reducing agents like 2-mercaptoethanol or dithiothreitol are applied to reduce disulfide bridges. Chelating agents such as ethylenediaminetetraacetic acid are added to prevent metal-catalyzed oxidation of cysteines and methionines. By disruption of disulfide and noncovalent bonds, the proteins are unfolded and dissolved in the buffer. Mild dissolution allows retention of secondary structures intact and thus improving subsequent refolding. In the next step, the concentration of the denaturants is substantially reduced. Different methods to do this are possible, for example, dilution, electrodialysis, or diafiltration. At low concentrations of the denaturant, the proteins can refold to their native form and be further purified. Low concentration of proteins promotes the fidelity of the refolding, whereas at high concentration the formation of aggregates is favored. A successful strategy is the slow addition of solubilized protein to the renaturation buffer. This keeps the concentration of unfolded protein low and the renatured protein does not form new aggregates.

8.4.8 Final Product Processing

After most of the impurities have been removed from the product solution, the product has to be prepared for final formulation. This can include crystallization, stabilization, drying, and final formulation with materials to assure stability.

8.4.8.1 Crystallization

In a crystallization step, the desired product is converted from its soluble form into its crystallized (solid) form. After crystallization, the crystals are separated from the liquid solution, for example, by filtration. The mother liquor is often recycled to the crystallization tank to increase the yield. Crystallization is usually done at the very end of the downstream processing when only a very few impurities remain. However, crystallization also can be used as a first purification step right after the bioreaction if other components of the broth do not precipitate and are not incorporated into the crystals. Crystallization is initiated either by a volume reduction of the solution or by reducing the solubility of the target molecules by the addition of a crystallizing agent, or by changing the physical or chemical conditions (pH, temperature, etc.). Often, crystallization is a combination of both approaches. Key parameters are the crystallization yield, the crystallization heat, and the necessary residence time. The purity and shape of crystals are dependent on many parameters including rate of crystallization. Crystallization is difficult to predict and to scale up. Therefore, well-designed experiments to map the experimental space are very important.

8.4.8.2 Product Stabilization

For products such as therapeutic proteins, it is necessary to stabilize the product to avoid premature degradation or denaturation. The shelf life of the product is usually extended by the addition of stabilizing agents or a complete buffer exchange before final filling into vials.

8.4.8.3 Drying

In a drying operation, water or another solvent is removed from a solid product. It is commonly used if the product is to be sold as powder. Two classes of dryers are used: contact dryers and convection dryers. For instance, in a drum dryer, an example of a contact dryer, the heat necessary to vaporize the water is provided via the drum wall from hot water, air, or steam that flows at the outer side of the wall. The drying agent and the product do not come into direct contact. Convection dryers are used more often. Here, the preheated drying gas is mixed with the solid and the solvent evaporates into the drying gas. Fluidized-bed and spray dryers are regularly used in bioprocesses. Both are characterized by a short residence time. In a spray dryer, the feed is sprayed as small droplets into a stream of hot gas. In a fluidized-bed dryer, the wet solid is transported through the dryer and is fluidized by the drying gas that is led in cross flow through the powder. The discharged air is usually saturated with solvent vapor. The specific air consumption depends on the exit temperature of the drying gas. At 50°C, typically 13 kg of air is required per kg of evaporated water, at 70°C around 5 kg/kg. A gentle way to dry heat-sensitive products, like proteins and vitamins, is freeze-drying, also known as *lyophilization*. In a first step, the wet product is frozen. The frozen material is introduced into a vacuum chamber and water starts to sublime. Owing to the heat required for sublimation, sublimation is usually accelerated by controlled heating.

8.4.8.4 Filling, Labeling, and Packing

The final step of a process is to get the product ready for the customer or patient. This part can be readily considered in a process model. It should be included if enough information is available as to how the product is formulated and packed, and if the product is traded as discrete entities. Then, the price of a pharmaceutical is quoted as $/100 vials or similar. In the filling step, the product is filled in containers of a defined volume. Labels are attached in the labeling steps, and they are put into boxes or on a pallet in the final packaging step.

8.4.9 Waste Treatment: Reduction and Recycling

Waste treatment is an important operation in today's industrial processes and requires compliance with the local Occupational Safety and Health Administration requirements as well as compliance with National Institutes of Health Guidelines for the disposition of contaminants.

In this section, we look briefly at methods for waste reduction. Figure 8.2 shows the different steps for waste prevention and treatment in an integrated process development. The first step is always to avoid the formation of waste. If this is feasible and cost-effective, subsequent treatment is unnecessary. If waste formation cannot be prevented completely, one should try to reduce it as much as useful. The reuse of material is one approach; for example, if a chromatography resin can be used for multiple cycles, the annual amount of waste is significantly reduced. The recycling of an organic solvent used in an extraction step is a good example of cost-effective recycling. To decide if the recycling is really

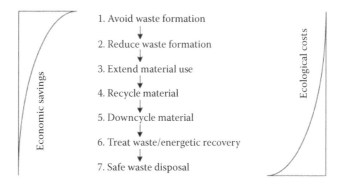

Figure 8.2 Steps of waste avoidance and treatment.

environmentally and economically favorable, the amount recycled and the amount of materials and energy necessary for the recycling should be compared. If the material cannot be recycled because the purification becomes too expensive, it might be used for another purpose that requires less purity (downcycling). The materials that remain after waste reduction and recycling steps have to be treated or disposed of safely. Thereby, treatment should be preferred to disposal. Ideally, some energy is produced during the treatment (e.g., incineration). There are a number of books recommended to further study pollution prevention and integrated waste reduction. The waste created in bioprocesses is often less a problem than in chemical processes. However, the amount can be quite large. The waste leaves the process boundaries as solid, liquid, and gaseous streams. The exhaust air from a bioreactor is the most common gaseous waste stream in bioprocesses. It usually contains air, carbon dioxide, and water. A filtration of the stream prevents the release of aerosols that might contain spores or other forms of the biocatalyst. This is especially relevant if pathogenic or recombinant organisms are used, even if considered as harmless. Gaseous waste streams are also formed in distillation and evaporation steps, for example, associated with crystallization. Most of the vapor is liquefied in a condensation step and then further processed. The exhaust air from a drying operation does not require treatment as long as water is the solvent that is removed. However, if organic solvents are removed, they have to be separated from the air stream to avoid volatile organic emissions. Solid waste is categorized as hazardous and nonhazardous waste. Hazardous waste, for example, containing heavy metals or highly toxic substances, needs special treatment or disposal with high-safety measures. Both cause higher costs. Compared with chemical processes, hazardous wastes are generated much less in bioprocesses. Wet biomass is the most common solid waste in bioprocesses. If a recombinant organism is used, sterilization of the material is necessary, usually by heat. The biomass can be used as animal feed or organic fertilizer or disposed as landfill. Owing to its high water content, it often can be added to a waste-water treatment plant. This is especially useful if the plant lacks organic carbon, nitrogen, or phosphorus, for example, when processing mainly chemical wastewater. Most bioreactions take place in an aqueous system and the product is dissolved in a liquid throughout most of the downstream processing. Thus, it is not a surprise that most waste streams in bioprocesses are liquid. They are treated in a biological sewage treatment plant at the production site of the bioprocesses, or they are released to the municipal sewer system. Under certain conditions, a pretreatment is necessary. At a high or low pH, the liquid waste has to be neutralized by adding base or acid. Besides sterilization, as discussed above, pretreatment is necessary if the stream contains specific contaminants such as pharmaceutically active substances that cannot be handled in a standard sewage plant. The raw materials used in the bioreaction and downstream processing influence the composition and complexity of the waste, which can cause higher costs and thus have to be considered when one compares different raw material alternatives. For example, molasses contains a wide range of impurities. If it is used as a carbon source in fermentation, the waste streams are much more complex when compared with the use of pure glucose or starch hydrolysates. Recycling of materials is regularly applied in bioprocesses. Biocatalysts are often immobilized to reuse them several times. Similar to other industrial processes, organic solvents are recycled to a high degree because they are relatively expensive and often environmentally critical. They usually have to be purified, for example, by distillation, before reentering the process. Water can also often be partly recycled. However, it is usually more economic to discharge an aqueous waste stream. Whenever a material stream is recycled, one has to validate whether there is a possible enrichment of undesired substances in the recycling loop or whether hygiene problems may arise.

Questions

1. What are the steps of a bioprocess?
2. What techniques can be used for sterilization?
3. Propose a strategy for sterilization of an input stream containing a heat-sensitive protein necessary for production of the product.
   Answer: Filtration sterilization would effectively remove potential bacterial contaminants without affecting the input protein because bacteria are considerably larger than proteins.
4. Why can prokaryotic cells be used with a higher volume fraction than eukaryotic cells?
5. What mass of steam is required to heat a 3L bioreactor containing a liquid suspension of yeast from ambient temperature, 70°F, to an operating temperature of 90°F?
6. What methods can be used to concentrate a biomass after completion of a bioreaction?
   Answer: Solvent evaporation, filtration, and precipitation can all be used to concentrate a biomass.
7. Compare and contrast chromatography processes.
8. If pharmaceutical production involves viral transfection of eukaryotic cells, what must be done prior to the distribution of the resulting pharmaceutical?
9. Why are postprocessing steps leading to protein refolding necessary?
   Answer: Oftentimes, the tertiary structure of a protein is not maintained throughout the process but is required for appropriate function of the protein as a therapeutic.
10. How can premature degradation of a protein therapeutic be mitigated?

9

Genetically Modified Organisms

LEARNING OBJECTIVES

1. Identify the possible species for production of recombinant proteins through genetic modification.
2. Understand the key elements necessary to incorporate into the expression vector design.
3. Recognize the significant advances that genetic modification brings in the production of therapeutic proteins.
4. Realize the improvement that fusion proteins provide over typical recombinant proteins.

9.1 INTRODUCTION

The choice of species and cell line used as expression system for a given protein is probably one of the most important strategic decisions taken in the bioprocess program. The primary choices include use of bacteria (*Escherichia coli*, *Bacillus subtilis*, *Lactococcus lactis*), yeast (*Saccharomyces cerevisiae*, *Pichia pastoris*), and mammalian cells (Chinese hamster ovary, CHO; baby hamster kidney). The baculovirus expression system in insect cells (sf9) is used (e.g., to express beta-glucosidases) but remains to be fully exploited; transgenic animal products are still not approved for human use though one application for an antibody derived from goat milk is pending approval.

The cell line (cell substrate) selected often requires a long time to produce the desired products because strict regulatory demands to cell line history, safety, genetic stability, expression levels, cell densities, and viability must be met in order to assure its acceptance by the regulatory authorities. Cell line optimization and safety demonstration require additional time. In practice, serially sub-cultivated cells (the working cell bank, WCB) are used as a starting source for each production batch. The WCB derives from the master cell bank (MCB), which is made first, usually from an initial clone or from a preliminary cell bank derived from an initial clone. The MCB and WCB may differ from each other in certain respects (e.g., culture components and culture conditions). The MCB and WCB are also tested differently. The safety issues include test for adventitious agents, which may be present in the donor of cells, serum used to propagate cells, and other culture media components. Especially mammalian cells are prone to contamination because of their complexity and the duration of culture. Mammalian cells may have latent or persistent virus infection or endogenous retrovirus. Or the virus can be introduced into the cells by derivation of cell lines from infected animals, use of virus to establish the cell line, or use of contaminated reagents such as serum. The genetic stability of the cells must be assured during fermentation and it must be shown that no mutations or loss of recombinant DNA is taking place during the cell culture period. In early development phase, the characteristic of expressed proteins is not well understood; other factors like protein stability, batch-to-batch variations, cell mutation rates, fermentation process variables, and process economy are also uncertain. The factors, however, that can be considered at this early stage include intellectual property issues, genetic stability, productivity, quality, impurities, yield, and host-cell toxicity.

9.2 CELL LINE CHARACTERIZATION

The cell line history includes information about the source and identity of cell line, the nucleotide sequence that codes for the target protein, the method used to prepare DNA for genetic engineering, a detailed component map, all inserts and deletions, integration sites, complete sequence of the expression vector used, vector transfer methods, and criteria for selection of cell clones. The cultivation history of the cells should be documented together with information of culture medium and possible exposure to infectious agents during handling.

For microbes, the species, strain, known genotype and phenotype characteristics, organism, pathogenicity, toxin production, and other biohazard information should be provided.

For animal cell lines, donor characteristics such as tissue or organ of origin, geographic origin, age, sex, species, strains, breeding conditions, and general physiological condition of the original donor should be described.

9.3 CHARACTERIZATION OF CELL AND VIRUS BANKS

The International Conference on Harmonisation of Technical Requirements for Registration of Pharmaceuticals for Human Use guideline describes characterization of cells used in recombinant DNA work (www.emea.eu.int/pdfs/human/ich/029495en.pdfA). A cell bank is a collection of vials containing cells stored under defined conditions, with uniform composition, and obtained from pooled cells derived from a single cell clone, such as bacteria or mammalian tissue. The cell bank system usually consists of an MCB and a WCB, although more tiers are possible. The MCB is produced in accordance with current good manufacturing practices (cGMP) and preferably obtained from a qualified repository source (source free from adventitious agents) whose history is known and documented. The WCB is produced or derived by expanding one or more vials of the MCB. The WCB, or MCB in early trials, becomes the source of cells for every batch produced for human use. Cell bank systems contribute greatly to consistency of the production of clinical or licensed product batches, because the starting cell material is always the same. Mammalian and bacterial cell sources are used for establishing cell bank systems. The master virus bank (MVB) is similar to the MCB in that it is derived from a single production run and is uniform in composition. The working virus bank (WVB) is derived directly from the MVB. As with the cell banks, the focus of virus bank usage is to have a consistent source of virus, shown to be free of adventitious agents, to use in the production of clinical or product batches. In keeping with cGMP guidelines, testing of the cell bank to be used for the production of the virus banks, including quality assurance testing, should be completed prior to the use of this cell bank for the production of virus banks. Virus banks are used to provide testing of various therapeutic proteins such as interferon.

Cell and viral bank characterization is an important step toward obtaining a uniform final product with lot-to-lot consistency and freedom from adventitious agents. Testing to qualify the MCB or MVB is performed once and can be done on an aliquot of the banked material or on cell cultures derived from the cell bank. Specifications for qualification of the MCB or MVB should be established. It is important to document the MCB and MVB history, methods and reagents used to produce the bank, and storage conditions. All the raw materials required for the production of the banks, namely, media, sera, trypsin, and the like, must also be tested for adventitious agents.

Testing to qualify the MCB includes the following: (1) testing to demonstrate freedom from adventitious agents and endogenous viruses and (2) identity testing. The testing for adventitious agents may include tests for nonhost microbes, mycoplasma, bacteriophage, and viruses. Freedom from adventitious viruses should be demonstrated using both in vitro and in vivo virus tests, and appropriate species-specific tests such as the mouse antibody production (MAP) test. Identity testing of the cell bank should establish the properties of the cells and the stability of these properties during manufacture. Cell banks should be characterized with respect to cellular isoenzyme expression and cellular phenotype and genotype, which could include the expression of a gene insert or the presence of a gene-transfer vector. Suitable techniques, including restriction endonuclease mapping or nucleic acid sequencing, should be used to analyze the cell bank for vector copy number and the physical state of the vector (vector integrity and integration). The cell bank should also be characterized for the quality and quantity of the gene product produced.

Testing of the MVB is similar to that of the MCB and should include testing for freedom from adventitious agents in general (e.g., bacteria, fungi, mycoplasma, or viruses) and for organisms specific to the production cell line, including Replication Competent Viruses. Identity testing of the MVB should establish the properties of the virus and the stability of these properties during manufacture. Characterization of the WCB or WVB is generally less extensive, requiring the following: (1) testing for freedom from adventitious agents that may have been introduced from the culture medium; (2) resting for Replication Competent Viruses, if relevant; (3) routine identity tests to check for cell line cross-contamination; and (4) demonstration that aliquots can consistently be used for final product production.

9.3.1 Cell Banks

An MCB is a homogeneous pool of the production cell line dispensed in multiple containers, by which each aliquot is representative for each other vial, stored under defined conditions (liquid nitrogen). A tested and released MCB provides material for the WCB using one more tubes from MCB. The MCB and WCB may differ from each other in certain respects (e.g., culture components and culture conditions) but generally there is no need to extensively characterize WCB unless records indicate wide variability between MCB and WCB. The methods used to characterize cell banks are derived from the WHO requirements for the use of in vitro substrates for the production of biologicals (Requirements for biological substances No 50; Dev Biol Stand 1998; 93:141-171 and the International Conference on Harmonisation of Technical Requirements for Registration of Pharmaceuticals for Human Use guidelines Q5A, B, and D) (Tables 9.1 and 9.2).

Table 9.1 Suggested Methods for Test of Microbial Cell Banks (Bacteria and Yeast)

Test	Comments
Auxotrophic markers	Conformation of key markers (yeast)
Characterization	Characterization of insert by Southern blot and eventually DNA sequence of the integrated expression cassette
Identity	Phenotyping or genotyping may be used to confirm species and strain. Growth on selective media is considered adequate to confirm host cell identity for most microbial cells. For *E. coli* phage typing should be considered as a supplementary test
Purity	Freedom from adventitious microbial agents and adventitious cellular contaminants must be assessed (bacteria, bacteriophages, fungi). Visual examination of the characteristics of the isolated colonies using different media is suggested
Resistance to antibiotics	When antibiotic selection markers have been used
Stability	It must be demonstrated that the cell line produces the desired product in a consistent quality and quantity. Studies shall be performed to determine whether manipulation of the cell line changes it characteristics significantly

Table 9.2 Suggested Methods for Test of Insect and Metazoan Cell Banks

Test	Comments
Identity	Phenotyping or genotyping may be used. In most cases isoenzyme analysis is sufficient to confirm the species of origin. Other technologies include banding cytogenetics and use of species-specific antisera An alternative strategy is to demonstrate the presence of unique markers
Purity	Freedom from adventitious microbial agents and adventitious cellular contaminants must be assessed. Test for the presence of bacteria, fungi, and mycoplasma should be performed. Freedom of contaminating cell lines of the same or different species must be demonstrated
Purity, Viral agents using cell cultures	Monolayer cultures of the following cell types: • Cultures of the same species an tissue type as the cell line • Cultures of a human diploid cell line • Cultures of another cell line from a different species The PCR technology is receiving increasing attention from regulatory authorities especially after new validated quantitative tests have emerged

(Continued)

Table 9.2 (*Continued*)   Suggested Methods for Test of Insect and Metazoan Cell Banks

Test	Comments
Purity, viral agents using animals and eggs	Test for pathogen viruses not able to grow in cell cultures in both animals and eggs (e.g., suckling mice, adult mice, guinea pigs, fertilized eggs). The cell banks are suitable for production if none of the animals or eggs show evidence of presence of any viral agent (European Pharmacopoeia V.2.2.12)
Purity, test for retroviruses, endogenous viruses, or viral nucleic acid	Test shall include infective assays, transmission electron microscopy (TEM)4, and reverse transcriptase (Rtase) of cells cultured up to or beyond in vitro cell age. Induction studies have not been found to be useful
Purity test for selected viruses	Murine cell lines shall be tested species-specific using mouse, rat, and hamster antibody production tests (MAP, RAP, HAP). In vivo testing for lymphocytic chorimeningitis virus is required. PCR techniques may be used as well. Human cell lines shall be screened for human viral pathogens (Epstein–Barr virus, cytomegalovirus, human retroviruses, hepatitis B/C viruses with appropriate in vitro techniques)
Stability	It must be demonstrated that the cell line produces the desired product in a consistent quality and quantity. Studies shall be performed to determine whether manipulation of the cell line changes it characteristics significantly
Serum	Freedom from cultivable bacteria, fungi, mycoplasma, and infectious viruses must be demonstrated. Human serum should not be used and use of bovine serum shall meet specified requirements for biological substances
Trypsin	Trypsin shall be tested and found free of cultivable bacteria, fungi, mycoplasma, and infectious viruses, especially bovine or porcine parvoviruses, as appropriate
	Contaminating viruses are of major concern. Viruses can be introduced into the cell bank by several routes such as derivation of cell lines from infected animals, use of viruses to establish the cell line, use of contaminated reagents (e.g., animal serum), and contaminants during handling of cells. Although continuous cell lines are extensively characterized, viral contaminants will not be cytolytic. However, chronic or latent viruses may be present. Examples of viruses harbored in cell substrates are retroviruses (oncogenic), hantaviruses (CHO cells), hepatitis viruses (human cells), human papillomavirus (human cells), and cytomegalovirus (human cells). Additionally, cell line establishment or cell transformation is achieved using Epstein–Barr or Sendai viruses

9.3.2 Cell Line Selection

Of the currently approved products, the largest numbers of these products are expressed in three hosts: *E. coli,* followed by CHO cells and *Saccharomyces cerevisiae* (Table 9.3). There are clear advantages and disadvantages of each of the host system described above. These are summarized in Table 9.4.

Table 9.3 Most Popular Hosts for Approved Drugs

Host	Number of Approved Products
Escherichia coli	37
Chinese hamster ovary cell	29
Saccharomyces cerevisiae	11
Baby hamster kidney cells	2
Other mammalian	2
Mouse C 127	2
African monkey kidney cells (COS-1)	1
Lymphocyte activated	1
Mouse myeloma	1
Myeloma NSO	1
Prostate epithelium cell	1

Note: May include repetitive entry for a molecule in case of multiple approvals.

Despite the listed disadvantages, the ease of use of *E. coli* and their generally high expression yields for most proteins often have resulted in the continued preferential use of these bacteria, where feasible and continuous improvements in the bacterial systems to obviate the described disadvantages. The use of yeast strains such as *Saccharomyces cerevisiae* for production has been extensively explored. The production of proteins in yeast offers many theoretical advantages over *E. coli* while raising certain new concerns. Like *E. coli*, yeast can maintain stable plasmids extrachromosomally; however, unlike *E. coli*, yeast possesses the ability to produce glycoproteins.

The development of eukaryotic cell culture for the production of vaccines has long been established in the pharmaceutical industry and an extensive database has been developed to ensure the suitability of such protein products in humans. The extension of this technology to rDNA products was primarily a response to the limitations in the use of *E. coli*. Particularly with respect to large proteins or glycoproteins, eukaryotic cell expression is an attractive alternative to a bacterial system because eukaryotic cells can secrete proteins that are properly folded and identical in primary, secondary, and tertiary structure to the natural human protein. Concerns about the economics of this production system originally hindered its development. Recent advances, however, in improved expression levels, in large-scale cell culture using CHO cells, and in the formulation of more highly defined growth media have combined to dramatically improve the economic feasibility of eukaryotic cell substrates. The number of cell passages required for cloning, selection, amplification, and cell banking prior to production generally necessitates the use of immortal cell lines because nonimmortalized strains (i.e., diploid cultures) cannot be propagated long enough to provide an economically useful time in the production stage. Initial questions regarding the safety of such immortal cell lines were based on concerns over potential oncogenes and potential viral and retroviral contamination. These concerns have been minimized by the exhaustive analysis and characterization of MCBs for adventitious (accidentally introduced) agents, by effective process validation studies, and by the safety data gathered to

Table 9.4 Comparison of Host Systems Advantages and Disadvantages

Host	Advantages	Disadvantages
Bacteria (e.g., *E. coli*)	Many reference and experience available, wide choice of cloning vectors, gene expression easily controlled; easy to grow with high yields, product forming up to 50% of total cell protein, can be designed for secretion into growth media allowing for the removal of unwanted N-terminal methionine groups	No posttranslational modification, biological activity, and immunogenicity may differ from natural proteins; high endotoxin content in gram negative. The expressed protein product may cause cellular toxicity; inclusion bodies difficult to process
Bacteria (e.g., *S. aureus*)	Secretes fusion proteins into the growth media	Does not express such high levels as *E. coli*; pathogenic cells can be difficult and expensive to grow, cells grow slowly; manipulated cells can be genetically unstable; low productivity as compared to microorganisms
Mammalian cells (e.g., CHO cells)	Same biologic activity as native proteins, mammalian expression vectors available, can be grown in large-scale cultures	
Yeasts (e.g., *S. cervisiae*)	Lack detectable endotoxin, generally regarded as safe (GRAS), fermentation relatively inexpensive, facilitates glycosylation and formation of disulfide bonds, only 0.5% native proteins are secreted so isolation of secreted product is simplified, well established large-scale production and downstream processing	Gene expression less easily controlled; glycosylation not identical to mammalian systems
Cultured insect cells (baculovirus vector)	Facilitates glycosylation and formation of disulfide bonds, safe since few anthropods are adequate host for baculovirus; baculovirus vector received FDA approval for a clinical trial, virus stops host protein amplification, high level of expression of product	Lack of information on glycosylation mechanism, product not always fully functional; few differences in functional and antigenic properties between product and native protein
Fungi (e.g., *Aspergillus* sp.)	Well established system for fermentation of filamentous fungi; growth inexpensive	High level of expression not yet achieved; genetics not always characterized
Fungi (e.g., *A. niger* sp.)	This is also GRAS, can secrete large quantities of product into growth media, source of many industrial enzymes	No cloning vectors available
Transgenic plants		Low transformation efficiency, long generation time; often commercially not viable

date for products produced by this method. The resultant thoroughly characterized MCB is used for full-scale production. Other eukaryotic cell lines, such as those derived from insect cells, may be useful in achieving many of the conformational and posttranslational advantages that have been described for mammalian cell culture.

A large number of cell lines of animal origin are currently in use including the attachment cell lines such as MRC-5: human lung fibroblasts, HELA: human cervix epithelial cells, VERO: African green monkey kidney epithelial cells, NIH 3T3: mouse embryo fibroblasts, L929: mouse connective tissue fibroblasts, CHO: CHO fibroblasts, BHK-21: Syrian hamster kidney fibroblasts, HEK 293: human kidney epithelial cells, HEPG2: human liver epithelial cells, and BAE-1: bovine aorta endothelial cells. The suspension animal cell lines mainly comprise of NS0: mouse myeloma lymphoblastoid-like cells, U937: human histiocytic lymphoma lymphoblastoid cells, *Namalwa*: human lymphoma lymphoblastoid cells, HL60: human leukemia, lymphoblastoid-like cells, WEHI 231: mouse B-cell lymphoma lymphoblastoid cells, YAC 1: mouse lymphoma lymphoblastoid cells, U 266B1: human myeloma, lymphoblastoid cells, and SH-SY5Y: human neuroblastoma neuroblasts.

Animal cell culture development is faster than transgenics production, and it has a solid regulatory track record. It takes about one month (for insect cell processes) to five months (for mammalian cells) to go from genetic engineering to a production culture. Compare this with six months to a year for transgenic plants (from inserted genes to harvestable plants) and one to three years for transgenic animals (from gene to milk-producing mammals, although developing egg-laying hens is faster).

Animal cells by their nature are more fragile, do not have the strong cell wall of microbes, and are much larger than microbes, and as a result, they disrupt too easily, if for example, subjected to the conditions of fermenters; newer *airlift* designs incorporate forced air and liquid flow designs that replace impellers with pumps for more gentle treatment of animal cells in culture. The complex metabolism of animal cells requires complex mixture of nutrients. As a result, fetal bovine serum obtained as a by-product of the dairy and beef industries has been is a common additive to cell culture media. However, recently concerns about transmissible spongiform encephalopathies and blood-borne pathogens have led to the development of many serum-free, animal-product-free, and even protein-free media formulations. Recombinant insulin, transferrin, and bovine serum albumin (usually made by bacterial fermentation), and also human serum albumin made by yeast fermentation, take the place of serum in many modern cell culture processes.

Animal cells are also sensitive to culture conditions, often overreacting to small changes in temperature or pH. Animal cells propagate more slowly than microbes do, doubling their numbers during the log phase in 15–48 h They require less oxygen, which is a good thing because getting air to them can be difficult. Stirring the liquid medium by traditional impellers can break up the fragile cells. Even the impellers with rounded blades (based on the three-bladed type used to propel motorboats) designed to produce lower shear forces may be too dangerous. Bioreactors for animal cell culture use forced-air sparging or other means to introduce air into the mixture. Some animal cell lines will proliferate in suspension culture, floating about in their liquid medium. Others require a solid substrate: stuck on the insides of roller bottles, within gas-permeable polymer tubes in *hollow-fiber* bioreactors, or attached to plastic microcarrier beads or flat disks. Anchorage-dependent cells historically exhibited higher protein expression levels, but now optimized cell lines (such as NS0, CHO,

HeLa, and HEK-293) are used in suspension culture. Generally, the primary cell lines are attachment dependent and the development scientists are divided on the issue whether it will be possible to create high-yielding suspension cell lines in the future. Other techniques such as hybridomas are immortalized by fusion with myeloma tumor cells to secrete monoclonal antibodies. Established cell lines such as those mentioned above are available from numerous sources, such as, the American Type Culture Collection (ATCC). Cryopreservation allows companies to *bank* cells rather than running all cell lines in constant culture.

Many mammalian cell lines undergo apoptotic death in the bioreactor environment. The high susceptibility to apoptosis partially explains many of the technical problems associated with large-scale animal cell culture. Factors such as nutrient and oxygen deprivation, virus-based protein expression systems, and cytostatic agents have been identified as potent inducers of apoptosis in industrial cultivation. They limit culture duration and productivity. Suppressing apoptosis under such conditions leads to highly robust cell lines with improved production characteristics.

Insect cell culture offers the advantages of cost and ease of culturing over mammalian cells. The expression levels of heterologous proteins achieved using this system are generally variable and fall within the range of 1–600 mg/L culture medium. Some collagens have been produced in insect cells at 10–40 mg/L. One problem with insect cells is that they tend not to secrete recombinant proteins, maintaining them instead in the intracellular cytoplasm. This is a side effect of the transfection method involved, and it can complicate downstream processing. Baculovirus (which is not infectious to humans) expression vectors are widely used for expressing heterologous proteins in cultured insect cells. Recent advances include production of multisubunit protein complexes, coexpression of protein-modifying enzymes to improve heterologous protein production, and additional applications of baculovirus display technology. The application of modified baculovirus vectors for gene expression in mammalian cells continues to expand. (Kemp Biotechnologies Inc. [Frederick, MD; www.kempbiotech.com] is working on several insect cell projects.) Insect cell lines (with Baculovirus Expression Vector System) have, to date, not produced any approved therapeutics. A number of products are in advanced clinical trials: Dendreon Corp (Seattle, WA) has a prostate cancer vaccine in phase III stage, GlaxoSmithKline (London) is developing a human papilloma virus vaccine, and Protein Sciences Corporation is working on a flu vaccine (phase III) and has scaled up their process to 600 L and is looking at a variety of other vaccines. The United States Department of Agriculture has developed an immortal insect cell line from *Spodoptera* sp.

9.4 CELL LINE CONSTRUCTION

9.4.1 Endogenous Proteins Expression

The human body cellular functions are governed by a large number of proteins produced endogenously. Given below is a broad listing of these proteins:

Chaperones: Proteins involved in protein folding.
Conjugated proteins: Covalently bonded to prosthetic groups such as glycoprotein and metalloprotein.

Table 9.5 Types of Interleukins

Interleukins	Major Source	Major Effects
IL-1	Macrophages	Stimulation of T cells and antigen-presenting cells B-cell growth and antibody production Promotes hematopoiesis (blood cell formation)
IL-2	Activated T cells	Proliferation of activated T cells
IL-3	T lymphocytes	Growth of blood cell precursors
IL-4	T cells and mast cells	B-cell proliferation IgE production
IL-5	T cells and mast cells	Eosinophil growth
IL-6	Activated T cells	Synergistic effects with IL-1 or TNF α
IL-7	Thymus and bone marrow stromal cells	Development of T cell and B cell precursors
IL-8	Macrophages	Chemoattracts neutrophils
IL-9	Activated T cells	Promotes growth of T cells and mast cells
IL-10	Activated T cells, B cells, and monocytes	Inhibits inflammatory and immune responses
IL-11	Stromal cells	Synergistic effects on hematopoiesis
IL-12	Macrophages, B cells	Promotes TH1 cells while suppressing TH2 functions
IL-13	TH2 cells	Similar to IL-4 effects
IL-15	Epithelial cells and monocytes	Similar to IL-2 effects
IL-16	CD8 T cells	Chemoattracts CD4 T cells
IL-17	Activated memory T cells	Promotes T-cell proliferation
IL-18	Macrophages	Induces IFN-γ production

Cytokines: Regulate immunity, inflammation, apoptosis, and hematopoiesis.

Interleukins: They are the cytokines that act specifically as mediators between leukocytes. Table 9.5 shows the major source and effects of various types of interleukins.

Interferons: They are the cytokines that can *interfere* with viral growth. They also have the ability to inhibit proliferation and modulate immune responses. Four types of interferons have been identified: IFN-α, IFN-β, IFN-ω, and IFN-γ. The first three are Type I IFNs, which have relatively high antiviral potency. IFN-γ is the Type II IFN, also called *immune IFN*. Type I IFNs are produced by macrophages, neutrophils, and other somatic cells in response to infection by viruses or bacteria. After they are released, they may bind to their receptors that are expressed on most cell types, resulting in the production of over 30 different proteins in the target cell. Among them, two enzymes play a critical role in the inhibition of viral replication: RNA-dependent protein kinase and 2'–5' oligoadenylate synthetase (2–5A synthetase). Both enzymes can be activated by double-stranded RNA, which may be present in some viruses. The activated RNA-dependent protein kinase can phosphorylate a protein (eIF2) to inhibit protein synthesis. The 2–5A synthetase produces oligoadenylate that can bind and activate a cellular endonuclease to degrade mRNA. IFN-γ is produced in activated TH1 and NK cells, particularly in response to IL-2 and IL-12. Its production is suppressed by IL-4, IL-10, and TGF-β. Binding of IFN-γ to its receptor increases the expression of class I MHC on all somatic cells. It also enhances the expression of class II MHC on antigen-presenting cells. IFN-γ may also activate macrophages, neutrophils, and NK cells.

Tumor necrosis factors (TNF): TNFs are the cytokines produced mainly by macrophages and T lymphocytes that help regulate the immune response and hematopoiesis (blood cell formation). There are two types of TNFs.

TNFα: Also called *cachectin*, produced by macrophages

TNFβ: Also called *lymphotoxin*, produced by activated CD4+ T cells

Chemokines: They are the cytokines that may activate or chemoattract leukocytes. Each chemokine contains 65–120 amino acids, with molecular weight of 8–10 kD. Their receptors belong to G-protein-coupled receptors. Since the entry of HIV into host cells requires chemokine receptors, their antagonists are being developed to treat AIDS.

Hormones: Examples include insulin, growth hormone, and prolactin.

Prions: Toxic proteins that enter brain cells and there convert the normal cell protein PrPC to the prion form of the protein, called *PrPSC*. When normal cell proteins transform into prions, amino acids that are folded tightly into alpha helical structures relax into looser beta sheets. More and more PrPC molecules transform into PrPSC molecules, until eventually prions completely clog the infected brain cells. Mad cow disease is purported caused by prions.

Structural proteins: Collagen and myosin.

Transcription factors: Regulate gene transcription.

Ubiquitin: The marker for protein degradation. If a protein binds to ubiquitin, it will be degraded by proteasome.

Several proteins listed above have direct therapeutic application, wherein a break in the chain of endogenous production of these proteins produces a disease state. Most relevant proteins include cytokines and hormones. Figure 9.1 shows the structure of the most widely expressed therapeutic protein, human insulin.

On a commercial scale, these therapeutic proteins are manufactured using recombinant DNA techniques. A number of different genetic strategies are available for the design of processes for the production of recombinant proteins mostly developed during the past couple of decades. The focus of microbiological processing is to manufacture industrially and pharmaceutically significant substances using organisms, which either do not initially have genetically coded information concerning the desired product included in their DNA

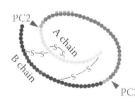

Figure 9.1 Amino acid sequence of proinsulin; chains A and B are separated from the third chair to active insulin.

or (in the case of mammalian cells in culture) do not ordinarily express a chromosomal gene at appreciable levels. To do so, a gene that specifies the structure of a desired polypeptide product is either isolated from a *donor* organism or chemically synthesized and then stably introduced into another organism, which is preferably a self-replicating unicellular organism such as bacteria, yeast, or mammalian cells in culture. Once this is done, the existing machinery for gene expression in the *transformed* or *transfected* microbial host cells operates to construct the desired product, using the exogenous DNA as a template for transcription of mRNA which is then translated into a continuous sequence of amino acid residues.

The production apparatus to manufacture therapeutic proteins consists of genetically modified cells (GMCs), which include bacteria, yeast, and animal-derived cells. The construction of GMCs is a complex process that follows the pathway given below (Figure 9.2).

Whereas the literature is rich in the microbiological techniques and relevant technology used to manufacture recombinant products, the most pertinent information for manufacturers of these drugs can be found in the patents that describe these proprietary methods. This includes the methodologies for the isolation, synthesis, purification, and amplification of genetic materials for use in the transformation of selected host organisms, which are amply described in various patent instruments. For example, the U.S. Patent No. 4,237,224 to Cohen et al. describes the transformation of unicellular host organisms with *hybrid* viral or circular plasmid DNA, which includes selected exogenous DNA sequences. The procedures of the Cohen patent first involve manufacture of a transformation vector by enzymatically cleaving viral circular plasmid DNA to form linear DNA strands. Selected foreign (*exogenous* or *heterologous*) DNA strands usually including sequences coding for desired product are prepared in linear form through use of similar enzymes. The linear viral or plasmid DNA is incubated with the foreign DNA in the presence of ligating enzymes capable of effecting a restoration process and *hybrid* vectors are formed, which include the selected exogenous DNA segment *spliced* into the viral or circular DNA plasmid. Transformation of compatible unicellular host organisms with the

Identification and characterization of target protein to be expressed
Isolation of the gene of interest (i.e., the DNA sequence coding that expressed the desired protein)
Full characterization of gene
Insertion of gene into a suitable vector such as a plasmid
Insertion of the plasmid into the host cell
Cloning of the transformed host cell line
Isolation of cells that produce the protein of interest in the desired quantities
Scale up of cloned cells in a fermentation or cell culture process to produce the protein product
Downstream processing to yield pure target protein

Figure 9.2 Process flow of GMC construction.

hybrid vector results in the formation of multiple copies of the exogenous DNA in the host cell population. In some instances, the desired result is simply the amplification of the foreign DNA and the *product* harvested is DNA.

9.5 DESIGNING GMCs

9.5.1 Gene Construct

The design of GMCs begins with a clear understanding of the genetic material found in the cells. The genetic materials comprise of those chemical substances that program and guide the manufacture of natural constituents of cells (and viruses) and direct the normal biological responses of these cells. The elements of genetic material include a long chain polymeric substance known as *deoxyribonucleic acid* (DNA), the genetic material of all living cells and viruses (except for certain viruses that are programmed by *ribonucleic acids* [RNA] and are thus called *RNA viruses*). The repeating units in DNA polymers are four different nucleotides, each of which consists of either a purine (adenine or guanine) or a pyrimidine (thymine or cytosine) bound to a deoxyribose sugar to which a phosphate group is attached. Attachment of nucleotides in linear polymeric form is by means of fusion of the 5′ phosphate of one nucleotide to the 3′ hydroxyl group of another. Functional DNA occurs in the form of stable double strands made up of single strands of nucleotides (known as *deoxyoligonucleotides*) attached to each other by hydrogen bonding between purine and pyrimidine bases (i.e., *complementary* associations existing either between adenine [A] and thymine [T] or guanine [G] and cytosine [C]). By convention, nucleotides are referred to by the names of their constituent purine or pyrimidine bases, and the complementary associations of nucleotides in double-stranded DNA (i.e., A–T and G–C) are referred to as *base pairs*. Figure 9.3 shows a drawing of DNA's two strands.

Ribonucleic acid is a polynucleotide comprising adenine, guanine, cytosine, and uracil (U), rather than thymine, bound to ribose and a phosphate group. The programming function of DNA is served through a process wherein specific DNA nucleotide sequences (genes) are *transcribed* into relatively transient messenger RNA (mRNA) polymers. The mRNA, in turn, serves as a template for the formation of structural, regulatory, and catalytic proteins from amino acids. This mRNA *translation* process involves the operations of small RNA strands (tRNA) that transport and align individual amino acids along the mRNA strand to allow for formation of polypeptides in proper amino acid sequences. The mRNA *message* derived from DNA and providing the basis for the tRNA supply and orientation of any given one of the twenty amino acids for polypeptide *expression* is in the form of triplet *codons* (sequential groupings of three nucleotide bases). The formation of a protein is the ultimate form of *expression* of the programmed genetic message provided by the nucleotide sequence of a gene. Figure 9.4 shows a typical transcription process.

There are other sequences of importance that control the process of transcription and these include the following:

Promoter DNA sequences usually *precede* a gene in a DNA polymer and provide a site for initiation of the transcription into mRNA.

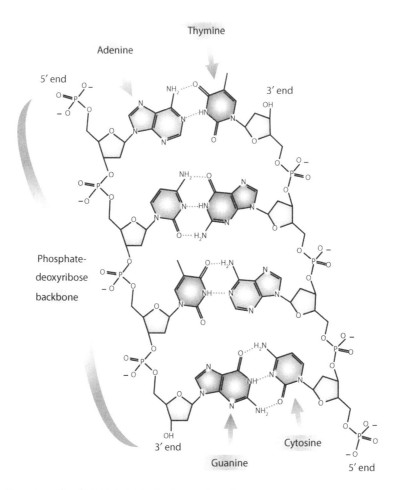

Figure 9.3 Two strands of DNA held by hydrogen bonds.

Regulator DNA sequences, also usually *upstream* of (i.e., preceding) a gene in a given DNA polymer, bind proteins that determine the frequency (or rate) of transcriptional initiation. Collectively referred to as *promoter/regulator* or *control* DNA sequence, these sequences that precede a selected gene (or series of genes) in a functional DNA polymer cooperate to determine whether the transcription (and eventual expression) of a gene will occur.

Terminator DNA sequences follow a gene in a DNA polymer and provide a signal for termination of the transcription into mRNA.

The development of specific DNA sequences for splicing into DNA vectors is accomplished by a variety of techniques, depending to a great deal on the degree of *foreignness* of the *donor* to the projected host and the size of the polypeptide to be expressed in the host. In general terms, three methods are used:

The *isolation* of double-stranded DNA sequence from the genomic DNA of the donor

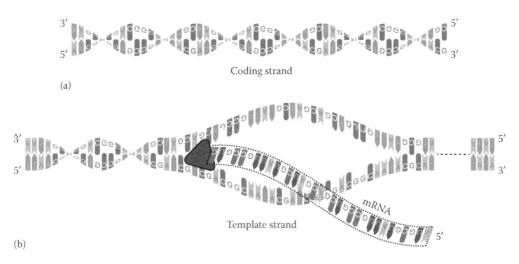

(a)

Coding strand

(b)

Template strand

mRNA

Figure 9.4   Transcription process. (a) DNA before transcription. (b) During transcription, the DNA unwinds so that one of its strand can be used as a template to synthesize a complementary RNA.

The chemical manufacture of a DNA sequence providing a code for a polypeptide of interest

The in vitro synthesis of a double-stranded DNA sequence by enzymatic *reverse transcription* of mRNA isolated from donor cells. The last-mentioned methods, which involve formation of a DNA *complement* of mRNA, are generally referred to as *cDNA* methods.

Manufacture of DNA sequences is frequently the method of choice when the entire sequence of amino acid residues of the desired polypeptide product is known. Developments in the methods include the following:

Providing for the presence of alternate codons commonly found in genes which are highly expressed in the host organism selected for expression (e.g., providing yeast or *E. coli preference* codons)

Avoiding the presence of untranslated *intron* sequences (commonly present in mammalian genomic DNA sequences and mRNA transcripts thereof) which are not readily processed by prokaryotic host cells

Avoiding expression of undesired *leader* polypeptide sequences commonly coded for by genomic DNA and cDNA sequences but frequently not readily cleaved from the polypeptide of interest by bacterial or yeast host cells

Providing for ready insertion of the DNA in convenient expression vectors in association with desired promoter/regulator and terminator sequences

Providing for ready construction of genes coding for polypeptide fragments and analogs of the desired polypeptides

When the entire sequence of amino acid residues of the desired polypeptide is not known, direct manufacture of DNA sequences is not possible and isolation of DNA sequences

239

coding for the polypeptide by a cDNA method becomes the method of choice despite its many drawbacks. Among the standard procedures for isolating cDNA sequences of interest is the preparation of plasmid-borne cDNA *libraries* derived from reverse transcription of mRNA abundant in donor cells selected as responsible for high-level expression of genes (e.g., libraries of cDNA derived from pituitary cells which express relatively large quantities of growth hormone products).

Where substantial portions of the polypeptide's amino acid sequence are known, labeled, single-stranded DNA probe sequences duplicating a sequence putatively present in the *target* cDNA may be employed in DNA/DNA hybridization procedures carried out on cloned copies of the cDNA, which have been denatured to single-stranded form (see, e.g., U.S. Patents 4,394,443 and 4,358,535).

Among the more significant recent advances in hybridization procedures for the screening of recombinant clones is the use of labeled mixed synthetic oligonucleotide probes, each of which is potentially the complete complement of a specific DNA sequence in the hybridization sample including a heterogeneous mixture of single-stranded DNAs or RNAs. These procedures are acknowledged to be especially useful in the detection of cDNA clones derived from sources that provide extremely low amounts of mRNA sequences for the polypeptide of interest. Use of stringent hybridization conditions directed toward avoidance of non-specific binding can allow, for example, for the autoradiographic visualization of a specific cDNA clone upon the event of hybridization of the target DNA to that single probe within the mixture which is its complete complement.

The use of genomic DNA isolates is the least common of the three above-noted methods for developing specific DNA sequences for use in recombinant procedures. This is especially true in the area of recombinant procedures directed to securing microbial expression of mammalian polypeptides and is due principally to the complexity of mammalian genomic DNA. Thus, while reliable procedures exist for developing phage-borne libraries of genomic DNA of human and other mammalian species origins relating to procedures for generating a human genomic library commonly referred to as the *Maniatis Library*, there have been relatively few successful attempts at use of hybridization procedures in isolating genomic DNA in the absence of extensive foreknowledge of amino acid or DNA sequences.

9.6 VECTOR

The key element in rDNA technology is the recombinant plasmid, which contains the gene that codes for the protein of interest, as described above. Plasmids are simple and small circular extrachromosomal segments of bacterial DNA that are isolated from a bacterium and are self-replicating. The basic technology involves the specific enzymatic cleavage of a plasmid using endonucleases followed by the insertion of a new piece of DNA that contains the gene of interest. The resultant recombinant plasmid is considered the key raw material of rDNA technology. The recombinant plasmid is introduced into the host organism through a process called *transformation*, where it passes on its new genetic information and results in the production of the protein product.

The vector (plasmid) generally contains a selectable marker that can be used to identify cells that contain this gene. This is in addition to the gene coding for the protein of interest and the regulatory nucleotide sequences necessary for plasmid replication and mRNA transcription (the first step in protein synthesis). Selection of the desired cells is simplified because only properly transformed cells containing the selectable marker gene will survive under the growth conditions used to identify and propagate the transformed cells. Typically, the bacterial and eukaryotic selectable markers may include both antibiotic resistance and genes that complement an auxotrophic host mutation. There are numerous examples of both types of markers in each system.

Significant differences exist in the rDNA production process between prokaryotic and eukaryotic cells. In general, bacterial cells express greater concentrations of protein product and require relatively simple media components. However, prokaryotic cells do not perform many important posttranslational modifications such as glycosylation, and historically, it was not possible to express large proteins in *E. coli*. These limitations necessitate the use of eukaryotic cells in many cases. The production differences between eukaryotic and prokaryotic host cells have significant impacts that are reflected in the requirements for process validation, purification, and analytical methodology.

In order to clone the gene of interest, all engineered vectors have a selection of unique restriction sites downstream of a transcription promoter sequence. The choice of vector family is governed by the host. Once the host has been selected, many different vectors are available for consideration, from simple expression vectors to those that secrete fusion proteins. However, as for the selection of a suitable host system, the final choice of vector should take into consideration the specific requirements of the application and the behavior of the target protein. One key factor that has led to the increased use of fusion protein vectors is that amplification of a fusion protein containing a tag of known size and biological function can greatly simplify subsequent isolation, purification, and detection. In some cases, the protein yield can also be increased. Maintenance and cloning protocols are highly specific for each vector and the instructions provided by the supplier should be followed carefully. This topic is further elaborated elsewhere in the book.

The most commonly used vectors include the following:

pTrc 99: A *E. coli* vector for expression of proteins encoded by inserts lacking a start codon, inducible by isopropyl β-D-thiogalactopyranoside (IPTG)

pKK223-3: For overexpression of proteins under the control of the strong *tac* promoter in *E. coli*

pSVK 3: For in vivo expression in mammalian cell lines

pSVL SV40: For high-level transient expression in mammalian cells

pMSG: For inducible expression in mammalian cells

The ATCC (http://www.atcc.org/Products/vectors.cfm) provides a large number of vectors. ATCC is also an official depository for the U.S. Patent and Trademark Office; GMCs subject to U.S. patents are deposited here. Figure 9.5 shows a typical scheme how plasmids are made and Figure 9.6 shows a plasmid for *E. coli*.

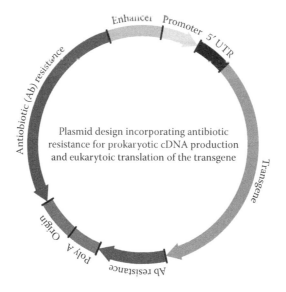

Figure 9.5 Plasmid design.

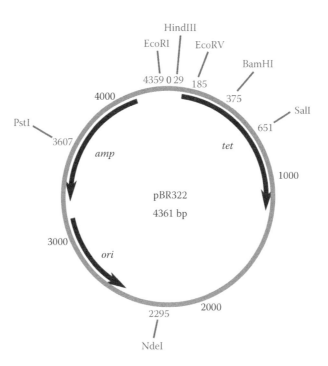

Figure 9.6 pBR322 plasmid for use in *E. coli*.

242

9.7 HOST SYSTEMS

Several expression host systems are available including bacteria, yeast, plants, filamentous fungi, insect or mammalian cells grown in culture, and transgenic animals. The rDNA products are presently produced in prokaryotic (bacteria) or eukaryotic systems (e.g., yeast and mammalian cell culture). The choice of the production organism is generally a direct function of the molecular complexity of the protein that is to be produced as well as the economics and efficiency of the fermentation or cell culture process. The earliest biotechnology-derived products were produced in *E. coli* based on the high degree of understanding of its molecular biology. Within the last few years, however, the use of large-scale eukaryotic cell culture has become relatively commonplace. The choice of host system depends on many factors, such as the size, structure, and stability of the product, and the requirements for posttranslational modifications for biological activity, the necessary production yields, acceptable cost and quality specifications of the final product also have to be considered. The choice of host generally depends on many factors:

1. Properties and the final use of the expressed protein. If the protein consists of multiple subunits or requires substantial posttranslational modifications, the preferred host usually is of higher eukaryotic origin, for example, CHO cells.
2. Regulatory considerations in reducing the immunogenic potential and endotoxin loading. These considerations make yeast as one of the most ideal host.
3. Cost considerations dictate that large amounts of proteins (e.g., required in the case of insulin even though it requires multiple subunits) be expressed in bacteria such as the *E. coli*, which has been successfully used for the production of several relatively complex proteins.

The final yield is critical and as a result continuous efforts are made to modify bacterial strains such as deletion of protease genes or engineered for over expression of rare-codon tRNAs, foldases, or chaperones. It has also been demonstrated that gene-multimerization strategies can be beneficial in improving production yields. A consequence of the fragile and finicky nature of animal cells is that very large quantities of them are often needed. In the 1980s, yields approaching 100 mg/L were considered remarkable; now companies like MedImmune® produce 200–700 mg/L of an immunoglobulin-M MAb using hybridomas cultured in a hollow-fiber bioreactor. The highest reported CHO cell yields of heterologous proteins 20 years ago were 5–50 mg/L, 50–500 mg/L 10 years ago, and now we are approaching almost 5 g/L in special circumstances; apparently, we are able to reach a 10-fold increase every 10 years. The question of a workable yield should be considered in light of the regulatory impact of using a new and novel system. For biogeneric drug manufacturers, this is an important consideration as they are likely to emulate the approved process, a process that may have been approved decades ago.

Suitability of extraction of intracellular accumulation of protein versus secretion into periplasm or cell culture medium is important. However, genetic-design approaches are frequently applied to influence the targeting of the gene product. The recent developments in the use of gram-negative bacteria that secrete the product in the periplasm is of significance. Genetic design are also altered to facilitate the recovery of recombinant proteins by using gene fusion techniques that simplify the recovery process in such a way that it

243

might be possible to integrate several unit operations, increasing the overall efficiency in the downstream purification process. In this realm, affinity fusions have been commonly used, but also other principles, such as modified pI or hydrophobic properties, have been successfully investigated. A general drawback with fusion strategies is that the fusion partner often has to be removed to release a native gene product. Futuristic techniques like the introduction of combinatorial protein engineering to generate tailor-made product-specific affinity ligands allows highly specific recovery of a recombinant protein that can be expressed in its native form and this novel type of protein ligand (e.g., the protein A-based affibodies) can be sanitized using common industrial cleaning-in-place procedures (CIP).

9.8 EXPRESSION SYSTEM IN *E. COLI*

In any new development of a host system, *E. coli* remains the primary choice to begin with and alternate systems are tried only if this one fails if the product is biologically inactive after production due to lack of essential posttranslational modifications, incorrect folding, or when the recovery of the native protein is too low. Successful production of a recombinant protein in *E. coli* involves the following:

- Transcriptional and translational efficiency
- Stability of the expression vector and of the transcribed mRNA
- Localization
- Proteolytic stability
- Folding of the gene product
- Cell growth

An *E. coli* expression vector should contain the following:

- The gene of interest
- An origin of replication
- A gene that confers antibiotic resistance (or an alternative selectable marker)
- A promoter
- A transcription terminator

The hybrid *tac* promoter (P) consists of the 35 and 10 sequences, which are separated by a 17-base spacer. The arrow indicates the direction of transcription. The ribosome-binding site (RBS) consists of the Shine–Dalgarno (SD) sequence followed by an AT-rich translational spacer that has an optimal length of approximately 8 bases. The SD sequence interacts with the 3 end of the 16S rRNA during translational initiation, as shown. The three start codons are shown, along with the frequency of their usage in *E. coli*. Among the three stop codons, UAA followed by U is the most efficient translational termination sequence in *E. coli*. The repressor is encoded by a regulatory gene (R), which may be present on the vector itself or may be integrated in the host chromosome, and it modulates the activity of the promoter. The transcription terminator (TT) serves to stabilize the mRNA and the vector, as explained in the text. In addition, an antibiotic resistance gene, for example, for tetracycline, facilitates phenotypic selection of the vector, and the origin of replication (Ori) determines the vector copy number.

9.9 CONFIGURATION OF EFFICIENT EXPRESSION VECTORS

The essential architecture of an *E. coli* expression vector is shown in Figure 9.7. The promoter is positioned approximately 10 to 100 bp upstream of the RBS and is under the control of a regulatory gene, which may be present on the vector itself or integrated in the host chromosome. Promoters of *E. coli* consist of a hexanucleotide sequence located approximately 35 bp upstream of the transcription initiation base (35 region) separated by a short spacer from another hexanucleotide sequence (10 region). There are many promoters available for gene expression in *E. coli*, including those derived from gram-positive bacteria and bacteriophages. A useful promoter exhibits several desirable features: it is strong, it has a low basal expression level (i.e., it is tightly regulated), it is easily transferable to other *E. coli* strains to facilitate testing of a large number of strains for protein yields, and its induction is simple and cost-effective.

Downstream of the promoter is the RBS, which spans a region of approximately 54 nucleotides bound by positions 35 and 19 to 22 of the mRNA coding sequence. The SD site interacts with the 3′ end of 16S rRNA during translation initiation. The distance between the SD site and the start codon ranges from 5 to 13 bases (93), and the sequence of this region should eliminate the potential of secondary-structure formation in the mRNA transcript, which can reduce the efficiency of translation initiation. Both 5′ and 3′ regions of the RBS exhibit a bias toward a high adenine content.

The transcription terminator is located downstream of the coding sequence and serves both as a signal to terminate transcription and as a protective element composed of stem-loop structures, protecting the mRNA from exonucleolytic degradation and extending the mRNA half-life.

In addition to the above elements that have a direct impact on the efficiency of gene expression, vectors contain a gene that confers antibiotic resistance on the host to aid in plasmid selection and propagation. Ampicillin is commonly used for this purpose; however, for the production of human therapeutic proteins, other antibiotic resistance markers are preferable to avoid the potential of human allergic reactions. Finally, the copy number of plasmids is determined by the origin of replication. In specific cases, the use of runaway

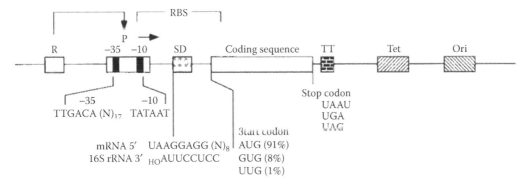

Figure 9.7 Sequence elements (not to scale) of a prokaryotic expression vector. (Reprinted from Makrides, S.C., *Microbiol. Rev.*, 60, 512–538, 1996. With permission.)

replicons results in massive amplification of plasmid copy number concomitant with higher yields of plasmid-encoded protein. In other cases, however, there appeared to be no advantage in using higher-copy-number plasmids over pBR322-based vectors. Furthermore, increasing the copy number of the plasmid decreases the production of trypsin in *E. coli* and the presence of strong promoters on high-copy-number plasmids severely impaired cell viability.

The origin of replication determines the vector copy number, which could typically be in the range of 25–50 copies/cell if the expression vector is derived from the low-copy-number plasmid pBR322, or between 150 and 200 copies/cell if derived from the high-copy-number plasmid pUC. The copy number influences the plasmid stability, that is, the maintenance of the plasmid within the cells during cell division. A positive effect of a high copy number is the greater stability of the plasmid when the random partitioning occurs at cell division. On the other hand, a high number of plasmids generally decreases the growth rate, thus possibly allowing for cells with few plasmids to dominate the culture, their being the faster growing. Generally, there appears to be no significant advantage of using higher-copy-number plasmids over pBR322-based vectors in terms of production yields.

The gene coding for antibiotic resistance is necessary both for identifying transformants and to ensure antibiotic selective pressure, that is, only cells that harbor an expression vector will divide, thus preventing plasmid loss. Genes conferring ampicillin, tetracycline, or kanamycin resistance are commonly used in expression vectors. Ampicillin resistance is mostly used only on a laboratory scale because the lactamase, which confers the resistance, degrades ampicillin and thus the selective pressure is lost after a few generations of cell growth. Furthermore, ampicillin has been thought to be potentially allergenic and is therefore usually not the antibiotic of choice in the production of biotherapeutics intended for human use. Another approach in preventing plasmid loss is to use a mutated *E. coli* strain deficient in a gene encoding an essential protein and include that crucial gene in the plasmid instead.

A number of strong promoters are available for high-level expression in *E. coli*. An important criterion of a promoter is its ability to be efficiently downregulated under non-induced conditions, that is, tightly regulated. An early overproduction of the heterologous protein, due to a non-silent promoter, might impair cell growth. It is therefore desirable to be able to repress the promoter during a cell growth phase to achieve high cell densities, after which the high-rate protein production would be initiated by induction of the promoter. Another important characteristic of a promoter is that it should be simple and inexpensive to induce. For laboratory-scale production, the isopropyl IPTG-inducible promoters, which are regulated by the product of the lacI gene, the lac repressor, are widely used. They include the lac promoter, the lac–trp hybrid promoter tac, and the trc promoter. A disadvantage with these promoters is that they are not completely downregulated under non-induced conditions and thus are not suitable if the target-gene product is toxic to the cell. The pET vector has a T7 promoter, which is transcribed only by T7 RNA polymerase, and must be used in a strain carrying a chromosomal T7 RNA polymerase gene, which is under the control of a lac promoter. The use of IPTG for induction of these promoters might not still be optimal for the large-scale production of human therapeutic proteins because of the cost of IPTG.

Lactose has been shown to be an inexpensive, but somewhat weaker, alternative for induction of the lac promoter in some applications. For large-scale cultivations, either the trp promoter or heat-induced promoters are commonly used. The trp promoter is induced by starvation of tryptophan or by the addition of β-indoleacrylic acid. One potential problem with the trp promoter is that it is difficult to completely downregulate under non-induced conditions, a problem which, however, can be minimized by the addition of fructose to the cultivation medium. Examples of heat-induced promoters are PL(λ), PR(λ), and the thermosensitive lac promoter lac (TS), which was constructed by mutation of the lacI gene. One drawback with these promoters is that the thermal induction could also induce the production of heat-shock proteins, including certain proteases that can cause enhanced degradation. Constitutive promoters, such as the *Staphylococcus aureus* protein A (SPA) promoter (PSPA), have also been used for recombinant-protein production. Promoters induced by cultivation conditions such as pH, oxygen levels, stationary growth, and osmolarity, as well as weak and moderately strong promoters, are also available.

A transcription termination downstream of the coding sequence enhances plasmid stability by preventing transcription through the replication region and through other promoters located on the plasmid. In addition, the transcription terminator enhances the stability of the mRNA transcript by a stem–loop formation at the 3′ end. The tandem T1T2 transcription terminator, derived from the rrnB ribosomal RNA operon of *E. coli*, is an efficient and commonly used transcription terminator.

9.10 PROTEIN PRODUCTION

Translation is initiated by the binding of the ribosomes at the SD sequences located within the RBS in the mRNA sequence. Optimal translation initiation is obtained for mRNAs with the SD sequence UAAGGAGG. Also the space between the binding site and the initiation codon, ideally four to eight nucleotides in length, is important for efficient translation initiation. Furthermore, the secondary structure around the RBS and in the sequence immediately downstream of the start codon has been described to influence the translational initiation efficiency, and an enrichment of A and T residues in those regions has been shown to improve the efficiency of translation. It has recently been suggested that the codon that follows the AUG initiation triplet (the + 2 codon) is of particular importance for the translation initiation efficiency and that there is a preference for adenine residues in this codon in highly expressed gene products.

The frequencies with which the different codons appear in genes in *E. coli* are different from those in genes of human origin. The amount of specific tRNAs is also reflected by the frequency of the codon, which means that a tRNA which recognizes a rarely used codon is present in low amounts. Therefore, human genes that contain codons which are rare in *E. coli* may be inefficiently expressed. This problem can be solved either by exchanging codons in the target gene for codons, which are more frequently used in *E. coli*, or, alternatively, by co-production of the rare tRNAs. The most abundant codons in *E. coli* have been determined by examination of sets of genes, and lists of codon usage can be found in several publications. The effect on expression levels by substitution of rare codons with optimal ones has been extensively studied, but general conclusions have been difficult to draw. The preferred stop codon in *E. coli* is UAA, while the prolonged UAAU stop codon can be used for more efficient translational termination.

9.10.1 Strategies for Production

A major consideration when designing a process for production of a recombinant protein in *E. coli* is whether the gene product should be produced intracellularly or if a secretion system could be used. Different genetic design strategies, together with the inherent properties of the target protein, decide which expression route will be the most successful. Upon intracellular expression, the product can either accumulate as a soluble gene product or precipitate in the form of inclusion bodies. If a secretion system is used, and the product is found to be secretable, the gene product will be accumulated in the periplasm or in some cases even be translocated also through the outer membrane to the extracellular culture medium. Every production strategy has its advantages and disadvantages (Table 9.6).

Table 9.6 Advantages and Disadvantages of Different Strategies for the Production of Recombinant Proteins in *E. coli*

Production Strategy	Advantages	Disadvantages
Secretion/leakage to the extracellular medium	Disulfide formation possible. Extensive proteolysis might be avoided. Possible to obtain authentic N-terminus. Significantly reduced levels of contaminants. No need for cell disruption	Secretion to the medium usually not possible. Dilution of the product
Periplasmic production	Disulfide formation possible. Possible to obtain authentic N-terminus. Reduced levels of contaminants	Secretion to the periplasma not always possible. No large-scale procedure for selective release of periplasmic proteins available. Periplasmic proteases can cause proteolysis
Intracellular production as inclusion bodies	Inclusion bodies easy to isolate. Protection from proteases. Protein is inactive and cannot harm host. High production yields usually obtained	Solubilizing and in vitro folding necessary which usually result in lower yields and higher cost. Normally no authentic N-terminus
Intracellular and soluble production	No need for solubilization and refolding	High levels of intracellular product can be harmful to the cells. Complex purification. Proteolysis might occur. Disulfide formation usually not possible. Normally no authentic N-terminus

9.10.2 Production by Secretion

The periplasm contains only about 100 proteins as compared with about 4,000 proteins in the cytoplasm. Thus, considerable purification and concentration effects are achieved by the targeting of the gene product to the periplasm. Additional beneficial effects achieved through the secretion of the gene product include enhanced disulfide-bond formation, possibility to obtain gene products with authentic N-termini, decreased proteolysis, and minimization of harmful action of recombinant proteins which are deleterious to the cell. The specific release of the periplasmic protein content is simple and commonly used at the laboratory scale by different osmotic-shock procedures. However, on an industrial scale, efficient methods for selective release of periplasmic proteins are lacking. Nevertheless, it has been shown that treatment at an elevated temperature after completed cultivation can improve unspecific leakage to the culture medium. It would be even more attractive to obtain translocation of the gene product to the growth medium, since this would lead to a significantly simplified purification scheme for the gene product. Protection against proteolysis might also be achieved using this strategy, because E. coli has very low extracellular proteolytic activity under normal conditions.

9.10.2.1 Secretion into the Culture Medium

There are no efficient pathways available for specific translocation of proteins through the outer membrane of E. coli. Instead, the secretion of some recombinant proteins to the periplasm is suggested to cause a destabilization of the outer membrane, which becomes leaky and allows the protein to diffuse into the extracellular medium in a semi-specific manner. Examples of proteins that have been efficiently secreted to the culture medium include different heterologous proteins fused to SPA domains to calmodulin and to the OmpA signal sequence. Another strategy is to use leaky E. coli mutants, which constitutively release periplasmic proteins into the culture medium due to loss of outer-membrane integrity. However, these mutants are fragile and revert readily to the non-leaky phenotype, a fact which makes these strains unsuitable for large-scale protein production. Alternatives to the use of leaky mutants are co-expression of the bacteriocin release protein or of the third topological domain of the transmembrane protein TolA, whereby a leaky phenotype is induced by disrupting the integrity of the outer membrane causing periplasmic proteins to leak into the growth medium. Supplementation of the growth medium with glycine has also been shown to enhance the release of periplasmic proteins into the cultivation medium.

9.10.2.2 Secretion to the Periplasmic Space

Many recombinant proteins have been successfully secreted to the periplasm by fusion of a signal sequence or a normally secreted protein N-terminally to the target protein. Frequently used signal sequences include those derived from the E. coli periplasmic proteins PhoA and MalE, the outer membrane proteins OmpA and LamB, β-lactamase and DsbA. Interestingly, the gram-positive signal sequence derived from SPA has shown to efficiently direct recombinant proteins to the periplasm of E. coli.

Proteolysis caused by envelope proteases is one of the most severe problems encountered when directing a recombinant protein to the periplasm of E. coli. The proteolysis can be minimized by different approaches, for example, by using protease-deficient strains or by genetic design of the gene product. Proteases that degrade many heterologous proteins in the periplasm are DegP, Tsp (denoted Prc in some publications), protease III (also named Pi), and OmpT. *E. coli* strains with single, double, and triple mutants of these proteases have been shown to efficiently decrease the degradation of different heterologous proteins secreted to the periplasm. One problem in using hosts deficient in multiple proteases is that viability, and thus growth, is impaired. Growth condition parameters such as temperature, pH, and medium composition also affect the periplasmic proteolysis. Genetic design approaches include in vitro mutagenesis in order to specifically eliminate protease cleavage sites in the target protein gene and different fusion protein strategies to protect the target protein from proteolysis. For example, the two IgG-binding domains ZZ, derived from SPA (Nilsson et al., 1987), and the albumin-binding protein BB from streptococcal protein G have successfully been used as fusion partners serving this purpose. They have either been fused to the N-terminus, the C-terminus, or to both termini of the target protein. The most pronounced stabilization effect has been obtained using the dual-affinity fusion strategy, which, in addition, allows recovery of the full-length product by two subsequent affinity-purification steps.

The environment in the periplasm is less reducing than that of the cytoplasm and favors the correct folding of recombinant proteins containing disulfide bonds. The periplasmic space also harbors foldases involved in the formation of disulfide bonds and isomerization of the proline imide bonds.

9.10.3 Intracellular Production

An intracellularly produced recombinant protein can be accumulated in a soluble form in the cytoplasm, precipitate and form inclusion bodies, or, alternatively, be partly in the form of inclusion bodies and partly in soluble form. It is usually impossible to predict whether the gene product will be soluble or if it will precipitate, and empirical investigations are therefore necessary. Among the most important factors influencing the inclusion-body formation are protein expression rate and presence of disulfide bonds, but hydrophobicity and choice of fusion partner have also been shown to have a significant impact.

9.10.3.1 Production of Soluble Gene Products

If the gene product is stable against proteolysis and not harmful to the host cell, it might be desirable to keep the protein soluble in the cytoplasm and thereby avoiding the solubilization and refolding steps that have to be performed if inclusion bodies are formed. There are several different approaches to minimize the formation of inclusion bodies when producing heterologous proteins intracellularly in *E. coli*. Reduction of the rate of protein synthesis, which can be achieved by using a moderately strong or weak promoter, or partial induction of a strong promoter, has been found to result in a higher amount of soluble protein. Other means of reducing the protein-synthesis rate is by growing the culture at lower temperature or to add non-metabolizable carbon sources at the time of induction. Substitution of amino acid residues, for example, replacement of multiple hydrophobic phenylalanine residues in respiratory-syncytial-virus (RSV) G protein or replacement of cysteine residues in S1 dihydrofolate reductase, has been shown to dramatically improve the solubility. However, this approach is limited to applications where the substitutions do not alter the desired function or activity of the recombinant protein. Fusion of the target protein to a highly soluble fusion partner, thereby increasing the overall solubility of the fusion protein, is a convenient and efficient method to increase the fraction of soluble gene product in the cytoplasm. Proteins used as solubilizing fusion partners include thioredoxin, ubiquitin, NusA the IgG-binding domains ZZ from SPA, the albumin-binding BB from Protein G, the maltose-binding protein, and a mutant form of DsbA. The overexpression of intracellular chaperones has in many studies resulted in an increased accumulation of soluble gene products. However, as for co-expression of foldases, this approach is protein-specific and is not a universal means of preventing inclusion-body formation. Usually, the redox potential in the cytoplasm prevents disulfide formation. In order to generate a less reducing environment in the cytoplasm, thereby facilitating disulfide-bond formation, strains deficient in thioredoxin reductase have been used.

For soluble gene products accumulated intracellularly in the *E. coli* cytoplasm, the first step in downstream processing is the release of the recombinant protein. On a laboratory scale, the cells are typically lysed by enzymic treatment, by chemical treatment, or by mechanical-disruption techniques such as sonication. High-pressure homogenization or bead mills are used in large-scale processing. Such treatment effectively liberates the desired protein, but it also releases the bulk of host-cell proteins and nucleic acids. If the expressed recombinant protein is thermostable, a convenient method to reduce the amounts of the contaminating host-cell proteins is heat precipitation. Additional advantage with heat precipitation is the thermal deactivation of the *E. coli* cell and of its proteases, reducing the potential risk of degradation of the target protein. It has also been shown that heat-treatment procedures performed on undisrupted cells efficiently can release recombinant proteins accumulated in a soluble form in the cytoplasm, thus combining the product-release step with the benefits of heat precipitation of host-cell proteins.

Such a heat-treatment procedure was recently successfully used in the recovery of an intracellularly accumulated fusion protein, BB-C7, in a production process for human pro-insulin C-peptide, where the heat treatment actually functioned as an initial purification step, giving a purity of ~70%, as compared with a purity of 10% obtained after conventional cell-disruption procedures.

9.10.3.2 Production as Inclusion Bodies

Many heterologous proteins expressed in *E. coli* are prone to precipitate, which in many cases is an advantage. The formation of inclusion bodies normally protects the gene product from host-cell proteases. The product is inactive and cannot harm the host cell, often giving high expression levels. Furthermore, the dense inclusion bodies can be readily recovered by centrifugation and a relatively high purity and degree of concentration of the gene product are thus normally obtained after solubilization. The main disadvantage with inclusion-body formation is the need for solubilization and refolding steps, necessary for regaining a correct protein structure and activity. These steps can reduce the yield and be costly, especially on a large scale. Different strategies have been utilized to enhance the tendency for the formation of inclusion bodies, for example, increasing the rate of protein synthesis by using strong

251

promoters such as the T7, trp or lac promoters, fusion of the target protein to certain other proteins, such as TrpLE, and cultivation at elevated temperatures or at a pH other than 7.0.

In vitro refolding inclusion bodies have an increased density and can easily be recovered by centrifugation after the disruption of the cells. The resulting inclusion-body-containing pellet consists mainly of the overexpressed recombinant protein, but contaminants originating from the host cells are also present. To remove these contaminants, the pellet can be washed with low concentration of denaturants or with detergents. After washing, the inclusion bodies are solubilized by using high concentration of denaturants. If the recombinant protein contains cysteine residues, a reducing and chelating agent should also be included in the solubilization buffer.

Renaturation of the solubilized gene product is initiated by the removal of the denaturant and, where appropriate, also the reducing agent, by dialysis or dilution. During the refolding procedure, it is important to limit product aggregation. This can be done by performing the refolding at low protein concentration, typically in the range of 10–50 mg/L. However, refolding at such low concentrations requires very large volumes, which becomes difficult and expensive when performed in industrial-scale applications. Therefore, other methods to keep the concentration of the unfolded protein low in the refolding buffer have been developed. Stepwise addition of the denatured recombinant protein and different dialysis approaches are examples of such methods. Different strategies have been developed to increase the refolding yield, either by stabilizing the native state, by destabilizing incorrectly folded molecules, or by increasing the solubility of folding intermediates and of the unfolded state. By performing the refolding at non-denaturing concentrations of denaturant, a high refolding yield has been obtained at high protein concentrations. Other low-molecular-mass additives have also successfully been used to enhance the refolding yield of a variety of different recombinant proteins. Molecular chaperones and foldases, monoclonal antibodies, and specific binding proteins have also been shown to increase the yield of correctly folded protein.

If the recombinant protein contains disulfide bonds, the renaturation buffer also has to contain a redox system, which provides the appropriate redox potential and enables formation and reshuffling of disulfides. The most common redox system is that of glutathione and its oxidized variant glutathione disulfide, but other low-molecular-mass thiol-based redox systems have also been utilized. Typically, a 1:1–5:1 molar ratio of reduced to oxidized thiol is used. For certain proteins, the yield of renaturation is increased if the thiol groups in the denatured protein are first completely oxidized by formation of mixed disulfides with glutathione. Disulfide bond formation is promoted by the addition of catalytic amounts of a reducing agent in a following renaturation step. In another method, the thiol groups in the denatured protein are sulfonated by treatment with Na_2SO_3 and a reducing agent. Under renaturating conditions, the protein is thereafter refolded in the presence of small amounts of reducing agent.

9.10.3.3 Purification of the Gene Product

After a successful production of a recombinant protein, different purification steps will be needed in order to recover a biologically active protein at high purity. The downstream process for the recovery and purification of a gene product depends on the production strategy used, but it consists typically of product release and clarification steps, an initial purification step and different chromatographic purification steps. During recent years, the major challenge in designing downstream processes has been to simplify and improve the overall efficiency by combination and elimination of unit operations to cut production costs. This has been achieved both by the development of new separation techniques and by genetic design of the produced recombinant protein.

9.10.4 Initial Recovery Methods

The aim of an initial recovery step is to rapidly remove or inactivate proteases, which can degrade the product, to remove impurities and particles, which have a negative effect on subsequent chromatographic purification steps, and to concentrate the sample. An ideal initial recovery step also gives a high degree of purification. Furthermore, it is essential that the equipment used is compatible with robust cleaning and sanitizing methods when considering industrial-scale production.

The expanded-bed adsorption (EBA) technology represents an initial recovery step that allows the capture of proteins from particle-containing feedstock without prior removal of the particulates. EBA has shown to be suitable for industrial production scale and the technology can also withstand harsh cleaning procedures. Precipitation is another simple approach for recovery of a gene product from a cultivation broth or homogenate. Various methods exist by which precipitation can be achieved: addition of salts, organic solvents, or organic polymers, or varying the pH or temperature. These precipitation methods are non-specific and give a low degree of purification. By using affinity pre-cipitation, increased specificity can be obtained. Different aqueous two-phase extraction systems have been extensively studied as an initial recovery step. An aqueous two-phase extraction system can also be combined with affinity precipitation combining the benefits of both methods.

9.11 GENETIC MANIPULATIONS TO IMPROVE YIELD

In recent years, a number of genetic strategies have designed to improve production yields, to simplify the recovery processes, to facilitate in vitro refolding, to provide site-specific cleavage of gene fusion product, and to create tailor-made product-specific affinity ligands.

9.11.1 Gene Fusion

Currently, there are two types of expression vector in *E. coli* for expressing mammalian genes. One is the non-fusion expression vector (as described above in detail) and the other is the fusion expression vector. The former is easier to use, however, certain genes are not expressed well or even not expressed at all in non-fusion expression vectors. In such cases, the only choice for expressing genes is to use a fusion expression vector. The features of fusion protein amplification that may influence the final choice of vector are listed below:

Fusion proteins
- Targeting information can be incorporated into a tag, provides a marker for expression, simpler purification using affinity chromatography under denaturating and non-denaturating conditions, easy detection, and refolding achievable on a chromatography column ideal for secreted proteins as the product is easily isolated from growth media
- Tag may interfere with protein structure and affect folding and biological activity, cleavage site is not 100% specific if tag needs to be removed

Nonfusion proteins
- No cleavage steps necessary
- Purification and detection not as simple reducing potential yield, problem with solubility may be difficult to overcome

Several kinds of fusion expression vectors have been constructed, characterized and commercialized. The fusion partners include glutathione *S*-transferase (GST), maltose-binding protein, staphylococcal protein A, and thioredoxin. The greatest advantage of fusion expression vectors is that the inserted genes can usually be expressed well. The major shortcoming of current fusion expression vectors is that chemicals, such as IPTG, are expensive and in short supply. The two most commonly used tags are GST tag and 6× histidine residues $(His)_6$ tag. As for the selection of host and vectors, the decision to use either a GST or a $(His)_6$ tag must be made according to the needs of the specific application. Table 9.7 provides the key features of these tags that should be considered. Polyhistidine tags such as $(His)_4$ or $(His)_{10}$ are also used. They may provide useful alternatives to $(His)_6$ if there are specific requirements for purification.

When choosing an affinity-fusion system, it is important to remember that all systems have their own characteristics, and no single system is ideal for all applications. For example, if secretion of the gene product is desired, it is necessary to choose a system with a secretable affinity tag. If the gene product needs to be purified under denaturated conditions, a system which has a tag that can bind under those conditions must be chosen, for example, the polyhistidine affinity tag. The polyhistidine tag is suitable for purification of gene products accumulated as inclusion bodies, because the fusion protein can be directly applied to an immobilized-metal-ion-affinity-chromatography (IMAC) column after being solubilized with a suitable denaturing agent. An additional advantage with the small polyhistidine affinity tag is that it can easily be genetically fused to a target protein by PCR techniques. It is also important to choose an affinity-fusion system with elution conditions under which the target protein does not get denaturated. For large-scale pharmaceutical production, however, affinity fusions have not been as extensively utilized, despite the ability to replace multiple steps with one step. The main reason is most probably that, for most applications, the affinity tag needs to be removed afterward. Furthermore, proteinaceous ligands may leak from the column during elution, making it necessary to remove the ligand from the eluate. If the ligand originates from a mammalian source, there is also risk of viral contamination. Questions concerning the possibility of column sanitation, and column lifetime, capacity and cost must also be considered. Table 9.8 provides examples of vectors for fusion proteins together with suggested purification products.

Table 9.7 Key Features of GST and (His)$_6$ Tags

GST Tag	(His)$_6$ Tag
Can be used in any expression system	Can be used in any expression system
Purification procedure gives high yields of pure product	Purification procedure gives high yields of pure product
Selection of purification products available for any scale	Selection of purification products available for any scale
pGEX6P PreScission™ protease vectors enable cleavage and purification in a single step	Small tag may not need to be removed, for example, tag is poorly immunogenic so fusion partner can be used directly as an antigen in antibody production
Site-specific proteases enable cleavage of tag if required	Site-specific proteases enable cleavage of tag if required. Note: Enterokinase sites that enable tag cleavage without leaving behind extra amino acids are preferable
GST tag easily detected using an enzyme assay or an immunoassay	(His)$_6$ tag easily detected using an immunoassay
Simple purification. Very mild elution conditions minimize risk of damage to functionality and antigenicity of target protein	Simple purification, but elution conditions are not as mild as for GST fusion proteins. Purification can be performed under denaturing conditions if required. Note: Neutral pH but imidazole may cause precipitation. Desalting to remove imidazole may be necessary
GST tag can help stabilize folding of recombinant proteins	(His)$_6$-dihydrofolate reductase tag stabilizes small peptides during expression
Fusion proteins form dimers	Small tag is less likely to interfere with structure and function of fusion partner; mass determination by mass spectrometry not always accurate for some (His)$_6$ fusion proteins

Table 9.8 Examples of Fusion Protein Vectors

Vector Family	Tag
pGEX	Glutathione *S*-transferase
PQE	6× Histidine
pET	6× Histidine
pEZZ 18 (non-inducible expression)	IgG-binding domain of protein A
pRIT2T (expression inducible by temperature change)	IgB-binding domain of protein A

9.11.1.1 Cleavage of Fusion Proteins

It is necessary to remove the affinity tag after the affinity-purification step. There are several methods, based on chemical or enzymic treatment, available for site-specific cleavage of fusion proteins. Advantages with the chemical cleavage methods are that the reagents used are inexpensive and widely available, and the reactions are generally easy to scale up. However, the harsh reaction conditions often required can lead to amino-acid-side-chain modifications or denaturation of the target protein. Furthermore, the selectivity is

255

often rather poor, and cleavage can occur on additional sites within the target protein. Therefore, chemical cleavage methods are usually only suitable for release of peptides and smaller proteins. For many applications, enzymic cleavage methods are preferred to chemical ones, because of their higher selectivity, and because the cleavage often can be performed under physiological conditions. Disadvantages of enzymic cleavage methods are that some enzymes are very expensive and that not all enzymes are widely available. Furthermore, if the enzyme is of mammalian origin, virus-removal and virus-clearance validations need to be performed if the target protein is to be used as a pharmaceutical. Recombinant proteases, produced in bacteria or yeast, are for that reason preferred.

9.11.1.2 Improved Recovery

Examples of gene fusions that have been used to improve initial recovery steps include fusions of hydrophobic tails to the target proteins to favor the partitioning into the top phase in aqueous two-phase systems and fusions of aspartic acid residues to the protein to enhance polyelectrolyte precipitation efficiency. Increased efficiency in anion-exchange chromatography in the EBA format was achieved by fusion of the target protein to the ZZ domains from Protein A, whereby the pI was lowered. By fusion of a stretch of arginine, glutamic acid, and phenylalanine residues, the efficiency of ion-exchange chromatography and hydrophobic-interaction chromatography was increased. One example of a tailor-made fusion partner is the engineered basic variant of the Z domain (Z_{basic}), enabling cation-exchange-chromatography separations to be performed at high pH values. Since almost no other host-cell proteins were found to bind under such conditions, very efficient purification could be achieved. Utilizing the features of the charged Z_{basic}, an integrated production strategy for Klenow DNA polymerase was developed. The Klenow DNA polymerase was produced as a Z_{basic}–Klenow fusion protein that could be efficiently recovered by cation-exchange chromatography in the EBA mode. The Z_{basic}–Klenow fusion was subsequently cleaved to release free Klenow polymerase, with the help of a Z_{basic}-tagged viral protease 3C, whereafter fused Klenow could be recovered from the reaction mix by separating Z_{basic}-protease 3C and Z_{basic} fusion partner using cation-exchange chromatography.

9.11.1.3 Facilitated In Vitro Refolding

Fusions of target proteins to highly soluble fusion tags have been shown to enhance in vitro refolding. For example, a high refolding yield at high protein concentration was obtained by fusion of a moderately soluble target protein to ZZ from protein A. By fusion of a target protein to a histidine tag, immobilization of the fusion protein on an IMAC column can be made under denaturing conditions. A subsequent on-column refolding step typically gives high yield of renatured target protein. A related example, in which a hexa-arginine polypeptide extension was fused to the target protein, the fusion protein was immobilized on a cation-exchange column and renatured target protein was obtained after on-column refolding.

9.11.1.4 Gene Multimerization

When expressing peptides in *E. coli*, low yields are often obtained. One reason could be the susceptibility of the peptides to proteolysis. A common strategy to improve the stability is to produce the peptide as a fusion. A major disadvantage with this strategy is that the desired product only constitutes a small portion of the fusion protein, often resulting in low yields of the target peptide. One way of increasing the molar ratio, and hence increase the amount of peptide produced, is to produce a fusion protein with multiple copies of the target peptide. An additional beneficial effect is often obtained by this strategy, since the gene multimerization has also been shown to increase the proteolytic stability of the produced peptides. When the gene multimerization strategy is employed to increase the production yield, subsequent processing of the gene product to obtain the native peptide is needed. By flanking a peptide gene with codons encoding methionine, CNBr cleavage of the fusion protein, containing multiple repeats of the peptide, has successfully been used for obtaining native peptide at high yield. Takasuga and co-workers produced a pentapeptide multimerized to 3, 14, and 28 copies, fused to dihydrofolate reductase, engineered to be separated by trypsin cleavage. A similar strategy was used to produce a peptide hormone of 28 residues. Eight copies of the peptide gene were linked in tandem, separated by codons specifying lysine residues flanking the peptide, and the construct was fused to a gene fragment encoding a portion of β-galactosidase. Endoproteinase Lys-C, an enzyme which specifically cleaves on the C-terminal side of lysine residues, was used instead of trypsin, together with carboxypeptidase B, to release the native peptide. Similarly, a multimerization strategy was used to improve the yields of the 31-amino-acid human proinsulin C-peptide. The C-peptide was expressed intracellularly in *E. coli* as one, three or seven copies as parts of fusion proteins. Since it was found that the three different fusion proteins were expressed at equal levels and that they all were efficiently processed by trypsin/carboxypeptidase B treatment to release native C-peptide, the seven-copy construct was used to generate a recombinant production process.

9.11.1.5 Simplified Site-Specific Removal of Fusion Partners

Genetically designed recombinant proteases have been used to simplify the removal of proteases after site-specific cleavage of fusion proteins. By fusing the protease to the same affinity tag as the target protein, an efficient removal of the affinity-tagged protease, the released affinity tag, and uncleaved fusion protein can be achieved using affinity chromatography. This principle is commercially available, examples being the systems based on His-tagged tobacco-etch-virus protease and human rhinovirus 3C protease fused to a glutathione *S*-transferase tag (PreScission™ protease). An affinity-tagged protease can, as an alternative to covalent coupling, also be immobilized to an affinity matrix and be utilized for on-column cleavage. On-column cleavage, in which the produced fusion proteins are site-specifically cleaved while still immobilized on the affinity column, has also been described. An affinity-fusion system, consisting of a protein splicing intein domain from *S. cerevisiae* and a chitin-binding domain, allows simultaneous affinity purification and on-column cleavage. Different immobilizing approaches are especially important for large-scale applications, since they can reduce the protease consumption and help to avoid additional contamination by the added protease.

9.11.1.6 Tailor-Made Product-Specific Affinity Ligands

Powerful in vitro selection technologies, such as phage display, have proven efficient for the isolation of novel binding proteins from large collections (libraries) of peptides or proteins constructed, for example, by combinatorial protein engineering. One example of such binding proteins is the so-called *affibodies*, selected from libraries constructed by random mutagenesis of the Z domain derived from SPA. The Z domain, used as scaffold during library constructions, is proteolytically stable, highly soluble, small (6 kDa), and has a compact and robust structure devoid of intramolecular disulfide bridges, making it an ideal domain for ligand development. Using phage-display technology, affibody ligands to a wide range of targets have been successfully selected. Recently, such affibody ligands showed selective binding in authentic affinity-chromatographic applications involving the purification of target proteins from *E. coli* total cell lysates. Such tailor-made product-specific affinity ligands have also been generated and used for highly efficient recovery of recombinant human Factor VIII produced in CHO cells and a recombinant vaccine candidate, derived from the RSV G protein, produced in baby hamster kidney cells.

The obvious advantage of using a ligand selected to bind to the target protein instead of fusing the target protein to an affinity tag is that no cleavage step to obtain the native protein is needed. The disadvantage is that a new high-affinity ligand must be selected and produced for every new recombinant protein needed to be purified. It is nevertheless likely that this strategy will be attractive in recombinant bioprocesses, since highly selective affinity matrices can be created that potentially even could discriminate between different folding forms of the target protein and could thus replace several other chromatographic steps in the recovery process. Interestingly, no loss of column capacity or selectivity for the target protein was obtained even after repeated cycles of low pH elution and column sanitation protocols, including 0.5 M NaOH. This might suggest that affinity chromatography using protein ligands could become increasingly used also in industrial-scale recombinant-proteins recovery processes in the future.

9.11.1.7 Molecular Chaperons

It is now well established that the efficient posttranslational folding of proteins, the assembly of polypeptides into oligomeric structures, and the localization of proteins are mediated by specialized proteins termed molecular chaperones. The demonstration that efficient production and assembly of prokaryotic ribulose bisphosphate carboxylase in *E. coli* require both GroES and GroEL proteins led to an increasing interest in the use of molecular chaperones for high-level gene expression in *E. coli*. In addition to their utility in purification and detection, specific fusion peptides may confer advantages to the target protein during expression, such as increased solubility, protection from proteolysis, improved folding, increased yield, and secretion. The engineering of specific protease sites in many fusion proteins facilitates the cleavage and removal of the fusion partner(s).

Normally, protein folding proceeds toward a thermodynamically stable end product. Proteins that are drastically destabilized will probably fold incorrectly, even in the presence of chaperones. Thus, the truncation of polypeptides, the production of single domains from multisubunit protein complexes, the lack of formation of disulfide bonds which ordinarily contribute to protein structure, or the absence of posttranslational modifications such as glycosylation may make it impossible to attain thermodynamic stability. Moreover, it is now clear that different types of chaperones normally act in concert. Therefore, the overproduction of a single chaperone may be ineffective. For example, the overproduction of DnaK alone resulted in plasmid instability which was alleviated by the coproduction of DnaJ. Similarly, the coexpression of three chaperone genes in *E. coli* increased the solubility of several kinases. In some cases, it may be necessary to coexpress chaperones cloned from the same source as the target protein. Still another variable to consider is growth temperature. For example, GroES-GroEL coexpression increased the production of β-galactosidase at 30 but not 37 or 42C, whereas DnaK and DnaJ were effective at all temperatures tested. Finally, the overexpression of chaperones can lead to phenotypic changes, such as cell filamentation, that can be detrimental to cell viability and protein production.

9.11.1.8 Codon Usage

Genes in both prokaryotes and eukaryotes show a nonrandom usage of synonymous codons. The systematic analysis of codon usage patterns in *E. coli* led to the following observations:

- There is a bias for one or two codons for almost all degenerate codon families.
- Certain codons are most frequently used by all different genes irrespective of the abundance of the protein; for example, CCG is the preferred triplet-encoding proline.
- Highly expressed genes exhibit a greater degree of codon bias than do poorly expressed ones.
- The frequency of use of synonymous codons usually reflects the abundance of their cognate tRNAs. These observations imply that heterologous genes enriched with codons that are rarely used by *E. coli* may not be expressed efficiently in *E. coli*.

The minor arginine tRNA has been shown to be a limiting factor in the bacterial expression of several mammalian genes, because the codons AGA and AGG are infrequently used in *E. coli*. The coexpression of the *argU* (*dnaY*) gene that codes for tRNA results in high-level production of the target protein. The production of β-galactosidase decreases when AGG codons are inserted before the 10th codon from the initiation codon of the *lacZ* gene. To date, however, it has not been possible to formulate general and unambiguous *rules* to predict whether the content of low-usage codons in a specific gene might adversely affect the efficiency of its expression in *E. coli*. Nevertheless, from a practical point of view, it is clear that the codon context of specific genes can have adverse effects on both the quantity and quality of protein levels. Usually, this problem can be rectified by the alteration of the codons in question, or by the coexpression of the cognate tRNA genes.

Questions

1. Why do mammalian cell strategies require a long time prior to generation of commercial product?
2. What is a cell bank?
3. What are the differences between a master cell bank and a working cell bank?
   Answer: The master cell bank is the source from which the working cell bank is derived. By having a master cell bank, problems that arise with the working cell bank can be mitigated by having a *backup*. The working cell bank does not require extensive characterization because it is derived from the master cell bank.

4. Are the master and working cell banks ever the same?
   Answer: Yes, often early production proceeds with a singular cell bank that serves as both the master and working cell banks.
5. What are the most common genetically modified organisms based on currently approved products?
6. What disadvantages and advantages are present in using mammalian cells for recombinant protein production?
   Answer: Advantages are they are often faster than plant and transgenic animals; disadvantages are they are often more fragile and require more complicated culture systems.
7. What role does the plasmid play in developing genetically modified cells?
8. What were the first genetically modified organisms that lead to biotechnology-derived products?
9. Why are there often two antibiotic resistances incorporated into a vector?
   Answer: One provides selection during bacterial expansion of the vector and the other provides positive selection for mammalian cells that have incorporated the vector.
10. What decisions go into selection of a host for recombinant protein production?
11. What advantage do fusion proteins provide and what are the complications these advantages bring?

10

Manufacturing Overview

LEARNING OBJECTIVES

1. Identify the processes involved in recombinant protein production.
2. Understand the unique advantages and disadvantages of microbial culture systems for product production.
3. Recognize the appropriate governmental regulatory agencies for each aspect of product production.

10.1 INTRODUCTION

Macromolecular (large molecules) substances (e.g., therapeutic proteins) are manufactured by a number of methods including extraction from natural sources (as done in the past to extract erythropoietin from urine), modification of naturally occurring protein, mammalian cell culture in vitro, mammalian cell culture in vivo, and production by microorganisms, and chemical syntheses. The overall regulatory scheme for biotechnology-derived products is the same as for products in the same category produced by traditional manufacturing methods, with the addition of specific requirements suited to the biotechnology-derived product. As an example, somatropin (human growth hormone) was approved by the U.S. Food and Drug Administration (FDA) on July 30, 1976, derived from natural sources (Asellarcin of Serono) and in April 1979 (Crescormon of Genentech); both these products are discontinued now and instead replaced with recombinantly produced somatropin in 1993. The entire technical package relating purity and characterization of somatropin remains the same for the recombinantly produced somatropin except there are additional production steps. Generally, manufacturing recombinant therapeutic proteins involves the following:

1. Cloning of a specific gene in the laboratory, or the construction of a synthetic gene
2. Insertion into a host cell and subcloning in a microorganism or cell culture
3. Process development on a pilot scale to optimize yield and quality
4. Large-scale fermentation or cell culture processes
5. Purification of the macromolecular proteins
6. Animal testing, clinical testing, regulatory approval, and marketing

This applies to both rDNA-derived products as well as monoclonal antibody products. Biotechnology-derived products are therefore readily differentiated from proteins or peptides that have been obtained by isolation from natural source materials such as plasma, serum, or tissue, or by chemical synthesis even though the nature of the product is same and even labeled as such, for example, hEPO (human erythropoietin) or hIFN (human interferon); except for the undesirable changes that may arise as a result of processing, these products are indeed exact replica of what the body produces.

The manufacturing processes follow similar basic requirements for process validation, environmental control, aseptic manufacturing, and quality control/quality assurance systems as required for pharmaceutical products, though with a great deal more complexity, as the processes of cell propagation, purification methods, and analytical controls are significantly different and more detailed. Most pharmaceutical companies are not likely to have in-house expertise to handle this new requirement slanted toward biological rather than chemical aspects. It is always inevitable not to recruit specialized manpower for the manufacturing of biological products. This applies not just to the recombinant phase of manufacturing but also the formulation aspects that offer unique handling and therefore validation problems.

Overall, the process of manufacturing comprises of *upstream, downstream,* and *formulation* processing. Upstream refers to cell culture, leading to fermentation. Downstream segment of process begins with the harvest step where the cells are separated, separation of target proteins from host and process-related impurities, an intermediate purification step (or further separation from host), a polishing step to separate target protein from impurities. The yield at this point is called drug substance. Formulation step involves preparing a dosage form ready for administration to humans by converting drug substance into drug product. This is an equally important step as studies show that protein structures can be significantly altered depending on how the batch is handled. For example, a recent change in the label for erythropoietin indicates that the vial should *not* be shaken prior to administration to protect the protein structure. In upstream the major strategic issue is whether the cell culture should be run in the batch, fed-batch or in continuous mode, the latter being very attractive at low expression levels because of higher yields in continuous processing. Whereas the recombinant process outline is to some extent determined by the expression system used, but most recombinant processes are following identical patterns. The target protein is expressed in cellular systems (bacteria, mammalian cells, and insect cells), transgenic animals or plants (upstream part). The harvest is purified by means of several purification unit operations divided into capture, intermediary purification, and polishing (downstream) resulting in the purified bulk material (drug substance). Finally the drug substance is transformed into a product acceptable for use in humans (drug product). Upstream refers to protein expression and harvest; downstream refers to capture, intermediate purification, and polishing; and formulation refers to conversion of drug substance to drug product.

The entire manufacturing process must be tightly connected at each unit operation of upstream and downstream processing. Yield variation, impurity diversity, and potency achieved are the factors that can significantly affect all steps. As a result, the manufacturing process is carefully laid out in a lengthy exercise of process definition and development, a flowchart that identifies slacks as well as sizing issues.

10.2 CELL CULTURE EXPRESSION SYSTEMS

The starting material for manufacturing therapeutic proteins are the bacterial, yeast, insect, or mammalian cell culture which expresses the protein product or monoclonal antibody of interest. The cell seed lot system is used by manufacturers to assure identity and purity of the starting raw material. A cell seed lot consists of aliquots of a single culture. The master cell bank (MCB) is derived from a single colony (bacteria, yeast) or a single eukaryotic cell, stored cryogenically to assure genetic stability and is composed of sufficient ampoules of culture to provide source material for the working cell bank (WCB). The WCB is defined as a quantity of cells derived from one or more ampoules of the MCB, stored cryogenically and used to initiate the production batch.

The most common cellular expression systems used to manufacture therapeutic proteins include bacteria (*Escherichia. coli, Bacillus subtilis, Lactococcus lactis*), yeast (*Saccharomyces cerevisiae, Pichia pastoris*) and mammalian cells (Chinese hamster ovary [CHO], baby hamster kidney [BHK]) and insect cells where the baculovirus expression system is used to some extent and may prove itself as a future biopharmaceutical expression system; currently, there are no products approved using insect cell lines or transgenic animals, though several are under development (Table 10.1).

Table 10.1 Cell Lines Used for Commercially Produced Recombinant Products as Approved by the U.S. FDA

Cell Lines	Commercial Recombinant Products
African monkey kidney cells (COS-1)	Antihemophilic factor (Advate®)
Baby hamster kidney cells	Antihemophilic factor (Helixate® and Kogenate®FS)
Chinese hamster ovary cell	Adalimumab (Humira®)
	Alefacept (Amevive®)
	Alemtuzumab (Campath®)
	Algasidase beta (Fabrazume®)
	Alteplase (Activase®, Cathflo®)
	Antihemophilic factor (Bioclate®, Recombinate® Kaht®, ReFacto®)
	Choiogonadotropin alfa (Ovidrel®)
	Coagulation factor IX (BeneFix®)
	Darbepoetin alfa (Aranesp®)
	Dornase alfa (Pulmozyme®)
	Drotrecogin alfa (Xigris®)
	Efalizumab (Raptiva®)
	Epoietin alfa (Epogen®, Procrit®)
	Etanercept (Enbrel®)
	Follitropin alfa (Gonal-F®)
	Follitropin beta (Follistim®)
	Ibritumomab tiuxetan (Zevalin®)
	Imiglucerase (Cerezyme®)
	Interferon beta 1-alpha (Avonex®)
	Laronidase (Aldurazyme®)
	Omalizumab (Xolair®)

(Continued)

263

Table 10.1 (Continued) Cell Lines Used for Commercially Produced Recombinant Products as Approved by the U.S. FDA

Cell Lines	Commercial Recombinant Products
	Rituximab (Rituxan®)
	Tenecteplase (TNKase®)
	Thyrotropin alfa (Thyrogen®)
	Trastuzumab (Herceptin®)
E. coli	Aldesleukin Proleukin, IL-2®
	Alpha interferon+ribavarin Reberon®
	Alpha-interferon (Intron A®)
	Anakinra (Kineret®)
	Bone morphogenetic protein [rhBMP-2-] device (Infuse®Bone Graft/LT-CAGE®)
	Coagulation factor VIIa (NovoSeven®)
	Denileukin difitox (Ontak®)
	Filgrastim (Neupogen®)
	Growth hormone (BioTropin®)
	Insulin (Humalog®, Humulin®, Velosulin®, BR Novolin®, Novolin L®, Novloin R®, Novolin® 70/30, Novloin N®)
	Insulin aspart (Novolog®)
	Insulin glargine (Lantus®)
	Insulin glulisine (Apidra®)
	Interferon alfa-2a (Roferon-A®)
	Interferon alfacon-1 (Infergen®)
	Interferon beta 1-a (Rebif®)
	Interferon beta 1-B (Betaseron®)
	Interferon gamma-1b (Actimmune®)
	Nesiritide (Natrecor®)
	Oprelvekin (Neumega®)
	Pegfilgrastim (Neulasta®)
	Peginterferon alfa-2z (Pegasys®)
	Pegvisomant (Somavert®)
	Pegylated interferon alfa-2b (PEG-Intron®)
	Reteplase (Retavase®)
	Somatotropin (Humatrope®)
	Somatrem (Protropin®)
	Somatropin (Norditropin®, Nutropin®/ Nutropin AQ®®) Nutropin (Depot®GenoTropin® Geref®)
	Teriparatide (Forteo®)
Lymphocyte activated	Daclizumab (Zenapax®)
Mouse C 127	Growth hormone (Saizen®, Serostim®)
Mouse myeloma	Basiliximab (Simulect®)
Myeloma NSO	Gemtuzumab ozogamicin (Mylotarg®)
Mammalian	Tositumomab with I-131(Bexxar®)
	Abciximab (ReoPro®)

(Continued)

Table 10.1 (*Continued*)   Cell Lines Used for Commercially Produced Recombinant Products as Approved by the U.S. FDA

Cell Lines	Commercial Recombinant Products
Prostate epithelium cell	Capromab pendetide with In-111 (ProstaScint®)
Saccharomyces cerevisiae	Becaplermin gel (Regranex® Gel)
	Glucagon (GlucaGen®)
	Granulocyte macrophage colony-stimulating factor (Leukine®)
	Haemophilus B conjugate (Comvax®)
	Hepatitis A inactivated and hepatitis B vaccine (Twinrix®)
	Hepatitis B and inactivated polio-virus vaccine (Pediarix®)
	Hepatitis B vaccine (Engerix-B®, Recombivax-HB®)
	Lepirudin (Refludan®)
	OspA lipoprotein (LYMErix®)
	Rasburicase (Elitek®)

The choice of expression system depends on factors such as type of target protein, posttranslational modifications, expression level, intellectual property rights, and economy of manufacture. The *E. coli* expression system offers rapid and cheap expression, but cannot express complex proteins, and include in vitro folding and tag-removal into the downstream process. Yeast generally expresses the target protein in its native form to the medium, but expression levels are very low. Insect cells provide many advantages of the mammalian cell characteristics. Table 10.2 lists the advantages and disadvantages of each of these systems.

10.2.1 Bacterial Systems

The bacterial expression system make use of gram-negative (e.g., *E. coli*) and gram-positive host cells (*Bacillus* and *Lactococcus*) allow both intra- and extracellular expression of target protein, however, without posttranslational modifications. It takes about five days from introduced gene to protein production at acceptable levels of a few hundred mg/L to g/L. Bacterial systems are easy to scale up from culture flask to fermenters with capacity into thousands of liters because of simpler nutrition and aeration requirements and the ability to take carrying shear force. Several types of culture process are used such as batch and fed-batch, making this system highly flexible. The major adventitious agents are host cell proteins and endotoxins from *E. coli*; viruses are of little concern, except what may be required to control general exposure during processing. Critical steps including control of impurities arising out of released proteolytic enzymes and endotoxins, besides the handling of inclusion bodies, in vitro folding and cleavage of the N-terminal extension introduced to overcome the problem with expression of Met-protein. As a result, the downstream processing is often complicate which can limit the choice of this expression system. However, the regulatory record is impressive (Table 10.2); at this stage only gram-negative organisms have been approved.

Table 10.2 Comparison of Various Expression Systems, Advantages and Disadvantages

Qualifier	Bacteria	Yeast	Insect Cells	Mammalian Cells	Transgenic Animals
Example	*E. coli*	*Saccharomyces cerevisiae, Pichia pastoris*	Lepidopteran	Chinese hamster ovary cells	Cattle
Level of expression	High	Medium	Medium	Medium	Very high
Time to produce expression system	Fast	Fast	Medium	Slow	Very slow
	5 days	14 days	4 weeks	4–8 weeks	6–33 months
Cost	Low	Low	High	High	Medium
Extracellular expression	No	Yes	Yes	Yes	Yes
Met-protein expression	Yes	No	No	No	No
Posttranslation modifications	No	No	Yes	Yes	Yes
Major impurities	Endotoxins	Glycosylated products	Viruses	Viruses	Viruses and prions
In vitro protein refolding	Yes	No	No	No	No
Unintended glycosylation	No	Possible	Possible	Possible	Possible
Host cell protein expression	No	No	No	No	Yes
Regulatory track record	Good	Good	N/A	Good	N/A

10.2.2 Yeast Systems

The yeast species *Saccharomyces cerevisiae* and *Pichia pastoris* are also used and their use growing fast (Tables 10.1 and 10.2) as these systems offer high efficiency (short doubling times, high cell densities, high yields from better mass transfer of nutrients in unicellular growth morphology) and low fermentation costs. The media cost and scale-up considerations are similar to those encountered in bacterial systems; however, the development time frame is a bit longer, about 14 days from gene construct to production. Both batch and fed-batch culture methods are used. The target protein is usually expressed directly to the medium in its native form, although some proteins tend to undergo degradation upon expression (e.g., proinsulin). A low redox potential of the medium/harvest is sometimes observed resulting in cleavage of disulfide bonds. Yeast has GRAS (generally regarded as safe) FDA status and host-related impurities are very low since the organism has rigid cell wall and the expressed protein is secreted to the medium. Like the bacterial cultures, viruses are of little significance as contaminants. The purification process is usually simpler compared to the bacterial system (since the product is secreted in yeast) and no extra host cell-related operations are required. However, the disadvantages include lack of posttranslational modifications and unexpected formation of mono- and di-glycosylated forms of the target proteins that may be difficult to remove.

10.2.3 Insect Cells

Insect cells constitute a promising, yet unproven, alternative to bacterial and yeast expression systems for a wide range of target proteins requiring proper posttranslational modifications. The difficulties in scale up arise because of difficulties in aeration and type of infection needed for high-level expression. The use of baculovirus system is becoming accepted very fast; it has been used to transform *lepidopteran* insect cells into high-level expression systems in the range of 1–600 mg/L. Preparation and purification of the recombinant virus is faster than the process in mammalian cells and can be completed in about 4 weeks. In the fermentation cycle, the insect cells grow 50-fold in about a week but only in single batches or in semicontinuous batches because of the sensitivity of the cells to shear force. The costs for culture media are moderate (serum-free media) to expensive compared to bacteria and yeast media. The system is suited for expression of cell toxic products since the cells can be grown in a healthy state before infection. Insect cells lack the ability to properly process proteins that are initially synthesized as larger inactive precursor proteins (e.g., peptide hormones, neuropeptides, growth factors, and matrix metalloproteases). Baculoviruses are not infectious to vertebrates and therefore do not pose a health threat, though the risk of adventitious viruses is still not settled requiring virus inactivation and active filtration. Also, the cyclic killing and lysis of the host cell releases intracellular proteins and nucleic acids into the medium severely straining the downstream purification steps (like in the case of bacterial cells with inclusion bodies). The regulatory record of insect cells remains poor as no products have been approved by the U.S. FDA yet.

267

10.2.4 Mammalian Cells

Mammalian cells like CHO, human cervix (HeLa), African green monkey kidney (COS), BHK cells, and hybridomas are widely used for the production of monoclonal antibodies and complex posttranslational eukaryotic proteins. The target protein is generally expressed directly to the medium in its native form. The development timeline from gene construct to production is 4–5 months and the yields obtained range from a few mg/L to g/L. Since the protein is expressed to the low viscosity medium and the content of host cell proteins is usually low, the purification processes are relative simple, however these must remove components like peptone, anti-foam reagents, growth factors, and so on when used and the released host cell proteins and nucleic acids due to apoptosis and cell sensitivity to sheer forces, and the process of virus inactivation/removal. Mammalian cells are difficult and slow to grow and are more fragile than microbial cells making them very sensitive to sheer forces; batch or fed-batch cultures are often used for antibody production, while other recombinant protein also may be produced in continuous cultures over 4–8 weeks. Culture media are expensive relative to those used for microbial and yeast protein expression. Since viral contamination is a real risk, inactivation and removal must be designed into the downstream process and extensive control procedures established (e.g., end of production testing and virus validation). The relative low expression levels combined with high prices on culture media and expensive quality control programs makes it generally more expensive to produce recombinant proteins in animal cells than in microbial systems. However, complex proteins cannot be expressed in microbial systems leaving transgenic animals or plants as the only alternative. The regulatory record of the use of mammalian cells is very good (Table 10.2).

10.3 TRANSGENIC ANIMALS

Transgenic animals are one of the most promising recombinant protein expression systems in the biopharmaceutical industry. The first product, an antibody expressed in goats is about to be approved by the U.S. FDA. In this system, even complex posttranslational modified proteins are successfully expressed in their native biologically active form, thus making it possible to produce plasma proteins, human antibodies, and other proteins not easily derived from other sources at industrial scale. It takes 6 to 33 months (depending on host organism) from gene construct to product expression, usually in the mammary gland, often at high protein concentrations (50 mg/mL), resulting in a yearly production of up to 10–100 kg per animal (cows). Transgenic animals co-express species-specific target protein, which can be difficult to separate from the recombinant target protein. Virus inactivation and removal procedures must be included. Even though rarely recorded, prions as well as the most likely viruses undergo virus inactivation and removal and with extensive control procedures must be established (e.g., end-of-production test and virus validation). The skim milk fraction is an excellent starting material after capture of fat and casein. For large-scale production (>100 kg/y), the costs of raw products are one-tenth for transgenic animals compared to mammalian cell cultures, mainly because of reduction in capital investment. The regulatory record in the use of transgenic animals is poor (Table 10.2).

10.4 CELL LINES AND CHARACTERIZATION

Because genetic stability of the cell bank during storage and propagation is a major concern, it is important to know the origin and history (number of passages) of both the MCB and WCB. A MCB ampoule is kept frozen or lyophilized and only used once. Occasionally, a new MCB may be generated from a WCB. The new MCB should be tested and properly characterized. For biological products, a product license application or amendment must be submitted and approved before a new MCB can be generated from a WCB. Information about the construction of the expression vector, the fragment containing the genetic material that encodes the desired product, and the relevant genotype and phenotype of the host cell(s) are submitted as part of a product application. The major concerns of biological systems are genetic stability of cell banks during production and storage, contaminating microorganisms, and the presence of endogenous viruses in some mammalian cell lines. As part of the application document, manufacturers are required to submit a description of all tests performed to characterize and qualify a cell bank.

It must be emphasized that the tests required to characterize a cell bank will depend on the intended use of the final product, the host/expression system and the method of production including the techniques employed for purification of the product. In addition, the types of tests may change as technology advances. The MCB is rigorously tested using the following tests, though the testing may not be limited to these tests:

- Genotypic characterization by DNA fingerprinting
- Phenotypic characterization by nutrient requirements, isoenzyme analysis, and growth and morphological characteristics
- Reproducible production of desired product
- Molecular characterization of vector/cloned fragment by restriction enzyme mapping, sequence analysis
- Assays to detect viral contamination
- Reverse transcriptase assay to detect retroviruses
- Sterility test and mycoplasma test to detect other microbial contaminants

It is not necessary to test the WCB as extensively as the MCB; however, limited characterization of a WCB is necessary. The following tests are generally performed on the WCB, but this list is not inclusive:

- Phenotypic characterization
- Restriction enzyme mapping
- Sterility and mycoplasma testing
- Testing the reproducible production of desired product

The MCB and WCB must be stored in conditions that assure genetic stability. Generally, cells stored in liquid nitrogen (or its vapor phase) are stable longer than cells stored at −70°C. In addition, it is recommended that the MCB and WCB be stored in more than one location in the event that a freezer malfunctions.

10.5 MEDIA

Media must be carefully selected to provide the proper rate of growth and the essential nutrients for the organisms producing the desired product. Raw materials should not contain any undesirable and toxic components that may be carried through the cell culture, fermentation, and the purification process to the finished product. Water is an important component of the media and the quality of the water will depend on the recombinant system used, the phase of manufacture and intended use of the product. Raw materials considered to be similar when supplied by a different vendor should meet acceptance criteria before use. In addition, a small-scale pilot run followed by a full-scale production run is recommended when raw materials from a different vendor are used, to assure that growth parameters, yield, and final product purification remain the same.

Most mammalian cell cultures require serum for growth. Frequently, serum is a source of contamination by adventitious organisms, especially mycoplasma, and firms must take precautions to assure sterility of the serum. There is an additional concern that bovine serum may be contaminated with bovine spongiform encephalopathy (BSE) agent. Because there is no sensitive in vitro assay to detect the presence of this agent, it is essential that the manufacturers know the source of the serum and request certification that the serum does not come from areas where BSE is endemic. Other potential sources of BSE may be proteases and other enzymes derived from bovine sources. Biological product manufacturers have been requested to determine the origin of these materials used in manufacturing.

The media used must be sterilized generally by sterilizing in place (SIP) or a using a continuous sterilizing system (CSS) process. Any nutrients or chemicals added beyond this point must be sterile. Air lines must include sterile filters. The following checklist, though not totally inclusive, should be used frequently:

- Confirm the compliance of the source of serum
- Confirm that the sterilization cycle has been properly validated to ensure that the media will be sterile
- Verify that all raw materials have been tested by quality control. Determine the origin of all bovine material
- Document instances where the media failed to meet all specifications
- Verify that expired raw materials have not been used in manufacture
- Check that media and other additives have been properly stored

10.6 CULTURE GROWTH

Cell cultures are run in batch, fed-batch, or continuous mode depending on expression system used. Continuous systems may take weeks to complete and several harvest pools often result making it necessary to clearly define the batch strategy. Bioreactor inoculation, transfer, and harvesting operations must be done using validated aseptic techniques. Additions or withdrawals from industrial bioreactors are generally done through steam-sterilized lines and steam-lock assemblies. Steam may be left on in situations for which the heating of the line or bioreactor vessel wall would not be harmful to the culture.

It is important for a bioreactor system to be closely monitored and tightly controlled to achieve the proper and efficient expression of the desired product. The parameters for the fermentation process must be specified and monitored. These may include growth rate, pH, waste by-product level, viscosity, addition of chemicals, density, mixing, aeration, and foaming. Other factors that may affect the finished product include shear forces, process-generated heat, and effectiveness of seals and gaskets.

Many growth parameters can influence protein production. Some of these factors may affect deamidation, isopeptide formation, or host cell proteolytic processing. Although nutrient-deficient media are used as a selection mechanism in certain cases, media deficient in certain amino acids may cause substitutions. For example, when *E. coli* is starved of methionine and/or leucine while growing, the organism will synthesize norleucine and incorporate it in a position normally occupied by methionine, yielding an analogue of the wild-type protein. The presence of these closely related products will be difficult to separate chromatographically; this may have implications both for the application of release specifications and for the effectiveness of the product purification process.

Computer programs used to control the course of fermentation, data logging, and data reduction and analysis should be validated (see Section 10.11).

Bioreactor systems designed for recombinant microorganisms require not only that a pure culture is maintained, but also that the culture be contained within the systems. The containment can be achieved by the proper choice of a host-vector system that is less capable of surviving outside a laboratory environment and by physical means, when this is considered necessary. The *National Institutes of Health (NIH) Guidelines* described under Section 10.21 discusses the details further.

10.7 EXTRACTION, ISOLATION, AND PURIFICATION

Several techniques have been used to condition the sample for the first chromatographic capture step: centrifugation, filtration, and microfiltration. In some cases, the harvest and capture steps have been united by means of expanded bed technology. Due to the large volumes handled, major changes in ionic strength or pH are not recommended. Instead, a purification principle matching the characteristics of the application sample should be selected. The recovery process begins with isolation of the desired protein from the fermentation or cell culture medium, often in a very impure form. The advantage of cell culture and yeast-derived products is that many of these proteins are secreted directly into the medium, thus requiring only cell separation to obtain a significant purification. For *E. coli*-derived products, lysis of the bacteria is often necessary to recover the desired protein. It is important in each case to achieve rapid purification of the desired protein because proteases released by the lysed organisms may cleave the desired product. Such trace proteases are a major concern in the purification of biotechnology-derived products because they can be very difficult to remove, may complicate the recovery process, and can significantly affect final product stability. The recovery process is usually designed to purify the final product to a high level. The purity requirement for a product depends on many factors, although chronic use products may be required to have much higher purity than those intended for single-use purposes. Biotechnology-products contain certain impurities that the recovery processes are specifically designed to eliminate or minimize. These impurities include trace amounts of DNA, growth factors, residual host proteins, endotoxins, and residual cellular proteins from the media.

10.8 CAPTURE

Once the fermentation process is completed, the desired product is separated, and if necessary, refolded to restore configuration integrity, and purified. The first part of the downstream process is capture.

- It separates the expressed protein from major impurities (water, cell debris, lipoproteins, lipids, carbohydrates, proteases, glycosidases, colored compounds, adventitious agents, fermentation additives, and fermentation by-products).
- It conditions the sample for further intermediary purification steps.

The target protein should be concentrated and transferred to an environment, which will conserve the biological activity. The main purpose of the capture step is to get rid of water, host, and process-related impurities. Due to the large volumes handled, and the nature of the application sample, the first chromatographic purification step is built on the on/off principle aiming for selective binding of the protein to the matrix. Large particle sizes are used to avoid clotting of the column and low resolution should be expected. One of the fundamental principles for capture operations is to focus on the target protein properties to achieve effective binding and pay less attention toward contaminants, since purity is not the issue at this stage. The high selectivity of affinity chromatography can be an attractive approach for capture provided that the affinity ligand stability does not put severe restrictions on the use of efficient cleaning and sterilization regimes. The most frequent purification principles used are packed bed or expanded bed affinity, and ion exchange chromatography (IEC). In expanded bed technology, direct application of the cell culture is possible, thereby reducing the number of unit operations. Capture operations should make use of simple technologies, broad parameter intervals, high flow rates, cheap chromatographic media, and large particle sizes to assure process robustness, consistency, and economy. The outcome of the capture operation is a severe reduction in sample volume; reduction of the amount of impurities; and a sample, which is conditioned for the next step.

For recovery of intracellular proteins, cells must be disrupted after fermentation. This is done by chemical, enzymatic, or physical methods. Following disruption, cellular debris can be removed by centrifugation or filtration. For recovery of extracellular protein, the primary separation of product from producing organisms is accomplished by centrifugation or membrane filtration. Initial separation methods, such as ammonium sulfate precipitation and aqueous two-phase separation, can be employed following centrifugation to concentrate the products. Further purification steps primarily involve chromatographic methods to remove impurities and bring the product closer to final specifications. Extraction and isolation requires either filtration or centrifugation, which are listed as follows:

- *Filtration*: Ultrafiltration is commonly used to remove the desired product from the cell debris. The porosity of the membrane filter is calibrated to a specific molecular weight, allowing molecules below that weight to pass through while retaining molecules above that weight. It is an integrated part of every downstream process in order to condition the sample for chromatographic purification and to perform sterile filtrations. The filtration techniques comprise conventional filtration, microfiltration, ultrafiltration, and the use of specific filters for removal of defined impurities such as endotoxins, viruses, or prions. In-depth filtration consists of separation of particles from the solute using large pore size filters. Most samples are filtered before entering the chromatographic column to prevent increase in backpressure. Microfiltration consists of separation of particles from the solute using specifically designed tangential flow-over membranes with pore sizes ranging from 0.1–0.3 Pm. Sheer forces may destabilize the protein. Ultrafiltration separates the protein from low molecular solvent molecules using specifically designed tangential flow-over membranes with a cutoff range from 1 to 100,000 kDa. Sheer forces may destabilize the protein. Filters with specific ligands are used a specific filters for virus and prion removal are entering the market. They may be used in future processes to increase product safety. Filtration is used throughout for sample conditioning. Microfiltration is used for clarification of the harvest. Ultrafiltration is used for buffer exchange and/or sample concentration. It is not recommended to use the technique as the final step in the downstream process, as the sheer forces may affect protein stability.

- *Precipitation:* This process is rarely used as a purification technique, but rather as an intermediary step between two chromatographic unit operations. The trend is to avoid precipitation for reasons of economy, time, compliance issues, and convenience. However, it may be useful to precipitate the protein for the purpose of storage. Precipitation is rarely used in capture due to the large volumes handled.
- *Centrifugation*: It can be open or closed. The environment where centrifugation is performed must be controlled. It is commonly applied to remove cells, cell debris, and precipitates from the harvest. The technique is labor demanding and is today sought replaced with microfiltration techniques or expanded bed technology.
- *Crystallization:* This process is protein specific. It offers both purification and the ability to store the protein in a convenient way. Crystallization may be used for some intermediary products.
- *Virus inactivation and/or active filtration*: This process is added as an extra unit operation when using mammalian cells or transgenic animals as the expression system.

10.9 PURIFICATION

Chromatography is one of the most powerful protein purification techniques. Over the years, the technique has been developed into an industrial tool, where most biopharmaceutical processes comprise at least three different chromatographic steps carefully adjusted to the capture, intermediary, and polishing principle. Table 10.3 gives an overview of the application areas for different chromatographic purification methods. The selection of chromatographic medium depends on the composition of the sample. Table 10.3 lists

Table 10.3 Relative Importance of Various Chromatographic Methods in Various Downstream Processes

Principle	Capture	Intermediary Purification	Polishing
Affinity	+++	+	+
Crystallization	+	++	+++
Filtration	+++	+++	+++
HAC	+	+++	+
HIC	++	+++	+
IEC	+++	+++	+++
IMAC	+++	++	+
Microfiltration	+++	+	+
Precipitation	+	+++	+++
RPC	+	+	+++
SEC	+	+	+++
Ultrafiltration	+++	+++	+++

some of the general features of the different chromatographic principles. Co-solvents mentioned will, generally, not affect the binding of the protein to the column. For every chromatographic technique used, there is a balance between resolution, speed, capacity, and recovery. Choose logical combinations of chromatographic techniques, based on the main benefits of the technique and the condition of the sample at the beginning or end of each step. Techniques may be combined but mainly when they are complimentary to each other. Given below is an explanation of various types of chromatography practices:

The purification process is primarily achieved by one or more column chromatography techniques.

Affinity chromatography (AC)

AC works on the basis of structural epitome recognition. Low protein concentration; large application volumes; any pH that applies; low to medium ionic strength. Affinity chromatography is a selective technique wherein the on/off principle fits very well into the capture mode, where large amounts of impurities are removed. Proteins normally elute from the column at low pH; common practice to apply the sample at neutral to slightly alkaline pH.

Anion exchange chromatography (AEC)

AEC works on the principle of electrostatic interactions. Low protein concentration; large application volumes; pH > pI; low ionic strength; ethanol, urea, and non-ionic detergents tolerated. IEC is the most common chromatographic technique in use. It suits capture, intermediate purification, and polishing, making use of the highly specific media developed with defined particle sizes, spacers, and ligands. HIC offers, generally, less resolution than IEC, but selectivity can be high when the proper ligand has been defined.

274

Cation exchange chromatography (CEC)
>   Low protein concentration; large application volumes; pH<pI; low ionic strength; ethanol, urea, and non-ionic detergents tolerated.

Hydroxyapatite chromatography (HAC)
>   Low protein concentration; large application volume; pH > 7.0; the matrix does not tolerate acidic pH; low-to-medium ionic strength; medium-to-high ionic strength; ethanol tolerated. HAC often provides excellent solutions to purification challenges. The high resolution RPC technique is primarily used for proteins of molecular weight lower than 25 kDa, as the binding constant for higher molecular weight proteins is too high. Elution in organic solvents is common and protein stability in these buffers is a major issue.

Hydrophobic interaction chromatography (HIC)
>   Low protein concentration; large application volume; any pH that applies; medium-to-high ionic strength. HIC is often used in combination with ion exchange, making use of the binding of proteins at high salt concentrations and elution at low salt concentrations. The presence of hydrophobic antifoam agents in fermentation broth and cell cultures may lower the binding capacity if HIC is used in the capture step. It may also be a less attractive capture technique if the feed volume is large and addition of salt is needed in order to increase the ionic strength of the solution. The large salt quantities thus needed add to the manufacture costs and causes a waste disposal problem.

Immobilized metal affinity chromatography (IMAC)
>   IMAC work on complex binding between metal-ligand and proteins. Low protein concentration; large application volumes; neutral pH; high ionic strength; denaturants, detergents, and ethanol tolerated. IMAC is rarely exploited in industrial downstream processing. It is a powerful capture technique for a number of proteins and a unique tool for histidine-tagged proteins. It is also a salt-tolerant technique being a useful feature considering typical ionic strength in biological starting materials Selectivity can be very high and depends on the combined efforts of primary, secondary and tertiary structure of proteins.

Reversed phase chromatography (RPC)
>   Hydrophobic interaction; silica-based matrices do not tolerate alkaline pH. Low protein concentration; large application volumes; any pH that applies; organic solvents can be used.

Size exclusion chromatography (SEC)
>   Steric exclusion from the intra particle volume; sample volume restricted to maximum 5% of the column volume; high protein concentration; small application volumes; any pI, any ionic strength; any solvent. SEC is recommended as the final purification step. Although the sample volume rarely exceeds 5% v/v of the column volume, the technique offers removal of di- and polymeric compounds, transfer to a well-defined buffer and, in many cases, enhanced protein stability. Relative importance of each of the unit operations is given in Table 10.3.

10.10 IMPURITY REMOVAL

A variety of impurities that these chromatographic techniques are expected to remove and the testing methods used to ascertain this removal include

- *Aggregated proteins*: SDS-PAGE, HPSEC
- *Amino acid substitutions*: Amino acid analysis, peptide mapping, MS, Edman degradation analysis
- *Deamidation*: Isoelectric focusing (IEF), HPLC, MS, Edman degradation analysis
- *DNA*: DNA hybridization, UV spectrophotometry, protein binding
- *Endotoxin*: Bacterial endotoxins test (pyrogen test)
- *Formyl methionine*: Peptide mapping, HPLC, MS
- *Host cell proteins*: SDS-PAGE, immunoassays
- *Microbial (bacteria, yeast, fungi)*: Microbial limit tests, sterility tests, microbiological testing
- *Monoclonal antibodies*: SDS-PAGE, immunoassays
- *Mycoplasma*: Modified 21 CFR method, DNAF
- *Other protein impurities (media)*: SDS-PAGE, HPLCb, immunoassays
- *Oxidized methionines*: Peptide mapping, amino acid analysis, HPLC, Edman degradation analysis, MS
- *Protein mutants*: Peptide mapping, HPLC, IEF, MS
- *Proteolytic cleavage*: IEF, SDS-PAGE (reduced), HPLC, Edman degradation analysis, MSS
- *Viruses (endogenous and adventitious)*: CPE and HAd (exogenous virus only), reverse transcriptase activity, mouse antibody production (MAP)

10.11 VALIDATION

Chemicals used in chromatography methods, either in the stationary (bonded) phase or in the mobile phase, may become impurities in the final product and the burden of validation (i.e., demonstrating removal of potentially harmful chemicals) lies on the manufacturer. A column material supplier certification regarding leaching of chemicals is not sufficient since the contamination is process and product dependent. Validation is necessary when isolating end product monoclonal antibodies or using a technique that contains a monoclonal antibody purification step. The process must demonstrate removal of leaching antibody or antibody fragments. It is also required to ensure the absence of adventitious agents such as viruses and mycoplasmas in the cell line that is the source of the monoclonal antibodies. The main concern is the possibility of contamination of the product with an antigenic substance whose administration could be detrimental to patients. Continuous monitoring of the process is necessary to avoid or limit such contamination. The problem of antigenicity related to the active as well as host proteins is one that is unique to biotechnology-derived products in contrast to traditional pharmaceuticals. Manufacturing methods that use certain solvents should be monitored if these solvents are able to cause chemical rearrangements that could alter the antigenic profile of the drug substance. The manufacturer is also obligated to produce evidence regarding performance consistency of novel chromatographic columns. Considerations for single-use products such as vaccines may differ because they are not administered continuously and, in this case, antigenicity is desirable. On the other hand, validating the removal of ligand or extraneous protein contamination is necessary. Unlike drugs derived from natural sources, manufacturers of biotechnology-derived products have been required to provide validation of the removal of nucleic acids during purification. Vaccines may again be different in this regard because of the accumulated clinical history on these products.

10.12 INTERMEDIATE PURIFICATION

The intermediate purification step

- Removes the majority of key impurities cellular proteins, culture media components, DNA, viruses, endotoxins, and so on.
- Is the first stage purification.
- Uses *medium size* particles in a variety of chromatographic techniques.
- Is used for chemical and/or enzymatic modifications of the protein.
- Is used for higher resolution between related compounds by
  - Applying more selective desorption principles such as multistep or continuous gradient elution procedures.
  - More specific chromatographic matrices, using smaller particles (offering better resolution) and technically more advanced solutions (gradients); made possible by higher purity and generally lower viscosity of the samples applied.
- Is ideal for packed bed technology.

10.13 POLISHING

The polishing step(s)

- Are high-resolution chromatographic methods to separate even closely related compounds (des-amido forms, oxidized forms, etc.).
- Require expensive, small uniform media particles with reversed phase, and IEC as the dominant chromatographic principles.
- Involve recommended SEC or desalting operation as the final polishing step. Use of SEC as the final step may serve a number of purposes:
  - Removal of di- and polymers
  - Possible buffer exchange to any buffer requested for formulation of drug substance bulk
  - Increase of protein stability
  - Uniform composition of the bulk material

The eluent from the polishing operation should be a stable well-defined bulk material (drug substance) meeting specifications and with a composition acceptable for further formulation.

10.14 FORMULATION

The formulation of the drug product is a crucial step; most therapeutic proteins are either packaged in a liquid form or in lyophilized form, both requiring a certain minimum volume to contain the final drug product. As a result, it may be necessary to include a size-exclusion or desalting step to reduce the volume, whereas much attention has been paid to the upstream and downstream step determining the final characterization of the product, the formulation step can significantly affect the safety and efficacy of the product. In the case of a lyophilized product, there are likely to be no added ingredients but in a liquid formulation, there could be several common ingredients. Examples include albumin, sucrose, polysorbates, buffer salts, and so on. Given below is the composition of a few such examples (Tables 10.4 through 10.16).

Table 10.4 Oprelvekin Injection (Interleukin IL-11)

Bill of Materials (Batch Size 1 L)					
Scale/mL		Item	Material	Quantity	UOM
1.00	mg	1	Oprelvekin (interleukin IL-11)	1.00	g
4.60	mg	2	Glycine	4.60	g
0.32	mg	3	Dibasic sodium phosphate heptahydrate	0.32	g
0.11	mg	4	Monobasic sodium phosphate monohydrate	0.11	g
qs	mL	5	Water for injection, qs to	1.00	L

Table 10.5 Interleukin Injection (IL-2)

Bill of Materials (Batch Size 1 L)					
Scale/mL		Item	Material	Quantity	UOM
0.25	mg	1	IL-2	0.25	g
0.70	mg	2	Sodium laurate	0.70	g
10.00	mM	3	Disodium hydrogen phosphate	10.00	M
50.00	mg	4	Mannitol	50.00	g
Qs	mL	5	Hydrochloric acid for pH adjustment 1 M	qs	
qs	mL	6	Water for injection, qs to	1.00	L

Table 10.6 Interferon Alfa-2a Injection

Bill of Materials (Batch Size 1 L)					
Scale/mL		Item	Material	Quantity	UOM
3 MM	IU	1	Interferon alfa-2a	3B	IU
7.21	mg	2	Sodium chloride	7.21	g
0.20	mg	3	Polysorbate 80	0.20	g
10.00	mg	4	Benzyl alcohol	10.00	g
0.77	mg	5	Ammonium acetate	0.77	g
qs	mL	6	Water for injection, qs to	1.00	L

Table 10.7 Interferon Beta-1b Injection

Bill of Materials (Batch Size 1 L)					
Scale/mL		Item	Material	Quantity	UOM
0.30	mg	1	Interferon beta-1b	0.30	g
15.00	mg	2	Albumin (human)	15.00	g
15.00	mg	3	Dextrose	15.00	g
5.40	mg	4[a]	Sodium chloride	5.40	g
qs	mL	5	Water for injection, qs to	1.00	L

[a] This item is packaged separately as 0.54% solution (2 mL diluent for lyophilized product).

Table 10.8 Interferon Beta-1a Injection

Bill of Materials (Batch Size 1 L)					
Scale/mL		Item	Material	Quantity	UOM
33.00	mcg	1	Interferon beta-1a	33.00	mg
15.00	mg	2	Albumin (human)	15.00	g
5.80	mg	3	Sodium chloride	5.80	g
5.70	mg	4	Dibasic sodium phosphate	5.70	g
1.20	mg	5	Monobasic sodium phosphate	1.20	g
qs	mL	6	Water for injection, qs to	1.00	L

Table 10.9 Interferon Alfa-n3 Injection

Bill of Materials (Batch Size 1 L)					
Scale/mL		Item	Material	Quantity	UOM
5 MM	U	1	Interferon alpha-n3	5B	U
3.30	mg	2	Liquefied phenol	3.30	g
1.00	mg	3	Albumin (human)	1.00	g
8.00	mg	4	Sodium chloride	8.00	g
1.74	mg	5	Sodium phosphate dibasic	1.74	g
0.20	mg	6	Potassium phosphate monobasic	0.20	g
0.20	mg	7	Potassium chloride	0.20	g
qs	mL	8	Water for injection, qs to	1.00	L

279

Table 10.10 Interferon Alfacon-1 Injection

Bill of Materials (Batch Size 1 L)					
Scale/mL		Item	Material	Quantity	UOM
0.03	mg	1	Interferon alfacon-1	0.03	g
5.90	mg	2	Sodium chloride	5.90	g
3.80	mg	3	Sodium phosphate	3.80	g
qs	mL	4	Water for injection, qs to	1.00	L

Table 10.11 Interferon Gamma-1b Injection

Bill of Materials (Batch Size 1 L)					
Scale/mL		Item	Material	Quantity	UOM
200.00	mcg	1	Interferon gamma-1b	200.00	mg
40.00	mg	2	Mannitol	40.00	g
0.72	mg	3	Sodium succinate	0.72	g
0.10	mg	4	Polysorbate 20	0.10	g
qs	mL	5	Water for injection, qs to	1.00	L

Table 10.12 Infliximab for Injection

Bill of Materials (Batch Size 1 L)					
Scale/mL		Item	Material	Quantity	UOM
10.00	mg	1	Infliximab	10.00	g
50.00	mg	2	Sucrose	50.00	g
0.05	mg	3	Polysorbate 80	0.05	g
0.22	mg	4	Monobasic sodium phosphate monohydrate	0.22	g
0.61	mg	5	Dibasic sodium phosphate dihydrate		
qs	mL	6	Water for injection, qs to	1.00	L

Table 10.13 Daclizumab for Injection

Bill of Materials (Batch Size 1 L)					
Scale/mL		Item	Material	Quantity	UOM
5.00	mg	1	Daclizumab	5.00	g
3.60	mg	2	Sodium phosphate monobasic monohydrate	3.60	g
11.00	mg	3	Sodium phosphate dibasic heptahydrate	11.00	g
4.60	mg	4	Sodium chloride	4.60	g
0.20	mg	5	Polysorbate 80 (Tween®)	0.20	g
qs	mL	6	Water for injection, qs to	1.00	L
qs	mL	7	Sodium hydroxide for pH adjustment	qs	
qs	mL	8	Hydrochloric acid for pH adjustment	qs	
qs	cuft	9	Nitrogen gas	qs	

Table 10.14   Coagulation Factor VIIa (Recombinant) Injection

Bill of Materials (Batch Size 1,000 vials)					
Scale/vial		Item	Material	Quantity	UOM
1.20	mg	1	rFVIIa	1.20	g
5.84	mg	2	Sodium chloride	5.84	g
2.94	mg	3	Calcium chloride dihydrate	2.94	g
2.64	mg	4	Glyglycine	2.64	g
0.14	mg	5	Polysorbate 80	0.14	g
60.00	mg	6	Mannitol	60.00	g

Table 10.15   Reteplase Recombinant for Injection

Bill of Materials (Batch Size 1,000 vials)					
Scale/vial		Item	Material	Quantity	UOM
18.10	mg	1	Reteplase	18.10	g
8.32	mg	2	Tranexamic acid	8.32	g
136.24	mg	3	Dipotassium hydrogen phosphate	136.24	g
51.27	mg	4	Phosphoric acid	51.27	g
364.00	mg	5	Sucrose	364.00	g
5.20	mg	6	Polysorbate 80	5.20	g

Table 10.16   Alteplase Recombinant Injection

Bill of Materials (Batch Size 1,000 vials)					
Scale/vial		Item	Material	Quantity	UOM
58MM	IU	1	Alteplase	100.00	g
3.50	g	2	L-Arginine	3.50	kg
1.00	g	3	Phosphoric acid	1.00	kg
11.00	mg	4	Polysorbate 80	11.00	g
Qs	mL	5	Water for injection, qs to	1.00	L

Several formulations require an added component for stabilization of proteins, for example, darbopoietin alpha, interferon beta 1a and 1b, interferon alpha 2b, antihemophilic factor, epoetin alpha (also available without albumin), recombinant factor VIII (also available without albumin), and laronidase. Extra care is needed as albumin is a known carrier of viruses; validated sources must be used to supply human albumin.

10.15 PROCESS OVERVIEW

10.15.1 Process Maturity

As soon as a project enters into the development phase the time of delivery of material for preclinical and clinical trials becomes a major issue. The amounts needed far exceed what can be produced in a development laboratory and material for clinical trials must be produced according to current good manufacturing practice (cGMP). The process designers face a dilemma: how much should process design be compromised in order to produce the material needed in shortest possible time? An immature process will lead to process redesign late in the project resulting in tedious repeats of analytical and biological testing. A too long process development period will—on the other hand—not be accepted by upper management due to tight project time constraints. It is important to understand the depth of the dilemma. Imagine a mammalian pilot-scale process being used to produce material for initial drug substance/product stability studies, references, tox studies, and virus validation studies. A major process change will raise doubt of all the data obtained with the original process, although much can be accomplished with comparability studies, stability and virus validation studies have to be repeated severely delaying the project. Project management must also consider other issues such as process economy, which does not compromise safety but can result in a no-go decision (Table 10.17).

Obviously, there is a need to define the process maturity level before scale up or in other words to define *a priori* process maturity criteria. Ideally, criteria listed in the

Table 10.17 Process Overview for Different Expression Systems

Expression System	Process	Protocol
General	Cell culture	Batch, fed batch, or perfusion; 3–40 days.
	Harvest	Centrifugation/filtration; omit if using expanded bed.
	Capture	Chromatographic unit operation is typically based on affinity or IEC. Remove major host and process-related impurities and water.
	Variable unit operation	The unit operation may be refolding (if *E. coli* is used) or virus inactivation if insect cells, mammalian cells, or transgenic animals are used.
	Intermediate purification	Chromatographic unit operation typically based on HIC, IEC, or HAC stepwise gradient technology used to remove host-and process-related impurities.
	Variable unit operation	This unit operation may include tag removal (if *E. coli* is used) or virus removal by filtration if insect cells, mammalian cells, or transgenic animals are used.
	Polishing	Chromatographic unit operation typically based on HP-IEDC or HP-RPC stepwise/linear gradient technology used to remove product-related impurities.
	Variable unit operation	SEC or ultrafiltration to assure proper drug substance formulation.

(Continued)

Table 10.17 (*Continued*)   Process Overview for Different Expression Systems

Expression System	Process	Protocol
	Drug substance	The conversion of the drug substance to drug product typically include change of buffer, precipitation, or crystallization.
	Formulation	Batch manufacturing often including stabilizers such as albumin.
	Finished drug product	Filling in appropriate containers such as vials or pre-filled syringes.
E. coli (gram negative)	Fermentation	Expression of N-terminally extended target protein to overcome formation of Met-protein.
	Harvest	Harvest of cells by centrifugation prior to cell disruption.
	Cell disruption	Disruption with French press or like; wash out inclusion bodies.
	Extraction	Extraction under reducing and denaturing conditions (e.g., 0.1 M cysteine, 7 M urea pH 8.5).
	Capture	Purification under reducing and denaturing conditions (e.g., IEC or IMAC if protein is His-tagged).
	Renaturation	Controlled folding of the target protein using hollow fiber, SEC, dilution, or buffer exchange.
	Intermediate purification	Purification of the folded target protein (e.g., IEC, HIC, and HAC).
	Enzyme cleavage	Cleavage of the N-terminal extension with exo- or endoproteases.
	Polishing 1	Purification of the target protein (e.g., HP-IEC and HP-RPC).
	Polishing 2	Purification of the target protein by SEC (not always included).
	Drug Substance	The purified bulk product.
	Formulation	Re-formulation of the drug substance preparing for administration to humans.
	Drug product	The final product.
Gram-positive bacteria	Fermentation	Expression the target protein to the periplasmatic room or medium.
	Harvest	Harvest of cells by centrifugation prior to cell disruption. This step may be bypassed by means of expanded bed technology.
	Capture	Purification of the target protein from the supernatant.
	Intermediate purification	Purification of the target protein (e.g., IEC, HIC, and HAC).
	Polishing 1	Purification of the target protein (e.g., HP-IEC and HP-RPC).
	Polishing 2	Purification of the target protein by SEC (not always included).
	Drug substance	The purified bulk product.
	Formulation	Re-formulation of the drug substance preparing for administration to humans.

Table 10.17 (Continued)   Process Overview for Different Expression Systems

Expression System	Process	Protocol
	Drug substance	The final product.
Yeast	Fermentation	Expression the target protein to the medium.
	Harvest	Harvest of cells by centrifugation prior to cell disruption. This step may be by-passed by means of expanded bed technology.
	Capture	Purification of the target protein from the supernatant or by expanded bed technology.
	Intermediate purification	Purification of the target protein (e.g., IEC, HIC, and HAC).
	Polishing 1	Purification of the target protein (e.g., HP-IEC and HP-RPC).
	Polishing 2	Purification of the target protein by SEC (not always included).
	Drug substance	The purified bulk product.
	Formulation	Re-formulation of the drug substance preparing for administration to humans.
	Drug product	The final product.
Insect cells	Cell culture	Expression the target protein to the medium.
	Harvest	Harvest of cells by centrifugation prior to cell disruption. This step may be bypassed by means of expanded bed technology.
	Capture	Purification of the target protein from the supernatant or by expanded bed technology.
	Virus inactivation	Inactivation by means of low pH, high temperature, detergents, and so on.
	Intermediate purification	Purification of the target protein (e.g., IEC, HIC, and HAC).
	Virus filtration	Nanofiltration.
	Polishing	Purification of the target protein (e.g., HP-IEC, HP-RPC, and SEC).
	Drug substance	The purified bulk product.
	Formulation	Re-formulation of the drug substance preparing for administration to humans.
	Drug product	The final product.
Mammalian cells	Cell culture	Expression the target protein to the medium.
	Harvest	Harvest of cells by centrifugation prior to cell disruption: This step may be bypassed by means of expanded bed technology.
	Capture	Purification of the target protein from the supernatant or by expanded bed technology.
	Virus inactivation	Inactivation by means of low pH, high temperature, detergents, and so on.
	Intermediate purification	Purification of the target protein (e.g., IEC, HIC, and HAC).
	Virus filtration	Nanofiltration.
	Polishing	Purification of the target protein (e.g. HP-IEC, HP-RPC, and SEC).

(Continued)

Table 10.17 (*Continued*)   Process Overview for Different Expression Systems

Expression System	Process	Protocol
	Drug substance	The purified bulk product.
	Formulation	Re-formulation of the drug substance preparing for administration to humans.
	Drug product	The final product.
Transgenic animals	Raw milk	Milking of animals according to Good Agricultural Practices.
	Skim milk	Centrifuged raw milk with low fat content.
	Capture	Purification of the target protein from the skim milk.
	Virus inactivation	Inactivation by means of low pH, high temperature, detergents, and so on.
	Intermediary purification	Purification of the target protein (e.g. IEC, HIC, and HAC).
	Virus filtration	Nanofiltration.
	Polishing	Purification of the target protein (e.g., HP-IEC, HP-RPC, and SEC).
	Drug substance	The purified bulk product.
	Formulation	Re-formulation of the drug substance preparing for administration to humans.
	Drug product	The final product.

Table 10.18 should be accomplished before tech transfer, but the real world is not perfect and certain task may remain unfinished at scale up with the risk of major adjustments and perhaps process redesign at a later stage. Some companies do plan with a process redesign between phases 2 and 3 as a compromise between time to market and extra development costs. Maturity criteria for technology transfer and scale up is described in Table 10.18.

10.15.2 Process Optimization

Once the process has been scaled up, the process design is locked, but there is room for optimization within the parameter intervals stated (proven acceptable range). The optimization process involves adjustment of the process to improve yields, process economy, process robustness, column lifetime, use of raw materials, and labor savings.

10.16 TECH TRANSFER AND DOCUMENTATION

Several factors should be considered before transferring the process from the development laboratory to the pilot facility. Culturally, there are huge differences between the two areas. The development staff tends to concentrate on the protein chemistry striving for maximal resolution and scientifically elegant solutions while the pilot staff tends to focus on engineering issues and optimal use of the equipment. It is therefore important

Table 10.18 Maturity of Process

Maturity Criteria	Comments
Cell line	QA release of the MCB required prior to transferring cells into the cGMP facility
Process design	Design should be robust with provisions for removal of host-, process-, and product-related impurities. Where refolding is involved, include a well-defined renaturation step; where virus contamination can be an issue, integrate virus removal and inactivation steps with due consideration for denaturation of protein.
Raw materials	A list of raw materials should be provided; do not use materials not qualified to be used in cGMP manufacturing.
Intermediary compounds	Data from three small-scale batches should be provided; critical parameters and their interaction should be defined. Holding times of relevance to large-scale operations should be provided.
Drug substance	Short-term stability of the intermediary compounds to be documented.
Drug product (DP)	Formulation to be flexible enough to change composition of the bulk; short-term stability documented.
In-process control	Parameters stated in intervals (validated and proven acceptable ranges) and monitored; analytical method description plus data for in-process analyses to be provided.
Specifications	Acceptance criteria for DS and DSP provided where possible.
Quality control	DS and DSP quality control plan defined and analytical method description plus typical data provided.

to assure excellent communication between the two areas and to stress the importance of *design in*. The size of the tech transfer package very much reflects the quality and maturity of the process and its associated activities. Below are listed issues of relevance for the tech transfer between the development laboratory and the pilot facility.

The technology transfer package for recombinant protein manufacturing is a comprehensive document that addresses various issues in sufficient detail to allow the transferee to replicate the process. Following is an example of typical items included in the tech transfer package.

Overview: Process rationale and brief strategy of production

Molecule: Physical and chemical properties of target protein

Cell line: History of cell line; MCB vials, WCB vials, WCB release documentation; safety profile; reworking and propagation documentation

Process: List of raw materials and equipment; hazardous element identification; development history documentation; description of unit operations; manufacturing process protocol; small batch data; critical parameters; related impurities description: host-, process-, and product-related; process flow sheet; major impurity removal steps; batch production plan

Fill and finish: Master production document; batch record; formulation deviation parameters; development history document; compliance record

Storage: Conditions for all in-process materials, drug substance, and drug product

Shipping: Conditions and instructions, packaging specifications for both drug substance and drug product

In-process control: Required tests and when needed; parameter intervals (tolerance and specifications) for pH, conductivity, redox potential, protein concentration, temperature, holding time, load, transmembrane pressure, linear flow, and so on

Specifications: Acceptance criteria for appearance, identity, biological activity, purity and quantity; pharmacopeial specifications where applicable

Analytical methods: Description, typical data, method qualification level, methods transfer protocols, and reference material

Stability: Real-time data and extrapolated data on both drug substance and drug product

Virus validation: Documentation and protocol; compliance report

Master validation plan: Update

Training: Employee training protocol, end of training objectives, and on-going support

10.17 VALIDATION

The economy of the manufacturing process (facility depreciation, raw material costs, quality control, and quality assurance) must match the expected results. As a rule of thumb, the expenses on manufacture should not exceed 15% of the price per dose (vial). Some of the factors influencing the process economy are manpower, chromatographic media, filters and membranes, buffers, other raw materials, number and type of in-process control analyses, and the overall yield obtained. Additional cost comes from complying with environmental requirements. Where organic solvents are used, their disposal is further costly. Waste disposal, particularly the requirement that all material in contact with the genetically modified cells (GMCs) must be properly sterilized and disposed, adds considerable overheads to the overall production costs.

Typically, manufacturers develop purification processes on a small scale and determine the effectiveness of the particular processing step. When scale up is performed, allowances must be made for several differences when compared with the laboratory-scale operation. Longer processing times can affect product quality adversely, since the product is exposed to conditions of buffer and temperature for longer periods. Product stability, under purification conditions, must be carefully defined. It is important to define the limitations and effectiveness of the particular step. Process validation on the production size batch should then compare the effect of scale up, whereas the data on the small scale can help in the validation, it is important that validation be performed on the production size batches. There are specific situations such as where columns are regenerated to allow repeated use; this requires proper validation procedures performed and the process periodically monitored for chemical and microbial contamination.

Where batches are rejected, it is important to identify the specific manufacturing and control systems that resulted in the failure and thus appropriated action plan brought in place to prevent reoccurrence of the mistake.

10.18 SCALE UP

The downstream process is designed such (in a linear manner) where most parameters are fixed and only column diameter in chromatographic unit operations, and the membrane area in filtration operations. The perpetual conflict between the pilot-scale mentality and the commercial-sale requirements continue to be the greatest impediment—the human factor. The initiative at the U.S. FDA in process analytical technology (PAT) initiative (http://www.fda.gov/cder/OPS/PAT.htm) discussed in detail elsewhere offers an ideal solution adopting the concept of *design in*, where issues related to process safety, robustness, cGMP compliance, facility constraints, economy, and time to market is built into the process at small-scale development. The process is tested in small scale before transfer against predefined process maturity factors, such as parameter intervals, in-process control points, critical parameters and their interactions, robustness, yield, documentation level, raw material qualification, and maturity of analytical procedures. This concept challenges the classic stepwise scale up (a short-cut approach to accommodate unrealistic timelines), where cell culture and initial purification steps (e.g., capture) are scaled up before the process is developed in small scale. The stepwise scale-up procedure creates much confusion, is time consuming, and invites to late process redesign. It is also common to outsource this stage of work and particularly if the company plans to outsource manufacturing as well. Transferring an immature process into the pilot environment may result in delayed phase 1–2 clinical material manufacture as process changes may raise doubt of the stability, virus validation, and preclinical data. Any signs of an immature process should therefore be dealt with immediately. Immature process indicators include the following:

- Yields are low or vary from batch to batch
- Target protein instability
- Changing impurity profiles
- UV diagrams are not superimposable
- Too many batches are discarded or do not meet specifications
- Manufacture is terminated during processing
- Reworking of unit operations is necessary
- The process is frequently being redesigned

10.18.1 Specific Scale-Up Issues

The optimal scale up and the choice of the scale is influenced by several factors in an integrated model. Given below is a cost estimation model.

10.18.2 Cost Calculations

The costs of producing a batch of recombinant-derived product can be calculated from the input figures listed in Table 10.19. It is recommended to use an excel spreadsheet for cost calculations including specific costs not mentioned in the table.

The cost contributions at various steps are given below. Opportunities should be recognized where costs can be cut, particularly in deciding the magnitude of scale up. The relative contribution of each of the step should be the first criterion of selection on which

Table 10.19   Input Figures for Cost Calculations

Category	Issue	Index	Comments
General	Expression level	A1	Amount in g/L expressed
	No. of batches	A2	
	Process yield	A3	% of purified protein (drug product)
	Dose	A4	mg/dose
	Pack size	A5	mg/vial
	Vials needed	A6	No. of vials/dose
Upstream	Facility	B1	Yearly cost ($) of using upstream component of cGMP facility (including maintenance and manpower)
	Utilization	B2	No. of months the upstream component is used for given project
	Culture volume	B3	Volume in liters in a given batch
	Media cost	B4	Price in $/L of culture media
	Utensils	B5	Price in $ for utensils used (e.g., filters, and bags)
Downstream	Facility	C1	Yearly cost ($) for using downstream component of the cGMP facility (including maintenance and manpower)
	Utilization	C2	No. of months the downstream component is used for a given project
	Chromatography steps	C3	Number of chromatography steps
	Binding capacity	C4	Average binding capacity in mg/mL
	Media cost	C5	Chromatography media cost in $/L
	Buffer volume	C7	Total consumption in L (on an average 15 column volumes are used/step)
	Buffer cost	C8	$/L
	Utensils	C9	Cost in $ for components used (filters, membranes, bags, etc.)
	Raw materials	C10	Cost in $ for expensive reagents, enzymes etc
	Formulation	C11	Cost in $ for formulation of drug substance
Fill and Pack	Number of vials	D1	Vials/batch
	Price	D2	Price/vial
	Shipping cost	D3	
In-process control	No. of analyses	E1	Total number per batch
	Cost of analysis	E2	Average in $/IPC analysis
DS quality control	No. of analyses	F1	Total number of drugs substance quality analysis per batch
	Cost	F2	$/analysis
DP quality control	No. of analyses	G1	Total number per batch of drug product
	Cost	G2	$/analysis
QA release	Cost	H1	$/batch

step to be reworked to reduce costs. The relative costs should be considered in terms of long-term impact. For example, a 1% recurring cost can add a substantial savings if reduced.

$$\text{Upstream cost} = \frac{(B1 * B2)}{12} + B3 * B4 + B5 \ \left(\text{asterisk is used for multiplier}\right) \tag{10.1}$$

$$\text{Downstream} = \frac{(C1 * C2)}{12} = \frac{(B3 * A1 * C5 * C3)}{(C4 * C6 * 1,000)} + (C7 * C8) + C9 + C10 \ C11 \tag{10.2}$$

$$\text{Fill and pack} = D1 * D2 * + D3 \tag{10.3}$$

$$\begin{aligned}\text{Total cost/batch} = &\ \text{upstream} + \text{downstream} + \text{fill and pack} \\ &+ E1 * E2 + F1 * F2 + G1 * G2 + H1\end{aligned} \tag{10.4}$$

$$\text{Yield per batch} = \frac{(B3 * A1 * A3)}{100,000} \tag{10.5}$$

$$\text{Cost/G} = \frac{\text{Total cost}}{\text{Yield}} \ \left(\text{per batch}\right) \tag{10.6}$$

$$\text{Cost per vial} = \frac{\text{Cost per batch}}{D1} \tag{10.7}$$

$$\text{Cost per dose} = \left(\frac{\text{Cost per batch}}{D1}\right) * A6 \tag{10.8}$$

Based on this model we can study what components of the entire process can be altered to achieve the best possible production costs.

- *Quantity required*. The cost is inversely proportional to quantity produced, ranging from about \$85/mg for insulin to \$1,000+/mg for some cytokines. For expensive products, it may be worthwhile not to look at production cost optimization as timely entry may be more relevant.
- Batch is defined as the *batch* or fed-batch cell culture volume processed in downstream as a combined amount of material resulting in the drug substance. In continuous cell cultures or by transgenic animal technology, the harvest or milk may be pooled in sub-fractions making it more difficult to define the batch and the batch scheme must provide information about the flow, the harvest procedures, pools, analytical in-process control programs, and intermediary compounds. Also included here are details if several columns are used or where parallel processing or splitting of processing is envisioned. Fact that inclusion bodies can be combined from several fermentation batches and then processed together requires clear identification of starting sub-batches.
- Batch variations document specifies variability and lack of reproducibility; this may be due to scale-up procedure due to formation of concentration gradients in large reactors or containers.

- Buffer preparation at large scale cannot be handled require automation and robotics management creating an entirely different set of validation requirements and tools including computer validation (see Section 211.68 [a, b] of the U.S. FDA cGMP for validation of automated systems, mechanized racks and computers).
- Column life when prolonged reduces cost significantly; remember that almost 70% of total production cost goes into downstream processing, mainly in the cost of chromatographic media. Measure taken to prolong column life include longer usage, recharging, and so on, must be properly validated and documents.
- Environmental issues relate to disposal of large waste; for example, use of ammonium sulfate will severely affect the environment in large-scale operations.
- Equipment interaction can determine the choice of chemicals used; sodium chloride is a corrosive agent to stainless steel; whereas sodium acetate is not. These issues should be addressed as early as possible in process development.
- Facility costs can be very high because of specialize area requirements, specialized manpower required, environment controls and waste disposal needs, and so on. A prospective biogeneric marketer would be wise to look into outsourcing manufacturing specially if several products are involved that may require separate processing suites. One of the control areas that is often not given full budgeting is the monitoring of environment; a 5,000 sq ft facility may cost upward of $2 million per year only to comply with the monitoring standards. As the regulatory environment is still evolving, the area requirements are likely to change that may cost substantial redesigning, another reason to outsource manufacturing until such time that the market is firmly established. The price per gram drug substance is significantly reduced by linking process design, scale-up factor, and batch logistics to the facility design and thereby reducing the occupancy time. This requires several levels of set up, one for transfer of technology to pilot scale, from pilot scale to first-stage manufacturing and from first-stage manufacturing to full-scale manufacturing.
- Validation of biological processes is an expensive exercise that continues throughout the commercial manufacturing operations. Typically, validation steps are initiated when all separation and purification steps are described in detail and presented with flowcharts. Adequate descriptions and specifications should be provided for all equipment, columns, reagents, buffers, and expected yields. The U.S. FDA defines process validation in the May 1987 "Guideline on General Principles of Process Validation" as: "validation—establishing documented evidence which provides a high degree of assurance that a specific process will consistently produce a product meeting its predetermined specifications and quality attributes." As a result, there is a need to establish comprehensive documentary proof to justify the process and demonstrate that the process works consistently. Validation reports for the various key processes would be dependent on the process involved; for example, if an ion-exchange column is used to remove endotoxins, there should be data documenting that this process is consistently effective as done by determining endotoxin levels before and after processing. It is important to monitor the process before, during, and after to determine the efficiency of each key purification step. One method commonly used to demonstrate validation is to *spike* the preparation with a known amount of a contaminant and then demonstrate its absence.

- Harvesting can be programmed to store inclusion bodies for longer time (even two years) and most large-scale operations should validate this storage step.
- Holding times can be long and add cost in commercial production; these are often not considered in developing processes; it is advisable that in the initial phases, realistic times should be validated. This aspect is related more to logistics than to science. It takes much longer to empty a 4,000 L tank than it does to dump a 2 L flask. Often the practical considerations of shift-change (if the process requires more than 8 h) are necessary in designing the process.
- Cleaning, sanitization, and storage of columns, equipment, and utensils are an integrated part of the manufacturing program. Whereas liberties are routinely taken in small-scale production, these issues can add substantial costs in a poorly designed process and facility but also raise contamination risks that may not be acceptable by the regulatory authorities.
- Analytical assays to test quality may soon become less expensive, if manufacturers are able to avoid them in processes that are well developed. This is particularly important as large-scale manufacturing require larger testing protocols. Recently the U.S. FDA released a draft on PAT at http://www.fda.gov/cder/guidance/5815dft.htm. This extended approach, taken during the development phase, not only includes traditional analytical testing, but also real-time monitoring of the process parameters and responses. A better monitoring of parameters and responses may result in a reduced analytical in-process control program.
- Labor-intensive processes are expensive and costs may be reduced by reducing the number of unit operations and by automation. Each unit operation adds to cost and reduces yield. However, there is a limit to the number of process steps involved because of requirement for effective impurity removal and virus inactivation, if insect cells, mammalian cells, or transgenic animals have been used for protein expression. There is an extensive effort to automate systems as generic companies, which have reasons to adopt more cost-effective systems, enter the market. From robotics to continuous processing systems to wave bioreactors are all efforts to reduce human resource cost. A prospective manufacturer must look at all available and soon to be available alternates in designing the process. However, the U.S. FDA requirements for validating automated process and computer systems should be implemented as early as possible.
- Monitoring through online data collection systems is needed to control and adjust parameters critical to processes. This creates a problem because small-scale instruments may not have the same level of monitoring potential as do the large ones (which can be ordered with custom features).
- Process design depends on the nature of the target protein; the expression system used; and the demand for safety, robustness, and compliance with cGMP. In order to produce a safe product qualified raw materials must be used and host-, process-, and product-related impurities removed. Although variations in process design may occur, certain general rules apply such as use of at least three chromatographic principles, virus inactivation, and filtration in process based on insect cells, mammalian cells, or transgenic animals. Target protein stability must be documented throughout processing and upon storage. Process design is a small-scale

activity and in principle no process should be transferred for scale up before it is reasonably tested in small scale. The major process maturity criteria are linked to specifications, robustness, and cGMP compliance. Although drug substance and drug product specifications and their accept criteria are not fully defined at this early stage, data from at least three small-scale batches must be provided and tested against available specifications and accepts criteria. The process must be robust and to some extent provide the expected outcome. Knowledge of critical parameters and their interactions is valuable information prior to scale up. The process should be tested with respect to cGMP to make sure that the process complies with the facility design and manufacturing procedures. Difficulties should be expected if the expression yield is low, the protein unstable, the purification yield is low or the process comprises too many steps.

- Process economy determines the scale-up factor adopted as there is always a certain maximum capacity to which a process can be scaled with economic advantage. A good example of this would be the manufacturing of insulin, which is produced in quantities of tons rather than grams. If a scale-up process moves from 100 L fermenter to 30,000 L, the cost is not necessary proportional to the capacity and may render the project commercially not feasible. Also, when outsourcing, it is always a good idea to adjust the process to available bioreactor size as not all CMOs carry all sizes of bioreactors. When processing bacterial cultures, it may be worthwhile to take advantage of pooling inclusion bodies when only smaller-size fermenters are available. However, as the batch size decreases, the costs for analytical assays increases, so batch size and analytical programs should be carefully balanced.

- Quality control testing is required for both drug substance and drug product; reduced test programs should be reconsidered upon scale up. Some test analyses introduced in an early development phase may be skipped from the batch release program as combined data have confirmed process robustness. The rationale for removing a given analytical assay should be given. The PAT initiative at the U.S. FDA may reduce the testing of products.

- Quality assurance systems should assure that the process scale up does not alter process safety, robustness, or compliance with regulatory demands. If the process is redesigned during scale up, the validity of preclinical data should be considered. Robust systems introduce strict control of unit operation parameters and define parameters in intervals rather than set points. The parameter intervals are tested and justified in small scale (proven acceptable range) making room to adjust the intervals according to large-scale needs. In the linear-scale concept these parameter intervals are kept constant upon scale up. Other factors, such reactor volumes, sample loads, and column diameters are increased—all in a linear fashion.

- Cell cultures offer most opportunities and most problems in scale up. For example, large-scale animal cell cultures are fundamentally different from conventional microbial fermentation due to the fragility of mammalian cells. The cells are easily damaged by mechanical stress making it impossible to use conditions of high aeration and agitation; this includes the use of the newly introduced Wave bioreactors. Fortunately animal cells grows slowly and at less cell densities and therefore do not require the high oxygen inputs typical of microbial cultures. Cell culture scale

293

up often result in changes in the cell culture supernatant composition, which may affect the downstream process. However, except for reactor volume, other parameters like culture medium, pH, temperature, redox potential, osmolality, agitation rate, flow rate, ammonia, glucose, glutamine, lactate concentrations, pCO_2, and OUR remain constant within the prescribed interval limits.

- Precipitation step scale up involves only change in the amount of sample and the volume of reagent as all other parameters like sample pH, conductivity, temperature, concentration, redox potential, holding time, reagent concentration, and precipitation time remain constant within interval limits. The procedure of precipitation also remains identical.
- Chromatography scale up produces more problems than any other operation in the process. Larger equipment may cause extra-column zone broadening due to different lengths and diameters of outlet pipes, valves, monitor cells, and so on. An increase in column diameter may result in decreased flow rate due to a reduction in supportive wall forces (at constant pressure drop). For example, a decrease in flow of 30%–45% is observed for a column packed with sepharose 6 FF when the diameter is increased from 2.6 to 10 cm. Prolonged sample holding times on column may result in precipitation of material resulting in clotting of pipes, valves, or chromatographic columns. Parameters which are changed proportionally (linear scale up) include sample volume, sample load, column diameter, column area and column volume, flow rate; residence time remains constant (an alternate method would keep residence time constant allow for variations in both column area and height). Parameters that remain constant within the interval limits include sample pH, conductivity, temperature, concentration, redox potential, holding time, bed height, residence time, linear flow rate, binding capacity, back pressure, buffers, equilibration procedure, wash procedure, elution procedure, and cleaning-in-place (CIP) procedure remain unchanged. Gradients should not be changed linearly but step-wise.
- Filtration step scale up does not change the interval limits for pH, redox potential, temperature, concentration, conductivity, holding time, membrane type, transmembrane pressure, retentate pressure, feed pressure, cross-flow velocity, filtrate velocity, wall concentration, flux, and CIP procedures. Parameters that are increased linearly include sample volume and membrane area.
- Equipment change is the most significant aspect of scale up from laboratory scale to production scale. Not all equipment is available in scalable type. This consideration should be the prime deciding factor in laboratory-scale development. Manufacturers like New Brunswik, Amersham, and Pall offer a broad line of products in terms of capacity and are always preferred to single source suppliers, even if the initial cost is higher to use this equipment. Large-scale hardware often has a different design, for example, pump design may change from high precision piston or displacement pumps to rotary, diaphragm, or peristaltic pumps. Similarly, low volume multi-port valves are replaced by simple one-way valves, which combined with large-scale tubing, may expand volumes of equipment accessories substantially and lead to extra dispersion of the target protein molecules. Large-scale equipment is often build of stainless steel and does not withstand high

concentrations of sodium chloride. The scale-up issues to consider in relation to large-scale equipment include differences in chromatographic column physics of movement, the choice and placement of tubing, valve and reservoir, chemical resistance of construction material, the choice of CIP and SIP, and so on.

10.19 SPECIFIC ECONOMY ISSUES

Economy considerations start already with the choice of expression system, culture conditions, and demand for process robustness, hence this is part of the *design in* strategy recommended. A rule of thumb tells that manufacturing comprising upstream, downstream, formulation, fill and pack, quality control, and documentation should add up to 15% of the vial price, but no more. Since a cGMP facility is expensive, outsourcing is highly recommended for new entrants to biogeneric field. This advice is not merely a cost-saving measure but also offers only logistic solutions. For example, where a transgenic animal is involved, few pharmaceutical manufacturers would know how to handle farming of animals and comply with good cattle-raising practices. The costs of upstream, downstream, and quality control are closely interrelated not only by variations in process design but also in respect to batch sizes versus in-process control and analytical control programs. A robust process will allow for large batches, thus reducing the demand for manpower and the number of samples to be analyzed.

Process design should be distinguished from process optimization, where factors such as labor, automation, lean management, column life-time, re-use of utensils, and batch planning affect the process economy. The latter issues are dealt with at a later development stage, typically when the process design has been locked.

- Expression system selection and eventually cell line takes place early in the process and is the most important decision. The choice depends on the nature of the target protein (glycosylation, phosphorylation, acylation, size, etc.), expected expression levels, expression system development time, risk of batch failure, safety considerations, amount needed, and regulatory record.
  - The target proteins without posttranslational modifications can be expressed in all expression system (bacteria, yeast, insect cells, mammalian cells, transgenic animals or transgenic plants); bacterial system is historically preferred for cost considerations but better expression yields have been obtained with yeast, mammalian cell cultures, and the introduction of transgenic animals and plants over the past 10 years challenge the bacterial systems, where intracellular expression of Met-protein and in vitro folding increases the complexity of the downstream process. Posttranslational modified proteins or more complex proteins are expressed in insect cells, mammalian cells, and transgenic animals or plants. Microbial systems cannot be used.
  - Expression level varies with the host organism used and the nature of the target protein. Typical expression levels vary widely. In most hosts these range at less than 1 g/L; *E. coli* generally gives a better yield of 1–4 g/L, while mammalian cells when used for antibodies generally produce much higher levels; transgenic animals provide the highest yield of 5–40 g/L; the yield in transgenic

plants is uncertain and not widely available for evaluation. The nature and quality of the expressed protein influences the purification yield. Although expression levels of *E. coli* usually are high, expression of N-terminal extended target protein and the need for in vitro refolding significantly influences the overall process yield. Further, stressed cells tend to express less stable protein resulting in great losses during purification or production of drug substance/product with shortened lifetime.

- Expression system development time vary widely between various expression systems. However, for most hosts, 4–6 months are required to develop the system. Once developed, the time to target protein expression depends on the bioreactor system deployed but generally range from a few days, for example, 5 days for *E. coli* and other bacteria, two weeks for yeast, four weeks for inset cells and 2–16 weeks for mammalian cells. The longer development time for transgenic goats and cows (18–24 months) is partly compensated for by the relative high expression levels and the fast access to target protein, once the system has been developed.
- Risk of batch failure is mainly due to infections; large-scale mammalian cell cultures, having long cell expansion times including several bioreactors and running over long time intervals, are associated with higher risk factors than other expression systems. Due to the high cell culture media cost, the economic loss can be substantial.
- Safety considerations add to cost significantly. Insect, cells, mammalian cells and transgenic animals can be infected with viruses. Costly virus testing, virus reduction unit operations, and validation programs are needed to assure product safety. The potential prion infection risk of sheep, goats, and cows is being debated emphasizing the need for controlled herds.
- Amount needed. A 1,000 L bioreactor with an expression level of 1 g/L produces 1 kg of target protein per reactor volume. A batch or fed-batch culture typically runs for 7 days offering a productivity of 100 g/day. A 1,000 L perfusion bioreactor with a $2 \times$ flow per 24 h and with an expression level of 1 g/L produces 200 g/day. A transgenic cow expressing 20 g/L milk produces 400 g/day assuming a volume of 20 L milk per day. In terms of output, the transgenic cow is a far more efficient expression system than the cell culture-based systems and probably less risky. Animal-based expression systems should therefore seriously be considered for large-scale operations.
- Regulatory record of insect cells, transgenic animals, and transgenic plants is poor. This is an important consideration when selecting a system to assure that favorable regulatory review is forthcoming.
- Raw materials vary in price between culture media used for microbial, insect, and mammalian cell cultures and commercial-scale fermenter media, the former being the most expensive per liter. Unfortunately, mammalian cell cultures usually offer relatively low expression levels compared to microbial systems, making expenses to culture media a major cost contributor. An expression system yielding 1,000 g/L with 40% yield, the contribution of the cost of media is about $25/g of protein; when the expression level drops to 10 g/L, the cost contribution of

media rises to \$2,500/g of protein. Obviously, low mammalian cell expression levels adversely affect the process economy.

- Cell growth is normally achieved in batch, fed-batch, or continuous mode, the latter mainly being used for mammalian cell bioreactors up to a volume of maximum 300 L, at present. A bioreactor run in the batch mode has a fixed working volume and the cell culture is grown to a defined cell density before harvest. The harvest volume defines the batch and the yield is the expression level × harvest volume. For example, a bioreactor of 100 L working volume with an expression level 300 mg/L results in a batch yield of 30 g. The productivity is thus 30 g/week or 0.3 g/L culture medium assuming it takes one week to complete the batch. A bioreactor run in fed-batch mode may result in a final volume of 130 L equivalent to a productivity of 39 g/week or 0.3 g/L culture medium assuming identical culture time and expression level. A 100 L working volume bioreactor run in continuous mode at a flow of 2 reactor volumes per day and an expression level of 100 mg/L produces $100 \times 2 \times 7 \times 100 = 140$ g/week or $140/1,400 = 0.1$ g/L culture medium or one-third of the batch culture. The increased overall productivity may compensate for the decreased productivity per liter culture medium.

- In-process control is less expensive for batch and fed-batch systems compared to continuous cultures, but the overall cost may not be too different and is worth considering in light of the PAT initiative of the U.S. FDA. Milking procedures may result in production of small volume bags increasing the cost for analytical control programs. The insect and mammalian cell end-of-production test comprising sterility, fungi, mycoplasma, and virus testing should be included in the cost calculations.

- Yield is the composite of each purification step's output. A downstream process comprising 10 unit operations with an average recovery of 95% will result in an overall yield of 57%, which is acceptable. However, an average recovery of 80% will result in a total yield of 11%, which in most circumstances is not acceptable. In several cases more than 10 unit operations are needed to guarantee a safe product, making it fair to conclude that one should aim for more than 95% recovery in most if not all unit operations. Some of the most recent trends to alter the molecular structure, for example, PEGylation has met with lower yields. Because of the mathematical nature of proportional reduction, small changes in step yields result in dramatic changes in the total yield. For example, a step yield of 95% where 15 steps are involved gives 46% total yield; the same 15 steps in 75% step yield would give only 1% of the total yield. In most instances 5–10 steps are minimally involved; for example at ten steps, the total yield ranges from 60% to 6% for 95% to 75% step yield transition.

- Batch size is decided on a variety of consideration, not all of them have economic optimization. Large batches require automated facilities, but results in relative small number of samples to analyze.

- Chromatographic media costs are a minor fraction of the entire manufacturing costs and it may be wise to select media from other criteria than price per liter. Service, troubleshooting, linking media, column and equipment to the same supplier, and regulatory support files may be far more important aspects as the number of failed batches can be reduced by such actions. Suppliers like Amersham or others with wide range of offering and validation should be the first choice as media vendors. The major factors influencing the economy of chromatographic unit operations are media cost, binding capacity, recovery, column lifetime, linear flow, and shelf life.

- Utensils are bags, filters, or any other equipment exchanged at regular intervals. It has become common practice to use bags, filters, tubes, and so on only once in order to reduce cost and time to CIP procedures.
- Number of steps in a process directly affect cost and yield; however, reducing the number of steps process can affect robustness and safety and even later costs in additional testing as may be required by the regulatory authorities. For example, a choice may have to be made whether to add an additional adventitious agent removal process of validate the system.
- In-process control testing should be minimal and this is only possible with a well-defined system, which may incur higher costs initially. The trend is to reduce the number of in-process analytical methods and to expand on monitoring of parameters and responses, thereby keeping strict control of the process in real time. The number of samples to analyze is inversely related to the batch size; large batches reduce the cost for in-process control.
- Formulation, fill, and pack operations of the API can also be subject to cost reduction depending on the formulation. Obviously, a lyophilized product will cost more and if a ready-to-inject formula can be developed, which should be a better choice. The components such as syringes, pen systems, and so on, added at this stage add substantially to the cost of the product.
- In-process and quality control testing is extensive (see U.S. Pharmacopoeia [USP], European Pharmacopoeia [EP], or British Pharmacopoeia [BP]) and expensive because of the nature of tests involved, notwithstanding other requirements of validation common to all types of testing. The assays used for in-process control are justified as they provide essential process information during development or are used to monitor a given outcome important for in-process control in manufacturing processes. Thus, reducing the cost would mean reducing the number of in-process analyses without compromising process control. It is a common practice to revise the program as more and more data become available and the process matures. Another way to reduce costs is to use the PAT approach recently suggested by the U.S. FDA (http://www.fda.gov/cder/guidance/5815dft.htm). PAT is considered to be a system for designing, analyzing, and controlling manufacturing through time measurements of critical quality and performance attributes of raw and in-process materials and processes with the goal of ensuring final product quality. The goal of PAT is to understand and control the manufacturing process as quality cannot be tested into products but should be built in. This approach can be taken during the development phase extending the in-process control program to include not only traditional analytical testing but also real-time monitoring of the process parameters and responses. A desired goal of the PAT framework is to

design and develop processes that can consistently ensure a predefined quality at the end of the manufacturing process. Such procedures would be consistent with the basic tenet of quality by design and could reduce the risks to quality and regulatory concerns while improving efficiency. A third way to reduce costs is to lower the price per sample by assuring a continuous flow of samples, thereby reducing time spent on method set up and calibration.

- Quality control testing is performed on both, the drug substance (DS) and the drug product (DP) (see DP/EP/USP). The testing typically comprises from 10 to 15 different analytical methods with an average price between $500 and $3,000 per sample. If outside laboratories are inducted to provide additional testing, the cost can skyrocket. For example, National Institute of Biological Standards and Control (NIBSC) would typically charge about $20,000 to test one sample; animal assays and viral assays can be extremely expensive when outsourced; yet, outsourcing is still the preferred way of doing these assays to obviate the large cost of maintaining animal houses or viral containment systems and validating the methods.

10.20 PROCESS MATERIALS

The quality of water should depend on the intended use of the finished product. For example, CBER requires water for injection (WFI) quality for process water. On the other hand, for in vitro diagnostics purified water may suffice. For drugs, the quality of water required depends on the process. Also, because processing usually occurs either at cold or at room temperature, the self-sanitization of a hot WFI system at 75°C–80°C is lost.

For economic reasons, many of the biotech companies manufacture WFI by reverse osmosis rather than by distillation, which may result in contaminated systems because of the nature of processing equipment that is often difficult to sanitize. Any threads or drops in a cold system provide an area where microorganisms can lodge and multiply. Some of the systems employ a terminal sterilizing filter. However, the primary concern is endotoxins, and the terminal filter may merely serve to mask the true quality of the WFI used. The limitations of relying on a 0.1 ml sample of WFI for endotoxins from a system should also be recognized. The system should be designed to deliver high purity water, with the sample merely serving to assure that it is operating adequately. As with other WFI systems, if cold WFI water is needed, point-of-use heat exchangers can be used.

Buffers can be manufactured as sterile, non-pyrogenic solutions and stored in sterile containers. Some of the smaller facilities have purchased commercial sterile, non-pyrogenic buffer solutions.

The production and/or storage of non sterile water that may be of reagent grade or used as a buffer should be evaluated from both a stability and microbiological aspect.

WFI systems for biotechnology-derived pharmaceuticals are the same as WFI systems for other regulated products. As with other heat-sensitive products, cold WFI is used for formulation. Cold systems are prone to contamination. The cold WFI should be monitored both for endotoxins and microorganisms.

10.21 ENVIRONMENT CONTROL

Microbiological quality of the environment during various processing is very important, particularly as the process continues downstream, more intensive control and monitoring is recommended. The environment and areas used for the isolation of the BDP should also be controlled to minimize microbiological and other foreign contaminants. The typical isolation of BDP should be of the same control as the environment used for the formulation of the solution prior to sterilization and filling.

10.21.1 NIH Guidelines for Handling DNA Material

The recombinant technology is associated with a number of safety issues related to the expression system used, cell banking, fermentation and cell cultures, raw materials used, downstream processing, and unintended introduction of adventitious agents (bacteria, viruses, mycoplasma, prions). One of the major purposes of the purification process is to provide a rational design assuring the removal of the said adventitious agents and other harmful impurities. A rule of thumb says that at least three different chromatographic principles should be used in a biopharmaceutical downstream process. If insect cells, mammalian cells, or transgenic animals have been used, a virus inactivation step and an active virus filtration step should be considered. The adventitious agents and their relation to the expression system used is simply understood as endotoxins, nucleic acids, bioburden, viruses, and prions be an issue in all systems of expression except that viruses and prions are not an issue in microbial systems; prions are also not an issue in other systems except in transgenic animals. The use of raw materials should be carefully investigated. Only raw materials suited for biopharmaceutical processing should be accepted, based on solid documentation on safety and quality.

The purpose of the *NIH Guidelines* is to specify practices for constructing and handling (1) recombinant deoxyribonucleic acid (DNA) molecules and (2) organisms and viruses containing recombinant DNA molecules. Any recombinant DNA experiment, which according to the *NIH Guidelines* requires approval by NIH, must be submitted to NIH or to another Federal agency that has jurisdiction for review and approval. Once approvals, or other applicable clearances, have been obtained from a Federal agency other than NIH (whether the experiment is referred to that agency by NIH or sent directly there by the submitter), the experiment may proceed without the necessity for NIH review or approval. For experiments involving the deliberate transfer of recombinant DNA, or DNA or RNA derived from recombinant DNA, into human research participants (human gene transfer), no research participant shall be enrolled until the recovery audit contractor (RAC) review process has been completed.

In the context of the *NIH Guidelines*, recombinant DNA molecules are defined as either (1) molecules that are constructed outside living cells by joining natural or synthetic DNA segments to DNA molecules that can replicate in a living cell or (2) molecules that result from the replication of those described in (1) above. Synthetic DNA segments that are likely to yield a potentially harmful polynucleotide or polypeptide (e.g., a toxin or a pharmacologically active agent) are considered as equivalent to their natural DNA counterpart. If the synthetic DNA segment is not expressed in vivo as a biologically active polynucleotide or polypeptide product, it is exempt from the *NIH Guidelines*.

Genomic DNA of plants and bacteria that have acquired a transposable element, even if the latter was donated from a recombinant vector no longer present, are not subject to the *NIH Guidelines* unless the transposon itself contains recombinant DNA.

Risk assessment is ultimately a subjective process. The investigator must make an initial risk assessment based on the risk group (RG) of an agent. Agents are classified into four RGs according to their relative pathogenicity for healthy adult humans by the following criteria: (1) RG1 agents are not associated with disease in healthy adult humans; (2) RG2 agents are associated with human disease which is rarely serious and for which preventive or therapeutic interventions are *often* available; (3) RG3 agents are associated with serious or lethal human disease for which preventive or therapeutic interventions *may be* available; and (4) RG4 agents are likely to cause serious or lethal human disease for which preventive or therapeutic interventions are *not usually* available.

Considerable information already exists about the design of physical containment facilities and selection of laboratory procedures applicable to organisms carrying recombinant DNA. The existing programs rely upon mechanisms that can be divided into two categories: (1) a set of standard practices that are generally used in microbiological laboratories and (2) special procedures, equipment, and laboratory installations that provide physical barriers that are applied in varying degrees according to the estimated biohazard.

There are six categories of experiments defined in the *NIH Guidelines* involving recombinant DNA that require the following:

1. Institutional Biosafety Committee (IBC) approval, RAC review, and NIH Director approval before initiation. Experiments considered as *major actions* would include: The deliberate transfer of a drug resistance trait to microorganisms that are not known to acquire the trait naturally, if such acquisition could compromise the use of the drug to control disease agents in humans, veterinary medicine, or agriculture, they will be reviewed by RAC.

2. NIH/OBA and Institutional Biosafety Committee approval before initiation. Experiments involving the cloning of toxin molecules with LD50 of less than 100 ng/kg body weight. Deliberate formation of recombinant DNA containing genes for the biosynthesis of toxin molecules lethal for vertebrates at an LD50 of less than 100 ng/kg body weight (e.g., microbial toxins such as the botulinum toxins, tetanus toxin, diphtheria toxin, and *Shigella dysenteriae* neurotoxin). Specific approval has been given for the cloning in *E. coli* K-12 of DNA containing genes coding for the biosynthesis of toxic molecules which are lethal to vertebrates at 100 ng to 100 µg/kg body weight.

3. Institutional Biosafety Committee and Institutional Review Board approvals and RAC review before research participant enrollment. Experiments involving the deliberate transfer of recombinant DNA, or DNA or RNA derived from recombinant DNA, into one or more human research participants. For an experiment involving the deliberate transfer of recombinant DNA, or DNA or RNA derived from recombinant DNA, into human research participants (human gene transfer), no research participant shall be enrolled until the RAC review process has been completed. In its evaluation of human gene transfer proposals, the RAC will consider whether a proposed human gene transfer experiment presents characteristics

that warrant public RAC review and discussion. The process of public RAC review and discussion is intended to foster the safe and ethical conduct of human gene transfer experiments. Public review and discussion of a human gene transfer experiment (and access to relevant information) also serves to inform the public about the technical aspects of the proposal, meaning, and significance of the research, and any significant safety, social, and ethical implications of the research.

4. Institutional Biosafety Committee approval before initiation. Prior to the initiation of an experiment that falls into this category, the principal investigator must submit a registration document to the Institutional Biosafety Committee which contains the following information: (1) the source(s) of DNA; (2) the nature of the inserted DNA sequences; (3) the host(s) and vector(s) to be used; (4) if an attempt will be made to obtain expression of a foreign gene, and if so, indicate the protein that will be produced; and (5) the containment conditions that will be implemented as specified in the *NIH Guidelines*.

   a. Experiments using RGs 2 through 4 or restricted agents as host-vector systems. Experiments involving the introduction of recombinant DNA into RG2 agents will usually be conducted at biosafety level (BL) 2 containment. Experiments with such agents will usually be conducted with whole animals at BL2 or BL2-N (animals) containment.

   b. Experiments involving the use of infectious DNA or RNA viruses or defective DNA or RNA viruses in the presence of helper virus in tissue culture systems caution: Special care should be used in the evaluation of containment levels for experiments that are likely to either enhance the pathogenicity (e.g., insertion of a host oncogene) or to extend the host range (e.g., introduction of novel control elements) of viral vectors under conditions that permit a productive infection. In such cases, serious consideration should be given to increase physical containment by at least one level.

   c. Experiments involving whole animals. This section covers experiments involving whole animals in which the animal's genome has been altered by stable introduction of recombinant DNA, or DNA derived there from, into the germ line (transgenic animals) and experiments involving viable recombinant DNA-modified microorganisms tested on whole animals. For the latter, other than viruses which are only vertically transmitted, the experiments may *not* be conducted at BL1-N containment. A minimum containment of BL2 or BL2-N is required.

   d. Experiments involving whole plants. Experiments to genetically engineer plants by recombinant DNA methods, to use such plants for other experimental purposes (e.g., response to stress), to propagate such plants, or to use plants together with microorganisms or insects containing recombinant DNA.

   e. Experiments involving more than 10 L of culture. The appropriate containment will be decided by the Institutional Biosafety Committee. Where appropriate, Appendix K of the *NIH Guidelines*, "Physical Containment for Large Scale Uses of Organisms Containing Recombinant DNA Molecules," shall be used. Appendix K describes containment conditions of good large-scale practice through BL3-large scale.

5. Institutional Biosafety Committee notification simultaneous with initiation. Examples include experiments in which all components derived from non-pathogenic prokaryotes and nonpathogenic lower eukaryotes and may be conducted at BL1 containment.

    a. Experiments involving the formation of recombinant DNA molecules containing no more than two-thirds of the genome of any eukaryotic virus. Recombinant DNA molecules containing no more than two-thirds of the genome of any eukaryotic virus (all viruses from a single family being considered identical) may be propagated and maintained in cells in tissue culture using BL1 containment. For such experiments, it must be demonstrated that the cells lack helper virus for the specific families of defective viruses being used. The DNA may contain fragments of the genome of viruses from more than one family but each fragment shall be less than two-thirds of a genome.

    b. Experiments involving whole plants.

    c. Experiments involving transgenic rodents.

6. Are exempt from the *NIH Guidelines*. The following recombinant DNA molecules are exempt from the *NIH Guidelines* and registration with the Institutional Biosafety Committee is not required:

    a. Those that are not in organisms or viruses.

    b. Those that consist entirely of DNA segments from a single nonchromosomal or viral DNA source, though one or more of the segments may be a synthetic equivalent.

    c. Those that consist entirely of DNA from a prokaryotic host including its indigenous plasmids or viruses when propagated only in that host (or a closely related strain of the same species), or when transferred to another host by well-established physiological means.

    d. Those that consist entirely of DNA from an eukaryotic host including its chloroplasts, mitochondria, or plasmids (but excluding viruses) when propagated only in that host (or a closely related strain of the same species).

    e. Those that consist entirely of DNA segments from different species that exchange DNA by known physiological processes, though one or more of the segments may be a synthetic equivalent. A list of such exchangers will be prepared and periodically revised by the NIH Director with advice of the RAC after appropriate notice and opportunity for public comment.

    f. Those that do not present a significant risk to health or the environment as determined by the NIH Director, with the advice of the RAC, and following appropriate notice and opportunity for public comment.

10.21.2 Biosafety Levels

There are four BLs are described. These BLs consist of combinations of laboratory practices and techniques, safety equipment, and laboratory facilities appropriate for the operations performed and are based on the potential hazards imposed by the agents used and for the laboratory function and activity. BL4 provides the most stringent containment conditions, BL1 is the least stringent. Experiments involving recombinant DNA lend themselves to a third containment mechanism, namely, the application of highly specific biological barriers. Natural barriers exist that limit either (1) the infectivity of a vector or vehicle (plasmid or virus) for specific hosts or (2) its dissemination and survival in the environment. Vectors, which provide the means for recombinant DNA and/or host cell replication, can be genetically designed to decrease, by many orders of magnitude, the probability of dissemination of recombinant DNA outside the laboratory.

Since these three means of containment are complementary, different levels of containment can be established that apply various combinations of the physical and biological barriers along with a constant use of standard practices. Categories of containment are considered separately in order that such combinations can be conveniently expressed in the *NIH Guidelines*.

Physical containment conditions within laboratories may not always be appropriate for all organisms because of their physical size, the number of organisms needed for an experiment, or the particular growth requirements of the organism. Likewise, biological containment for microorganisms may not be appropriate for all organisms, particularly higher eukaryotic organisms. However, significant information exists about the design of research facilities and experimental procedures that are applicable to organisms containing recombinant DNA that is either integrated into the genome or into microorganisms associated with the higher organism as a symbiont, pathogen, or other relationship. This information describes facilities for physical containment of organisms used in non-traditional laboratory settings and special practices for limiting or excluding the unwanted establishment, transfer of genetic information, and dissemination of organisms beyond the intended location, based on both physical and biological containment principles. Research conducted in accordance with these conditions effectively confines the organism.

Revision of Appendix K of the *NIH Guidelines* revised in April 2002 (http://www4.od.nih.gov/oba/rac/guidelines/guidelines.html) reflects a formalization of suitable containment practices and facilities for the conduct of large-scale experiments involving recombinant DNA-derived industrial microorganisms. Appendix K replaces portions of Appendix G when quantities in excess of 10 L of culture are involved in research or production. For large-scale research or production, four physical containment levels are established: GLSP, BL1-LS, BL2-LS, and BL3-LS.

- *GLSP (Good large-scale practice)*: Level of physical containment is recommended for large-scale research of production involving viable, nonpathogenic, and nontoxigenic recombinant strains derived from host organisms that have an extended history or safe large-scale use. The GLSP level of physical containment is recommended for those organisms that have built-in environmental limitations, which permit optimum growth in the large-scale setting but limited survival without adverse consequences in the environment.
- *BL1-LS(BL1-large scale)*: Level of physical containment is recommended for large-scale research or production of viable organisms containing recombinant DNA molecules that require BL1 containment at the laboratory scale.

- *BL2-LS*: Level of physical containment is required for large-scale research or production of viable organisms containing recombinant DNA molecules that require BL2 containment at the laboratory scale.
- *BL3-LS*: Level of physical containment is required for large-scale research or production of viable organisms containing recombinant DNA molecules that require BL3 containment at the laboratory scale.
- *BL4-LS*: No provisions are made at this time for large-scale research or production of viable organisms containing recombinant DNA molecules that require BL4 containment at the laboratory scale.

There should be no adventitious organisms in the system during cell growth. Contaminating organisms in the bioreactor may adversely affect both the product yield and the ability of the downstream process to correctly separate and purify the desired protein. The presence or effects of contaminating organisms in the bioreactor can be detected in a number of ways such as growth rate, culture purity, bacteriophage assay, and fatty acid profile.

To assure compliance with the NIH guidelines, the following needs to be followed:

- Verify that there are written procedures to assure absence of adventitious agents and criteria established to reject contaminated runs.
- Maintain cell growth records and verify that the production-run parameters are consistent with the established pattern.
- Establish written procedures to determine what investigations and corrective actions will be performed in the event that growth parameters exceed established limits.
- Assure proper aseptic techniques during cell culture techniques and appropriate in-process controls in their processing.

The U.S. FDA is responsible under the National Environmental Policy Act (NEPA) for ascertaining the environmental impact that may occur due to the manufacture, use, and disposal of the U.S. FDA-regulated products. The U.S. FDA makes sure that the product sponsor is conducting investigations safely. Typically, a product sponsor describes environmental control measures in environmental assessments (EAs) that are part of the product application. When the product is approved, the EA is released to the public. Of particular importance are the NIH guidelines for recombinant DNA research and particularly the Appendix K (2002), regarding the establishment of guidelines for the level of containment appropriate to good industrial large-scale practices. It must be assumed that the equipment and controls described in the EA as part of the biocontainment and waste processing systems are validated to operate to the standards; the equipment is in place, is operating, and is properly maintained. Such equipment may include, for example, HEPA filters, spill collection tanks with heat or hypochlorite treatment, and diking around bioreactors and associated drains. SOPs should be established for the cleanup of spills, for actions to be taken in the case of accidental exposure of personnel, for opening and closing of vessels, for sampling and sample handling, and for other procedures that involve breaching containment or where exposure to living cells may occur.

10.22 GOOD MANUFACTURING CONTROLS OF ACTIVE PHARMACEUTICAL INGREDIENTS

The good manufacturing practices prescribed for the active pharmaceutical ingredient (API) depend to a great degree on the type of API manufactured; for example, Table 10.20 shows the increasing compliance requirement in various API manufacturing types.

10.23 MANUFACTURING SYSTEMS AND LAYOUT

Each unit operation will require careful adjustment of the sample parameters (pH, conductivity, protein concentration, redox potential, load). In some cases, desalting, ultrafiltration, or addition of co-solvents are needed in order to assure proper conditions. One should be aware that ion exchange generally requires samples of low ionic strength, while hydrophobic interaction chromatography is generally used for samples of high ionic strength. Such observations can be used in the design of the process, thus reducing the number of unit operations. The particle size of the media will decrease from capture to polishing to accommodate the need for resolution by decreasing zone spreading on the column. The manufacturing layout will depend on the unit operations included in the manufacturing system.

A biopharmaceutical manufacturing process must fulfill the criteria of consistency and robustness, meaning that the outcome of each of the unit operations and the entire process shall be the same from lot to lot. Not only shall the acceptance criteria of the drug substance specification program be met, but also in-process acceptance criteria must be specified and met. Each parameter of each of the unit operations should be defined as a proven acceptable range within which the operation has to take place. It is a common practice to qualify and validate the downstream process unit operations by means of statistical factorial design analysis. Small variations in handling procedures or in parameter set points must not influence the outcome of the manufacturing process. Most proteins are unstable in aqueous solutions and the demand for robustness is not easily obtained. Procedures that are easy to carry out in a laboratory scale (pH adjustment, chromatographic gradients, fraction collection) are technically complicated in large scale. Much can be gained if the process designers think ahead by, for instance, defining broad parameter intervals.

Where multiple products manufacturing is envisioned, the manufacturer is faced with the dilemma of design parameters that would comply with the regulatory requirements internationally. Given the cost of establishing such facilities, global compliance, rather than a regional approval, is recommended. It is well established that the U.S. FDA follows certain strict requirements, whereas the EU requirements of cGMP compliance often exceed the U.S. FDA requirements. The U.S. FDA has moved therapeutic proteins from the CBER to CDER, these remain pretty much covered under the same regulations as are the biological products, including the timely visits and approvals by the agency, of the manufacturing facility. Biologics License Applications 357 provides details of this inspection schedule. The fundamental question whether a facility can be used to manufacture a multitude of molecules needs examination. If we broadly classify

Table 10.20 Application of the cGMP Guidance in API Manufacturing

Type of Manufacturing	Application of cGMP to Steps Used in This Type of Manufacturing				
Chemical manufacturing	Production of the API starting material	Introduction of the API starting material into process[a]	Production of intermediate(s)[a]	Isolation and purification[a]	Physical processing and packaging[a]
API derived from animal sources	Collection of organ, fluid, or tissue	Cutting, mixing, and/or initial processing	Introduction of the API starting material into process[a]	Isolation and purification[a]	Physical processing and packaging[a]
API extracted from plant sources	Collection of plant	Cutting and initial extraction(s)	Introduction of the API starting material into process[a]	Isolation and purification[a]	Physical processing and packaging[a]
Herbal extracts used as API	Collection of plants	Cutting and initial extraction		Further extraction[a]	Physical processing and packaging[a]
API consisting of comminuted or powdered herbs	Collection of plants and/or cultivation and harvesting	Cutting/ comminuting			Physical processing and packaging[a]
Biotechnology: fermentation/cell culture	Establishment of MCB and WCB	Maintenance of WCB[a]	Cell culture and/or fermentation[a]	Isolation and purification[a]	Physical processing and packaging[a]
Classical fermentation to produce an API	Establishment of cell bank	Maintenance of cell bank	Introduction of the cells into fermentation[a]	Isolation and purification[a]	Physical processing and packaging[a]

[a] Application of cGMP to steps.

the processes involved based on the type of fermenter required, the decision can be relatively straightforward. Bacterial and yeast fermentation requires a faster agitating fermenter requiring at least two sets of line of production, one for mammalian cells (which require slow and more gentle stirring) and the other type that require relatively more agile stirring. Many newer systems now offer an opportunity for a closed system of transfer of culture to the larger fermenting vessels reducing the environment definition, say from 100,000 area classification to pharmaceutical-grade (unclassified) conditions. With computerized CIP and SIP available on most equipment, such systems are highly recommended. However, where closed systems are not utilized, the rooms where fermentation is installed should be at least of 100,000 class. In all areas where the product is exposed such as in the cell culture transfer and downstream processing purification, the rooms must be class 10,000 with separation equipment placed under class 1,000 laminar flow curtains. Most regulatory authorities will not allow GMCs be let out in the environment. This requires an elaborate setup to sterilize the media prior to its discharge. A word of caution applies here where bacterial inclusion bodies are involved. Most of the cells are ground, whereas some remain, requiring an equally intensive treatment of media.

Figure 10.1 shows a typical layout for a biotechnology manufacturing unit. The manufacturing layout of biological products is determined by two major factors: (1) the size of

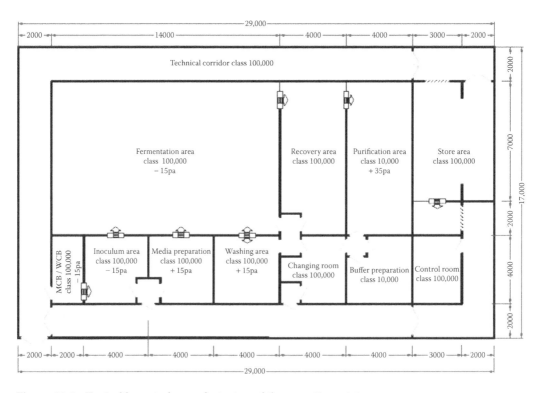

Figure 10.1 Typical layout of manufacturing of therapeutic proteins.

production and (2) the type of production; in most cases the conditions of containment described above and the need to process products under clean room conditions are similar to the processing of sterile products otherwise. As a rule of thumb, the environment should be comparable to preparation room environment for sterile products. There are four major types of work performed in a biological product manufacturing and given below are the requirements for each of these phases:

1. *MCB and WCB*: A dedicated room is to be made available for each GMC; this room includes a cold storage system (often a liquid nitrogen system) and a cold (–70°C) cabinet. The cells in the MCB are used to create WCB and both of these are kept under high security. It is recommended that this be a vaulted area with class 100,000 environment; generally a 100–200 sq ft area would suffice for this purpose. Some manufacturers divide the room into two, one for MCB and one for WCB with restricted entrance to each. In some designs a direct transfer from WCB to the inoculum/culture room (see below) is allowed through a transfer window under negative pressure. (However, this practice is questioned on the basis of need to maintain a certain area classification; as a result, the MCB/WCB is to be considered as supply center at the time of use, processed through materials dispensing.) In all instances a duplicate MCB shall be maintained off site from the immediate manufacturing area. These rooms should have a backup supply of electricity to assure no power breakdown losses along with alarms to record temperature variations in the cabinets storing the GMCs; an electronic recording device that would transmit the temperature at which the GMCs are stored should be installed. The room should also be equipped with an automated system of pressure differential; the room to be maintained negative with respect to the corridor. This room is dedicated to each GMC; the reason being to avoid mixing up of cultures, access restrictions to different personnel, and the storage requirements.

2. *Inoculum room*: This is the first room where the culture tubes are opened for the purpose of making WCB, or for making the inoculum for fermentation the room should be a class 10,000. If the fermentation system used is a closed inline system then this room will also have a 4–8 L fermenter to make the starter culture; the culture will then be directly transferred to larger size fermenters. Where roller bottles are used, this room will serve as the staging room to prepare the culture for inoculation into the bottles, which would be done in another room because of the size of operation involved. The culture is handled under a biosafety laminar flow hood (biosafety hoods prevent exposure of operator). The room should have a 10,000 classification with class 100 under the laminar flow hood. Generally, this room will be connected to the fermentation area, the recovery area, and the roller bottle preparation area, preferably through a negative pressure passing carousel. The room should be of smallest size possible (100–200 sq ft).

3. *Fermentation room*: This generally being the largest room of the facility may comprise a series of rooms depending on the size of production. Where larger fermenters such as 25,000 L sizes are involved, this may take a three-stage fermenting. A facility of this size would likely be a 20,000+ sq ft facility that may comprise several floors to accommodate large fermenters. However, for many therapeutic

proteins of low dosing, fermenters of 500 L should be sufficient and these can be accommodated on a single floor basis. The area classification for this room is 100,000 unless a complete closed system is use (which is recommended) wherein general pharmaceutical-grade classification (unclassified) may be used.

4. *Roller bottle room*: Where mammalian cell cultures are used in roller bottles, the fermentation room (above) is replaced with two rooms, one for staging the roller bottles and the other a 37°C room to roll the bottles. The classification of both rooms is 100,000 with bottles being opened under a class 100 biosafety laminar flow hood. There are several issues involved in using roller bottles, the most important being the cost and time constraints in processing large number of bottles. Newer systems offer robotic controls and also recently, a multiple bottle automated continuously flowing system; these will be discussed later in the manufacturing details. Where large quantities are involved, manufacturers will be advised to develop a ferementation-based system; much progress has been made in this area and it would be discussed later as well. The size of roller bottle room will depend on the number of rolling racks involved and the size of staging room will depend on the type of process involved (robotics, manual, continuous flow, etc.). For a medium-scale operation, the 37°C room is about 150 sq ft and the staging area about 400 sq ft.

5. *Recovery room*: The product of fermentation (either from fermenters or from roller bottles) is brought to this room for the first stage of processing. Where inclusion bodies are involved (such as in the use of bacterial cultures) this room will house cold centrifuge and cell disrupters; for the mammalian culture systems where the protein is secreted, the first stage of reduction of volume through filtration will be done. This room is also used to store the product where refolding is involved at 2°C–8°C environment generally (provided by walk in refrigerators). This area classification of this room remains 100,000. A room of about 500 sq ft is required for this purpose.

6. *Downstream processing room*: This is the second 10,000 classification room with large square footage under laminar flow hoods for the purification process. It is noteworthy that dedicated contact equipment (columns, vessels, etc.) are required for each product. A room of about 500 sq ft is required as a minimum; the size of the room will depend on the volume of production and the steps involved; in some instances this may take more than 5,000 sq ft where large-scale filtration equipment is involved and may comprise several floors. Some manufacturers do their downstream processing in different facilities; in such instance, there should be proper SOPs describing the packaging and transportation of the fermentation product.

7. *Media and buffer preparation rooms*: Each process requires a specific buffer and media; depending on the size of operation the quantity of these liquids can be substantial. For example, where using large fermenters (1,000 L or up), it may be advisable to switch to closed systems of media preparation and transfer to fermenters; however, for most medium-and small-scale operations, a large media preparation room is required (500 sq ft) with 10,000 classification and work under class 100 hood; the media prepared is then transferred to storage area and issued a specification code; the same applies to buffers used in downstream processing. Buffers should be prepared in a separate room and transported in closed containers to the storage area prior to dispensing.

8. *Storage rooms*: Incoming material is stored in special environment-controlled areas; large refrigerated space is required for many components including media and buffer. This room is also a 100,000 classification room of about 1,000 sq ft. A part of the room is dedicated to staging of supplies at the time of batch issue for production wherein material will be gathered from the WCB, media, and buffer rooms.
9. *Finished product storage room:* This is a relatively smaller room, about 100 sq ft where concentrate is stored at refrigerated temperature. The classification remains 100,000.

10.24 CLEANING PROCEDURES

Validation of the cleaning procedures for the processing of equipment, including columns, should be carried out. This is especially critical for a multiproduct facility. The manufacturer should have determined the degree of effectiveness of the cleaning procedure for each BDP or intermediate used in that particular piece of equipment. Validation data should verify that the cleaning process will reduce the specific residues to an acceptable level. However, it may not be possible to remove absolutely every trace of material, even with a reasonable number of cleaning cycles. The permissible residue level, generally expressed in parts per million (ppm), should be justified by the manufacturer. Cleaning should remove endotoxins, bacteria, toxic elements, and contaminating proteins, while not adversely affecting the performance of the column. There should be established a written equipment cleaning procedure that provides details of what should be done and the materials to be utilized. Some manufacturers list the specific solvent for each BDP and intermediate. For stationary vessels, often CIP is used and in these instances necessary diagrams should be drawn to identify specific parts (e.g., valves) that are part of the cleaning protocol.

After cleaning, there should be some routine testing to assure that the surface has been cleaned to the validated level. One common method is the analysis of the final rinse water or solvent for the presence of the cleaning agents last used in that piece of equipment. There should always be direct determination of the residual substance.

The efficiency of the cleaning system would depend to a large degree on the robustness of the analytical system used to characterize the cleaning end points. The sensitivity of modern analytical apparatus has lowered some detection thresholds below ppm, even down to parts per billion (ppb). The residue limits established for each piece of apparatus should be practical, achievable, and verifiable. There should be a rationale for establishing certain levels which must be documented to prove their scientific merit. Another factor to consider is the possible non-uniform distribution of the residue on a piece of equipment. The actual average residue concentration may be more than the level detected.

10.25 PROCESSING AND FILLING

The products of biotechnology are proteins and peptides that are relatively unstable molecules compared to most organic pharmaceuticals. Most biotechnology processes involve the transfer of proteins from one stabilizing or solubilizing buffer to another during the purification process. Ultimately, the protein is exchanged into its final solution dosage form where long-term stability is achieved. In addition, these products often require lyophilization to achieve long-term stability because of the potential for degradation by a variety of mechanisms, including deamidation, aggregation, oxidation, and possible proteolysis by trace levels of host cell proteases. The final dosage form of the protein usually contains stabilizing compounds that result in the optimal pH and solution conditions necessary for long-term product stability and/or the desired properties for administration of the product (tonicity). These compounds include proteins, polyhydric alcohols, amino acids, carbohydrates, bulking agents, inorganic salts, and nonionic surfactants. In addition, these excipients may be required for stable lyophilized cake formation. There are special requirements for lyophilized products, such as the control of moisture levels, that generally are defined in the individual USP monograph and that may be important to product stability. Significantly, the assessment of protein stability usually requires the use of multiple analytical methods, each of which may be used to assess a specific mode of protein degradation. The use of accelerated stability studies to predict the shelf life of protein formulations is often complicated by the effects of temperature on protein conformation, resulting in non-Arrhenius behavior. Thus, reliance on real-time, recommended storage condition stability studies is often required for establishing the expiration dating of biotechnology-derived products.

Most BDP cannot be terminally sterilized and must be manufactured by aseptic processing. The presence of process-related contaminants in a product or device is chiefly a safety issue. The sources of contaminants are primarily the cell substrate (DNA, host cell proteins, other cellular constituents, and viruses), the media (proteins, sera, and additives), and the purification process (process-related chemicals and product-related impurities).

Because of stability considerations, most BDP are either refrigerated or lyophilized. Low temperatures and low moisture content are also deterrents to microbiological proliferation. For the validation of aseptic processing of the non-preserved single dose biopharmaceutical (that is aseptically filled) stored at room temperature as a solution, the limitations of 0.1% media fill contamination rate should be recognized.

Media fill data and validation of the aseptic manufacturing process should be well documented. Some BDP may not be very stable and may require gentle mixing and processing. Whereas double filtrations are relatively common for aseptically filled parenterals, single filtration at low pressures are usually performed for BDP. It is for this reason that manufacturing directions be specific, with maximum filtration pressures given.

The environment and accessibility for the batching of the non-sterile BDP should be controlled. Because many of these products lack preservatives and inherent bacteriostatic or fungistatic activity, bioburden before sterilization should be low and this bioburden should be determined prior to sterilization of these bulk solutions and before filling. Obviously, the batching or compounding of these bulk solutions should be controlled in order to prevent any potential increase in microbiological levels that may occur up to the time that the bulk solutions are filtered (sterilized). One concern with any microbiological level is the possible increase in endotoxins that may develop. Good practice for the compounding of these products would also include batching in a controlled environment and in sealed tanks, particularly if the solution is to be stored prior to sterilization. Good practice would also include limitations on the length of manufacturing time between formulation and sterilization.

In-process testing is an essential part of quality control and ensures that the actual, real-time performance of an operation is acceptable. Examples of in-process controls are stream parameters, chromatography profiles, protein species and protein concentrations, bioactivity, bioburden, and endotoxin levels. This set of in-process controls and the selection of acceptance criteria require coordination with the results from the validation program.

The filling of BDP into ampoules or vials presents many of the same problems as with the processing of conventional products. In established companies these issues are addressed using adequate documentation; however, for the new BDP facility, attempting to develop and prove clinical effectiveness and safety along with validation of sterile operations, equipment, and systems can be a lengthy process, particularly if requirements are not clearly understood.

The batch size, at least when initially produced, likely will be small. Because of the small batch size, filling lines may not be as automated as for other products typically filled in larger quantities. Thus, there is more involvement of people filling these products, particularly at some of the smaller, newer companies. This can bring quality inconsistencies. Problems during filling include inadequate attire; deficient environmental monitoring programs; hand-stoppering of vials, particularly those that are to be lyophilized; and failure to validate some of the basic sterilization processes. Because of the active involvement of people in filling and aseptic manipulations, the number of persons involved in these operations should be minimized, and an environmental program should include an evaluation of microbiological samples taken from people working in aseptic processing areas.

Another concern about product stability is the use of inert gas to displace oxygen both the during processing and filling of the solution. As with other products that may be sensitive to oxidation, limits for dissolved oxygen levels for the solution should be established. Likewise, validation of the filling operation should include parameters such as line speed and location of filling syringes with respect to closure, to assure minimal exposure to air (oxygen) for oxygen-sensitive products. In the absence of inert gas displacement, the manufacturer should be able to demonstrate that the product is not affected by oxygen.

Typically, vials to be lyophilized are partially stoppered by machine. Where an operator places stopper manually, serious problems can arise. Another major concern with the filling operation of a lyophilized product is assurance of fill volumes. Obviously, a low fill would represent a subpotency in the vial. Unlike a powder or liquid fill, a low fill would not be readily apparent after lyophilization, particularly for a product where the active ingredient may be only a milligram. Because of the clinical significance, subpotency in a vial potentially can be a very serious situation, clinically.

10.26 LABORATORY TESTING

The following tests may be applicable to component, in-process, bulk, and/or final product testing. The tests that are needed will depend on the process and the intended use of the product.

- *Quality*
  - Color/appearance/clarity
  - Particulate analysis
  - pH determination

313

- Moisture content
- Host cell DNA
- *Identity*: A single test for identity may not be sufficient. Confirmation is needed that the methods employed are validated. A comparison of the product to the reference preparation in a suitable bioassay will provide additional evidence relating to the identity and potency of the product.
  - Peptide mapping (reduced/non-reduced)
  - Gel electrophoresis
  - SDS PAGE
  - IEF
  - Immunoelectrophoresis
  - Two-dimensional electrophoresis
  - Capillary electrophoresis
  - HPLC (chromographic retention)
  - Immunoassay
  - ELISA
  - Western blot
  - Radioimmunoassay
  - Amino acid analysis
  - Amino acid sequencing
  - Mass spectroscopy
  - Molecular weight (SDS PAGE)
  - Carbohydrate composition analysis (glycosylation)
- *Protein concentration/content*:
  - Tests that may be encountered are as follows:
    - Protein quantitations
    - Lowry
    - Biuret method
    - UV spectrophotometry
    - HPLC
    - Amino acid analysis
    - Partial sequence analysis
- *Purity*: *Purity* means relative freedom from extraneous matter in the finished product, whether or not harmful to the recipient or deleterious to the product. Purity includes, but is not limited to, relative freedom from residual moisture or other volatile substances and pyrogenic substances. Protein impurities are the most common contaminants. These may arise from the fermentation process, media, or the host organism. Endogenous retroviruses may be present in hybridomas used for monoclonal antibody production. Specific testing for these constituents is imperative in in vivo products. Removal of extraneous antigenic proteins is essential to assure the safety and the effectiveness of the product.
  - Tests for protein impurities:
    - Electrophoresis
      - SDS PAGE
      - IEF

- Two-dimensional electrophoresis
- Peptide mapping
- Multiantigen ELISA
- HPLC, size exclusion HPLC, reverse phase HPLC
- Tests for non-protein impurities:
  - Endotoxin testing
  - USP rabbit pyrogen test
  - Limulus amebocyte lysate (LAL) E
  - Endogenous pyrogen assay
- *Pyrogen contamination*: Pyrogenicity testing should be conducted by injection of rabbits with the final product or by the LAL assay. The same criteria used for acceptance of the natural product should be used for the biotech product. The presence of endotoxins in some in vitro diagnostic products may interfere with the performance of the device. Also, it is essential that in vivo products be tested for pyrogens. Certain biological pharmaceuticals are pyrogenic in humans despite having passed the LAL test and the rabbit pyrogen test. This phenomenon may be due to materials that appear to be pyrogenic only in humans. To attempt to predict whether human subjects will experience a pyrogenic response, an endogenous pyrogen assay is used. Human blood mononuclear cells are cultured in vitro with the final product, and the cell culture fluid is injected into rabbits. A fever in the rabbits indicates that the product contains a substance that may be pyrogenic in humans.
  - USP rabbit pyrogen test
  - LAL
  - Assay endogenous pyrogen assay
- *Viral contamination*: Tests for viral contamination should be appropriate to the cell substrate and culture conditions employed. Absence of detectable adventitious viruses contaminating the final product should be demonstrated.
  - Cytopathic effect in several cell types
  - Hemabsorption embryonated egg testing
  - Polymerase chain reaction (PCR)
  - Viral antigen and antibody immunoassay
  - MAP
- *Nucleic acid contamination*: Concern about nucleic acid impurities arises from the possibility of cellular transformation events in a recipient. Removal of nucleic acid at each step in the purification process may be demonstrated in pilot experiments by examining the extent of elimination of added host cell DNA. Such an analysis would provide the theoretical extent of the removal of nucleic acid during purification. Direct analyses of nucleic acid in several production lots of the final product should be performed by hybridization analysis of immobilized contaminating nucleic acid utilizing appropriate probes, such as nick-translated host cell and vector DNA. Theoretical concerns regarding transforming DNA derived from the cell substrate will be minimized by the general reduction of contaminating nucleic acid.
  - DNA hybridization (dot blot)
  - PCR

- *Protein contamination*
  - SDS PAGE
  - PLC
  - IEF
- *Foreign protein contamination*
  - Immunoassays
  - Radioimmunoassays
  - ELISA
  - Western blot
  - SDS PAGE
  - Two-dimensional electrophoresis
- *Microbial contamination:* Appropriate tests should be conducted for microbial contamination that demonstrates the absence of detectable bacteria (aerobes and anaerobes), fungi, yeast, and mycoplasma, when applicable.
  - USP sterility test
  - Heterotrophic plate count and total yeasts and molds
  - Total plate count
  - Mycoplasma test
  - LAL/pyrogen
- *Chemical contaminants:* Other sources of contamination must be considered, for example, allergens, petroleum oils, residual solvents, cleaning materials, and column leachable materials.
- *Potency (activity):* Potency is interpreted to mean the specific ability or capacity of the product, as indicated by appropriate laboratory tests or by adequately controlled clinical data obtained through the administration of the product in the manner intended, to produce a given result. Tests for potency should consist of either in vitro or in vivo tests, or both, which have been specifically designed for each product so as to indicate its potency. A reference preparation for biological activity should be established and used to determine the bioactivity of the final product. Where applicable, in-house biological potency standards should be cross-referenced against international (World Health Organization [WHO], NIBSC) or national (NIH, National Cancer Institute U.S. FDA) reference standard preparations, or USP standards. Validated method of potency determination include the following:
  - Whole animal bioassays
  - Cell culture bioassays
  - Biochemical/biophysical assays
  - Receptor-based immunoassays
  - Potency limits
    - Identification of agents that may adversely affect potency
    - Evaluation of functional activity and antigen/antibody specificity
    - Various immunodiffusion methods (single/double)
    - Immunoblotting/radio or enzyme-linked immunoassays
    - HPLC-validated to correlate certain peaks to biological activity

- *Stability*: It is the capacity of a product to remain within specifications established to ensure its identity, strength, quality, purity, safety, and effectiveness as a function of time. Studies to support the proposed dating period should be performed on the final product. Real-time stability data would be essential to support the proposed dating period. Testing might include stability of potency, pH, clarity, color, particulates, physiochemical stability, moisture, and preservatives. Accelerated stability testing data may be used as supportive data. Accelerated testing or stress tests are studies designed to increase the ratio of chemical or physical degradation of a substance or product by using exaggerated storage conditions. The purpose is to determine kinetic parameters to predict the tentative expiration dating period. Stress testing of the product is frequently used to identify potential problems that may be encountered during storage and transportation and to provide an estimate of the expiration dating period. This should include a study of the effects of temperature fluctuations as appropriate for shipping and storage conditions. These tests should establish a valid dating period under realistic field conditions with the containers and closures intended for the marketed product. Some relatively fragile biotechnically derived proteins may require gentle mixing and processing and only a single filtration at low pressure. The manufacturing directions must be specific with maximum filtration pressures given in order to maintain stability in the final product. Products containing preservatives to control microbial contamination should have the preservative content monitored. This can be accomplished by performing microbial challenge tests (i.e., USP antimicrobial preservative effectiveness test) or by performing chemical assays for the preservative. Areas that should be addressed are as follows:
  - Effective monitoring of the stability test environment (i.e., light, temperature, humidity, and residual moisture)
  - Container/closure system used for bulk storage (i.e., extractables, chemical modification of protein, and change in stopper formulations that may change extractable profile)
  - Identify materials that would cause product instability and test for presence of aggregation, denaturation, fragmentation, deamination, photolysis, and oxidation
- Tests to determine aggregates or degradation products:
  - SDS PAGE
  - IEF
  - HPLC
  - IEC
  - Gel filtration
  - Peptide mapping
  - Spectrophotometric methods
  - Potency assays
  - Performance testing
  - Two-dimensional electrophoresis
- *Batch-to-batch consistency*: The basic criterion for determining that a manufacturer is producing a standardized and reliable product is the demonstration of lot-to-lot consistency with respect to certain predetermined release specifications.

- *Uniformity*: Identity, purity, functional activity
- *Stability*: Acceptable performance during shelf life, precision, sensitivity, and specificity. Like other small molecules, protein drugs are subject to demonstration of stability (providing a predetermined minimum potency) to the time of use and in addition, a safety profile since the degradation products of protein drugs can be immunogenic, compared to small molecules where the concern is mainly creation of toxic molecules. The stability studies for therapeutic proteins are conducted at three levels: preformulation, formulation development, and formal GMP studies. The preformulation studies determine basic stability properties of bulk protein or peptide and the accelerated studies at this stage are primarily intended to establish stability indicating assays and other analytic methods. The formulation development studies are intended for the candidate formulation and encompass large studies that evaluate the effects of excipients; container/closure systems; and where lyophilized, a study of myriad factors that can alter the characteristics of products. The data generated in the formulation development studies is used to select final formulation and to design the studies that follow formal GMP studies. The formal stability studies are used to support clinical use, IND, and then all the way through a Biological License Application (submitted to CDER; effective June 2003, therapeutic proteins are now handled by CDER). When preparing supplies for the clinical use, it is important to know that there is no need to demonstrate shelf life for the commercial dosage form and only stability demonstration is required during the testing phase, such as 6 months; many manufacturers used frozen product to assure adequate stability; this may create a logistics problem of assuring that the clinical sites can store the produce frozen. Obviously, for products which may be adversely affected by freezing will not be subject to this method of reducing the clinical startup time. Also, at this stage of initial clinical testing under an IND, the test methods need not be fully validated or having demonstrated robustness; as long as reproducibility and repeatability is demonstrated, this should be acceptable to the U.S. FDA. The formal GMP studies monitor commercial lots and clear ICH guidelines are available to follow the protocols of these studies (see ICH Stability Guidelines for Biologics, Federal Register July 10, 1996, Volume 61, No. 133, pp. 36466–36469).

10.27 LABORATORY CONTROLS

A quality control program for the drug substance and drug product must be defined and acceptance criteria set for each analysis. The setting of acceptance criteria is an ongoing activity throughout development (and scale up) as more and more data become available. A batch is released provided all analytical results are within the specified ranges. A high acceptance rate should be expected if the process is robust and in compliance, implying that both the regulatory authorities and the manufacturer often share identical views. The process designer is advised to carefully consider the above-mentioned issues when designing the purification process (the design in principle). Much of the design can be carried out before entering the laboratory due to the restrictions governing biopharmaceutical processing. The pre-design phase is called process modeling, thus preceding the experimental design phase for optimization and testing, which takes place in the laboratory.

In general, quality control systems for biotechnology-derived products are very similar to those quality control systems routinely employed for traditional pharmaceutical products in such areas as raw material testing and release, manufacturing and process control documentation, and aseptic processing. Biotechnology-derived products quality control systems incorporate some of the same philosophies applied to the analysis of low-molecular-weight pharmaceutical products. These include the use of chemical reference standards and validated methods to evaluate a broad spectrum of known and/or potential product impurities and potential breakdown products. The quality control systems for biotechnology-derived products are generally analogous to those established for traditional biologicals with respect to determining product sterility, product safety in experimental animals, and product potency. The fundamental difference between quality control systems for biotechnology-derived products and traditional pharmaceuticals is in the types of methods that are used to determine product identity, consistency, purity, and impurity profiling. Furthermore, in biotechnology quality control, it is frequently necessary to use a combination of final product and validated in-process testing and process validation to ensure the removal of undesired real or potential impurities to the levels suggested by regulatory agencies. Biotechnology-derived products generally require a detailed characterization of the production organism (cell), a complete assessment of the means of cell growth/propagation, and explicit analysis of the final product recovery process.

The complexity of the quality control systems for biotechnology-derived products is related to both the size and structural characteristics of the product and manufacturing process. In general, the quality control systems required for products produced in prokaryotic cells are less complex than the systems required for products produced in eukaryotic cells. The quality control systems for prokaryotic production organisms usually entail documentation of the origin of the producer strain and encompass traditional testing for adventitious organisms, karyology, phenotyping, and antibiotic resistance. In addition, newer techniques such as DNA restriction mapping, DNA sequence analysis, and routine monitoring that may include measurement of mRNA and/or plasmid DNA levels may be useful. The quality control of the MCB and WCB for eukaryotic production organisms generally includes testing for adventitious organisms, karyology, identity, and stability monitoring. All eukaryotic cell lines (except yeast) are generally tested for the presence of retroviruses, retroviral activity markers, and tumorigenicity, although many of these tests may be of limited value.

The laboratory controls are similar to what is expected in normal cGMP/GLP compliance for all pharmaceutical products with special consideration given to unique materials and their handling.

- *Training*: Laboratory personnel should be adequately trained for the jobs they are performing.
- *Equipment maintenance/calibration/monitoring*: Documentation and scheduling for maintenance, calibration, and monitoring of laboratory equipment involved in

the measurement; testing; and storage of raw materials, product, samples, and reference reagents.

- *Validation*: All laboratory methods should be validated with the equipment and reagents specified in the test methods. Changes in vendor and/or specifications of major equipment/reagents would require revalidation. Raw data should support validation parameters in submitted applications.
- *Standard/reference material*: Reference standards should be well characterized and documented, properly stored, secured, and utilized during testing.
- *Storage of labile components*: Laboratory cultures and reagents, such as enzymes, antibodies, test reagents, and so on, may degrade if not held under proper storage conditions.
- *Laboratory SOPs*: Procedures should be written, applicable and followed. Quality control samples should be properly segregated and stored.

10.28 DOCUMENTATION

The development program comprises a variety of activities comprising project planning, cell banking, process development, development of analytical procedures, scale up, manufacture, stability studies, preparation of reference materials, and quality assurance. The work will ultimately lead to a process for the manufacture and control of the licensed product. In order to obtain a license, extensive documentation must be provided (new drug application, biological license application). However, much of the work carried out during development and scale up is not included in the said applications, and it is up to the project owner to provide the development documentation upon inspection from regulatory authorities. The statement "if it is not documented, it has not been carried out" should be taken rigorously.

A major part of the documentation required, can be planned (e.g., cell banking reports, unit operation descriptions, development report, analytical method descriptions, and batch records). Other reports (e.g., summary reports) are written along with the experimental work. Although, such reports are not providing a description of the final work, they are very useful for informing coming users about the rationale for decision-making. It is therefore recommended to include summary reports in the tech transfer package.

The drug development program produces hundreds or even thousands of documents written by different people from different departments and often from different companies. Any of these documents may be needed at a later stage and it is necessary to set up an efficient documentation system to assure document tracking. An important part of the tracking procedure is to ensure efficient authentication of the document comprising information of author, date, version, company, facility, and so on.

10.29 TECHNICAL PACKAGE

The documents listed above serves as the basis for the tech transfer between laboratory scale, pilot scale up, and non-GMP manufacture and cGMP manufacture.

- According to the common technical document, ICH (www.nihs.go.jp/dig/ich/m4index-e.html) information about the nomenclature and the chemical/physical properties of the target protein should be given.
- The rationale and strategy for the process design should be documented.
- The process development work should be documented in laboratory notebooks, summary reports, unit operation descriptions, a development report, and a process protocol. Batch records should be included for test batches used for process evaluation in small scale.
- It is common practice to include a list of raw materials together with raw material information and qualification documentation.
- The manufacturer must ensure the quality and safety of the drug substance by a series of test procedures with established acceptance criteria to which the drug substance must conform. An important part of the total control strategy is to provide analytical batch data and compare these with the specified acceptance criteria. A complete set of acceptance criteria cannot be disclosed *a priori* as some acceptance criteria are established and justified during development and production of preclinical and clinical test batches. Acceptance criteria are linked to the total analytical program established as part of the quality control and drug substance characterization program. As more and more data are collected during development and early phase pilot production the acceptance criteria may be adjusted or changed, and thus making it difficult to establish defined batch release procedures in the development phase.
- Updated unit operation documents, raw material list, and process protocol should be included together with scale-up summary reports and batch records.
- Data collected during development, scale up, and manufacture comprises a valuable repository of information, which can be used for troubleshooting, comparability, and equivalence studies. Control should be exerted on all levels and should constitute an integrated part of the total quality assurance. Each analytical method used in the development and for in-process control, drug substance, and drug product release should be described in an individual report including relevant analytical data. The report will gradually develop into a validation document for the method of choice.
- Short- and long-term stability studies for intermediary compounds, drug substance, and drug product should be documented.
- Reference materials and standards are usually extensively characterized. The process protocol, analytical methods used, and the analytical data must be provided in an accompanying report.

10.30 OUTSOURCING IN BIOTECH MANUFACTURING

One of the major bottlenecks in the rapidly growing biotech industry is manufacture of drug products for clinical trials. Demands for safety, robustness, and compliance make it necessary to produce clinical material in highly specialized cGMP facilities making biopharmaceutical drug development and cGMP manufacture a complex multitask operation for experts only. With the steady increasing number of biotech companies entering this area and the huge costs involved in building cGMP facilities, outsourcing of development activities and manufacture to highly specialized contract research and manufacturing organizations has become a common practice. However, one thing, which cannot be outsourced, is the responsibility for the product and biotech companies are strongly advised to keep in control by proper management throughout the program. In deciding the nature and extent of outsourcing that can be practiced, several questions must be answered:

- Which contract manufacturer should the biotech company partner with?
- Which research organizations should the biotech company partner with?
- How does the biotech company negotiate the contracts?
- What are the liability issues?
- What does it cost?
- What is the timeline?

10.31 ISSUES TO DISCUSS

This chapter describes parameters that would be useful in answering these questions to assist the user in setting up a proper strategy for the activities to be outsourced (Table 10.21). Generally, a decision should be made of the level of outsourcing. The overall step layout includes the following:

Molecular biology (gene construct) → fermentation development (upstream) → purification (downstream) → protein characterization and analysis → preclinical testing → regulatory filing → clinical supplies (cGMP) → full-scale manufacturing.

Table 10.21   Example Strategy for Determining Items to Be Outsourced

Area	Items to Discuss
Management	Project plan
	Batch plans
	Budgets
	Work sheets
	Communication
	Gantt chart
Cell work	Cell line optimization
	Establish MCB
	MCB sterility
	MCB characterization
	MCB storage and stability
	Establish WCB
	WCB sterility
	WCB characterization
	WCB storage and stability

(Continued)

Table 10.21 (*Continued*) Example Strategy for Determining Items to Be Outsourced

Area	Items to Discuss
Upstream development	Media, conditions, holding times, etc. Process scale Critical parameters and interactions Production of three consecutive batches in small scale meeting specifications
Process development	Provide process rationale and strategy Process scale Process design aiming for cGMP production Production of three (consecutive) batches in small scale meeting specifications Critical parameters and interactions Protein stability during processing
Non-cGMP production of drug substance from preclinical tests	Amount of drug substance to be produced Batch size Time schedule
Formulation development	Drug product development
Reference material	Amount of reference standard to be produced Conditions for storage
In-process control	Protein concentration assays 1D-SDS PAGE High performance IEC High performance RPC Size exclusion chromatography Specific biological activity
Quality control	Protein concentration assays 1D-SDS PAGE High performance IEC High performance RPC Size exclusion chromatography Endotoxins Host cell proteins DNA Bioburden Viruses Leachables Contaminants Carbohydrate pattern Specific biological activity Specific immunological activity Toxicity Appearance
Drug substance characterization	The following analyses should be discussed: Mass spectrometry

(Continued)

Table 10.21 (Continued)   Example Strategy for Determining Items to Be Outsourced

Area	Items to Discuss
	Amino acid sequencing
	Amino acid analysis
	Peptide map
	2D-electrophoresis
	UV-scanning
	IR-spectroscopy
	Optical rotation
	Fluorescence
	Circular dichroism
	NMR
	Diffraction pattern
	FTIR
	Carbohydrate structure
Drug substance stability studies	3, 6, 12, and 24 months' stability study including HP-IEC, HP-RPC, SEC, and biological activity
Drug product stability studies	3, 6, 12, and 24 months' stability study including HP-IEC, HP-RPC, SEC, and biological activity
cGMP production of drug product: phase I and II	Specifications
	Amount of drug product to be produced
	Batch release procedures
	List of raw materials
	Fill and pack
	Documentation
	Data collection and storage
Documentation	Laboratory notebook system
	Cell work reports
	Fermentation reports
	Downstream processing: Strategy and rationale report
	Summary reports
	Unit operation reports
	Analytical reports, QC
	Drug substance characterization reports
	Report on the reference materials
	Development report
	Batch records
	Manufacturing protocols
	List of raw materials
	Change control and deviation reports
	Facility documentation
	Equipment documentation
	Utility documentation
Technology transfer	Discovery to development
	Development to pilot production
	Tech transfer packages
	Tech transfer plan

Questions

1. Name and define the three stages of recombinant protein production
   Answer:
   Upstream: It is a cell culture process where the protein of interest is produced.
   Downstream: It is a process of harvesting the produced protein and purifying it from host and process-related impurities.
   Formulation: It is a process of reparing the purified material to be a drug product that can be delivered to have the desired effect in the target population (i.e., a drug to be injected into humans).

2. Name two drawbacks and three advantages for using bacterial systems for expression.

3. Why is purification of yeast-produced products usually simpler than bacterially produced proteins
   Answer: Yeast products are usually secreted into the media, which does not require additional extraction techniques necessary when working with bacteria.

4. Although insect cells are an attractive model, what is the major hurdle that has yet to be overcome in the United States?

5. Mammalian cell models have many useful characteristics, name two drawbacks.

6. Why is it essential to use serum for cell culture that is certified to be free of bovine spongiform encephalopathy?

7. List the chromatography techniques that are generally compatible with high-ionic strength solutions and then list those that are generally compatible with organic solvents.
   Answer:
   High ionic strength solutions: Hydroxyapatite chromatography, hydrophobic interaction chromatography, immobilized metal affinity chromatography, size exclusion chromatography
   Organic solvents: Hydroxyapatite chromatography, reverse phase chromatography, size exclusion chromatography

8. When calculating cost of producing a new product, when might it be permissible to choose an increased cost?

9. *True or false*: Reducing the number of steps in a purification procedure for an unstable protein will ensure that all hurdles to successful production are overcome.
   Answer: False. An unstable protein will provide difficulties.

10. Why can it be important to investigate acceptable intervals for validation parameters before scale up?

11. List factors that are in the process optimization stage, only occurring after the process design is complete.

12. Considering the significant cost and time investment in transgenic animals, why would one still choose this production method?

13. A team has decided that to be cost effective to use a production facility, the yield for a low-dose protein will need to be 240 g/month. Knowing that the facility is equipped with batch bioreactors that have a volume of 50 L (up to 3 are

available), what expression level in grams per liter of culture medium will be required? (Assume 4 weeks/month and that a batch uses 1 week of reactor time.)

Answer:

240 g/month × 1 month/4 weeks = 60 g/week → 20 g/week per bioreactor

20 g/50 L = 0.4 g/L

14. As a rule of thumb, how many chromatographic principals should be used in downstream biopharmaceutical processing?

15. When moving to animal or human studies, list several regulatory groups or agencies from which approval may be required.

16. For open processing steps, work should be done in what kind of environment at a production facility?

17. In addition to virus and bacterial contaminates, what other contaminates can reduce purity of a final product?

    Answer: Proteins, nucleic acids, processing chemicals, and so on.

18. What method is useful in determining expiration dates when waiting for the expiration of a product at *normal* speed is prohibitive to bringing the product to market?

19. Describe some of the information that needs to be documented to transfer information between the stages of development.

11

Disposable Bioprocessing Systems

LEARNING OBJECTIVES

1. Recognize the advantages of disposable systems.
2. Understand the challenges that disposable systems present.
3. Identify the appropriate governmental regulatory protocols for disposable systems.

11.1 INTRODUCTION

Bioprocessing entails the use of a biologic entity to produce a target product as a by-product of the metabolic activity of the entity used. The science and the art of processing dates back to thousands of years, from the fermentation of grapes by yeast to today's mass-scale production of monoclonal antibodies (MAb) using Chinese hamster ovary (CHO) cells. Recombinant engineering has made it possible to manufacture hundreds of life-saving endogenous proteins at a cost that is now affordable. However, the manufacturing of biological drugs (e.g., proteins and vaccines) is a difficult art to practice because the toxicity of these drugs is not always related to their chemical purity but to the subtle variations in their structure, both three and four dimensional, that can produce serious immunologic reactions. Produced in recombinant cell lines and organisms, these proteins merely simulate and do not always mimic the human proteins despite the use of the known genetic code to express these in host cells and organisms. A key concern of regulatory agencies, therefore, lies in assuring that there is no cross contamination of the batches since it would not be possible to rely on any type of cleaning validation to assure that minute traces of substances would not affect the structure of the proteins. In most instances, we would not even know what the contaminants are.

The U.S. Food and Drug Administration (FDA) and European Medicines Evaluation Agency (EMEA) thus strongly urge manufacturers to create environments that would keep the contaminants out rather than trying to clean them, and to show by validation protocols the effectiveness of the cleanliness. This stance of regulatory authorities became sterner in the 1970s as the issue of viral contamination came to surface in the preparation of human and animal tissue-derived drugs. A large number of manufacturers who could not comply with the new requirements shut down, and a new awareness about the risks involved in the manufacturing of biological drugs arose. Companies that survived made huge investments in isolating manufacturing steps, continuous monitoring, and extensive viral clearance studies. The breakout of transmissible spongiform encephalopathy further compounded the complexity and, as a result, it became extremely costly to manufacture biological drugs in facilities that would be BLA-compliant.

To assure compliance with the new regulatory requirements, major suppliers of components in drug manufacturing, like Pall, Sartorius, and Millipore, took the lead and developed disposable products that would eliminate the need to conduct cleaning validation exercises. The earliest products in this category were as simple as filters, and soon these became the standard components: today, more than 95% of filters used in bioprocessing are of the disposable type.

Before moving further into the historical perspective of disposable components, it is necessary that we review the regulatory definition of the term *single-use*, which is only in context with devices: SEC. 201. (21 U.S.C. 321) Definitions states: (1) "The term 'single-use device' means a device that is intended for one use, or on a single patient during a single procedure." The term *disposable* is defined by the *Oxford English Dictionary* as: "made to be thrown away after use." Obviously, a single-use device is disposed of once its use comes to end. A good example is a paper cup, which is disposed after it is used, but is there no reason why it could not be used a few times before it is thrown away? Similarly, how long can one reuse a disposable filter if the same buffer is sterilized by filtration over several days? The fact is that regulatory agencies do not require the use of single-use or disposable items in manufacturing; it is the responsibility of the manufacturer to assure compliance with limits of cross-contamination. It is when the cost and time required to meet those requirements becomes onerous that the cost of single-use or disposable items becomes a serious consideration.

Whereas over the past few years, a greater number of components in bioprocessing are of a disposable type, these are still not in the mainstream of manufacturing for many reasons including the lingering questions about the quality of materials used, scalability, running costs, level of automation possible with these components, and the training of staff required to assimilate these components in an established bioprocessing system. The advantages are obvious: safer, greener, cheaper (particularly capital costs), and offering greater flexibility of operations. Perhaps the greatest impediment in the wider acceptance of disposable items comes from the inability of manufacturers to discard their large investments made, relatively recently (1970s and 1980s), in fixed equipment and systems. As a result, the changes that are taking place are at the level of smaller companies, research organizations, and contract companies. However, this is about to change rapidly. The high cost of production that was acceptable to large pharmaceutical companies must now be challenged as the patents of blockbuster recombinant drugs have begun to expire allowing smaller companies to compete on cost—the generic business in biological drugs should convince the industry to embrace the future of bioprocessing. There are also environmental considerations involved. For example, Amgen's facility manufacturing Etanercept in Rhode Island consumes 800,000 gal of water per day, most of which is to perform steam in place (SIP)/cleaning in place (CIP) and operate autoclaves—none of these would be needed in the new generation of disposable systems.

11.1.1 Evolution of the Bioprocessing Industry

While the barriers to develop new drugs keep getting higher because of the regulatory demands of assuring safety, the technological barriers to manufacturing these drugs have certainly come down. The current technology of bioprocessing can be traced back to the dawn of civilization, though mammalian cell culture technology—the expression system preferred for most known therapeutic proteins with desirable glycosylation patterns—is relatively new. It took two decades of trials and tribulations to bring cell culture from a bench technique at milligram scales to industrial production at kilogram scales. The era of biopharmaceuticals is manifested in the capability of producing large quantities of biologics in stainless-steel bioreactors. Today those large-scale stirred-tank bioreactors (usually >10,000 L in scale) represent modern mammalian cell culture technology, a major workhorse of the biopharmaceutical industry. Many blockbuster biologics—such as Enbrel (etanercept from Immunex Corporation, Seattle, WA), Avastin (bevacizumab from Genentech, San Francisco, CA [Roche]), and Humira (adalimumab from Abbott Laboratories, Rockville, MD)—are produced using large-scale bioreactors. The current state of manufacturing thus represents the peak of what we conveniently call the age of stainless steel.

The method of manufacture of biological drugs progressed through an expected route. Fermentation in large vats, whether it was done for wine or industrial chemicals or drugs like penicillin, was a well-established technique, so when the time came to manufacture recombinant drugs, the same systems were transported over to this new class of drugs around 30 years ago. Large stainless-steel fermenters suited well as their science and technology was well developed. However, lurking was a new inquiry by major regulatory agencies: the quest to control cross-contamination and viral clearance, the two most important causes of the side effects of these drugs. The quality guidelines by the U.S. FDA and EMEA began emphasizing the safety issues for cleaning validation and viral clearance, and the industry responded with more robust validation plans to prove compliance. The costs of manufacturing soared but that did not make any difference because all of these molecules were under patent and the companies were able to get whatever price they needed to justify these huge investments.

The first *disruptive* innovation came to the industry when the first disposable Wave bioreactor was introduced in 1996, which coincided with the highest ever number of biotechnology drugs approved in a single year between 1982 and 2007. Almost immediately, the biological manufacturing industry (and more particularly the stainless-steel industry) began a debate on the safety and utility of plastic bags to manufacture biological drugs and the greatest fear inculcated in the heart of prospective users was the issue of extractables and leachables, a topic that gets a detailed review in this book. Ironically, this issued had long been resolved when the U.S. FDA allowed the use of plastic bags to administer drugs of all types, of both aqueous and lipid origin and including hyperalimentation solutions. The risks to patients were minimal vis-à-vis the convenience of administration. In reality, the leachables in the biological manufacturing are of little importance as the exposure to these possible chemicals comes at a very early stage in the production and the robust downstream purification that removes even the isomers of the compounds is more than adequate to remove these contaminants. The greater risk lies in the interactions in the final dosage forms. A notable incidence was the reporting of pure red-cell aplasia (PRCA) in using erythropoietin and, while many causes were brought to attention, one was the interaction between the rubber stopper and the newly formulated drug containing a new surfactant that might have extracted some extractables from the rubber stopper.

The fear of leachables, the strong presence of a well-established stainless steel industry, and a user industry in no rush to learn how to reduce the cost of production that slowed down the implementation of plastic containers, more particularly of the disposable containers in drug manufacturing.

First came the changes in practice as the industry began using disposable filters, flexible containers, membranes, sampling devices, and now there has been a wave of disposable bioreactors to address the most critical barriers in biological drugs manufacturing. Disposable bioreactors have since evolved beyond the wave-based design and have been adopted for both research purposes and GMP production. Other disposable technologies, such as disposable filters, flexible containers, membranes, sampling devices, and chromatography columns, have also made a significant headway in being accepted as the standard of manufacturing.

As new technology became common, many companies found they did not have in-house expertise to manufacture these molecules and that resulted in an exponential growth of contract research organizations (CROs) and contract manufacturing organizations (CMOs) to fill the gap. However, CROs and CMOs could not afford the capacity of large stainless-steel technology since they would not know which product they would handling the next day: disposable became very popular (because they required so little capital investment) among the CRO/CMO groups as well as research organizations, even their need for regulatory compliance was less. Only recently, has the disposable system been recognized by the first approval of a product in Europe using totally disposable system and in 2012, Therapeutic Proteins International, LLC (Chicago, IL) was the first company to get clearance to use a proprietary disposable system for a product expressed in bacteria.

The improved efficiency of being able to switch over to different products and manufacturing methods pushed the equipment supplier industry to make some quick innovations. The list of disposable items expanded very quickly and we can readily classify them in three categories:

Category I includes well-established disposables that came a long time ago, and these include analyzer sample caps, culture containers, flasks, titer plates, petri dishes, pipette and dispensing tips, protective clothing, gloves, syringes, test tubes, and vent and liquid filters.

Category II includes line items that were necessitated by the problems in cleaning validation. These became fully accepted about a decade ago and included aseptic transfer systems, bags, manifold systems, connectors, tri-clamps, flexible tubing, liquid containment bags, stoppers, tank liners, and valves.

Category III includes the most recent trends within the past five years and includes bioprocess containers (though the first one was introduced in 1996 by Wave, it became mainstream only after GE Healthcare bought Wave), bioreactors, centrifuges, chromatography systems, depth filters and systems, isolators, membrane adsorbes, diafiltration devices, mixing systems, and pumps.

There are many published surveys of the industry reported in the literature and while these statistics can be tainted because the equipment suppliers support most of these, a few general trends that are established include (please refer to Bibliography on sources):

Current state of the use of disposable systems as of 2010 (BioProcess International Survey summary):

1. The use of disposable bioprocessing is growing at a rate of 30% per year.
2. The biopharmaceutical or biological manufacturing industry consumes almost one-third of all disposable products used, followed by the biodiagnostic industry.
3. The CROs are least likely to use disposables because of the capital cost investment and the fact that they are used to the adaptability of the hard-walled systems.
4. Most of the adaptations of the disposable technology are in the United States, comprising two-third of all worldwide use, and with Europe a far 50% of the United States.
5. The companies with less than 100 employees constitute about one-third of customers and so are the companies with more than 5,000 employees; the mid-size companies are taking longer to evaluate the merits of disposable systems.
6. Three-fourth of the companies using disposable systems are using these for manufacturing, with less than 10% of companies involved in drug discovery using disposable systems.
7. Companies with more than six products account for almost 60% of all disposables used.
8. More than 80% of new products utilize disposable system and almost 70% of existing manufacturing processes have been modified to include disposable systems.
9. The main concerns about the use of disposable systems in the order of importance are as follows:
   a. Capital investment
   b. Experience in using these systems
   c. Validation and environmental concerns
   d. Concern about leachables and extractables
   e. Integrity of systems
10. European regulatory agencies, as well as European companies, have greater concerns for leachables and extractables; and while the U.S. FDA allows greater flexibility in adopting newer systems, the EMEA has drifted away from common acceptance criteria.
11. The most widely used disposable components are bags and bioprocess containers, followed by filters (which constitute the main cost concern), connectors, bioreactors, mixing vessels, chromatography, and sensors. This trend shows that the simplest of the components, which require little problems in validation, are the easiest to adopt; obviously, chromatography and the use of disposable sensors would present a much high barrier to validation.
12. The unmet needs of the industry in adopting disposable processes include the following:
    a. Leachables
    b. GMP compliance of disposable sensors and calibration scale
    c. Robustness of sensors and chromatography equipment

     d. Reliable bioprocessors that are cheaper
     e. Scalability
     f. High volume and flow rates
     g. Lack of single pressure flow and temp transmitter
     h. Larger scale, greater than 100 L
     i. Standardization
     j. Lab scale, less than 3 L

13. Most companies have allocated less than U.S.$ 100 K for disposable products.
14. Main reasons for adopting disposable systems include the following:
     a. Cleaning/sterilization cycle
     b. Convenience
     c. Flexibility
     d. Operating cost
     e. Capital cost
     f. Turn-around time
     g. Reduced process steps
     h. Smaller foot print
     i. Rapid scale up
     j. Improved environment
15. Selection of specific disposable systems depends on the following:
     a. Availability
     b. Price
     c. Quality
     d. Approved supplier
     e. Documentation
     f. Customer service
     g. Product offering
     h. Past purchase history
     i. Engineering support
16. The disposable systems are disposed of 57% by incineration, 37% by landfill, 20% waste to energy, and 10% converted for alternate purposes.
17. Over 80% of users are satisfied with their adoption of disposable systems and have demonstrated savings in cost.
18. The main misconceptions in the use of disposable systems include the following:
     a. May be more costly over time, especially filtration
     b. Not sure of savings
     c. New investment needed
     d. Have no need to save cost
19. The main regulatory concerns about disposables include the following:
     a. Sterilization and extractables/leachables
     b. Leaking of containers
     c. Bag integrity
     d. Validation of sterility/manufacturing process
     e. Aseptic process validation
     f. Quality of multiple suppliers

g. Validation, lot-to-lot variability
h. Material compatibility
i. Reproducibility of batch process

Next to the total cost, which is significantly lower, is the attraction of timeliness in the use of disposable components. Ready and available components that require little preparation make it easier to switch over applications easily. The newest concept is to offer a complete line of solutions as offered by the major suppliers (GE Healthcare, Little Chalfont, UK; Sartorius Stedim, Gottingen, Germany; Pall, New York City, NY; and Millipore, Billerica, MA).

One way to look at the value of disposable system is to make comparisons of the time it takes to complete a batch. For example, it takes about 50 h for a batch of a MAb to reach from the end of upstream stage to purification; using disposable systems, this time can be reduced by at least 50% by using the GE ReadyToProcess system, an integrated system of disposable components. Similar systems are offered by Sartorius Stedim, Pall, and EMD Millipore, the details of which are provided in Section 11.1.2.

Another advantage of disposable technologies is their portability. The floor plan of a disposables-based facility can be changed much more easily than that of a traditional facility. Different process requirements can easily be addressed by moving equipment into or out of a production suite. Because of the disposable nature of disposable systems, contamination is of less concern (especially cross-contamination for multihost, multiproduct facilities).

11.1.2 Lines of Disposable Systems

11.1.2.1 Sartorius Stedim

Sartorius Stedim (www.sartorius-stedim.com) offers its disposable technology factory that includes the following:

1. FlexAct is a new system that enables one to custom-configure disposable solutions for entire biomanufacturing steps. The FlexAct system consists of the central operating module that offers the widest variety of configuration options so one can take complete control of practically any steps in upstream and downstream processing. FlexAct CDS offers configurable disposable solutions for buffer preparation (BP), cell harvest (CH), virus inactivation (VI), media preparation (MP), and virus removal (VR). Next in line are UF DF crossflow (UD), polishing (PO), form fill (FF), and form transfer (FT).
2. Biostat CultiBag STR Plus is used for cell culture at all levels from 50 to 1,000 L including single-use optical dissolved oxygen (DO) and pH measurements.
3. Flexboy is a flexible bag system.
4. Flexel 3D mixing bags.
5. Levmixer and Palletank for mixing bases.

11.1.2.2 Pall Corporation

Pall Corporation (www.pall.com) also offers an extensive range of disposable products including

1. Allegro™ 2D and 3D Biocontainers
2. Allegro™ Jacketed Totes

3. Allegro™ Disposable Systems—Recommended Capsule Filters and Membrane
4. Kleenpak™ Nova Sterilizing-grade and Virus Removal Capsule Filters (see Table 11.1)
5. Kleenpak™ Sterile Connectors
6. Kleenpak™ Sterile Disconnectors
7. Kleenpak™ TFF CapsulesStax™ Disposable Depth Filter Systems
8. Stax™ Disposable Depth Filter w/ Seitz® AKS Activated Carbon Media

11.1.2.3 EMD Millipore (www.millipore.com)

With Mobius FlexReady Solutions, one can install equipment, configure applications, and validate processes quickly and easily. Mobius FlexReady Solutions target key steps in the MAb processing/purification train, designed and optimized for the following processes:

- Clarification
- Media and BP
- Tangential flow filtration (TFF)
- Virus filtration

11.1.2.4 GE Lifesciences

GE Lifesciences (www.gelifesciences.com) offer a ReadyToProcess system to include all steps of upstream and downstream processing, These components include the following:

1. *Bioreactors*
   The Wave Bioreactor is a scalable, effective, cost-efficient rocking platform for cell culture. The culture medium and cells contact only a presterile, disposable Cellbag ensuring very short setup times. There is no need for cleaning or sterilization, providing easy operation and protection against contamination. The rocking motion of the platform induces waves in the culture fluid to provide efficient mixing and gas transfer, resulting in an environment well-suited for cell growth. The Wave system is completely scaleable across our platform ranging from 200 mL to 500 L.
2. *Disposable Bioreactor Bags*
   Manufactured from multilayered laminated clear plastic, Cellbag disposable bioreactors are suitable for specific cell culture process needs for research, development, or cGMP manufacturing operations. Cellbag components are similar to those used for biological storage bags and meet USP Class VI specifications for plastics. Validation data and Cellbag DMF are available to demonstrate biocompatibility. Cellbags can be highly customized to meet specific processing requirements.
3. *Fluid Management*
   ReadyCircuit assemblies comprise bags, tubings, and connectors. Together with ReadyToProcess filters and sensors, ReadyCircuit assemblies form self-contained bioprocessing modules that maintain an aseptic path and provide convenience by removing time-consuming process steps associated with conventional systems. Bags, tube sets, filters, and related equipment can be secured in appropriate orientations for efficient operation using the ReadyKart mobile processing station. With an array of features, and optional accessories, the ReadyKart is designed to support a variety of process-specific fluid, handling needs.
4. *ReadyToProcess Konfigurator*

Table 11.1 Features and Characteristics of Different Bioreactor Technologies

Application/unit operation	Mixers	FlexReady Solutions	CellReady Bioreactor	Assemblies	Tubes and Connectors	Drums	Novaseal Crimper	Lynx Sterile Connector	Bins
Buffer and media preparation		X		X		X			
Mixing	X			X					
Bioreactor			X						
Clarification		X							
Column protection				X					
Trace contaminant removal									
Virus removal		X							
Ultrafiltration/ diafiltration		X							
Sterile filtration				X					
Storage				X		X			X
Transport				X		X			X
Sampling				X					
Connectology					X		X	X	

ReadyToProcess Konfigurator lets one design fluid-handling circuits with ease online. Enter the parameters to generate the design needed; includes fast output of P&ID drawings and convenient Bill of Materials for simplified ordering.

5. *Connectivity*

   ReadyMate connectors are genderless aseptic connectors that allow simple connection of components maintaining secure workflows and sterile integrity. Additional accessories, such as tube fuser and sealer of thermoplastic tubing support, secure aseptic connectivity throughout the manufacturing process.

6. *Filters*

   ReadyToProcess filters are a range of preconditioned and ready to use cartridges and capsules for both cross flow and normal flow filtration operations. Factory prepared to water for injection quality for endotoxins, total organic carbon (TOC), and conductivity and sterilized via gamma radiation. They enable simpler and faster bioprocessing with maximum safety.

7. *Chromatography columns*

   ReadyToProcess columns are high-performance bioprocessing columns that come prepacked, prequalified, and presanitized. ReadyToProcess columns are designed for seamless scalability, delivering the same performance level as available in conventional processing columns such as AxiChrom and BPG.

8. *Chromatography system—ÄKTA ready*

   ÄKTA ready (www.gehealthcare.com) is a liquid chromatography system built for process scale up and production for early clinical phases. The system operates with ready-to-use, disposable flow paths and as a consequence, cleaning between products/batches and validation of cleaning procedures is not required. Äkta ready is a liquid chromatography system built for process scale up and production for early clinical phases. System meets GLP and cGMP requirements for Phases I–III in drug development and full-scale production, provides improved economy and productivity due to simpler procedures, single use eliminates risk of cross-contamination between products/batches, easy connection to and operation with prepacked ReadyToProcess columns and other process columns, scalable processes using UNICORN software.

11.2 SAFETY OF DISPOSABLE SYSTEMS

Disposable devices from filter housings to the lining of bioreactors make extensive use of plastic materials or elastomer systems. Today perhaps the most significant impediment in the wider acceptance of disposable systems is the controversy surrounding the possibility of contaminating the product from the chemicals in the plastic film. So, before entering a broad description the choices of disposables available, this topic should be examined in detail.

All final containers and closures shall be made of material that will not hasten the deterioration of the product or otherwise render it less suitable for the intended use. All final containers and closures shall be clean and free of surface solids, *leachable* contaminants and other materials that will hasten the deterioration of the product or otherwise render it less suitable for the intended use. (Biologics *21 CFR 600.11[h]*)

Leachables are chemicals that migrate from disposable processing equipment into various components of the drug product during manufacturing. Extractables are chemical entities (organic and inorganic) that can be extracted from disposables using common laboratory solvents in controlled experiments. They represent the worst-case scenario and are used as a tool to predict the types of leachables that may be encountered during pharmaceutical production.

The issue of chemicals leaching from plastic has been the hottest topic not just for the bioprocess industry but also for many other industries including the food industry where issues like the safety of bisphenol-A (BPA) in water bottles keep rising. A Google search of the topic results in millions of hits. How the use of plastic affects bioprocessing is of great interest to the stainless-steel industry.

While regulatory requirements pertain to the toxic effects of leachables, a risk unique to biological drugs arises in the effect of leachables on the three- and four-dimensional structure of protein drugs: such changes can render the drug more immunogenic if not less effective, and these side effects are, thus, of greater importance to the bioprocessing industry. The most well-known problem is the high incidence of PRCA reported in patients using commercial erythropoietin formulations leading to several deaths. While the source of the PRCA induction is not clearly settled, it is generally attributed to a change in the drug formulation that included a new surfactant, which caused unexpected leaching of an elastomer compound from the rubber stopper.

11.2.1 Polymers and Additives

The materials used to fabricate single-use processing equipment for biopharmaceutical manufacturing are usually polymers, such as plastic or elastomers (rubber), rather than the traditional metal or glass. Polymers offer more versatility because they are lightweight, flexible, and much more durable than their traditional counterparts. Plastic and rubber are also disposable, so issues associated with cleaning and validation can be avoided. Additives can also be incorporated into polymers to give them clarity of glass or to add color to labels or to code parts.

Unlike metals, where the risk lies mainly in oxidation, polymers are affected by heat, light, oxygen, and autoclaving and, thus, degrade over time if not stabilized, and this can adversely affect the mechanical properties. Polymers are thus stabilized by incorporating chemicals that are prone to leaching during the manufacturing process and storage of biological materials.

When a plastic resin is processed, it is often introduced into an extruder, where it is melted at high temperatures and its stability is influenced by its molecular structure, the polymerization process, the presence of residual catalysts, and the finishing steps used in production. Processing conditions during extrusion (e.g., temperature, shear, and residence time in the extruder) can dramatically affect polymer degradation. End-use conditions that expose a polymer to excessive heat or light (such as outdoor applications or sterilization techniques used in medical practices) can foster premature failure of polymer products as well, leading to a loss of flexibility or strength. If left unchecked the results often can be the total failure of the plastic component.

Polymer degradation is controlled by the use of additives, which are specialty chemicals that provide a desired effect on the polymer. The effect can be stabilization that allows a polymer to maintain its strength and flexibility or performance improvement that adds color or some special characteristic such as antistatic or antimicrobial properties. There are typically three classes of stabilizers, which are as follows:

- Melt processing aids, such as phosphites and hindered phenols, antioxidants that protect a polymer during extrusion and molding.
- Long-term thermal stabilizers that provide defense against heat encountered in end-use applications (e.g., hindered phenols and hindered amines).
- Light stabilizers that provide ultraviolet (UV) protection through mechanisms such as radical trapping, UV absorption, or excited state quenching.

One application in which an additive can improve or alter the performance of a polymer is a filler or modifier that affects its mechanical properties. Additives known as plasticizers can affect the stress–strain relationship of a polymer. Polyvinylchloride (PVC) is used for home water pipes and is a very rigid material. With the addition of plasticizers, however, it becomes very flexible and can be used to make intravenous (IV) bags and inflatable devices. Lubricants and processing aids are also used to reduce polymer manufacturing cycle times (e.g., mold-release agents) or facilitate the movement of plastic and elastomeric components that contact each other (e.g., rubber stoppers used in syringes).

Additives are not always single entities. Some are manufactured from naturally occurring raw materials such as tallow and vegetable oils that are themselves composed of many different components and can vary from batch to batch. Others are considered *products-by-process*, as they are formed during processing by adding several starting materials to affect the chemical reaction. The complexity of chemical reactions that take place in the manufacturing of plastic makes the analysis of extractables and leachables very complex and difficult. In testing extractables and leachables, those lesser-known minor chemical species may be the ones that leach into a drug product, but this is not predictable as it is to a greater degree a function of the characteristics of the product.

Stabilizers incorporated into plastics and rubbers are constantly working to provide much-needed protection to the polymer substrate. This is a dynamic process that changes according to the external stress on the system. For example, good stabilizers are efficient radical scavengers. Generally, a two-tiered approach is used to protect polymers from the heat and shear they encounter during processing: using primary antioxidants (e.g., hindered phenols such as butylated hydroxy toluene [BHT] or Ciba's Irganox) for protection during processing can provide long-term heat stability. Secondary antioxidants are also added as process stabilizers, typically hydroperoxide decomposers that protect polymers during extrusion and molding and protecting the primary antioxidants against decomposition. All the by-products of these reactions become available to leach from polymers into a drug product.

Elastomers are also used for special stabilization: acid scavengers are used to neutralize traces of halogen anions formed during the aging of halogen-containing rubbers (e.g., brominated or chlorinated isobutylene isoprene). If not neutralized, anions cause premature aging and a decrease in the performance of rubber articles over time. Metal oxides can be very efficient acid scavengers. Ions of copper (Cu), iron (Fe), cobalt (Co), nickel (Ni), and other transition metals that have different oxidation states with comparable stability are called *rubber poisons* because they are easily oxidized or reduced by one-electron transfer. They are very active catalysts for hydroperoxide decomposition and contribute to the degradation of rubber vulcanizates. Rubber poisons thus require a specific stabilizer: a metal deactivator like 2,3-bis[3-(3,5-di-tert-butyl-4-hydroxyphenyl)propionyl]propiono-hydrazide, which binds ions into stable complexes and deactivates them.

As a result of the need to add chemicals to elastomer systems, the extractables in a disposable system can include the following:

- Monomer and oligomers from incomplete polymerization reactions
- Additives and their transformation and degradation products
- Lubricants and surface modifiers
- Fillers
- Rubber curing agents and vulcanizates
- Impurities and undesirable reaction products such as polyaromatic hydrocarbons (PAHs), nitrosamines, and mercaptobenzothiazoles.

Unexpected additives can also be present in a polymer system because of the inconsistencies in the process of manufacturing elastomer systems whereby unpredictable reactions can take place.

Despite the risk in the use of additives added to polymers, the utility of polymers in disposable bioprocess equipment (and in all medical or pharmaceutical applications) far outweighs the risks associated with their use. These risks can be managed well by taking three steps: material selection, implementation of a proper testing program, and partnering with vendors.

11.2.2 Material Selection

The type of plastic used should match the needed physical and chemical properties and compatibility of the additives used for the product manufactured. For example, phenolic antioxidants, each with the same active site (the hindered phenol moiety) but with different nature of the remainder of molecule, makes them soluble or compatible with a given polymer substrate. An antioxidant that is compatible with nylon might not be the best choice for use in polyolefins, as an example.

Ensuring compatibility often lessens the amount of leaching that can occur. It is also important to select polymers and additives that are approved for use by the regulatory authorities for specific use. Such compounds have already undergone a fair amount of analytical and toxicological testing, so a good amount of information is often available for them. Because of this, most manufacturers are likely to continue using these additives and thus the user may not have to alter the composition at a later stage as these compounds and the art of using them is likely to survive obviating the need for a change control step as significant changes in the process need to be reported back to the U.S. FDA.

Commercially supplied plastic films are proprietary formulations and arrangements; for example, Advanced Scientific produces its bags utilizing two films. The fluid contact film is a 5.0 mm polyethylene. The outer is a 5-layer 7 mil co-extrusion film, which provides barrier and durability. A typical test report is given in Figure 11.1.

Biocompatibility			
	USP Acute Systemic Injection Test	Pass	USP<88>
	USP Intracutaneous Injection Test	Pass	USP<88>
	USP Intramuscular Implantation Test	Pass	USP<88>
	USP MEM Elution Method	Non-cytotoxic	USP<87>
	Physiochemical Test for Plastics	Pass	USP <661>

Extractables			
		TOC after 90 days (ppm)	pH shift after 90 days
	Purified Water (pH = 7)	<2	–0.79
	Acidic Water (pH < 2)	<3	+0.01
	Basic Water (pH > 10)	<4	+0.87

Physical Data				
	Water Vapor Transmission Rate (g/100 in^2/24 h)	0.017		ASTM F-1249
	Carbon Dioxide Transmission Rate (cc/100 in^2/24 h)	0.129		ASTM F-2476
	Oxygen Transmission Rate (cc/100 in^2/24 h)	0.023		ASTM F-1927
		Average Force	Average MOE	Average Elongation	
Tensile	32.73 lb	25110 psi	1084%	ASTM D 882-02
		Min Force	Average Force	Max Force	
Tear Resistance	6.77 lb	7.21 lb	7.74 lb	ASTM D1004-03
Puncture Resistance	16.42 lb	18.61 lb	19.51 lb	FTMS 101C

Figure 11.1 A representative table summarizing the tests carried out, and results obtained for a plastic film used to produce bioreactor bags. (Data from www.asisus.com.)

ATMI (Danbury, CT) offers its proprietary TK8 film, which is constructed from laminated layers of polyamide (PA), ethylene vinyl alcohol polymer (EVOH), and ultralow density polyethylene (ULDPE). The outer PA layer provides robust puncture resistance, strength, and excellent thermal stability. The EVOH layer minimizes gas diffusion across the film while maintaining a very good flex crack resistance. The ULDPE layers provide flexibility; integrity; and an ultra-clean, ultra-pure, low-extractables product-contacting layer.

The combination of these layers results in a film that has outstanding optical clarity, is easy to handle, and performs well in a broad range of bioprocess applications. The inner ULDPE layer used in TK8 is blow-extruded in-house by ATMI under clean room conditions (0.2 µm filtered air), ensuring the cleanest possible product-contacting surface. Lamination is also performed under controlled, ultra-clean conditions. Lastly, TK8 film is converted into ATMI bag products in an ISO Class 5 clean room. All of the layers in TK8 are made from medical-grade materials, meaning that they comply with industry standards and are subject to strict change controls. The entire structure of TK8 is totally free of any animal-derived components (ADCF). ATMI has also created TK8 with dual sourcing and contingency planning in mind, to ensure security of supply.

- TK8 film complies with USP Class VI (USP 87, USP 88, and USP 661)
- ULDPE resin complies with EP 3.1.3
- Shelf life is supported by aging validation studies
- Certified ADCF
- Bioburden evaluation available (ISO 11737)
- Particle count data available (EP 2.9.19 or USP 788)
- By performing blow extrusion in-house, ATMI maintains full control and traceability of the contact film composition, from resin to finished bag product.

11.2.3 Testing

Polymers used in medical and pharmaceutical applications should comply with the appropriate USP guidelines, and it is recommended that they meet USP Class VI testing as documented in USP 88. Appropriate extractables and leachables testing programs must be implemented for all bioprocessing materials that come into direct contact with the drug.

The best-practice guidelines for conducting such testing are provided by the Bio-Process Systems Alliance as a two-part technical guideline for evaluating the risk associated with extractables and leachables, specifically for single-use processing equipment. This organization is dedicated to encouraging the use of disposable systems and provides excellent support and assistance; the reader is highly encouraged to visit their website for newer information as well as participate in their many seminars and conventions to stay abreast of the developments in this fast-changing field.

The testing for leachables should not necessarily end once the materials have been qualified. It is necessary to have in place a quality control program instead of testing the product or equipment alone. The level of quality control testing will depend on risk tolerance. Fortunately, the manufacturing of recombinant drugs involves extensive purification steps that are likely to remove most of these leachables. Also, the final medium used for protein solutions is aqueous and many of the leachables are not soluble in water; this further reduces the risk. Greater risk can be seen in the final packaging components; for example, rubber stoppers used in packaging the final dosage form are more likely to be a risk to the protein formulation than any other component in the chain of disposables to which the drug is exposed during the manufacturing process.

While it is always a good idea to establish in-house testing of leachables, often it is neither possible nor recommended; several highly reputed laboratories have fully certified programs; given below is a short list of these laboratories:

- Product Quality Research Institute (www.pqri.org)
- Rapra Technology Ltd. (www.rapra.net)
- Impact Analytical (www.impactanalytical.com)
- Avomeen Analytical Services (www.avomeen.com)
- SGS North America (www.us.sgs.com)
- Cyanta (www.cyanta.com)
- Irvine Pharmaceutical Services (www.ialab.com)
- Pace Analytical Services, Inc. (www.pacelabs.com)
- American Society for Quality (www.asq.org)
- Intertek (www.intertek.com)

11.2.4 Partnering with Vendors

Reputable vendors often have extractables data already on hand to share with customers. In many cases, they will provide a certificate of analysis and toxicological information associated with materials used to fabricate their products. Vendors also should have well-established change control processes for the products they sell to allow sponsors to modify their applications with regulatory agencies accordingly.

11.2.5 Responsibility of Sponsors

Companies filing regulatory approval have the responsibility of complying with the requirements of validating the process to minimize the risk from leachables. Extractables and leachables evaluations are part of a validation program for processes using disposable biopharmaceutical systems and components. There is minimal regulatory guidance that directly addresses extractables and leachables in bioprocessing.

The extractables are evaluated by exposing components or systems to conditions that are more severe than normally found in a biopharmaceutical process, typically using a variety of solvents at high temperatures. The goal of an extractable study is to identify as many compounds as possible that have the potential to become leachables. A positive outcome is one where the list of extractables from a material is sizable. Although it is not expected that many of those extractables will actually leach into the drug product at detectable levels, a materials extractables profile provides critical information in pursuit of a comprehensive leachables test.

Not all leachables may be found during the extractables evaluation because drug formulation components or buffers may interact with a polymer or its additives to form a new *leachable* contaminant that was not previously identified during the extractables analysis. In addition, leachables that were not identified as extractables also will be found if the drug product formulation and processing conditions are unique and more severe than the conditions at which extractable tests were performed—or when the analytical methodologies used in the two types of studies are different.

11.3 REGULATORY MATTERS

There are as yet no specific standards or guidance that reference extractables and leachables from disposable bioprocessing materials. Many references that do apply were written to address the processing materials and equipment without regard to the materials of construction.

11.3.1 United States and Canada

The foundation for the requirement to assess extractables and leachables in the United States is introduced in Title 21 of the Code of Federal Regulations (CFR) Part 211.65, which states that

> Equipment shall be constructed so that surfaces that contact components, in-process materials, or drug products shall not be reactive, additive, or absorptive so as to alter the safety, identity, strength, quality, or purity of the drug product beyond the official or other established requirements.

This regulation applies to all materials, including metals, glass, and plastics.

Extractables and leachables generally would be considered *additive*, although it is also possible for leachables to interact with a product to yield new contaminants.

The U.S. FDA regulatory guidance for final container–closure systems, though not written for process contact materials, gives directions about the type of final product testing that may be provided regarding extractables and leachables from single-use process components and systems. The May 1999 guidance document from the U.S. FDA's Center for Drug Evaluation and Research (CDER) indicates the types of drug products and component dosage form interactions that the U.S. FDA considers to be the highest risks for extractables. Generally, the likelihood of the packaging component interacting with dosage form is the highest in injectable dosage forms, mainly because of the low level of leachables that can be allowed in such drug delivery systems.

Drugs that will be administered as injectables or inhalants will have higher levels of regulatory concern than oral or topical drugs. Similarly, liquid dosage forms will have higher regulatory concern than tablets because extractables migrate into liquids more easily than into solids.

In addition, pharmaceutical-grade materials are expected to meet or exceed industry and regulatory standards and requirements such as those listed in USP 87 and 88. The USP procedures test the biological reactivity of mammalian cell cultures following contact with polymeric materials. USP Chapters 87 and 88 are helpful for testing the suitability of plastics for use in fabricating a system to process parenteral drug formulations. However, they are not considered sufficient regulatory documentation for extractables and leachables because many toxicological indicators are not evaluated, including subacute and chronic toxicity along with evaluation of carcinogenic, reproductive, developmental, neurological, and immunological effects.

11.3.2 Europe

In the European Union (EU), a related statement to the U.S.C. 21 CFR 211.65 is found in the rules governing manufacture of medicinal products. The EU good manufacturing practice (GMP) document states: "Production equipment should not present any hazard to the products. The parts of the production equipment that come into contact with the product must not be reactive, additive or absorptive to such an extent that it will affect the quality of the product and thus present any hazard."

The EMEA published a guideline on plastic immediate packaging materials in December 2005 that also addresses container-closure systems and has been used to provide direction for single-use process contact materials. Data to be included relating to extractables and leachables come from extraction studies (*worst-case leachables*), interaction studies, migration studies (similar to leachable information for those components), identify what additional information or testing is required, and then set and execute a plan to fill in the gaps.

11.4 RISK ASSESSMENT

Risk assessment is based on the following considerations:

- *Compatibility of materials*: Most biological drugs formulations are aqueous-based and therefore compatible with the materials used in most disposable processing components. Still, a check to make sure that the process stream and/or formulation do not violate any of the manufacturer's recommendations for chemical compatibility, pH, and operating pressure/temperature is warranted before proceeding. A full analysis of data generated by the vendor should be completed upfront as a preparatory step.
- *Proximity of a component to the final product*: Product contact immediately before the final fill increases the risk of leachables in a final product. For example, tubing or connectors used to transfer starting buffers probably present a lower risk because of their upstream location. Processing steps such as diafiltration or lyophilization that could remove leachables from a process should also be considered because they may reduce associated risk. However, it cannot be assumed that a step that can potentially remove some leachables will remove all leachables. In such cases, supporting data should be obtained.
- *Product composition*: In general, a product stream or formulation that has higher levels of organics, particularly high or low pH, or solubilizing agents such as surfactants (detergents), will increase the regulatory and safety concern for potential leachables. Neutral buffers lower concern about potential leachables.
- *Surface area*: The surface area exposed to a product stream varies widely. It is relatively high for filters, in which the internal surface area is 1,000× the filtration area. Conversely, surface area is relatively small for O-ring seals.
- *Time and temperature*: Longer contact times allow for more potential leachables to be removed from a material until equilibrium is reached. Higher temperatures lead to more rapid migration of leachables from materials into a process stream or formulation.
- *Pretreatment steps*: Sterilization by steam autoclave and/or gamma irradiation may cause higher levels of extractables and leachables depending on the polymer formulation involved in a single-use component. On the other hand, rinsing may lower the concern for extractables and leachables (e.g., when filters are flushed before use).

The following are some highlights relating to risk assessment of extractables and leachables:

1. Regulatory responsibility for overall assessment and understanding of a finished product and process components involved in its production remains with the product sponsor. This includes evaluations of extractables and leachables. Regulatory agencies do not have a guideline available yet to help sponsors.

2. All elastomeric and plastic-based materials contain extractables specific to the formulated and cured material(s) from which they are constructed

3. Contaminants are also found in stainless-steel systems in the form of residues left after cleaning or traces of metals such as iron, nickel, and chromium salts from the stainless steel itself, so the problem of contamination from the container is not restricted to disposable containers.

4. Most polymers without certain additives would not work as materials of use in disposable processing: this includes stabilizing the polymer, extruding it, and preventing its oxidation and UV degradation; other additives include antistatic agents, impact modifiers, catalysts, release agents, colorants, brighteners, bactericides, and blowing agents. The choice of polymer or method of polymerization (by heat or chemical means) directly affects the levels and types of compounds found as extractables.

5. Fluoropolymers offer the best choice as they are typically processed without additives, stabilizers, or processing aids.

6. A DMF or BMF for process-contact equipment is not explicitly required by U.S. regulatory authorities. However, it represents a way for vendors to share proprietary information about a component or raw material with the U.S. FDA and to ensure that such information remains up to date. It is therefore important that sponsors work only with the most reputable suppliers of disposable components.

7. The levels and types of compounds found as extractable analytes are directly affected by the type and degree of sterilization performed (e.g., gamma irradiation, ethylene oxide gas, or autoclaving). The leachable analyte and concentration that may be of issue to one particular drug formulation may have no impact on another. It is for this reason that it is the responsibility of product sponsors to qualify and demonstrate the applicability of process components within their manufacturing systems. Leachables are always final-product–specific.

8. All component materials should be evaluated that have the potential to come into direct contact with a manufactured drug product. Of greater importance are the components that would contact the product in the post-purification stage.

9. Controlled extraction studies are designed to generate extractables; the presence of extractables is expected. This does not necessarily reflect the degree and concentration of leachables that will be found upon contact with a product stream: leachables are a result of the nature of the product, the length of exposure, and the environmental conditions for the storage of the product.

10. Detection of a toxic or otherwise undesirable extractable under aggressive conditions requires testing to ensure that migration to the product is below acceptable limits under actual processing conditions. It is done by controlled extraction using studies using multiple solvents of varying polarity to fully elucidate the

extractable analytes in question. Techniques such as Soxhlet extraction, solvent refluxing, microwave extraction, sonication, and/or acid washing at an elevated temperature may also be used. For extractables testing, the contact surface area can be maximized by mechanical methods such as cutting or grinding.

11. For leachables testing, it is most applicable to mimic actual process conditions by leaving test components intact. Controlled extraction studies should use extraction media of varying polarities and physical properties. Ideally, this would come from using two or three solvents that include analysis by high-pressure liquid chromatography (HPLC), GC-MS, and ICP-MS.

12. Toxicology of leachables should be performed using approved protocols. A Product Quality Research Institute (PQRI) document on extractables and leachables suggests an approach to address toxicology using LD50 with a 1,000× or 10,000× safety factor based on the dosage quantity. In addition, several structural activity relationship (SAR) databases are readily available to professional toxicologists. Examples include the "Carcinogenic Potency Database" (CPDB, http://potency.berkeley.edu/) and the U.S. Environmental Protection Agency's "Distributed Structure-Searchable Toxicity Network" (DSSTOX, http://www.epa.gov/ncct/dsstox/) database. Chances are that most sponsors will not be able to conduct these studies in-house, and it is advised to outsource these evaluations.

13. The classes of compounds that extractables include, more particularly, *N*-nitrosamines, polynuclear aromatics (sometime termed PHAs), and 2-mercaptobenzothiozole, along with biologically active compounds such as BPA. Individual extractable compounds are too numerous to list, but examples include aromatic antioxidants such as BHT, oleamide, bromide, fluoride, chloride, oleic acid, erucamide, eicosane, and stearic acid. Databases on extractables are widely available, such as by PQRI. Comprehensive extractable data for components can reduce the time and resources needed to qualify leachables from the systems where they are used. When comparing supplied extractables data for components constructed of like materials, end users should carefully review the methods used to generate the data. Less rigorous methods may under-represent the actual levels and extent of extractables, and a report describing more extractables may simply come from using more rigorous methods.

14. For determination of leachables in products, it is currently the industry standard to validate analytical methods according to ICH and USP criteria. This ensures appropriate levels of analytical precision and accuracy.

15. The overall quantity of extractables or leachables can be estimated using nonspecific methods such as TOC and non-volatile residue (NVR) analysis. Such nonspecific quantitation is especially useful in comparing materials before their final selection for a process. These analyses can be used individually or collectively to estimate amounts of extractable material present and to ensure that targeted methods are not missing a major extractable constituent. For instance, nonpolar compounds without chromophores can be identified using Fourier-transform infrared (FTIR) analysis of NVRs.

16. Organic extractables will leach into formulations at a higher level if the products have higher organic content or if surfactants are present.

17. The toxicity of leachables is frequently estimated based on the amount entering the human body in each dose. Thus, it is often not the quantity of leachables in a product but how much finds its way into the human body. This is somewhat analogous to the limits many regulatory agencies set on residual deoxyribonucleic acid (DNA) in a finished product.

18. The component used for an extractables study should be the same one that will be used in a process, and it should have the same pretreatment steps as is intended for that process. For instance, if a process uses gamma irradiation for sterilization, then the component used for extractables testing should be sterilized by this method. Often a vendor will provide a simulated data based on similar products by extrapolating the data from other components; this would not be acceptable.

19. The solvents used for leachables studies should include water and a low-molecular-weight alcohol such as ethanol or *n*-propanol. Where appropriate, an organic solvent with the appropriate solubility parameters will help identify additional extractables. Extractions should be performed at relatively extreme time and temperature conditions. However, the solvents or extraction conditions should not be so extreme as to degrade materials to a point at which they are not mechanically functional (e.g., melting or dissolving). Extreme conditions used should be relative to those under which a material is normally used. For example, one normally used at room temperature might be extracted at an elevated temperature of 50°C or 70°C.

20. Analytical methods should include HPLC and GC-MS methods to detect and identify specific, individual, extractable compounds. HPLC with an UV (HPLC-UV) or mass spectrometer (LC-MS) detector and GC-MS are the most scientifically robust methods for this purpose. When metals are a concern, inductively coupled plasma analysis is widely used, both with and without mass-spectrometric detection (ICP and ICP-MS).

21. While it is desirable to identify each extractable, for some extractables, such as siloxanes and oligomers of base polymers, precise identification is not feasible because of the large number of closely related isomers and oligomers. In such cases, a general classification can be used. Quantitation of identified extractables is informative, but it does not need to be performed at a high level of precision. This is different from recommendations for evaluating extractables for final containers or closures, for which analytical and toxicological limits should be set based on a measured level of extractables.

22. User-specific components, such as filters, connecters, tubing and bags, and so on, may be built by using subcomponents from different vendors. It is unlikely that the composite system would have complete data on extractables from the vendor assembling the component. Individual data for each subcomponent can be pooled but it may be easier for the sponsor to conduct the study on the entire component at one time. It is therefore advisable that sponsors use off the shelf products where possible.

23. Biocompatibility testing is a very complex issue. It is a material's lack of interaction with living tissue or a living system by not being toxic, injurious, or physiologically reactive, and not causing an immunological rejection. This testing is required, and two common test regimens are commonly used to measure biocompatibility: USP 88, Biological Reactivity Testing (USP Class VI), and ISO 10993, Biological Evaluation of Medical Devices, which has replaced the USP Class VI test.

24. The ISO 10993 has 20 parts and provides testing requirements in great detail. These parts include the following:
    a. Evaluation and testing (see Section 11.1.2)
    b. Animal welfare requirements
    c. Tests for genotoxicity, carcinogenicity, and reproductive toxicity
    d. Selection of tests for interactions with blood
    e. Tests for in-vitro cytotoxicity
    f. Tests for local effects after implantation
    g. Ethylene oxide sterilization residuals
    h. Clinical investigation of medical devices
    i. Framework for identification and quantification of potential degradation products
    j. Tests for irritation and delayed-type hypersensitivity
    k. Tests for systemic toxicity
    l. Sample preparation and reference materials
    m. Identification and quantification of degradation products from polymeric medical devices
    n. Identification and quantification of degradation products from ceramics
    o. Identification and quantification of degradation products from metals and alloys
    p. Toxicokinetic study design for degradation products and leachables
    q. Establishment of allowable limits for leachable substances
    r. Chemical characterization of materials
    s. Physicochemical, morphological and topographical characterization of materials
    t. Principles and methods for immunotoxicology testing of medical devices
25. The USP 88 protocols are used to classify plastics in Classes I–VI, based on end use, type, and time of exposure of human tissue to plastics, of which Class VI requires the most stringent testing of all the six classes. These tests measure and determine the biological response of animals to the plastic by either direct or indirect contact, or by injection of the specific extracts prepared from the material under test. The tests are classified as follows:
    a. Systemic toxicity test is used to determine the irritant effect of toxic leachables present in extracts of test materials
    b. Intracutaneous test is used to assess the localized reaction of tissue to leachable substances
    c. Implantation test is used to evaluate the reaction of living tissue to the plastic. The extracts for the test are prepared at one of three standard temperatures/times: 50°C (122°F) for 72 h, 70°C (158°F) for 24 h, and 121°C (250°F) for 1 h.
26. Typical testing data for disposable bioreactors (as supplied by GE Healthcare) would include
    a. Testing is performed on irradiated film (50 kGy)
    b. USP XXII plastic class VI and ISO 10993
    c. ISO 10993-4 Hemolysis study in vivo extraction method
    d. ISO 10993-5 Cytotoxicity study using ISO elution method
    e. ISO 10993-6 Muscle implantation study in rabbit

f.   ISO 10993-10 Acute intracutaneous reactivity study in rabbit

g.   ISO 10993-11 Acute systemic toxicity in mouse

11.5 DISPOSABLE CONTAINERS

Disposable containers form the heart of any comprehensive maximally disposable-system equipped facility. To replace dozens of hard-walled (steel or glass) containers that are used to store media, starting materials, and intermediate and finished products, whether kept at room temperature of kept frozen; there is a great need for containers. Fortunately, disposable bag systems have been very well adopted as alternates to hard-walled containers. And this is because, historically, pharmaceutical products, such as sterile IV solutions, blood, plasma, plasma expanders, and hyperalimentation solutions, have been stored and dispensed in these types of bags. For blood storage a disposable bag would have one-layer films made from polyvinyl chloride (PVC) or ethylene vinyl acetate (EVA).

Given below is a listing of major suppliers of disposable containers. Most major equipment suppliers have proprietary bags to fit only their equipment, and while generic bag manufacturers may have alternates to these proprietary bags, there are intellectual property issues involved as many of these bags may have patent protection.

11.5.1 Proprietary Bag Suppliers

The list of proprietary bag suppliers are as follows:

- Thermo Scientific (www.thermoscientific.com)
- Sartorius Stedim (www.sartorius-stedim.com)
- Pall (www.pall.com)
- GE (www.gelifesciences.com)
- Millipore (www.millipore.com)
- Xcellerex (www.xcellerex.com)
- LevTech by ATMI Life Sciences (http://www.atmi.com/lifesciences/)
- New Brunswick Scientific (www.nbsc.com)

11.5.2 Generic Bag Suppliers

11.5.2.1 Advanced Scientifics (ASI, www.advancedscientifics.com)

- PL-01077 polyethylene single-use bag is a 5 layer 7 mil co-extrusion film which provides barrier and durability. Utilized on smaller bag sizes up to 1 L, it maintains comparable, extra values to larger PE bags.
- PL-01026/PL-01077 polyethylene single-use bags are produced utilizing two films. The fluid contact film is a 5 mil polyethylene (PL-01026). The outer is a 5-layer 7 mil co-extrusion film which provides barrier and durability (PL-01077).
- PL-01028 ethyl vinyl acetate single-use bags are produced utilizing a single film. The film is a 4-layer 12.5 mil co-extrusion film which provides barrier and durability.
- Drums, protective containers, and tank liners.

- Containers/fill port automatic aseptic filling, when used in conjunction with good technique and a laminar flow hood, this yields an aseptic bag fill. The semiautomatic filling system utilizes a fixture and cap assembly developed and manufactured by ASI, and fully controls the filling interface with no user interaction required with the fill port. What is left after completion is a tamper-evident dispensing port. This results in a cleaner, more efficient, and cost-effective method of filling.

11.5.2.2 Charter Medical (www.chartermedical.com)

- Bio-Pak® Cell Culture Bio-Containers are designed for single-use bioprocessing applications, and incorporate Charter Medical's Clear-Pak® film which was chosen by Charter Medical for its superior clarity and excellent performance in promoting cell growth and viability. The Clear-Pak® film is a single-web, multilayer, co-extruded film which provides excellent gas barrier properties to minimize pH shift for greater product stability.
- Bio-Pak® 3D Gusset Bio-Containers are available in a range of sizes from 50 to 1,000 L. The 3D gusset design is ideal for preparation and storage of media and buffer solutions.
- Bio-Pak® Small Volume Bio-Containers are designed for bioprocessing applications, storage, and transport of sterile fluids. They are available in sizes ranging from 50 mL to 20 L. The boat port design provides flexibility in tubing interface options and facilitates maximum recovery of stored materials.
- Bio-Pak® XL & XLPlus Bio-Containers are an efficient, lightweight, and cost-effective alternative to large tanks and totes for sterile fluid containment and processing. The single-use Bio-Pak® XL bags eliminate the issues surrounding cleaning validation, storage, and sterilization of traditional biocontainers.
- Contour Tank Liners are a cost-effective alternative to dedicated tanks and totes. Contour liners reduce cleaning validation and sterilization of traditional containers. Most importantly, because they are single use, the potential of cross-contamination between different products is reduced.
- Bio-Pak® Totes are application-designed, mobile totes mounted on durable, non-marking wheels. These stainless-steel totes hold the flexible bag plus outlet tubing in a self-contained, wheeled unit that can be safely transported by forklifts. A unique bottom outlet system allows fast flow rates and minimal container holdup volume.
- Freeze-Pak™ Cryogenic Bio-Containers are designed for use in cryogenic temperature applications under liquid nitrogen conditions, and are used predominately for clinical and research applications. The Freeze-Pak™ cryogenic film is a single-web polyolefin monolayer of 12 mil thickness and is preferred based on the film's performance during the freeze-thaw process.

11.5.2.3 Applied Bioprocessing Containers (http://www.appliedbpc.com)

- Small volume containers, 50 mL to 20 L, with integrated handle, integrated hanging capability, and needle-free sampling port, which may be used with a sterile welder and is available as manifold system.

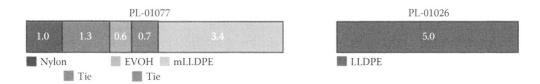

Figure 11.2 Layers of plastics in PL-01077 bag film offered by ASI. (Data from www.asius.com.)

- Containers for cylindrical tanks, 50 to 750 L, two-dimensional (2D) and three-dimensional (3D) designs, top or bottom drain, and available as liner, fit most cylindrical tanks and is available as manifold system.

Disposable bags are made from plastic films, whose composition is determined by the need for robustness, performance, and often the size of the container. These bags have multiple layers for strengthening the walls. Given below is the construction of ASI's typical bag design (Figure 11.2).

There is a wide choice available from 1 to 3,500 L bags with a variety of shapes, volume, available ports, tubing, in-line filters, and any other custom feature besides the standard offering by these manufacturers. Generally, it would be advisable to use an off-the-shelf item even though the generic manufacturers offer custom bags readily: the reason for this choice is that there is likely to be a larger volume of data available on off-the-shelf bags and also they are likely to be available on an as-needed basis. The typical applications in bioprocessing use tank liners and 2D and 3D bags.

11.6 TANK LINERS

Tank liners are simple, disposable bags used to line containers and transportation systems. In most cases, they are not gamma sterilized since these are used in open systems most of the time, such as in the preparation of buffer solutions and culture media at the first stage of preparation. The container within which the liner is inserted is there only to provide mechanical support.

Commercially available overhead mixers can readily be integrated because these systems are open. A broad choice of low-density polyethylene liners is available from vendors that supply to several industries reducing the cost of liners. Disposable equipment suppliers also offer these choices. For example, Thermo Scientific's HyClone tank liners are designed for use with commercially available overhead mixers. The chamber is constructed of CX3-9 film with dimensions optimized for Thermo Scientific HyClone standard drums and commonly used industry standard cylindrical tanks. Top entry standard products for maximum recovery using industry standard connection systems in unit volumes of 50, 100, and 200 L. Tanks are supplied sterile to minimize bioburden. A dolly is available to provide mobility of volumes up to 500 L.

The hard-walled containers are necessary in the preparation of buffers and media as this offers the cheapest alternative; however, these containers do not contact any formulation component and, as a result, the cheapest containers should be used. The most likely choice would be a plastic off-the-shelf drum, such as a 55 gal drum. Several major equipment suppliers provide a complete line of mixing systems and, while these do offer an advantage in handling large volumes consistently, one can readily put together a system from off-the-shelf components at a substantially lower cost. It is noteworthy that the more expensive systems come with programming elements that might make the process analytical technology (PAT) work easier but at the stages of BP and MP, the challenges are few and readily overcome by implementing the simplest and cheapest systems. This is what is intended in the max-dispo concept—to use only what adds value.

11.6.1 2D Fluid Containers

For smaller volumes, 2D bags work well, from less than 1 to 50 L, before they become difficult to handle. GE provides the largest 2D fluid container for bioreaction for their Cellbag operations (Wave Bioreactor) in 1,000 L size; other suppliers like Charter Medical can provide containers up to 3,500 L in size. These bags are produced from two-layer films, which are welded together at their ends. The result is a flat chamber, which has ports either face welded or end welded. The user determines the choice of ports and most suppliers have standard combinations that might work well in most instances. It is important to iterate here that any custom-designed bag or configuration would require new studies to establish the role of leachables; this may not be necessary if standard off-the-shelf items are used that have already gone into cGMP manufacturing and approval of products made using them.

Besides their use as bioreactors, the 2D bags are utilized in a reclining or hanging position as manifolds for sampling, dispensing, and holding the product.

11.6.2 2D Powder Bags

In some instances, it may be necessary to use bags to store powders (such as buffer salts, API, and excipients): these bags have a funnel shape and are equipped with large sanitary fittings or aseptic transfer systems, and are antistatic and free of additives. An example of such bag is the Thermo Scientific HyClone Powdertrainer. Large size powder bags are generally custom designed.

11.6.3 3D Bags

The 2D bags have an interesting problem in their design that at a larger scale it becomes difficult to maintain their integrity. The 1,000 L bag offered by GE is recommended to be used with no more than 500 L of media; beyond that, the seals may not hold since the weight of the fluid inside is transferred to the seams of these bags. This becomes particularly problematic when the 2D bags are rocked or shaken, which adds stress to the seams.

3D bags as liners in hard-walled containers obviate the problems of integrity with 2D bags; today, these bags are available in sizes of 3 to 4,000 L sizes. The 3D design also provides additional surface to install ports with complex functions and at both top and bottom. The 3D bags are made by welding films and are mostly offered in cylindrical, conical, or cube shapes. Often the shape is determined by the method how these containers are stored or stacked in outer containers that have the same shape which allows a snug fitting of the 3D bags. While a very large liner can always be brought into the manufacturing area, the outer containers are at times built before the facility is completed; companies offering modular construction of outer containers would do well in the future if they offer an option of assembling an outer container from smaller pieces.

To facilitate their use such as in DP, these outer containers may be equipped with weight sensors, recirculation/mixing fluid management, and temperature control if required. The temperature control can be achieved in several ways, the cheapest one being wrapping them in blankets that are temperature controlled, and the most expensive being to use jacketed containers with circulating fluids. The weight measurement is of greatest importance and, while most manufacturers would use a floor scale, large-scale production requires installation of load cells in the outer containers to avoid moving the containers for weighing.

11.6.4 Transportation Container

Products at different stages of manufacturing often need to be transported within the company or to remote locations to complete the process; finished products are also shipped out to customers and this requires the selection of safe, stable, and closed container systems that maintain sterility. Examples of these containers include

- Flexboy, Flexel 3D Palletank, and Celsius FFT products (www.sartorius-stedim. com).
- Nalgene (www.nalgene.com).
- Thermo Scientific (www.thermoscientific).
- BioShell™ container system designed to protect single-use bags during storage, handling, and shipping. High-purity, dual-density foam construction can withstand multiple impacts at $-70°C$ (www.bio-shell.com).

Disposable bags can be readily used to transport or store frozen products, from cell culture as WCB for direct introduction into a bioreactor to shipping biological API; while flexible bags can survive temperature variations, often it is difficult to detect damage to them during transportation and, thus, require a protective surface around them to obviate this risk.

11.6.5 Summary

- Plastic disposable containers offer the best solution in disposable components utilization as they remove the cleaning and validation requirements.
- Low density PE liners in a hard-walled plastic container and a standard mixer make the cheapest combination of pieces to prepare buffers and media.
- More complex mixing systems are not necessary, and neither are the expensive proprietary containers to hold these PE liners.
- 2D bags can be used only for smaller size volumes while 3D bags with an outer non-disposable container increase the limit of fluids that can be contained to thousands of liters.

- Several novel shapes and sizes are available to fit just about any need.
- Flexible bags can be used for the transportation of biological drugs and, while they survive freeze-thaw cycles, it is often difficult to record breaches in their integrity, thus requiring an outer protective surface.
- Custom-designed bags are readily available but these are very expensive and do not give the user the benefit of the large database provided by the vendors, so one should stick to off-the-shelf products whenever possible.
- Future novel uses of bags may include storage of WCB for direct addition to bioreactors.

11.7 MIXING SYSTEMS

The unit operation of mixing is extensively involved in bioprocessing systems. Some of the keys to mixing operations include mixing to dissolve components of a buffer, culture media, refolding solution, dispersion of cell culture in bioreactors, and heating or cooling of liquids.

All mixing operations must be fully validated as part of PAT to assure that optimal mixing has been achieved all the time. While the stainless-steel mixing vessels have long been used and the principles behind mixing and de-mixing of components with traditional mixing devices have long been studied, much remains to be understood about achieving homogenous mixtures in disposable bags.

In bioprocessing operations, two types of mixing are important: one that leads to the dissolution of solutes, and the other that provides a homogenous environment such as in a bioreactor or a refolding tank. How fast a mixture of powdered components in a buffer mixture dissolves will depend to a great degree on the solubility of individual components, the agitation applied, and the temperature and length of mixing. In theory, mixing involves distributive, dispersive (breaking of aggregates), or diffusive steps. All of these steps require energy which is provided by the mechanical motion induced in liquids. A laminar movement of liquid or a turbulent movement can achieve the mixing and the Reynolds number (Re) of mixing obtained can predict this.

In fluid mechanics, the Re is a dimensionless number that gives a measure of the ratio of inertial forces to viscous forces and consequently quantifies the relative importance of these two types of forces for given flow conditions. Laminar flow occurs at low Res, where viscous forces are dominant, and is characterized by smooth, constant fluid motion; while turbulent flow occurs at high Res and is dominated by inertial forces, which tend to produce chaotic eddies, vortices, and other flow instabilities. In a cylindrical vessel stirred by a central rotating paddle, turbine, or propeller, the characteristic dimension is the diameter of the agitator (D). The velocity is ND (where N is the rotational speed [revolutions per second]), μ is kinematic viscosity, and ρ is the density of fluid. Then Re is

$$\text{Re} = \frac{\rho N D^2}{\mu} \qquad (11.1)$$

The system is fully turbulent for Re values above 10,000.

In fluid dynamics, mixing length theory is a method attempting to describe momentum transfer by turbulent Re stresses within a fluid boundary layer by means of an eddy viscosity. The mixing length is the distance that a fluid parcel will keep its original characteristics before dispersing them into the surrounding fluid.

Laminar mixing, often encountered in fluids with high viscosities, originates from a longitudinal mixing where fluid motion is dominated by linear viscous forces. Fluid particles flow along parallel streamlines and, to obtain homogeneity, radial mixing is necessary, which can be achieved through mechanical forces such as using a stirring bar or an impeller or rocking the base. Thus turbulent mixing provides the greatest effectiveness as evidenced by the utility of high-speed stirrers.

Manufacturing processes are validated for their outcome in a cGMP environment; as a result, the desired mixing quality, which in most cases is a homogenous mixture, is obtained by mixing for a certain period of time (with a range) and with a certain force applied (such as rpm, rocking motions per minute, or other such parameters) and, in those instances where a demixing may occur, a time for which the mixture remains homogenous. Generally, for most of the mixing processes encountered in bioprocessing, these parameters are easy to study and validate: the most difficult one is the mixing of culture in a bioreactor, a topic that will receive greater discussion in the next chapter.

11.7.1 Types of Mixing

There are several distinct types of mixing systems currently available in bioprocessing where disposable mixing containers are used. These include

1. Stirrer systems
   a. Rotating stirrer
   b. Tumbling stirrer
2. Oscillating systems
   a. Rocker
   b. Vibrating disc
   c. Orbital shaker
   d. Pedal push
3. Peristaltic system
   a. Recirculating pump

The systems using stirrers can have the stirring element either driven magnetically or connected through a sealed shaft. Oscillating types mix by moving the liquid inside a bag (mostly 2D types) by rocking them or shaking using mechanical vibrations or ultrasonic vibrations. Generally, the mixing systems that do not involve any mechanical parts inside the bag (either 2D or 3D) are preferred to reduce the cost, the risk of damage to the bag from rotating devices, the grinding of bag or the stirrer inside the bag; those stirring systems that use a magnetic field provide better sterility compared to those which are magnetically coupled.

11.7.1.1 Stirring Magnetic Mixer

- XDM (Xcellerex), 100 to 1,000 L, the XDM Quad Mixing System comprises of an integrated magnetic stirrer with compact motor, a bottom-mounted disposable stirrer; the coupling between the motor and the disposable stirrer is magnetic. The square configuration offers enhanced mixing efficiency through a natural baffling effect and compact storage capability. The bottom is slanted to ensure a low residual volume after discharge.
- The Flexel 3D LevMix System for Palletank, 50 to 1,000 L, combines the LevTech levitated impeller licensed by ATMI and the Sartorius Stedim Flexel 3D Bag. It comprises a stainless steel, cube-shaped container with a door for ease of bag mounting. In addition, it has windows to enable observation of the mixing process, a drive unit for levitating or rotating the stirrer, and a disposable bag with a center-mounted magnetic stirrer.
- Magnetic Mixer (ATMI Life Sciences), 30 to 2,000 L.
- Jet-Drive (ATMI Life Sciences), 50 to 200 L.
- Mobius (Millipore), 100 to 500 L.
- LevMixer (ATMI Life Sciences), 30 to 2,000 L, ultraclean as it does not produce any residue from mechanical motion, suitable for downstream operations as well.

11.7.1.2 Stirring Mechanical Coupling Mixer

- Single-use mixers (SUM) (Thermo Fisher Scientific), 50 to 2,000 L; there are two types of magnetic stirrers driven by a stirring plate available for different mixing applications. Not intended for sterile applications, suitable applications include dissolving solid media and/or buffer components prior to sterile filtration.
- Thermo Fisher Scientific HyClone Mixtainer Systems with an impeller linked to an overhead drive and is coupled by a sealed bearing assembly, which maintains the integrity of the system. The mixing stirrer is installed off-center. This mixer is intended for powder–liquid and liquid–liquid mixing and has sterile disposable contact surfaces.

11.7.1.3 Tumbling Mixer

- Pad-Drive (ATMI Life Sciences), 25 to 1,000 L, uses a tumbling stirrer mounted from top, the wand rotates inside an inert polymer sleeve.
- WandMixer (ATMI Life Sciences), 5 to 200 L, uses a tumbling stirrer whose axle is built into the bag from the top of the bag.

11.7.1.4 Oscillating Mixer

- Wave (GE Healthcare), 20 to 1,000 L, horizontal oscillation on a rocker. The rocking motion is very efficient in generating waves, and the wave-induced motion in the bag causes large volumes of fluid to move facilitating the dispersion of solids. The optimum operating parameters depend on the combination of the container geometry, bag support, filling volume, rocking angle, rocking rate, and the characteristics of the mixture (solids, foam, etc.).

- HyNetics (HyNetics Corporation), 30 to 5,000 L, vertical oscillation of a disk or septum. The key feature is the mixing disk, which is fabricated from rigid, engineered polymers. Multiple, evenly distributed slots penetrate the disk. The underside of the disk incorporates pie-shaped flaps. These flaps open as the disk moves up from the bottom of the mixing bag on the drive's upstroke, allowing fluid to flow through the disk's slots. The flaps close on the down stroke, forcing the liquid toward the bottom of the vessel and subsequently up the walls of the vessel. The mixing disk, flaps, polymer mixing shaft, and the shaft rolling diaphragm seal, which attaches to the bag film, are disposable.
- SALTUS (Meissner), 5 to 2,000 L, vertical oscillation of a disk or septum; based on a vibrating disk with conical orifices. Due to the oscillating movement and the conical orifices, liquid jets develop at the tapered end of the holes. Thus, an axial fluid flow pattern is achieved. The frequency and amplitude of the vibration can be adjusted to provide either vigorous or gentle mixing. The bag is preassembled with the rigid high-density polyethylene (HDPE) vibrating disks and with tubes, filters, and a sampling port, in addition to a disposable sensor plate for pH, DO, and temperature measurement. Due to the frictionless, oscillating movement of the disk, it can be used where an ultraclean environment is required.
- PedalMixer (MayaBio, www.mayabio.com), 10 L to unlimited volume, no stirring device, uses a pedal outside of the bag to push the liquid to mix, and can be used with any generic bag; this is the lowest cost option. The newest type of oscillating system is a patented pedal system whereby the 2D bag remains stationary on a flat surface and a pedal pushes at one end of the bag creating waves inside the bag; a slight tilt of the platform imparts potential energy to the contents while the kinetic energy moves the liquid and provides a mixing profile identical to that obtained using a rocking platform or any other form of the use of mechanical energy. A significant advantage of this system is that it can accommodate any size (since no stress is produced on the bag) and can accommodate all shapes and sizes of bags, allowing the use of generic bags.

11.7.1.5 Peristaltic Mixer

- The Flexel3D Palletank for recirculation mixing incorporates one or two recirculation loops and can be equipped with Sartorius Stedim's Mechatronics load cells to facilitate fluid management

11.7.2 Summary

- A large number of unit operations in bioprocessing involve mixing; fortunately, these are relatively simple operations that are easily validated.
- The largest mixing operations involve BP and MP that can involve thousands of liters. Since these components are sterilized, likely by filtration, it is not necessary to use any special proprietary mixing system. An off-the-shelf plastic drum with a PE liner and industry-standard mixers can do the job well at a fraction of the cost. It is not necessary to use any proprietary liners as long as the user is able to

qualify a supplier; at this stage the qualification is relatively simple. Since all of unit operations in a cGMP operation are validated, once a system has been qualified, it can be used repeatedly.

- Open mixing of media and buffer may be provided with a laminar hood in those environments where there is a risk of cross contamination to reduce any additional burden on filter systems.
- The mixing systems available today are the same as used in disposable bioreactors: in some instances the platform can be used for both operations.
- While many reputable suppliers have developed highly sophisticated 3D systems, these are not necessary for BP and MP; the cost of 3D bags with built-in stirring systems can be prohibitive.
- The 2D bags offer many advantages including the ease of storage because they are horizontally expanded; the wave motion created inside these bags is extremely efficient.
- The newest entry in mixing technology, which is from MayaBio, makes it possible for users to use any generic bag for mixing, further reducing the cost as well as reducing the dependence on a proprietary supplier of components.
- The power requirements in operating the mixing systems are the lowest in non-stirring types, such as the oscillating mixers; however, this is not a major consideration in the overall cost of mixing.
- In the future, several novel systems and the utilization of existing systems will appear in the market, and there are likely to be greater integration of the various steps of bioprocessing.

11.8 DISPOSABLE BIOREACTORS

Hard-walled bioreactors have been used for centuries, from kitchen utensils to multistory stainless-steel behemoths; the field of bioreactor design has remained pretty much the same for a long time. The essential elements of a bioreactor, a utensil to contain a culture and media with sufficient mixing and aeration, are readily provided in the traditional designs of bioreactors. Today, we have multitude of options in the design of bioreactors and these came about once the use of bioreactors expanded in the manufacturing of biological drugs requiring many control features that were not needed or required in other industries. With the use of animal, human, and plant cells and viruses to produce therapeutic proteins, vaccines, antibodies, and so on, there arose a need to modify the traditional bioreactors to accommodate the growth needs of these new production engines: recombinant engineering put these new engines in the forefront of biological drug production. One major change in the design of bioreactors that is recent is the use of disposable bioreactors to avoid the challenges of cleaning validation reducing the regulatory barriers in drug production. Hundreds of new molecules are under development using disposable bioreactors and in many instances disposable bioreactors are used to manufacture clinical supplies, yet no drug has been approved for marketing that is manufactured on a commercial scale using a disposable bioreactor; however, this taboo would soon break as the new molecules under development move further in the approval cycle.

Almost all of recombinant drugs in the market today were developed by large pharmaceutical companies starting about 30 years ago when the only choice available was the traditional bioreactor; even though their process may be less efficient, it is not worth the effort to switch over to another manufacturing method because of the prohibitive cost of changeover protocols that need to be completed. A case in point is the use of roller bottles to manufacture erythropoietin: Amgen, the world's largest producer of erythropoietin continues to use roller bottles despite their inefficiencies and risks, but for new products Amgen will be using stirred bioreactors.

Disposable bioreactors have varied designs and purposes but all of them are made of Class VI plastic films, are sterilized by gamma radiation, and are disposed of after use; they may come with several attachments that allow the filtration of media, monitoring of pH, DO, OD, pCO_2, temperature, and other PAT-related parameters. Using stirrers, paddles, shaking, and rocking the bags by mechanical or hydraulic means achieve the method of mixing and aeration inside the bag. A choice of aeration systems may include surface aeration (e.g., in Wave Bioreactors) to forced sparging through proprietary ceramic tubes (e.g., MayaBioReactors). The host cell yields obtained using disposable bioreactors match or exceed those obtained in traditional reactors.

Disposable bioreactors come in many sizes from mL to thousands of liters; they can be equipped with bioinformatics systems from very simple to very complex; they can be manual or highly automated; they can be as inexpensive as a plastic bag to as expensive as the high-end traditional hard-walled bioreactors. The disposable bioreactor industry is still evolving with new inventions surfacing almost routinely. Here is a brief look at their historical development over the past 60 years:

1st Period—First 10 Years (1960s): Petri dishes, T- flasks, roller bottles, and shaken plastic bags. At first, the glass petri dishes were replaced by plastic plates, and the most significant development was the use of polypropylene and Teflon bags by Krolinska Institute in Sweden to grow bacteria and yeast cells, albeit at a very small scale.

2nd Period—Next 30 Years (1970s to 1990s): Disposable hollow fiber system, two-compartment system, multitry cell culture, static bags for cell expansion, pneumatic mixing (peristaltic recirculation), and rocking bags. The hollow fiber technology required recirculation of media to grow anchored or suspended animal cells using the Cellmax HFBS (FiberCell), the AcuSyst-HFBSs (BioVest), and the Xcell HFBS (BioVest). These bioreactors were able to operate continuously for months at a time and helped produce quantities from sub-gram to a few grams. Even though high cell densities could be achieved, the problems of scaling up these bioreactors caused their failure to stay as a viable option for commercial production and are used today to make small quantities of test substances.

The Cell Factory made of polystyrene was a flask-like culture system containing a number of trays stacked in parallel in a single unit. This was a good scale-up model for commercial production and replaced roller bottles used for adherent cells.

CellCube from Corning Costar is similar to the Cell Factory, runs in a perfusion mode, and proves useful for adherent cell lines; it was used for vaccine production on a limited scale and never showed a potential for commercial therapeutic protein manufacturing.

The LifeReactor was a peristaltic pump-driven bubble column bioreactor, where mass and heat transfer are achieved by direct sparging of a conical-shaped disposable culture bag (1 to 5 L). It was mainly used for the growth of plant origin organ cultures.

The two-compartment dialysis membrane bioreactors have a semipermeable membrane that separates the cells from the bulk of the medium and again permits continuous diffusion of nutrients into the cell compartment with simultaneous removal of waste products. The two models, the MiniPerm (Greiner Bio One) and the T-flask-based CELLine (INTEGRA Biosciences, Sartorius Stedim), must be kept in a CO_2 incubator, and achieve high cell density allowing antibody production.

3rd Period—Next 20 Years (1990s to current): Wave-mixed reactors, stirred 3D reactors, orbitally shaken reactors; used in clinical sample production, small-scale commercial manufacturing, comprehensive disposable systems. While the use of a shaken bag goes back to 1960s, it was not until around 1996 when Vijay Singh disclosed his invention of the Wave Bioreactor and marketed them in 1998 that the industry woke up to a new reality in biological drug manufacturing. While the original wave bioreactors served the purpose well, soon it was realized that many of the shortcomings, like inability to grow bacteria or scale up to larger volumes, were overcome recently (2010) by the disclosures of MayaBioReactors (www.mayabio.com) that all types of cells can be grown in 2D bags (Figure 11.3).

Given below is a description of the various methods used to induce motion inside a disposable bag (Figure 11.4).

Types of stirring mechanisms. From left, stirrer mechanically attached to a motor; stirrer magnetically levitating, no contact with motor; magnetic stirrer at bottom, rubs off the surface, mechanical stirrer inserted from top (Figure 11.5).

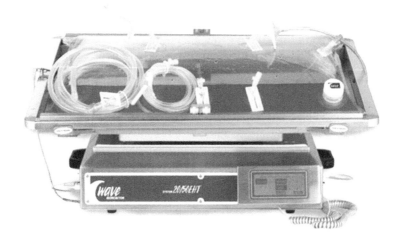

Figure 11.3 Wave bioreactor.

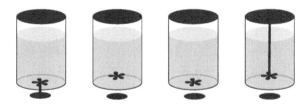

Figure 11.4 Comparison of various stirring systems in 3D disposable bioreactors.

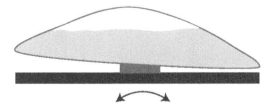

Figure 11.5 Liquid motion in wave-based mixing systems.

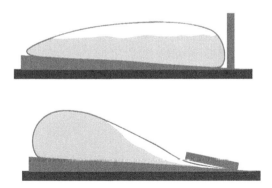

Figure 11.6 New concept of mixing in MayaBio reactors by pushing the liquid against an incline.

Rocking wave motion is the most commonly used; pioneered by Wave Bioreactor, several equipment suppliers have adopted this system (Figure 11.6).

Stationary bioreactor concept differs significantly from the usual wave motion that requires moving the base of plate; here the bag stays stationary and a flapper instead pushed down one edge of the disposable bag.

Somehow the concept of using 2D bags to grow host cells did not pan out widely, and most of the major equipment leaders, like Sartorius Stedim, Pall, EMD Millipore, New Brunswick Scientific, and Thompson Scientific, adopted 3D versions of disposable bioreactors. The recent entrant to the race is Xcellerex that has done well with its large-scale 3D bioreactors. The success of Xcellerex comes from its reputable customer support as they build out the equipment as client solutions while others positions themselves as equipment suppliers.

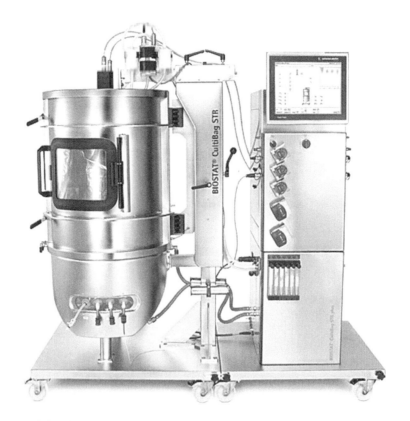

Figure 11.7 Cultibag bioreactor.

There is no doubt that the simplest and the most cost-effective bioreactors are the 2D or pillow types as they do not require an outer container and by design avoid any internal stirring. The wave-mixed bag systems represent one of the largest groups among single-use bioreactors and include the AppliFlex, the BIOSTAT CultiBag Rocking Motion, the BioWave, the CELL-tainer, the Wave Bioreactor, the Wave and Undertow Bioreactor (WUB), and the most recently introduced MayaBioReactors that have a stationary surface and require the least amount of energy input (Figure 11.7).

Perhaps the equipment suppliers' profit margins were not large enough or perhaps they understood the psychology of the industry well enough to know that it would not be easy for Big Pharma to come down from towering bioreactors to lay-flat bags with rocking motion as the manufacturing equipment. This caused the proliferation of 3D technologies. The stirring bag bioreactors were first introduced by Thermo Fisher's Single-Use Bioreactor (SUB), developed as a result of cooperation between Baxter and Hyclone and currently the market leader, and the XDR-Disposable Stirred Tank Bioreactor from Xcellerex were the only such systems available initially. This was followed by the Nucleo Bioreactor (ATMI Life Sciences), the BIOSTAT CultiBag Stirred (STR) (Sartorius Stedim),

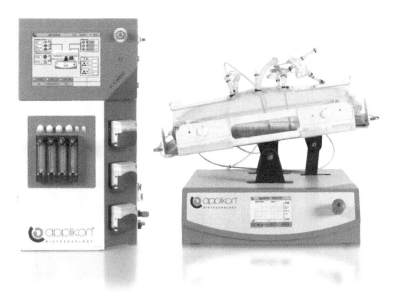

Figure 11.8 Applikon bioreactor.

the Mobius CellReady Bioreactor (EMD Millipore/Applikon), and the CelliGEN BLU Single-Use Bioreactor (Figure 11.8).

Xcellerex Bioreactor was recently acquired by GE Healthcare and now sells along with the Wave Bioreactors (Figure 11.9).

The non-stirring type 3D reactors include Sartorius Stedim's SuperSpinner D 1000, which is non-instrumented and its aeration comes from hollow fiber membranes wound around a tumbling stirrer, all features making it a simple reactor to operate and test expression of new cell lines.

Orbital shaker bioreactors comprise the third largest category after the wave and stirring types and promise high-throughput systems for scaling up to pilot scale. Screening systems such as the M24 Microbioreactor (Applikon, Pall Life Sciences), the BioLector (mp2-labs), and the Sensolux (Sartorius Stedim) are typically equipped with noninvasive single-use sensors useful for PAT work. Sine orbital shaking was first applied to flasks and plates, these can still be upgraded to reactor level by connecting them to a PreSens's Sensor Dish Reader (SDR) or a Shake Flask Reader (SFR) using precalibrated sensor patches for pH and DO. The CultiFlask 50 disposable bioreactor and the Disposable Shaken Bioreactor System (a cooperation between ExcellGene, Kiihner, and Sartorius Stedim) and the CURRENT Bioreactor (AmProteins) serve as mid-size reactors,

Zeta's bio-t (a proof-of-concept reactor) is a bag bioreactor with a Vibromixer, where the movement of a perforated disk fixed on a vertically oscillating hollow shaft causes an axial flow in the bag, which mixes and aerates the cells. The form, size, and position of the conical drill

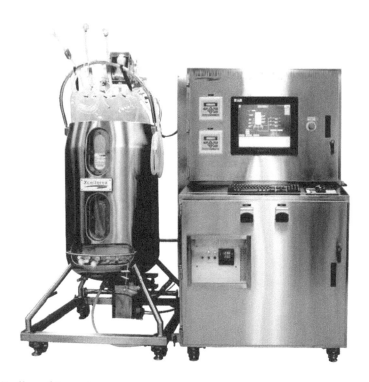

Figure 11.9 Xcellerex bioreactor.

holes on the disk affect the fluid flow and oxygen transfer efficiency in the bag and contribute to the elimination of vortex formation. Similarly, the BayShake Bioreactor achieves vertical oscillation wherein the culture broth oscillates in a surface-aerated cube-shaped bag.

The bubble bioreactors are exemplified by Nestle's Slug Bubble Bioreactor (SBB) that generates intermittent large, long, bullet-shaped bubbles termed *slug bubbles* that occupy nearly the entire cross section of a tube, are generated at the bottom of the bag and rise to the top. To provide a determined quantity of air at a given frequency, a solenoid valve is used to control bubble generation. Varying the air inlet pressure and the valve opening time controls the quantity of air and the bubble frequency.

The Pneumatic Bioreactor System (PBS) works with an air-wheel design and a dual sparger system for efficient mixing and aeration. In the case of the CellMaker systems (Cellexus Biosystems), the unique asymmetric shape of the culture bag is significant. The CellMaker Regular is a single-use bubble column. This system is preferable for microbial productions. The version specific to animal cell cultivations is the hybrid CellMaker Plus where pneumatic and mechanic drives are combined. Mixing and aeration is achieved by transverse liquid movement. While the airflow is induced by a sparger tube, the two magnetically driven propellers intensify the *riser* flow. Excessive foam formation, which is linked to flotation and a well-known problem in bubble columns, may be minimized or even eliminated by applying pressure to the headspace within the bag.

11.8.1 Cellexus Bioreactor

With exception of the WUB, the SBB, and the microbial versions of the XDR, CELL-tainer and CellMaker, all disposable bioreactors have been developed primarily for fed-batch operations with animal suspension cells. This kind of operation is most common in bio-manufacturing. Anchorage-dependent (adherent) cells are less widespread in today's processes; however, disposable bioreactors such as AmProtein's CURRENT Perfusion Bioreactor do allow the cultivation of adherent cells if they are grown on microcarriers. Microcarriers also support the cell attachment to a 3D structure, enabling a higher cell density and productivity, and culture conditions, which are nearly identical to an in vivo environment (Figure 11.10).

11.8.2 CELL-Tainer Cell Culture System

The fixed-bed bioreactors include the FibraStage (using FibraCel disks in four disposable bottles per bioreactor system, with maximum volume of 0.5 L column volume [CV] per bottle) from New Brunswick Scientific and Artelis's fixed-bed bioreactor (iCELLis bioreactor, with a maximum volume of 500 mL per packed bed). Both bioreactors, which require microcarriers, were specifically designed for the production of cell culture-based animal cells. The FibraStage is kept in an incubator and is suitable for production at a laboratory scale (Figure 11.11).

A novel small 3D bioreactor is Hamilton's BioLevitator operating with modified, surface-aerated 50 mL plastic tubes, which oscillate vertically. The fully automated SimCell MicroBioreactor System (with parallel disposable cassettes and six microbioreactors per plate) ensures efficient process optimizations for animal cell cultures, which can be transferred to stirred processes with high reproducibility.

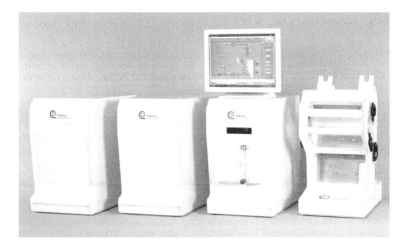

Figure 11.10   Celluxus bioreactor.

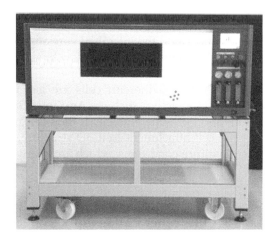

Figure 11.11 CELL-tainer culture system.

11.8.3 Wave-Mixed Bioreactors

These comprise a bag, which consists of a multilayer film; EVA is the contact layer in most cases. The mixing takes place in the bag by moving the platform sections. Oxygen is taken up from surface renewal of waves formed, leaving a bubble-free surface.

A variety of designs, degree of bioinformatics, and sizes are available in this category. Except for the WUB and CELL-tainer, the wave is caused by a one-dimensional horizontal oscillation of the culture broth in the bag located on a rocker unit. The intensity of the mass and energy transfer and, therefore, cell growth and product expression can be directly controlled through wave generation and propagation. These features are adjustable by modifying the rocking rate, the rocking angle, the filling level of the bag (up to 50% maximum), and the aeration rate of the Wave Bioreactor, the BioWave, its successor (the BIOSTAT CultiBag RM), the AppliFlex, the Tsunami Bioreactor, and the CELL-tainer.

Tsunami bioreactor, in which up to six rocker units integrated into one rack housing 5 bags (each with 160 L CV) or 64 bags (each with 5 L), moves in opposite directions. This is no longer available.

Oxygen transfer (which is described by the volumetric oxygen transfer efficiency rate [kLa] values) and its influence on the cultivation result have been investigated for the majority of the systems. For Newtonian culture broths, kLa values between 5 and 30/h were reported as typical for animal cell cultivations in the BioWave, the Wave, and the AppliFlex. Oxygen limitations may be virtually disregarded during such a process as increasing the rocking rate and angle is more effective in increasing the oxygen transfer than increasing the aeration rate.

The required high oxygen level can be achieved by operating a BIOSTAT CultiBag RM with low CV (50 L bag with 5 L CV) or the CELL-tainer. In contrast to the version for cell cultures (CELL-tainer Bioreactor) where kLa values exceed 100/h, values above 200/h are possible in the version for microbial cultures (CELL-tainer Microbial Bioreactor). This is attributed to the 2D movement of the CELL-tainer ensuring higher-oxygen-transfer rates for microorganisms.

In the WUB, the wave propagated inside the bag is generated by periodic upward movement of the movable head and/or foot section of the horizontal table (platform) on which the bag is located; the kLa values of the WUB are similar to those achieved with the BioWave. The parameters having the most impact on the kLa data are the angle of the platform, the percentage of the CV located on and lifted by the platform, the aeration rate, and the time taken for the platform to complete one oscillation.

The Wave Bioreactor, BioWave, and BIOSTAT CultiBag RM differ in their sensors and control units.

The wave-mixed bag bioreactors have secured a solid position in mammalian cell-derived seed train manufacturing and process developments aimed at producing therapeutic proteins. These bioreactors are run in a batch, fed-batch (feeding processes), or perfusion mode and are preferred reactors for transient transfections; they are becoming widely used in simple, medium-volume processes such as the production of viruses for gene therapies (e.g., recombinant adeno-associated virus vectors) and veterinary as well as human vaccines (e.g., Aujeszky's disease virus, porcine influenza virus, porcine parvovirus, mink enteritis virus, smallpox virus). Traditional disposable virus production bioreactors (roller flasks, Cell Factories) have been successfully replaced by wave-mixed bag bioreactors.

To date, wave-mixed bag bioreactors have proven acceptable for the cultivation of plant cell and tissue cultures in R&D. Focusing on biomanufacturing, secondary metabolite productions (taxanes, harpagosides, hyoscya-mine, alliin, ginsenosides, isoflavones) have been realized in the BioWave and the WUB. Suspension cells, embryogenic cells, and hairy roots were grown. In addition, the first proteins (e.g., human collagen/alpha, tumor-specific human antibody) were successfully produced with fast-growing suspension cells in the BioWave, the AppliFlex, and the WUB. However, up to now, wave-mixed bag bioreactors have not achieved the same importance for the production of plant cell culture-derived products as they have for animal cell-based target molecules. The same is the case for microbial products with pharmaceutical significance.

However, a recent modification of 2D bags by MayaBio has made it possible to use the wave-mixed systems for every type of cell and organism; studies reported by MayaBio show bacterial ODs of 70–80 in overnight cultures. The MayaBioReactor introduces a proprietary sparger in Wave Bioreactor bags that allows extensive aeration. Another major difference comes in the platform which is kept stationary and a pedal pushing up and down at one end of the bag creates wave motions inside the bag allowing mixing achieved by using rocking platform.

There is still interest in developing photo bioreactors and Applikon has recently made a disposable offering. A number of recent studies demonstrated that normal plants could be grown under light emitting diodes light sources very efficiently. These solid-state lamps (SSL) are tiny semiconductor chips that generate light when powered. The elements that the diode is made from determine the light spectrum it emits, these solid-state devices have been improved over the years and now have greatly increased light intensity and specific wavelengths. These developments have resulted in SSL as self-contained light source for plant growth. Applikon has chosen to develop light panel that are add-on modules for

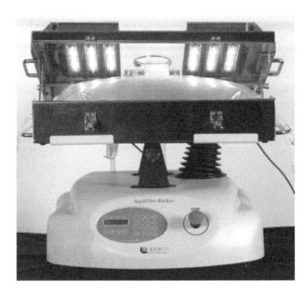

Figure 11.12   Applikon photo bioreactor.

our standard stirred tank and single-use bioreactors. This offer maximum flexibility and offer a very economical set-up for cultivating photosynthesizing organisms. The volume range covers 3 L up to 20 L autoclavable stirred tank bioreactors and 10 up to 50 L single-use bioreactors. SSL plant light has very unique characteristics which are useful for plant growth applications. An important characteristic is the spectral distribution of light in the wavelengths region of 450–500 nm and 630–700 nm, these bands are critical for normal plant growth as they fall within the Photo-synthetically active radiation, PAR, (400–700), which plants primarily use for biological processes and are also favorable for confined applications such as micropropagation. Another useful characteristic is long useful life of about 50,000 h and the high-energy conversion efficiency. This results in substantially cooler systems than other light sources. Systems also save energy by using less ventilation and cooling needs for growing plants in culture room. Second this provides new opportunities for enhancing growth of several hard to grow plants or plants that require a specific range of light spectrum (Figure 11.12).

11.8.4 Stirred Single-Use Bioreactors

The stirred systems sold by Thermo Fisher Scientific and Xcellerex, for use with animal cells and for volumes up to 1,000 and 2,000 L, offer challenges to stainless-steel bioreactors. Both of these bioreactors borrow their dimensions, proportions, sparging systems, and mixing systems from the traditional stainless-steel systems. In reality, these are standard stainless-steel systems wherein a liner has been installed. These bioreactors demonstrate that the way to attract Big Pharma is to offer expensive big machines. For example, the outer containers can be easily replaced with much cheaper plastic shell but that would make them less attractive and make it difficult to charge the high price these systems command. There is no savings in capital investment while there is a substantially higher expense involved in ongoing cost to operate these reactors. These reactors have also been converted to microbial versions and evaluation by many large companies who would not mind paying unjustified exorbitant prices of these reactors.

The BIOSTAT CultiBag STR of Sartorius Stedim is a closed system and demonstrates efficiencies close to reusable bioreactors. As an option, the bag is equipped with a sparger ring or a microsparger and two axial flow three-blade-segment impellers or a combination of one axial flow three-blade-segment impeller and one radial flow six-blade-segment impeller. Homogeneous mixing in the bag is achieved by the centered stirring system.

ATMI Life Science's Nucleo single-use bioreactors has a cube-shaped bag instead of a cylindrical bag, a tumbling (Pad-Drive) mixing system instead of a rotating impeller, and a dynamic sparging arrangement in place of a static structure and is available in 50 and 1,000 L volumes.

11.8.4.1 Integrity™ PadReactor™

The Integrity™ PadReactor™ system is a single-use bioreactor specifically designed to fulfill the needs of cell culturists. It is perfectly suited to laboratory environments, process development centers, clinical material supply, and flexible GMP. The PadReactor offers an open architecture controller platform, which gives the end user the opportunity to choose a preferred controller or use an existing control system.

The bioreactor vessel, which offers comparable functionality to classical stirred tank bioreactors, is a single-use bag integrating an internal paddle mixing and sparger system. This innovative bag design allows a non-invasive connection to the system. The paddle is enclosed in a medical grade ULDPE sleeve, made from the same contact material as the bag itself, and is coupled on top of the vessel with the mechanical mixing head.

As with all ATMI LifeSciences' single-use systems, the Integrity PadReactor utilizes disposable-mixing bags made from TK8 bioprocess film. The product-contacting layer of TK8 film is blow-extruded in-house by ATMI under clean room conditions using medical-grade ULDPE resin. It is then laminated to create a gas barrier film of exceptional cleanliness, strength, and clarity that is ADCF and complies fully with USP Class VI requirements

The Integrity PadReactor single-use bioreactor consists of the following:

Drive unit: The flexible drive unit allows the system to cultivate cells in disposable bags. One drive unit can allow the user to mix in multiple disposable mixing bags of various sizes. Each system comes with the appropriate mixing stick for your container.

Mobile retaining tank: The purpose of the retaining tank is to support the mixing bag and provide mobility before and after operation. Various tank sizes and options are available.

Bioreactor vessel: The reactor vessel uses an innovative bag design that allows a non-invasive connection to the mixer. Mixing is achieved when the integrated paddle/sparger inside the bag rotates within the bag.

Highlights and Benefits

- Superior mixing capabilities with highly reduced shear stress
- Innovative sparging device with better oxygenation and kLa
- Adapted for cultivation of suspended or adherent cells at very high densities
- Compatible with most cell culture processes
- Scalable customizable system
- No need for CIP/SIP (disposable bag technology)
- Avoid cross contamination risks
- Very low working volume

The Mobius CellReady 3 L bioreactor is equipped with a marine impeller (top driven), a microsparger or open-pipe sparger, standard sensors, and an Applikon ez-Control process control unit. Similar cell densities and antibody titers can be achieved in the Mobius CellReady, as in stirred 3 L glass bioreactors. A comparable approach to the Mobius CellReady represents New Brunswick Scientific's CelliGEN BLU Single-Use Stirred-Tank Bioreactor (Figure 11.13).

11.8.5 Orbitally Shaken Single-Use Bioreactors

Orbitally shaken bioreactors are very difficult to study because of the free movement of surfaces in the bioreactors. The surface-aerated CultiFlask 50 disposable bioreactor, a non-instrumented 50 mL centrifuge tube with a ventilated cap, can deliver kLa values of between 5 and 30/h at CVs of 10 to 20 mL and agitation speeds between 180 and 220 rpm.

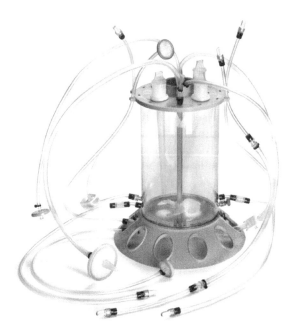

Figure 11.13   Mobius cell-ready reactor.

Systems with cylindrical bags include the Disposable Shaken Bioreactor System and the CURRENT Bioreactor. AmProtein utilizes EVA plastic bags in their CURRENT Bioreactor series. It was possible to demonstrate that the oxygen supply (critical for yield optimization) could be improved by the material of construction of the cultivation container in single-use bioreactors.

11.8.6 Bioreactor Selection

Factors to consider include the following:

1. Goal of production, biomass or cell production
2. Bioinformatic controls
3. Scale
4. Biosafety
5. Familiarity
6. Cost
7. Support

More choices are available for animal cell bioreactors. For all kinds of cell expansions and processes based on insect cells, wave-mixed bag bioreactors should be the design of choice. This is especially important if the culture medium used is serum free or protein free (i.e., it contains hydrolysates such as peptones from plants and yeasts), but not chemically defined, and consequently a strong foam formation could potentially be expected during cultivation. Because of the mechanical action hindering foam formation (the foam is continuously mixed into the medium by the wave action), the addition of antifoaming agents becomes unnecessary.

Non-instrumented small-scale systems, or systems with limited instrumentation, such as disposable T-flasks, spinner flasks, roller flasks, and their modifications, whose handling has been, to some extent, automated over the past few years, are regarded as routine workhorses in cell culture laboratories.

The application of noninvasive optical sensor technology to transparent cultivation containers for animal cells has resulted in highly automated or precisely monitored and/or controlled disposable micro-bioreactor systems. This has paved the way for a change in early stage process development from being unmonitored to being well characterized and controlled, and has made an important contribution to the accurate replication of larger-scale conditions.

In seed inoculum productions, process developments and GMP for mAB products and vaccines, wave-mixed and stirred bag bioreactors are increasingly replacing fixed-wall cell culture bioreactors. Furthermore, they are displacing the early disposable bioreactors such as roller bottles, Cell Factories, and hollow fiber bioreactors. This is due to the fact that the majority of animal and human cells grow serum free and in suspension, and also because cell culture bioreactor volumes are currently shrinking due to increased product titers.

When optimized cell densities and product titers must be achieved in the shortest possible time, cell culture technologists need to be willing to move away from their gold standard, that is, the use of stirring systems. In addition to highly instrumented, scalable wave-mixed and stirred single-use bioreactors, shaken disposable bioreactors, and novel approaches such as the PBS or the BayShake are on the increase.

It is assumed that the pharmaceutical industry's current drive toward safe, indi
vidualized medicines (e.g., personalized antibodies, functional cells for cancer, immune
and tissue replacement therapies) will contribute to the continuing growth of disposable
bioreactors.

Disposable bioreactors have not played an important role to date in the cultivation
of cells or tissues of plant origin and microorganisms. However, plant cell biomass, secondary metabolites for pharmaceutical use, cosmetics (e.g., PhytoCELLTec products from
Mibelle Biochemistry, Switzerland), and glycoproteins have already been successfully produced in satisfactory amounts in disposable bag bioreactors. They have been wave mixed,
stirred, or pneumatically agitated.

Similarly, for microorganism cultivations, where high-density growth is often desired,
disposable bioreactors ensuring higher power input and oxygen transfer efficiency should
be used. Currently, the user may have access to the first suitable types recommended for
microorganisms, for example, the CELL-tainer Microbial Bioreactor, the CellMaker Regular,
or the microbial version of the XDR-Disposable Stirred Tank Bioreactor. The Nucleo
Bioreactor represents another suitable bag bioreactor for microorganisms due to its high
kLa values of disposable bioreactors in plant cell-based and reaching 200/h (Figure 11.14).

Given below is a comparison of various commercial choices available to the bioprocessing engineer to select from (Table 11.3).

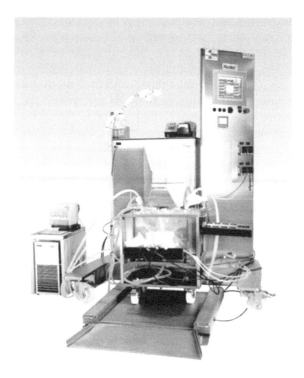

Figure 11.14 Nucleo bioreactor.

Table 11.3 Commercially Available Bioreactor Solutions

Bioreactor Brand	Vendor	Maximum Size	Main Applications
Mechanically Driven/Wave-Mixed (Horizontally Oscillation)			
BIOSTAT CultiBag RM (in the past Bio Wave)	Sartorius Stedim	300 L CV	Cultivation of animal cells, plant cells, and microorganisms having up to medium oxygen demands: screening, seed inoculum production, small and medium volume scale manufacture
Wave Bioreactor	GE Healthcare	500 L CV	Cultivation of animal cells, seed inoculum production
AppliFlex	Applikon	25 L CV	
Tsunami Bioreactor	Tsunami Bio	160 L CV per platform	No longer available
CELL-trainer Bioreactor, animal	Lonza	15 L CV	Cultivation of animal cells and plant cells: screening, seed inoculum production, sample production, small volume scale manufacture
CELL-trainer Bioreactor, microbial			Cultivation of microorganisms: screening, seed inoculum production, small volume scale manufacture
WUB	Nestlé	100 L CV	Cultivation of plant cells: small and medium volume scale manufacture
Mechanically driven/vertically Oscillation Bay Shake Bioreactor	Bayer Technology Services/Sartorius Stedim	1,000 L TV	Cultivation of animal cells: seed inoculum production, sample production, small and medium volume scale manufacture
Mechanically driven/orbitally shaken µ24 Microbioreactor	Applikon	7 mL TV	Cultivation of animal cells, plant cells, and microorganisms: screening
BioLector	Np2-labs	1.5 mL TV	
CulitFlask 50DBa	Sartorius Stedim	35 mL CV	
Sensolux		1 L TV	
SB-200X Disposable Shaken Bioreactor System	Kühner/Sartorius Stedim	200 L TV	Cultivation of animal cells: seed inoculum production, sample production, small and medium volume scale manufacture
CURRENT Bioreactor	AmProtein	300 L CV	
Mechanically driven/stirred S.U.B.	ThermoFisher Scientific	1,000 L CV	Cultivation of animal cells: seed inoculum production, small and medium volume scale manufacture

(*Continued*)

Table 11.3 (*Continued*) Commercially Available Bioreactor Solutions

Bioreactor Brand	Vendor	Maximum Size	Main Applications
BIOSTAT CultiBag STR	Sartorius Stedim	1,000 L CV	
Nucleo Bioreactor	ATMI Life Sciences	1,000 L CV	
XDR-DSTB, animal	Xcellerex	2,000 L CV	
XDR-DSTB, microbial		200 L TV	Manufacture of microbial HCD products
Mobius CellReady 3 L Bioreactor	Applikon/Millipore	3 L TV	Cultivation of animal cells: screening, seed inoculum production, sample production
CelliGen BLU SUB	New Brunswick	14 L TV	
SuperSpinner D1000a	Sartorius Stedim	1 L CV	
Pneumatically Driven			
SBB	Nestlé	100 L CV	Cultivation of plant cells: small and medium volume scale manufacture
PBS	PBS	250 L TV	Cultivation of animal cells: seed inoculum production, sample production small and medium volume scale manufacture
CellMaker Regular (in the past CellMaker Lite) Hybrid	Cellexus	50 L CV	Cultivation of microorganisms: seed inoculum production, sample production, small-volume-scale manufacture
CellMaker Plus	Cellexus	8 L CV	Cultivation of animal cells: seed inoculum production, sample production
MayaBio	MayaBioReactor	1–5000 L CV	2D bag on a stationary platform, wave motion induced by a flapper, or orbital motion, proprietary sparging system allows cultivation of every type of cell and organism

Source: R. Eibl, S. Kaiser, R. Lombriser, and D. Eibl. *Appl. Microbiol. Biotechnol.*, 86, 41–49, 2010.

Table 11.4 Different Types of Tube-to-Tube Fittings Available

Tube-to-Tube Fitting	Key Features
LuerLok	Male and female parts are connected securely via a thread; suitable for small-volume flow rates (hose barb: 1,116–3,116 in).
Sanitary fittings	Also known as tri-clamps (TC) genderless; a clamp connects both parts and secures a gasket between them. A connection with conventional sanitary fittings made of stainless steel is also possible (hose barb: 1/4 1 in).
Quick (dis)connect fittings	Male and female parts are connected securely via a click mechanism. An O-ring fitted to the male part provides the seal. Pressing a button on the female part breaks the connection (hose barb: 3/8–1.5 in also with sanitary termination).

11.9 DISPOSABLE CONNECTORS AND TRANSFERS

Disposable components came into use first in the field of connectors and lines, as it was difficult to clean them. Unlike hard piping, the flexible tubing incorporated into disposable transfer lines does not require costly and time-consuming cleaning and validation. This allows manufacturers to quickly change process steps or convert over to a new product. This is a key advantage for multiple product facilities in which process requirements change depending on the drug being produced. Innovative manufacturers now incorporate disposable tubing assemblies throughout the bioprocess from seed trains to final fill applications (Table 11.4). Additional cost savings result from reduced labor, chemical, water, and energy demands associated with cleaning and validation.

Modern bioprocessing facilities scale up inoculum from a few million cells in several milliliters of culture to production volumes of thousands of liters. This process requires aseptic transfer at each point along the seed train. Traditional bioprocessing facilities accomplish scale up using a dedicated series of stainless-steel bioreactors linked together with valves and rigid tubing. For these systems, to prevent contamination between production runs, a CIP system is designed into each bioreactor, vessel, and piping line to remove any residual materials. These CIP and SIP systems require extensive validation testing, and the valves and piping contained in these systems can create additional validation challenges.

Advances in disposable technology allow bioprocess engineers to replace most storage vessels and fixed piping networks with disposable storage systems and tubing assemblies. Disposables eliminate the need for CIP validation for many components and reduces maintenance and capital expense by eliminating expensive vessels, valves, and sanitary piping assemblies.

While total disposable systems are not always possible, there is a transition taking place and often there is a need to connect a disposable system with stainless-steel vessels. Disposable media storage systems are routinely manufactured for volumes from 20 to 2,500 L. Media storage systems arrive at the bioprocess facility sterilized by gamma irradiation and often are fitted with integrated filters, sampling systems, and connectors. Using an SIP connector like Colder Products' Steam-Thru® Connection (www.colder.com) allows operators to make sterile connections between these presterilized disposable systems and stainless-steel bioreactors for aseptic transfer of media.

Similarly, disposable tubing assemblies may be used to transfer inoculum between bioreactors using either a peristaltic pump or headspace pressure. Such transfer lines can reduce the number of reusable valves required for transfer and eliminate problem areas for CIP and SIP validation. Terminating each presterilized transfer line with a disposable SIP connector provides sterility assurance equal to that of traditional fixed piping at lower capital costs.

As disposable bioreactors are beginning to appear, companies are using them for both seed trains and small-scale production. These systems are connected to a cell culture media storage bag (either by aseptic welding or aseptic connectors such as Colder Products' AseptiQuik®) using flexible tubing. Flexible tubing with aseptic connectors are used as transfer lines between each reactor in the process.

There are also instances when liquids are transferred from a higher ISO environment to a lower ISO environment and assurance is needed that it does not result in cross-contamination; to assure this, a conduit can be installed in the walls connecting the two areas, with the cleaner room having a higher pressure. A pre-sterilized tube is then inserted from the lower ISO class side to the higher ISO class side and connected to the vessels between which the liquid is transferred by a peristaltic pump; upon completion of transfer, the tube is pulled into higher ISO class area and discarded. This method allows connection between downstream and upstream areas without the risk of transferring any contamination to a lower ISO class area such as downstream area.

11.9.1 Tubing

Flexible tubes are an essential part of all disposable systems and are subject to the safety concerns described in an earlier chapter with regard to the leachables and extractables. Several attributes of flexible tubing require evaluation such as their heat resistance, operating temperature range, chemical resistance, color, density, shore hardness, flexibility, elasticity, surface smoothness, mechanical stability, abrasion resistance, gas permeability, visible and UV light sensitivity, composition of layers, weldability, sealability, and sterilizability by gamma radiation or in an autoclave.

All tubes used in bioprocessing conform to USP Class VI classification, U.S. FDA 21 CFR 177.2600, and EP 3A Sanitary Standard. For cGMP manufacturing these are classified as bulk pharmaceuticals. Most common materials used for the tubing include the following:

- Thermoplastic elastomer (C-Flex, PharmaPure, PharMed BPT, SaniPur 60, Advanta Flex) is pump tubing, highly biocompatible, with easy sealability and low permeability. Thermoplastic tubes like C-Flex and PharMed (both from Saint Gobain, www.biopharm.saint-gobain.com/) are particularly suitable for aseptic biopharmaceutical applications because of moldability, being free of animal components, and sterilizability (while thermoplastic, which makes sealing and welding easy). C-Flex is a unique, patented thermoplastic elastomer specifically designed to meet the critical demands of the medical, pharmaceutical, research, biotech, and diagnostics industries. C-Flex biopharmaceutical tubing has been used by many of the world's leading biotechnological and pharmaceutical processing companies for over 20 years. Each coil of C-Flex tubing is extruded to precise ID, OD, and wall dimensions. All tubing is formulated to meet the standards of the biopharmaceutical industry and is QA tested before leaving the production facility.

11.9.1.1 Thermoplastic Elastomer Tubing
11.9.1.1.1 Features/Benefits

- Complies with USP 24/NF19, Class VI, U.S. FDA and USDA standards
- Manufactured under strict GMPs
- Non-pyrogenic, non-cytotoxic, non-hemolytic
- Chemically resistant to concentrated acids and alkalis
- Significantly less permeable than silicone
- Low platelet adhesion and protein binding
- Ultra-smooth inner bore
- Superior to PVC for many applications, with significantly fewer TOC extractables
- Longer peristaltic pump life
- Heat-sealable, bondable, and formable
- Remains flexible from −50°F to 275°F
- Sterilizable by radiation, ETO, autoclave or chemicals
- Available in ADCF, clear, and opaque formulations
- Lot traceable
- Safer disposal through incineration

11.9.1.2 Pharmed BPT Tubing
11.9.1.2.1 Typical Applications

- Cell culture media and fermentation
- Diagnostic equipment
- Pharmaceutical, vaccine and botanical product production
- Pinch valves
- High-purity water
- Reagent dispensing
- Medical fluid/drug delivery
- Dialysis and cardiac bypass
- Peristaltic pump segments
- Sterile filling and dispensing systems

PharMed® BPT biocompatible tubing is ideal for use in peristaltic pumps and cell cultures. PharMed® BPT tubing is less permeable to gases and vapors than silicone tubing and is ideal for protecting sensitive cell cultures, fermentation, synthesis, separation, purification, and process monitoring and control systems. PharMed® BPT tubing has been formulated to withstand the rigors of peristaltic pumping action while providing the biocompatible fluid surface required in sensitive applications. With its superior flex life characteristics, PharMed® tubing simplifies manufacturing processes by reducing production downtime due to pump tubing failure. The excellent wear properties of PharMed® BPT translate to reduced erosion of interior tubing walls, improving overall efficiency of filtering systems.

11.9.1.3 Features/Benefits

- Outlasts silicone tubing in peristaltic pumps by up to 30 times
- Low particulate spallation

- Autoclavable and sterilizable
- Temperature resistant from −60°F to 275°F
- Withstands repeated CIP and SIP cleaning and sterilization
- Meets USP Class VI and U.S. FDA criteria

11.9.1.4 Typical Applications

- Diagnostic test product manufacturing
- CH and media process systems
- Vaccine manufacturing
- Bioreactor process lines
- Production filtration and fermentation
- Sterile filling
- Shear-sensitive fluid transfer

Platinum-cured silicon: PureFit, SMP/SBP/SVP, Tygon 3350–3370, APST; biocompatible, no leachable additives, economical
Peroxide-cured silicon: Versilic SPX; biocompatible, no leachables
Modified polyolefin: Tygon LFL (www.tygon.com); chemically resistant, flexible, long-lasting
Modified PVC: Tygon LFL, chemical resistant, long-lasting

There are new products introduced routinely and the reader is recommended to refer to current information on these products. One of the best sources to meet just about all needs for tubing is Saint-Gobain Company; one ought to consult with them first.

11.9.2 Fittings and Accessories

Connections between bags or other process stages are done by fittings which come in a wide range of configurations, materials, and sterility. This includes straight couplers, Y-couplers, T-couplers, cross couplers, elbow couplers, and barbed plugs. This is necessary to allow ready solutions to go through the often complex routines of liquids in a bioprocessing facility. The size of these connectors ranges from 1/16 to 1 in in most instances; often-incompatible sizes are downgraded or upgraded by interim connectors called reduction couplers that are available for most types of connectors.

The barbed plug is the most convenient as it can be easily patented with ties to provide a very secure connection.

The tube-to-tube fittings can serve to change the size and are available in a variety of connection options. Also available are caps to close the tube end with the connector attached to transport the components.

Clamps are used for blocking or regulating flows and come in a variety of types, the most common being the inch clamp for quick starting and stopping flow; ratchet clamps adjust the flow rates. Special clamps with mechanical power transmission such as from Biovalves (www.biouretech.com), which maintain the contact pressure via a thread arbor, are available for larger tubes with thicker walls.

The BioPure BioValves is a precision restriction flow controller and shut-off valve for silicone tube for use in bioprocessing and pharmaceutical manufacturing applications. It is

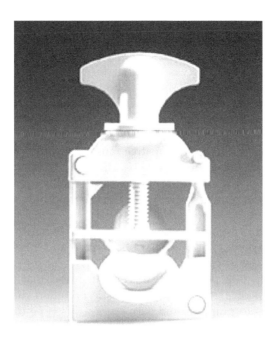

Figure 11.15 The aseptic connectors once installed cannot be disconnected to maintain patency of the process.

profiled to minimize flow path turbulence and can be used one handed. Its thread pitch is calibrated to 2 mm per turn, permitting accurate estimation of flow restriction. It is molded from glass reinforced Nylon USP Class VI. These can be repeatedly autoclaved at 134°C for 5 min or irradiated at 60 kGy (6 Mrad) with no detectable weakening (Figure 11.15).

11.9.3 Pumps

Pumps are used for fluid transfer by creating hydrostatic pressure or by differential pressure; the maximum allowed pressure would be determined by the weakest part of the bioprocess component exposed to the pressure. Peristaltic pumps, syringe pumps, and diaphragm pumps are all currently used to provide disposable pumping solutions. All of these are volume displacement pumps, are easy to use, and avoid contact with the product; they can, however, produce stress on the tubing especially when the operations are conducted for an extended period of time. It is for this reason that special peristaltic pump tubes are made available by Saint-Gobain Company. The stress on the tube may produce particles from erosion of the tube and contaminate the fluids being passed through.

High-end peristaltic dispensing pumps have benefited from improved pulsation-free pump head design, a precise drive motor, and a state-of-the-art calibration algorithm. They are exceptionally accurate at microliter fill volumes. Peristaltic pumps that incorporate disposable tubing eliminate cross-contamination and do not require cleaning because the tubing is the only part that comes into contact with the product. Likewise, the cleaning validation of peristaltic pumps with disposable tubing is significantly easier than for piston pumps. The cost of labor and supplies for writing and executing protocols, cleaning, and documenting the cleaning process is higher for a multiple use piston pump filling system. Adjusting the flow speed, and therefore preventing foaming or splashing, is easier for a peristaltic pump than for a piston pump. Operators can also use a ramp-up and ramp-down feature to determine how fast a peristaltic pump reaches its fill speed. This option helps optimize overall fill time and increase throughput.

Many biological drugs are shear-sensitive, and peristaltic pumps protect them by applying low pressure and providing gentle handling. In contrast, a piston pump's valve system generates fast flow through small orifices, potentially damaging biological products. Even valveless piston pumps apply high pressures and high shear factors that could harm a biological product.

On the other hand, viscous products can be problematic for peristaltic pumps. The pumps apply only approximately 1.3 bar of pressure, and their accuracy suffers when they handle products more viscous than 100 cP.

A diaphragm pump is a positive displacement pump that uses a combination of the reciprocating action of a rubber, thermoplastic or teflon diaphragm, and suitable non-return check valves to pump a fluid. Sometimes this type of pump is also called a membrane pump. The following are three main types of diaphragm pumps:

- Those in which the diaphragm is sealed with one side in the fluid to be pumped, and the other in air or hydraulic fluid. The diaphragm is flexed, causing the volume of the pump chamber to increase and decrease. A pair of non-return check valves prevents reverse flow of the fluid.
- Those employing volumetric positive displacement where the prime mover of the diaphragm is electromechanical, working through a crank or geared motor drive. This method flexes the diaphragm through simple mechanical action, and one side of the diaphragm is open to air.
- Those employing one or more unsealed diaphragms with the fluid to be pumped on both sides. The diaphragm(s) again are flexed, causing the volume to change.

When the volume of a chamber of either type of pump is increased (the diaphragm moving up), the pressure decreases, and fluid is drawn into the chamber. When the chamber pressure later increases from decreased volume (the diaphragm moving down), the fluid previously drawn in is forced out. Finally, the diaphragm moving up once again draws fluid into the chamber, completing the cycle. This action is similar to that of the cylinder in an internal combustion engine.

Diaphragm pumps have good suction lift characteristics, some are low pressure pumps with low flow rates, others are capable of higher flows rates, dependent on the effective working diameter of the diaphragm and its stroke length. They can handle sludges and slurries with a relatively high amount of grit and solid content. They are suitable for discharge pressure up to 1,200 bar and have good dry running characteristics. Like peristaltic pumps, they are low-shear pumps and can handle highly viscous liquids.

Mini diaphragm pumps operate using two opposing floating discs with seats that respond to the diaphragm motion. This process results in a quiet and reliable pumping action.

Higher efficiency of the pump is evident in the longer lifer of the motor pump unit. These DC motor diaphragm pumps have excellent self-priming capability and can be run dry without damage, rated to 160°F (70°C). No metal parts come in contact with materials being pumped; diaphragms and check valves are available in Viton, Santoprene, or Buna-N construction. So these mini diaphragm pumps are very chemically resistant. The mini diaphragm pumps prime within seconds of turning the pump on; prime is maintained by two check valves (one on either side). Separated from the motor, the pump body contains no machinery parts, so the pump can be in dry running condition for a short while. A built-in pressure switch inside the pump can automatically stop the pump when the pressure reaches a specified level.

The disposable diaphragm pump head must be integrated into the transfer line prior to sterilization. As the pump head is totally closed, no other part of the pump comes into contact with the fluid. After the process, the pump head is disposed of, together with the rest of the transfer line. Flow rates of 0.1–4,000 L/h can be achieved with disposable diaphragm pumps such as from Quattroflow (www.quattrowflow.com).

11.9.4 Aseptic Coupling

One of the most commonly method is to connect the tubes or components using sterile connectors under a laminar flow hood; however this is not always possible specially when the components like disposable bags are large and cannot be moved.

Some connectors require installation in a laminar hood followed by sterilization. These are called SIP connectors. Two aseptic systems go through sealing using these connectors following sterilization by autoclave, radiation, or chemical treatment. Examples of these SIP connectors are from Coler (www.coler.com) and EMD Millipore (www.millipore). The Lynx ST system from EMD Millipore comprises an integrated valve, which can be opened and closed after sterilization of the connection.

11.9.5 Aseptic Connectors

Critical to effective disposable processing operations are aseptic connection devices. Pharmaceutical manufacturers typically make about 25,000 aseptic connections each year, with some large manufacturers making as many as 100,000 aseptic connections annually

The most convenient connectors are aseptic connectors that allow aseptic connections in an open uncontrolled environment without using a laminar flow hood. Examples of these aseptic connectors include the offering from Pall, Sartorius Stedim, GE Healthcare, EMD Millipore, and Saint-Gobain. The aseptic parts on the connector side are sealed with sterile membrane filters or caps. After coupling, the sterile membrane filters must be withdrawn, and both parts have to be clamped or fixed. These connectors are secure and recommended to save time but offer an expensive choice and at times there is a limitation of sizes of tubes that can be connected. These connectors are also used as aseptic ports in bioreactors.

One of earliest entries in the field of aseptic filters was Pall Kleenpak Sterile Connector. AseptiQuik™ Connectors (www.colder.com) provide quick and easy sterile connections, even in non-sterile environments. AseptiQuik's *click-pull-twist* design enables users to transfer media easily with less risk of operator error. The connector's robust design provides reliable performance without the need for clamps, fixtures, or tube welders. Biopharmaceutical manufacturers can make sterile connections with the quality and market availability they expect from the leader in disposable connection technology.

The Opta® SFT Sterile Connector by Sartorius Stedim (www.sartorius-stedim.com) is a disposable device, composed of pre-sterilized female and male coupling body, that allows a sterile connection in biopharmaceutical manufacturing processes. The Opta® SFT-I Connector is supplied with Flexel® 3D, Flexboy® bags and transfer sets as part of integrated Sartorius Stedim Biotech Fluid Management assemblies. Opta® SFT-I is available with a 1/4, 3/8, and 1/2 in hosebarb. The Opta® SFT-D is available as individual device for end-user assembly with TPE tubing and autoclave sterilization. They are quick, easy to use, and are backed by extensive validation work as well as 100% in-house integrity testing.

Pall Corporation (www.pall.com) is expanding its line of Kleenpak™ Aseptic Connectors with two new sizes: 1/4 and 3/8 in. The new sizes enable vaccine manufacturers to apply the safety and efficiency benefits of instant aseptic connections throughout more of their disposable operations to help speed time to market and comply with GMPs. Pall revolutionized the aseptic connection process by shortening the time needed for connection from 15 minutes to seconds when it introduced its 1/2 in Kleenpak Connector. The addition of the two new Kleenpak Connector sizes increases flexibility to implement aseptic connections in more applications to improve disposable processing efficiency. This is especially important to complex vaccine production, which often requires a greater number of connection steps. The Kleenpak Connector is easy-to-use and projects an audible snap to signify that a sterile connection has been established.

ReadyMate Disposable Aseptic Connector (DAC) from GE Healthcare (www.gelifesciences.com) provides connections for high-fluid throughput and offers a secure, simple, and economical connection for upstream and downstream applications. DAC connectors can be autoclaved or gamma radiated, and can be part of a sterile circuit. The connectors can be used to connect unit operations and assemblies. DAC connectors and their components are manufactured in compliance with the cGMPs of the U.S. FDA and ISO 9000-2000. ReadyMate is a genderless, inter-size connectable disposable aseptic connector. There are four hose barb sizes (3/4, 1/2, 3/8, and 1/4 in), mini TC, and TC that all interphase. It has a genderless design, user-friendly sanitary coupling, easy to use with Tip'n'latch, complies with USP Class VI, and can be sterilized by radiation or autoclave. The main advantages of using the Bio Quate connector include simple set-up, rapid connection, direct connection of different tube sizes, direct connection of different tube materials, aseptic on-site manifold fabrication, large and smooth inside bore, no capital equipment to purchase, and no requirement for power or calibration or service. These connectors are supplied by Bioquate (www.bioquate.com) (Figure 11.16).

11.9.6 Welding

When it is possible to use a thermoplastic tube, welding offers an easy, inexpensive, and very secure solution. Examples of thermoplastic tubes include C-Flex, PharMed, and Bioprene. Both thermoplastic tubes must be aseptic, should have the same dimensions (inner diameter and OD), and should have their ends capped. The tubes are place parallel in opposite directions while a heated blade cuts through them and seals them

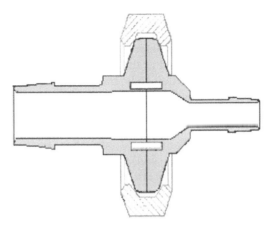

Figure 11.16 CellReady Bioreactor. (Data from www.theraproteins.com.)

simultaneously. Preheating of the blade is necessary both to achieve the welding tempera-ture and to sterilize and depyrogenize the blade itself prior to the welding process. The depyrogenize procedure normally lasts 30 s at 250°C or 3 s at 320°C. After being cut, the tubes are moved against each other so that the ends of each tube, which are con-nected to the aseptic systems, are positioned directly opposite each other on either side of the blade. A welding cycle can be between 1 and 4 min, depending on the material and the diameter of the tubes. The main welding systems available today include Sterile Tube Fuser (GE Healthcare), BioWelder (Sartorius Stedim), Aseptic Sterile Welder 3960 (SEBRA, www.Sebra.com), TSCD (Terumo, www.terumotransfusion.com), and SCD 11B (Terumo). (Terumo supplies its equipment mainly to blood transfusion industry.) Both GE Healthcare and Sartorius Stedim lead the installations in the bioprocessing industry.

The Hot Lips Tube Sealer by GE Healthcare is a portable device used to thermally seal thermoplastic tubing for the transport and setup of inoculums, culture, media, and buffers. The seal forms a tamperproof and leakproof closure. Preprogrammed for a wide range of tubing types, diameters, and wall thicknesses, a single button initiates the sealing opera-tion. The instrument is self-calibrating and a microprocessor-controlled motor ensures repeatable performance without the need for tubing adaptors.

The Sterile Tube Fuser also from GE Healthcare is an automated device for welding together a wide range of tubing types intended for aseptic operation. Operated via a single push-button operator interface, it connects tubing between sterile containers, Cellbag bioreactors, and process equipment for the aseptic transfer of large volumes of fluids such as inoculum, media, buffers, and process intermediates.

11.9.7 Aseptic Transfer Systems

Moving product across clean rooms may involve, at times, long distances; while transfer tubings between upstream and downstream areas and pass through autoclaves are common, larger volumes transfer systems are offered by Sartorius Stedim, ATMI Life Sciences,

Getinge, and LaCalhene, which essentially constitute double-door systems using disposable containers. In using these systems, the main, reusable port is always permanently fixed in the separating wall (in a clean room or isolator) and represents the containment barrier. The second connecting part is an integral part of the disposable container, which stores or conducts the components, fluids, and powders to be transferred. Both the connecting parts and the reusable containers and transfer systems can be coupled to the main port. After coupling, the ports are opened from inside the cleaner area and the transfer is started. The disposable container is normally the package for the fluid and the sterile barrier for the fluid conduction.

Biosafe® Aseptic Transfer Equipment: the Biosafe® range of aseptic transfer ports offers reliable and easy-to-use solutions for the secure transfer of components, fluids, and powders while maintaining the integrity of the critical areas (such as isolators, RABS, and clean rooms).

Biosafe® Aseptic Transfer Disposable Bag: a complete range of Biosafe® Aseptic Transfer Bags, either gamma sterile or autoclavable, and the Biosafe® RAFT System are designed to best fit requirements for aseptic transfer of components into clean rooms, isolators, or RABS and for contained transfer of potent powders.

Biosafe® RAFT System: the Biosafe® Rapid Aseptic Fluid Transfer (RAFT) system provides easy-to-use and reliable through-the-wall aseptic transfer of liquid between clean rooms of different environmental classification while ensuring a total confinement.

SART™ System: the SART System™ is designed to allow aseptic liquid transfer between two areas with different containment classifications.

Special bags have therefore been developed, for example, the Biosafe RAFT system by Sartorius Stedim, allowing aseptic coupling to larger fluid containers and ports in addition to fluid conduction.

11.9.8 Tube Sealers

When disconnecting an aseptic connection, the ends must be capped with aseptic caps and this can be done under a laminar hood or by using tube sealers, the examples of which include offerings from PDC (www.pdcbiz.com), Saint-Gobain (www.saint-gobain. com), Sartorius Stedim (www.sartorius-stedim.com), GE Healthcare (www.gelifesciences. com), Terumo (www.terumotransfusion.com), and SEBRA (www.sebra.com). Most of these sealers can seal from 0.25 to about 1.5 in tubes and take from 1–4 min to complete the seal. Most operate on electrical heating element but electrical and radio frequencies are also used for sealing tubes. There is no need for using a laminar flow hood for these operations. In most instances, applying a crimper in two places and cutting the tube between the crimps offers the cheapest solution.

11.9.9 Sampling

Sampling is a routine during manufacturing to assure compliance by obtaining these in process parameters like pH, DO, OD, pCO_2, and so on. Most disposable systems have one or more integrated sampling lines, which are partly equipped with special sampling valves, sampling manifolds, or special sampling systems. A popular disposable sample valve is the Clave connector from ICU-Medical (www.icumed.com), which is also used in intravascular catheters for medical applications. It allows a sample to be taken with a

LuerLok syringe. A dynamic seal inside the valve guarantees that the sample is not taken until the syringe is connected, thereby ensuring the sample only comes in contact with the inner, aseptic parts of the valve. However, the samples drawn do not remain sterile.

Manifolds consisting of sampling bags, sampling flasks, or syringes are appropriate for taking aseptic samples in disposable systems. These manifolds can be connected to the systems via aseptic connectors or tube welding. Sampling manifolds allow multiple sampling for quality purposes over a given period of time. The main feature of the manifold is that the number of manipulations in a process is significantly reduced. The manifold systems are delivered ready for process use, preassembled, and sterile. Only one connection has to be made to allow several bags to be filled.

Also used for sampling are manifold systems where sample containers of a manifold are arranged in parallel whereby the last one is used as a waste container. Through using Y-, T-, or X-hose barbs and tube clamps, the initial flow and the subsequent sample are guided to the appropriate containers. SIP connections, of course, also allow the connection of manifold systems to conventional stainless-steel processing equipment.

11.9.10 Conclusion

The complexity of bioprocessing makes it difficult to design systems that have any weak links; contamination is indeed the most significant risk that requires that all connectors, tubing, and implements to join various steps of a process and perform sampling remain patent. Disposable connectors and tubing were one of the first components that went disposable. Still, in hard-walled systems, SIP systems are in use only because there is steam for CIP/SIP operations. Even then, the risk of contamination remains. Since much of the disposable technology in these applications has come from the biomedical field, the device industry had always been ahead of the regulatory requirements. Biocompatibility issues have long been resolved and vendors are able to provide detailed information on their devices that might be needed by regulatory agencies. Since the manufacturing of these devices is complex, it is unlikely for a user to request custom devices; however, the diversity of choices available today are enough to modify any system that would be able to use an off the shelf item. As before, the emphasis on the important of off-the-shelf item over custom designs remains.

The tube connectors and sealers are a newer entry as disposable bags for mixing and bioreactors have becoming more popular; still, there is a limited choice of suppliers, mainly GE and Sartorius Stedim. The cost of this equipment is still high but then the alternative comes down to using expensive aseptic connectors. Generally, if a good choice of aseptic connectors is available, that should be preferred over tube connectors since it is always possible to make a poor connection using the heat-activated systems; also, the use of aseptic connectors allows connecting tubes that may not be thermolabile.

11.10 DISPOSABLE CONTROL AND MONITORING SYSTEMS

According to the U.S. FDA Guidance for Industry, PAT is intended to support innovation and efficiency in pharmaceutical development. PAT is a system for designing, analyzing, and controlling manufacturing through timely measurements (i.e., during processing) of critical quality and performance attributes of raw and in-process materials and processes with the goal of ensuring final product quality. It is important to note that the term analytical in PAT is viewed broadly to include chemical, physical, microbiological, mathematical, and risk analyses conducted in an integrated manner.

To fulfill process requirements, single-use sensors, which are either integrated in the single-use bioreactor or included in the cover and are disposed of with the bioreactor, are required. They provide a continuous signal and allow information about the status of the cell culture to be gathered at any time. The traditional batch analysis, such as HPLC, electrochemistry, and wet chemical analysis in place of disposable sensors increase the risk of contamination.

Since disposable bioreactors are new to the industry, the first attempt to monitor the product in the bioreactor was to use the traditional biosensors used in hard-walled systems to measure bioreactor temperature, DO, pH, conductivity, and osmolality. These probes must first be sterilized (via autoclaving) and then attached to penetration adapter fittings that are welded into bioreactor bags. Not surprisingly, this is a labor-intensive and time-consuming process that has the potential to compromise the integrity and sterility of single-use bioreactor bags, and has been largely discarded in favor of truly disposable sensors. Critical process parameters that are often monitored include pressure, pH, DO, conductivity, UV absorbance, flow, and turbidity. The packages that contain the traditional technologies for monitoring these parameters are not usually compatible with or effective when integrated into single-use assemblies for many reasons: cost, cross contamination, inability to maintain a closed system, and system incompatibility with gamma irradiation.

The practice of integrating bags, tubing, and filters into preassembled, ready-to-use bioprocess solutions is optimized if noninvasive sensing of critical process parameters is part of the package instead of using sensors that may require sterilization and cleaning validation, the core processes which are obviated in the use of disposable bioreactors.

Even though these obstacles do not always preclude the use of traditional measurement technologies, single-use solutions for monitoring process parameters eliminate the need for equipment cleaning and autoclaving small parts, reduce the risk and cost involved with making process connections, and may be more cost effective than tracking and maintaining traditional technologies. For example, a sanitary, autoclavable pressure transducer that is qualified for a certain number of autoclave cycles and requires recalibration may be more expensive to use versus a single-use pressure sensor.

The adoption of disposable sensors requires a keen understanding of their need and utilization. Their suitability would be determined by their material properties, sensor manufacturing, process compatibility, performance requirements, control system integration, compatibility with treatments before use, and regulatory requirements.

Several companies, including Finesse and Fluorometrix (recently acquired by Sartorius Stedim), have created single-use, membrane biosensors that can be added to or directly incorporated (during manufacturing) into single-use bioreactor bags.

There are two options in using disposable sensors: one where the sensors are placed in situ in contact with the liquid, and the other where the external sensors contact the medium either optically (ex situ) or via a sterile (and disposable) sample removal system (online). Disposable sensors must be sterilizable if they come in contact with media, these must also be cost-effective and reliable. Better designs use inexpensive sensing elements can be located inside a disposable bioreactor and combined with reusable (and more expensive) analytical equipment outside the reactor. Inexpensive, single-use sensors can also be placed on transistors and placed either in the headspace, inlet, outlet, or into the cultivation broth for liquid-phase analysis (temperature, pH, pO2). These can also be optical sensors, which allow noninvasive monitoring through a transparent window.

11.10.1 Sampling Systems

Continuous sampling from a bioreactor can be accomplished using a sterile filter and a peristaltic pump to obtain cell-free sample and where the dead volume of sample is of concern (as in smaller bioreactors), microfiltration (MF) membranes can be used which may be placed inside the bioreactor; disposable forms of these are not yet available. Suppliers include TraceBiotech (www.trace.de) and Groton (www.grotonbiosystems.com) (Figure 11.17).

11.10.1.1 TRACE System

Where removing cells proves cumbersome, the samples may be treated to stop their metabolic activity by freezing or using inactivation chemicals.

One way to solve the sampling problem is to use a presterilized sampling container, including a needleless syringe that can be welded to the sampling module of

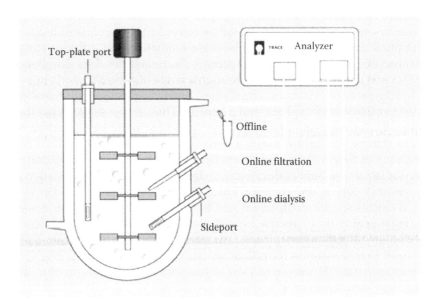

Figure 11.17 Groton BioSystems sampling method. (Data from www.theraproteins.com.)

the bag bioreactor. A sample is pumped into the container, the sampling containers can be removed, and the tube heat-sealed. Sartorius and GE use this method. Other fully sampling systems involve connecting to a bioreactor a presterilized Luer connection including a one-way valve to prevent the sample from flowing back into the reactor. The sample is withdrawn from the reactor by a syringe and directed through a sample line into a reservoir. Cellexus Biosystems (Cambridgeshire, UK) and Millipore (Billerica, MA) use this approach.

The Cellexus system is connected to the sample line are there are up to six sealed sample pouches. The sample from the reservoir can then be pushed into the pouches that are subsequently separated by a mechanical sealer resulting in sealed, sterile samples.

The proprietary Millipore system comprises a port insert that can be fitted to several bioreactor side ports and a number of flexible conduits that can be opened and closed individually for sampling and are connected to flexible, disposable sampling containers. Sampling is limited to the number of available conduits in each module.

These sampling systems allow aseptic sampling but are limited by the number of samples taken per module and the lack of automation. And while these methods come with good validation data, the risk of contamination cannot be removed since the bioreactor is indeed breached every time a sample is withdrawn. There is a need to develop other methods that will not require contact with media.

11.10.2 Optical Sensors

Optical sensors work on the principle of the effect of electromagnetic waves on molecules. It is an entirely noninvasive method and can provide continuous results of many parameters at the same time. It is relatively easy to use them through a transparent window in the bioreactors. The detector part of the system can be physically separated, allowing utilization of expensive analytical devices allowing optical sensors to be used in situ or online.

Fluorescence sensors can be optimized for measurements of nicotinamide adenine dinucleotide phosphate and are used for both biomass estimation and differentiating between aerobic and anaerobic metabolism. The 2D process fluorometry enables simultaneous measurement of several analytes by scanning through a range of excitation and emission wavelengths including proteins, vitamins, coenzymes, biomass, glucose, and metabolites such as ethanol, adenosine-5′-triphosphate, and pyruvate. Thus, it is possible to use fluorometry to characterize the fermentation process. Generally, a fiber optic light attached to the bioprocessor and shining the light through a glass window in the bioprocessor works very well. An example of this is the fluorometers from BioView system (www.delta.dk). The BioView sensor is a multichannel fluorescence detection system for application in the biotechnology, pharmaceutical, and chemical industries; food production; and environmental monitoring. It detects specific compounds and the state of microorganisms as well as their chemical environment without interfering with the sample. The BioView system measures fluorescence online directly in the process. An interference with the sample is eliminated. There is no need to take samples for offline analysis, which saves manpower and reduces the risk of contamination. However, in view of the complexity of spectra of multiple components, high-level resolution programming is required.

Finesse Solutions, LLC (www.fiesse.com), a manufacturer of measurement and control solutions for life sciences process applications, announced a live demonstration of its new

SmartBag product for rocker bioreactors at Interphex 2011 in New York, March 29–31. SmartBags are designed to be plug-and-play bio-processing containers having full measurement capability for at least 21 days.

The SmartBag SensorPak leverages TruFluor pH and DO phase fluorometric technology in a compact assembly that is pre-calibrated using a SmartChip and provides accurate, drift-free, in-situ measurements. The combined pH and DO optical reader uses advanced optical components including a large area photodiode that minimizes photodegradation of the active sensing elements. The SensorPak also leverages TruFluor temperature 316L stainless-steel thermal window for highly stable readings. The SensorPak is welded into the single-use vessel and eliminates the need for sterile connectors and their associated complications such as leakage and batch contamination. All wetted materials of the SensorPak are USP class VI compliant and, being identical to TruFluor, allow directly measurement comparisons and scale up from 10 L rocker bags to 2,000 L SUBs.

The biosensors manufactured by Fluorometrix are non-invasive, membrane sensors developed using optical fluorometric chemistries that can be directly incorporated into any disposable bioreactor bags. Because the sensors can be manufactured into any type of single-use bag, they are useful for both upstream and downstream applications. Also, these are compatible with the U.S. FDA's PAT initiative.

Many metabolic products in a bioreactor can be readily detected by IR spectroscopy but water-absorbed IR beam can only be NIR or SIR for biomass analysis when using in transmission mode. However, attenuated total reflectance spectroscopy (ATRIR) is based on the reflection of light at an interface of two phases with different indices of refraction, the light beam penetrates into the medium with the lower refraction index in the dimension of one wavelength. Absorption of IR results in decrease in the intensity of the reflected beam to detect the analyte. Probes for both types of IR spectroscopy are used. Hitec-Zang (www.hitec-zang.de) offers a large range of PAT devices including IR systems.

NIR transmission probes and ATR-IR probes for bioreactors are now commercially available. These are connected through silver halide fibers or radio-frequency connectors.

In addition to IR and fluorescence, optical methods based on photoluminescence, reflection and absorption are also used. The optical electrodes or *optodes* can be attached using glass fibers leaving the measurement equipment outside of the bioreactor as discussed above for fluorescence detectors allowing use of these chemosensors in situ or online.

Oxygen sensors work by quenching fluorescence by molecular oxygen; measurement requires a fluorescent dye (metal complexes) immobilized and attached to one end of an optical fiber, and the other end of the fiber is interfaced with an excitation light source. The duration and strength of fluorescence depend on the oxygen concentration in the environment around the dye. The emitted fluorescence light is collected and transmitted for reading outside of the bioreactor. These electrodes work better than the traditional platinum probe electrodes to detect oxygen, working in both liquid and gas phases. Examples of oxygen sensors include PreSens (www.presens.de) non-invasive oxygen sensors that measure the partial pressure of both dissolved and gaseous oxygen. These sensor spots are used for glassware and disposables. The sensor spots are fixed on the inner surface of the glass or transparent plastic material. The oxygen concentration can therefore be measured in a non-invasive and non-destructive manner from outside, through the wall of the vessel. Different coatings for different concentration ranges are available. It offers online monitoring of concentration ranges from 1 ppb up to 45 ppm DO, with dependence on flow velocity and measuring oxygen in gas phase as well; these can be autoclaved.

Ocean Optics (www.oceanoptics.com) offers world's first miniature spectrometer with a wide array of sensors for oxygen, pH, and in the gas phase.

The pH sensors work by fluorescence or absorption, and for fiber-optic pH measurements, both fluorescence-and absorbance-based pH indicators can be applied. For fluorescence, the most common dyes are 8-hydroxy1,3,6-pyrene trisulfonic acid and fluorescein derivatives; while phenol red and cresol red are used for absorption type measurements. Fluorescent dyes are sensitive to ionic strength limiting their use for broad pH measurement, more than 3 units.

The new Transmissive pH Probes from Ocean Optics use a proprietary sol-gel formulation infused with a colorimetric pH indicator dye. This material is coated onto the exclusive patches to reflect light back through the central read fiber or to transmit light through in order to sense the color change of the patch at a specific wavelength. While typical optical pH sensors are susceptible to drastic changes in performance in various ionic strength solutions, Ocean Optics' sensory layer has been chemically modified (esterified) to allow accurate sensing in both high and low salinity samples. The Transmissive pH Probes from Ocean Optics can be used with a desktop system as well as with the Jaz handheld spectrometer suite. The desktop system uses a module is SpectraSuite software that allows for simplified calibration, convenient pH readings, customizable data logging, and comprehensive exportation of data and calibration information.

- Proprietary organically modified sol-gel formulation engineered to maximize immunity to ionic strength sensitivity
- Compatible with some organic solvents (acetone, alcohols, aromatics, etc.)
- Sol-gel material chosen over typical polymer method, allowing for faster response time, versatility in the desired dopants, greater chemical compatibility, flexible coating and enhanced thermal and optical performance
- Indicator molecule allows high-resolution measurement in biological range (pH 5–9)
- Simplified algorithm takes analytical and baseline wavelengths into account to reduce errors caused by optical shifts

The TruFluor™ (www.finesse.com) DO and temperature sensor is a single-use solution consisting of a disposable sheath, an optical reader, and a transmitter. The single-use sheath can be pre-inserted in a disposable bioreactor bag port and irradiated with the bag, in order to both preserve and guarantee the sterile barrier. All wetted materials of the sheath are USP class VI compliant. The optical reader utilizes an LED and a large area photodiode with integrated optical filtering, that minimizes photodegradation of the acting sensing element. The design has been optimized to provide accurate in-situ measurement of DO using phase fluorometric detection in real time. The temperature measurement leverages a 316L stainless-steel thermal window embedded in the sheath, and provides a highly accurate temperature measurement that can be used as a process variable or for temperature compensation.

Carbon dioxide sensors work on the principle of measure pH of a carbonate buffer embedded in a CO_2-permeable membrane. The reaction time of the sensors is long and use of quarternary ammonium hydroxide has been made to achieve a faster response. Fluorescence-based sensors are attractive as they facilitate the development of portable and low-cost systems that can be easily deployed outside the laboratory environment. The sensor developed for this work exploits a pH fluorescent dye 1-hydroxypyrene-3,6,8-trisulfonic acid, ion-paired with cetyltrimethylammonium bromide (HPTS-IP), which has been entrapped in a hybrid sol-gel-based matrix derived from *n*-propyltriethoxysilane along with the liphophilic organic base. The probe design involves the use of dual-LED excitation in order to facilitate ratiometric operation and uses a silicon PIN photodiode. HPTS-IP exhibits two pH-dependent changes in excitation bands, which allows for dual excitation ratiometric detection as an indirect measure of the pCO_2. Such measurements are insensitive to changes in dye concentration, leaching and photobleaching of the fluorophore and instrument fluctuations unlike unreferenced fluorescence intensity measurements. The performance of the sensor system is characterized by a high degree of repeatability, reversibility, and stability.

The YSI 8500 CO_2 monitor measures dissolved carbon dioxide in bioprocess development applications. Engineered to fit within a variety of bioreactors, the unit delivers precise, real-time data that increase an understanding of critical fermentation and cell culture processes. This data can help in gaining insight into cell metabolism, cell culture productivity, and other changes within bioreactors.

An in situ monitor based on the reliable optochemical technology was developed by Tufts University and YSI Incorporated (www.ysilifesciences.com). The technology involves the use of a CO_2 sensor capsule consisting of a small reservoir of bicarbonate buffer covered by a gas permeable silicone membrane. The buffer contains hydroxypyrene trisulfonic acid (HPTS), a pH-sensitive fluorescent dye. CO_2 diffuses through the membrane into the buffer, changing its pH. As the pH changes, the fluorescence of the dye changes. The model 8500 monitor compares the fluorescence of the dye at two different wavelengths to determine the CO_2 concentration of the sample medium. The sensor can be autoclaved multiple times. It will measure dissolved CO_2 over the range of 1% to 25%, with an accuracy of 5% of the reading, or 0.2% absolute. Previously, CO_2 was measured either in the exit gases from the fermentation process or by taking a manual sample. The new optical-chemical technology uses a fiber-optic cable transfer light through a stainless-steel probe into a disposable sensor capsule, which contains a pH sensitive dye. The dissolved CO_2 diffuses through a polymer membrane to change the color of the dye which is then relayed by fiber optic cable back to a rack-mounted monitor which determines and displays the dissolved CO_2 level.

11.10.3 Biomass Sensors

Information about the biomass concentration can also be obtained via turbidity sensors. Generally, these sensors are based on the principle of scattered light. Most turbidity sensors have the disadvantage that there is only a linear correlation for low particle concentrations. But sensors that use backscattering light (180°) also have linear properties for high particle concentrations. A window that is translucent for the desired wavelength in the IR region is necessary for the use in disposable reactors. The S3 Mini-Remote Futura line of biomass detectors (www.applikonbio.com) make it possible to incorporate sensors inside disposable bioreactors. This system incorporates an ultra lightweight pre-amplifier for connecting to the ABER disposable probe. The main Futura housing can be mounted away from the single-use bioreactor vessel. Cells with intact plasma membranes in a fermenter can be considered to act as tiny capacitors under the influence of an electric field. The non-conducting nature of the plasma membrane allows a buildup of charge. The resulting capacitance can be measured: it is dependent upon the cell type and is directly proportional to the membrane bound volume of these viable cells. *The choice of* in situ steam sterilizable probes includes a single use, sterilizable flow through cell.

11.10.4 Electrochemical Sensors

Electrochemical sensors include potentiometric, conductometric, and voltammetric sensors. Thick- and thin-film sensors, as well as chemically-sensitive field-effect transistors (ChemFETs), possess potential as potentiometric disposable sensors in bioprocess control because they can be produced inexpensively and in large quantities.

Many pH sensing systems rely on amperometric methods but they require constant calibration due to instability or drift. The setups of most amperometric sensors are based on the pH-dependent selectivity of membranes or films on the electrode surface.

While turbidity sensors detect the total amount of biomass concentration, capacitance sensors provide information specifically about the viable cell mass. The electrical properties of cells in an alternating electrical field are generally characterized by an electrical capacitance and conductance. The integrity of the cell membrane exerts a significant influence on the electrical impedance, so that only viable cells can be estimated. The Biodis Series for monitoring viable biomass in disposables applications is available from Fogale (www.fogalebiotech.com) and Aber (www.aberinstruments.com), the latter now offers an integrated version with DASGIP (www.dasgip.de). The new Aber Futura Biomass Monitor has been designed so that multiple units can easily be incorporated into bioreactor controllers and SCADA systems.

The sensor CITSens Bio (http://www.c-cit.ch/) can monitor the consumption of glucose and/or the production of l-lactate during cultivation. The CITSens Bio utilizes an enzymatic oxidation process and electron transfer from glucose or lactate to the electrode (anode) via a chemical wiring process, which is catalyzed by an enzyme specific for ~-d-glucose or l-lactate and a mediator. The sensor function is therefore not affected by oxygen concentration and produces an exceptionally low concentration of side products, such as peroxide. The working principle of this sensor is in contrast to that of a number of well-known alternatives currently on the market, which depend on a sufficient supply of oxygen for their operation as they measure the hydrogen peroxide produced during the bioprocess. The principal feature of the CITSens Bio is a miniaturized, screen-printed electrode comprising a three-electrode system for amperometric detection of the current transmitted to the anode (working, counter, and reference electrode). This three-electrode system ensures a reliable electrical signal with long-term stability. The chemical components, including the enzyme, are deposited onto the active field of the working electrode, and the enzyme is cross-linked to form protein and hence is immobilized in this network. The immobilization process itself has an antimicrobial effect. A dialysis membrane is cast over the sensing head to create a barrier between the sensor and the cultivation medium.

11.10.5 Pressure Sensors

Another important process parameter that is frequently monitored during bioprocess unit operations like filtration, chromatography, and many others is pressure. Using a traditional stainless-steel pressure gauge in conjunction with a disposable experimental setup is possible, but has the drawback that the pressure gauge has to be sterilized separately. Furthermore, the connection of the sensor to the previously gamma-radiated disposable assembly can be problematic.

Many bioprocess unit operations are either controlled based on pressure or have significant pressure-related safety issues. Traditional stainless-steel reactors are monitored and controlled for pressure, as pressure is used as a means of influencing mass transfer and preventing contamination. In addition, a high-pressure event is a potentially hazardous situation. Single-use bioreactor systems, on the other hand, are frequently not monitored or controlled for pressure because stainless-steel pressure transducers are not compatible or cost effective when applied to disposable bioreactors. As a result, a clogged vent filter on a bioreactor can easily rupture bags, spilling the contents of the reactor and exposing the operators to unprocessed bulk.

Another application where pressure monitoring is central to process performance is depth and sterile filtration. A filter's capacity is primarily measured by either flow decay or pressure increases, although adding reusable traditional pressure transducers to a process train defeats the purpose of a single-use process set-up. Depending on the process application, the product contact surface of a traditional device requires either sanitization or moist heat sterilization.

There are traditional devices that are compatible with SIP, where only the product contact surface is exposed to steam, and even devices that can be placed in an autoclave where the entire device is exposed to steam. Many single-use process components, however, are not compatible with moist heat sterilization temperatures so there may be a requirement for separate sterilization of the stainless-steel device and possibly less than optimal connection to a pre-sterilized disposable assembly.

Single-use pressure sensing allows for rapid changeover of product contact parts in both development applications and especially in early phase clinical manufacture. For example, single-use pressure sensors from PendoTECH were designed to enable pressure measurement with single-use assemblies that have flexible tubing as the fluid path. These single-use pressure sensors are gamma compatible (up to 50 KGy), and the fluid-path materials meet USP class VI guidelines and are also compliant with EMEA 410 Rev 2 guidelines.

On a single-use bioreactor, a sensor can be installed on a vent line to measure headspace pressure. Even though the sensors are qualified for use up to 75 psi, the core sensor is accurate in the low-pressure range required for a single-use bioreactor.

A better solution with respect to ease of operation and compatibility are disposable pressure sensors, which are now available on the market. The single-use sensors from PendoTECH (www.pendotech.com) can be used with tubing of various sizes (0.25 to 1 in in diameter) and can be gamma radiated with tubing and bag assemblies. They are the alternative low-cost solution for use with tubing and bioprocess containers to the existing stainless-steel pressure sensors on the market. Available in caustic-resistant polysulfone so they can be in-line during caustic sanitization processes. The pressure sensors can be integrated for pressure measurement and control with a PressureMAT™ System (monitor/transmitter) or PendoTECH Process Control System and depending on the number of sensors and process requirements. The data collected by these systems can be output to a PC or another data monitoring device. They also can be integrated into other pre-qualified third party pumps and monitors (adapters for phone jacks can be made). The pressure sensors are very accurate in the pressure ranges typically used with flexible tubing and disposable process containers and are qualified for use to 75 psi. Applications include multistage depth filtration, TFF/cross-flow filtration, and bioreactor pressure monitoring.

NovaSensor's NPC-100 (www.ge-mcs.com) pressure sensor is specifically designed for use in disposable medical applications. The device is compensated and calibrated per the Association for the Advancement of Medical Instrumentation (AAMI) guidelines for industry acceptability. The sensor integrates a high-performance, pressure sensor die with temperature compensation circuitry and gel protection in a small, low-cost package.

The SciPres (www.scilog.com) combines pressure sensing capabilities and the convenience of disposability with easy setup. Each sensor is preprogrammed and barcoded with a unique ID for easy traceability and data documentation when combined with the SciLog SciDoc software. Factory calibration data is also stored on each sensor's chip for out-of-box, plug-and-play use. The SciPres comes in 5 different sizes to fit a variety of tubing sizes: Luer, 3/8″ barb, 1/2″ barb, 3/4″ TC (Tri-Clover), and 1.0″ TC (Tri-Clover).

The SciCon combines temperature sensing capabilities with conductivity sensing capabilities in a compact, disposable, single-use package at a low price point. Like the SciPres, each sensor is pre-programmed and barcoded with a unique ID for easy traceability and data documentation when combined with the SciLog SciDoc software, and factory calibration data is also stored on each sensor's chip for out-of-box, plug-and-play use. The SciCon comes in 5 different sizes to fit a variety of tubing sizes: Luer, 3/8″ barb, 1/2″ barb, 3/4″ TC (Tri-Clover), and 1.0″ TC (Tri-Clover).

11.10.6 Conclusions

The need to monitor the characteristics of a biomass goes across many industries and most notably in the fermentation industry such as wine-making, a method of online and in situ monitoring of just about every function that is needed to perform a full PAT work is available. In recent years, there have been significant breakthroughs in the technologies available for monitoring, including fluorescence, dye-base pH, and oxygen measurements. While most of the sensors were initially developed for the hard-walled bioreactor industry, the disposable versions of these sensors are appearing almost every day. The basic principle is that if a sensor is placed inside the bioreactor vessel, it should be sterile and preferably disposable; the cost of throwing away a sensor has come down significantly and it is now possible to readily monitor just about every function including cell mass, both total and live, using these disposable sensors. Alternately, many methods are available that work from outside of the bioreactor entirely, particularly those involving fluorescence and optical measurements.

It is anticipated that within the next five years as disposable bioreactors begin to replace large hard-walled systems, much improved systems will become available, especially those consolidating several monitoring functions into one.

11.11 DOWNSTREAM PROCESSING

The adoption of disposable components in downstream bioprocessing has been an evolutionary process with a few revolutionary peaks here and there. It started with buffer bags and devices for normal flow filtration, including virus filtration and guard filters for chromatographic columns, but gradually, more complex concepts have been introduced, including disposable devices for tangential flow filtration and chromatography in the downstream processing. Today, the consensus of the industry is that while many of the upstream operations can be converted to fully disposable systems, at least some elements of downstream processing will remain traditional and the reasons quoted for this assertion is that columns and resins will always be too expensive to throw away and, since columns can be of very large size, it will be difficult to find a suitable disposable substitution.

However, as history tells, these were the same arguments presented just 15 years ago opposing the conversion of bioreactors to disposable devices. Today, the downstream processing science is developing more rapidly than the upstream science; more recently, the use of membrane adsorbes has been recommended for large-scale purification of antibodies. These membranes are much cheaper than the classical resins.

For cell harvesting and debris removal, disposable filtration systems are available. Benefits include the ease of scale up and the availability of presterilized filter capsules that can be integrated directly into production lines. Though this stage is generally completed by centrifugation or lenticular filtration, the Millipore's Pod systems provide the first available alternative in disposable lenticular filters. This combines two distinct separation technologies in an adsorptive depth filter to enhance filter capacity and retention, while compressing multiple filtration steps into one efficient operation. Scale up is achieved by inserting multiple pods into a holder, with formats allowing 1–5 or 5–30 pods as required. Further disposable depth filter formats include the Stax-System from Pall Life Science, encapsulated Zeta Plus from Cuno, and the L-Drum from Sartorius Stedim.

The next step is cross-flow filtration to reduce the volume but the buildup of debris extends the time for filtration and while this process is not a sterile process, use of disposable filter prevents the problem of cross contamination.

For capturing and PO, a steel column is packed with a resin (stationary phase) comprising porous beads made of a polysaccharide, mineral, or synthetic matrix conjugated to specific functional groups exploiting different separative principles. The protein mixed with other components is loaded onto the column slowly and once it is bound to resin, the resin is eluted with appropriate pH and electrolyte solutions to separate the target protein from the mixture. The resin is cleaned and sanitized for repeated use that may involve dozens or perhaps hundreds of cycles. To overcome the time needed to pack resin and operate a column, several companies now offer columns such as GE's ReadyToProcess systems for use in AKTA machines. GE offers a wide range of resins and offer custom resins as well. These are high performance bioprocessing columns that come prepacked, prequalified, and presanitized. Designed for seamless scalability, delivering the same performance level as available in conventional processing columns such as AxiChrom™ and BPG™. Currently available with a range of BioProcess™ media in four different sizes, 1, 2.5, 10, and 20 L, these are designed for purification of biopharmaceuticals for clinical phase I and II studies. Depending on the scale of operations, they can also be used for full-scale manufacturing, as well as for preclinical studies. The columns can be used in a wide range of chromatographic applications for separation of various compounds such as proteins, endotoxins, DNA, plasmids, vaccines, and viruses.

Atoll offers the MediaScout MaxiChrom columns (www.atoll-bio.com), which are disposable and totally incinerable; they come packed with Amberlite XAD-4 as disposable item for removal of detergents after VI during production in completely incinerable columns, packed separation media for VR during production in completely incinerable columns, packed separation media for virus validation experiments during registration of a separation scheme in completely incinerable columns. MediaScout® MaxiChrom 100-X columns (X = 50 − 300 mm) are professionally packed with any resin or chromatography media chosen by the user, preferably with materials of particle size larger than 50 μm. They are individually flow-packed to take account of the varying compressibility of each resin. Bed heights are fixed to an accuracy of ±1 mm. MaxiChrom 100-X chromatography columns are designed for preparative applications and/or scale-up development work. The column hardware is fully incinerable, which makes the columns particularly useful for single use in bio-pharmaceutical production.

11.11.1 Case of Monoclonal Antibodies, a GE Report

To reduce costs and shorten time to market, the use of plug and play technology is increasing in process development as well as in later-stage production, the following study was conducted by GE and compared with their standard XK columns which can run all media types.

> ReadyToProcess™ columns are prepacked, prequalified, and presanitized columns ready for direct use. In this study, the performance of ReadyToProcess columns prepacked with MabSelect SuRe™, Capto™ Q, and Capto adhere media was compared with small-scale XK16/40 (XK) columns packed with the same media for the purification of a MAb in a three-step process in parallel experiments. Yield and contaminant levels were practically identical during all steps, demonstrating the comparable performance of the column types and that the process is scalable. In addition, ReadyToProcess columns can be used for repeated runs with retained performance.
>
> The increasing demand for MAbs as biopharmaceuticals has promoted the development of efficient processes for cell culturing, as well as for purification. Plug-and-play units make several time-consuming steps redundant, and therefore shorten time to market. Such solutions also reduce the risk of cross-contamination significantly. ReadyToProcess columns are prepacked, prequalified, and presanitized process chromatography columns, suited for purification of biopharmaceuticals (e.g., proteins, vaccines, plasmids, viruses) for clinical phase I and II studies. The columns

are ready for use and the design makes them easy to connect to chromatography systems and to dispose of after completed production. ReadyToProcess columns are available with a range of BioProcess™ media in several sizes. In this study, the performance of ReadyToProcess columns was compared with an established small-scale format. A MAb was purified from cell culture supernatant using a three-step, generally applicable process consisting of MabSelect SuRe, Capto Q, and Capto adhere. The BioProcess media in the ReadyToProcess columns are the same as those used in conventional process chromatography, thus allowing the use of a fully flexible mode in early production while keeping a conventional re-use option for later large-scale manufacturing open.

ReadyToProcess columns (2.5 L CV) and XK16/40 columns (40 ml CV) packed with the same media and having the same bed height (20 cm) were used to compare the performance of the column types and to demonstrate scalability. The three-step purification strategy involved capture using MabSelect SuRe, an affinity medium with an alkali-tolerant protein A-derived ligand. Further, intermediate purification using ion exchange was employed with Capto Q followed by a final PO step of the MAb with Capto adhere. The columns were connected to ÄKTAexplorer™ 100 (XK columns) and ÄKTAprocess™ (ReadyToProcess columns) chromatography systems. UNICORN™ software was used for control and evaluation. By using a platform approach, the development time and effort was kept to a minimum and the development work was concentrated on the third, PO step, where the multimodal anion exchanger Capto adhere was used.

The feed consisted of filtered CHO cell culture supernatant containing 2.7 mg MAb/ml. Sample volumes corresponding to 25 mg MAb/ml bed volume were applied to the XK 16/40 and RTP MabSelect SuRe 2.5 columns. Five cycles, each including CIP with 0.5 M NaOH, were run on each column, and the eluates were collected using an UV watch function. MAb purification at large scale typically contains a VI step at low pH after the protein A capture step, taking advantage of the low pH of the collected eluate. This step was omitted in this study. To match the buffer conditions of the equilibration buffer in the subsequent Capto Q step, pH of the collected eluates was immediately adjusted to 7.6.

The pH-adjusted eluates from the five MabSelect SuRe runs were pooled and applied to the Capto Q column in flowthrough mode. The flow through and part of the washing solution were collected and prepared for the Capto adhere step by adjusting the conductivity and pH to match the conditions of the equilibration buffer in the Capto adhere step.

All material from the Capto Q run was applied to Capto adhere in flow through mode. The flow through and washing solution were collected.

Samples were withdrawn for analysis at each stage of the purification process. The amount of dimer and aggregates in the samples was determined by gel filtration on a Superdex™ 200 10/300 GL column. Host cell protein (HCP) concentration was determined using the CHO-CM HCP ELISA kit (CM015, Cygnus Technologies). The concentration of leached MabSelect SuRe ligand was determined by a protein A ELISA method using purified ligand for the ELISA standard curve. The analyses were not optimized for this particular feed and MAb. Three-step monoclonal antibody purification was performed in parallel at two different scales. The overall yield was 88% for both processes, achieving contaminant levels acceptable for formulation. The three-step purification process is characterized by an overall good yield, low ligand leakage from MabSelect SuRe, and efficient contaminant and dimer/aggregate removal. It should be emphasized that the process development in this study was limited, since the conditions for the two first steps, MabSelect SuRe and Capto Q, are more or less generic, while the final Capto adhere step required some evaluation of operating conditions.

Both MabSelect SuRe columns were run five times each to investigate the effects of repeated runs on column performance, as well as to gather enough material for subsequent chromatography steps. The chromatograms obtained were similar. The uniform performance was confirmed by the analytical results. Yields were stable during all cycles, and the contaminant levels were comparable. The HCP level was efficiently reduced, and the ligand leakage low, which is characteristic for MabSelect SuRe. The higher level of ligand leakage in the first cycle, which was detected on both column types, is typical for protein A-based chromatography media. As a result of differences in scale, chromatography systems, and UV detectors, the relative eluate volumes measured in CV, were slightly different in the XK and ReadyToProcess runs. Each of the five eluates from the XK runs had volumes corresponding to 1.7 CV, while the five eluates from the ReadyToProcess runs had volumes corresponding to 2.0 CV. Therefore, the sample volumes in the subsequent Capto Q and Capto adhere steps were smaller for the XK runs compared to the ReadyToProcess runs. This difference becomes apparent when comparing the XK and the ReadyToProcess chromatograms from the Capto Q and Capto adhere runs.

The MAb-containing flowthrough and part of the wash were collected. Again, the comparable performance of the XK and ReadyToProcess columns was confirmed by the analytical results. The Capto Q step was characterized by high yield, reduction of HCP, and some reduction of leached ligand and dimer/aggregates. The MAb-containing flowthrough and all of the wash were collected. Again, the comparable performance of the XK and ReadyToProcess columns was confirmed by the analytical results. The Capto adhere step had a high yield and efficiently reduced the amount of dimers and aggregates in this study. With this particular MAb, it was necessary to run the column at low pH (5.0) and high salt (0.4 M NaCl) conditions. At these conditions the HCP removal is limited. Typically, when the MAb allows running at higher pH and lower salt conditions, Capto adhere also removes HCPs.

The performance of ReadyToProcess columns is comparable with established column formats as has been demonstrated in a three-step MAb purification process run in parallel at two different scales; small-scale XK columns and large-scale, prepacked ReadyToProcess columns. The ReadyToProcess columns behave similarly to the XK columns in all aspects studied, demonstrating that the purification process is directly scalable between XK and ReadyToProcess. Multiple cycles (five) have been performed on RTP MabSelect SuRe 2.5 without any detectable changes in column performance.

Smaller disposable columns are available from several sources including Bio-Rad (www.bio-rad.com) and Corning (www.corning.com). There is still an unmet need for inexpensive large disposable columns.

A disadvantage in using resin columns is the large footprint required in their use; compared to this, membrane chromatography employs thin, synthetic, porous membranes that are generally multilayered in a small cartridge, significantly reducing the footprint of the operation. Membranes have the same functional chemical groups to corresponding resins, but they do not need packing, checking, cleaning, refilling, or routine maintenance, and fouled or exhausted modules can be replaced with new ones with minimal process downtime. Sartorius offers a large choice in these membranes.

11.11.2 Membrane Chromatography

Purification of proteins from complex mixtures is a key process in pharmaceutical research and production. But chromatography based on particulate matrices involves lengthy procedures and separation times. Sartobind SingleSep® ion exchange capsules are designed to remove contaminants from therapeutic proteins at accelerated flow rates. This is a direct result of negligible mass transfer effects and is made possible by the >3 μm macroporous membrane. The design allows for robust chromatographic separations and drastically reduced validation costs. Sartobind SingleSep capsules are designed to remove charged contaminants from therapeutic proteins at accelerated flow rates by ion exchange membrane chromatography. The high throughput is a direct result of negligible mass transfer effects and is made possible by the >3 μm macroporous membrane with 4 mm (15 layer) bed height.

Sartobind replaces time-consuming tedious chromatographic steps for many protein and virus applications. The rapid purification on Membrane Adsorbers allows the isolation of protein with high yield up to 100 faster than conventional columns at a flow rate of 20–40 bed volumes per minute (Figure 11.18).

The micrograph shows some chromatographic gel beads (average particle size 90 μm) on the surface of the Sartobind Membrane Adsorber. Even at 500 fold magnification, pores

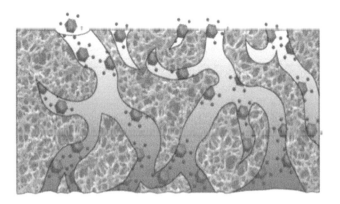

Figure 11.18   Schematic view of viruses binding to functional groups in the membrane pores.

of beads are invisible but the membrane displays a wide pore structure of 3–5 µm size (Figure 11.19).

Conventional beads keep more than 95% of the binding sites inside the particle. In Sartobind membranes the binding sites are grafted homogenously as an approximately 0.5–1 µm film on the inner walls of the reinforced and cross-linked cellulose network. Diffusion time in adsorbers is negligible because of the large pores and immediate binding of the target substance to the ligands. There is no pore diffusion as given in conventional beads but film diffusion on any place of the microporous membrane structure (Figure 11.20). At convective flow conditions the movement of the molecules of the mobile phase is directed by pump pressure only. That is why membrane adsorbers feature extremely short

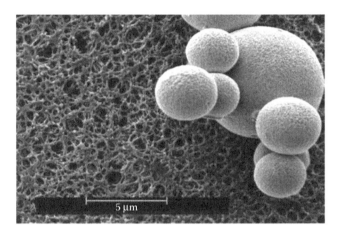

Figure 11.19   Sartobind Q membrane and a standard chromatographic matrix.

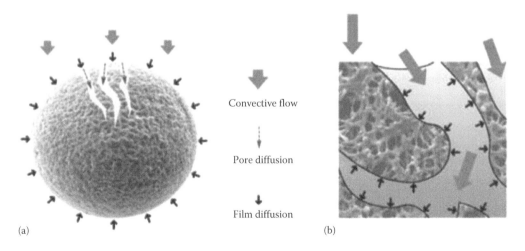

Convective flow

Pore diffusion

Film diffusion

(a)   (b)

Figure 11.20   Existing transport phenomena in (a) conventional beads and (a) membrane adsorbers.

Table 11.5 Different Types of Membrane and Ligands Available for Membrane Chromatography

Membrane Type	Description	Ligand	Pore Size (µm)
Sulfonic acid (S)	Strong acidic cation exchanger	$R\text{-}CH_2\text{-}SO_3-$	>3
Quaternary ammonium (Q)	Strong basic anion exchanger	$R\text{-}CH_2\text{-}N^+(CH_3)_3$	>3
Carboxylic acid(C)	Weak acidic cation exchanger	$R\text{-}COO-$	>3
Diethylamine (D)	Weak basic anion exchanger	$R\text{-}CH_2\text{-}N(C_2H_5)_2$	>3
Phenyl	Hydrophobic interaction (HIC)	Phenyl	>3
IDA	Metal chelate	Iminodiacetic acid	>3
Protein A	Affinity	Protein A	0.45
Epoxy-activated	Coupling	Epoxy group	0.45
Aldehyde-activated	Coupling	Aldehyde group	0.45

Source: Sartorius Stedim.

cycle times and exceptionally high flow rate and throughput. There are several available ligands including (Table 11.5).

A special advantage in the use of membrane adsorbes is the removal of high-molecular weight contaminants such as DNA and viruses in MAb manufacturing. Such molecules do not readily diffuse into the pores of traditional resins; thus, most PO steps relying on column chromatography require dramatically oversized columns. These hydrodynamic benefits provide the opportunity to operate membrane adsorber at much greater flow rates than columns, considerably reducing buffer consumption and shortening the overall process time by up to 100-fold.

Sartorius Stedim recently introduced single-use, disposable anion-exchange membrane adsorption cartridges which can be used for DNA and HCP removal or viral clearance. Likewise, Pall Corporation offers a similar disposable membrane product specifically designed for DNA removal. Other companies including GE Healthcare, Millipore, BioFlash Partners, and Tarpon Biosystems have developed prepacked and presanitized disposable-format chromatography columns. Most of these columns were designed for PO applications except Tarpon's, which can be also be used for the capture step in MAb purification. Capture of target remains a major challenge and contributes to the downstream bottlenecks plaguing many MAb manufacturers.

11.11.3 Virus Removal

Virus contamination is a risk to all biotechnology products derived from cell lines of human or animal origin. Contamination of a product with endogenous viruses from cell banks or adventitious viruses from personnel can have serious clinical implications. According to the EMEA, potential contaminants may have the following characteristics: enveloped or nonenveloped, small or large, DNA or ribonucleic acid, unstable or resistant viruses. Viral safety of licensed biological products must be assured by three complementary approaches, which are as follows:

- Thorough testing of the cell line and all raw materials for viral contaminants
- Assessing the capacity of downstream processing to clear infectious viruses
- Testing the product at appropriate steps for contaminating viruses

A combination of methods inactivation, adsorption, and size exclusion are available. The U.S. FDA requires demonstration of virus clearance by two methods. Examples of inactivation procedures are solvent and detergent, chemical treatments, low pH, or microwave heating. Methods of adsorption utilize chromatography, and removal by mechanical or molecular size exclusion uses normal (forward) and tangential flow filtration methods. The treatments with solvents/detergent, low pH, or microwave heating, all have significant limitations in their ability to inactivate small nonenveloped viruses. Low pH inactivation of murine retroviruses is reported to be highly dependent on time, temperature, and pH, and relatively independent of the recombinant protein type or conductivity conditions outlined. Heating is considered as one of the most reliable methods for VI because of the variation in stability of each virus genome to heat or temperature.

Ion exchange and Protein A chromatography is widely used to remove viruses and several key studies have been conducted in collaboration with the U.S. FDA, yet the responsibility of proving suitability of any method remains the responsibility of the developer.

Viral inactivation such as by UV exposure is also available, where the virus particles are physically or chemically altered but actually separated from the product.

Despite the clear demand for downstream processing steps that can provide high levels of viral reduction, few new techniques have surfaced to complement or replace those approaches common in today's biotechnology manufacturing processes. This is particularly true for smaller viruses, such as parvovirus, which often exhibit resistance to many inactivation strategies such as detergent and heat treatments.

Unfortunately, the risk of failing viral contamination is severe; Table 11.6 shows the action plan in various situations. Implementing UVC treatment as one of the orthogonal technologies for virus clearance both for animal cell culture media- and animal cell culture-derived biologicals is recommended. VI with UVivatec® CPV is an integral part of the orthogonal virus clearance technology platform at Sartorius Stedim Biotech (www.sartorius-stedim.com). This orthogonal technology platform features virus filtration, VI, and virus adsorption. UVivatec shows efficient (>4log) inactivation of both small nonenveloped viruses (20 nm) and large enveloped viruses (>50 nm) form biopharmaceutical feed stream by UVC irradiation (254 nm) while obtaining product integrity.

UVivatec, a newly developed VI technology, targets only small and nonenveloped viruses but offers a robust method for inactivating generous and enveloped viruses. This method uses low-dose radiation of UVC at 254 nm, more likely 260 nm (which is more specific to nucleic acids), to destroy the viral nucleic acid while maintaining the structural and functional integrity of the protein of interest. The efficiency of viral inactivation and product recovery is sensitive to the viscosity and absorption coefficient of the protein solution at 254 or 260 nm and its residence time in the radiation chamber. The key to a successful UVC intervention is to introduce it at an early stage of downstream processing so that most aggregates or variant species formed as a result of UVC exposure would be cleared in the subsequent PO steps.

Table 11.6 Action Plan for Process Assessment of Viral Clearance and Virus Tests on Purified Bulk

	Case A	Case B	Case C2	Case D2	Case E2
Status					
Presence of virus1	−	−	+	+	(+)3
Virus-like particles1	−				(1)3
Retrovirus-like particles1	−	+	−	−	(+)3
Virus identified	Not applicable	+	+	+	−
Virus pathogenic for humans	Not applicable	−4	−4	+	Unknown
Action					
Process characterization of viral clearance using nonspecific *model* viruses	yes5	yes5	yes5	yes5	yes7
Process evaluation of viral clearance using *relevant* or specific *model* viruses	no	yes6	yes6	yes6	yes7
Test for virus in purified bulk	Not applicable	yes8	yes8	yes8	yes8

Planova filters (www.planovafilters) are the world's first filters designed specifically for VR. The first Planova filter was launched in 1989 by Asahi Kasei Corporation, one of the world's leading filter manufacturers. Planova filters significantly enhance virus safety in biotherapeutic drug products such as biopharmaceuticals and plasma derivatives. They exhibit unparalleled performance in clearing viruses, ranging from human immuno-deficiency virus (HIV) to parvovirus B19, while providing maximum protein recovery. Planova filters contain a bundle of straw-like hollow fibers. When a protein solution with possible viral contamination is introduced into these hollow fibers, the solution penetrates the fiber wall and works its way to the outside of the fiber.

Within these walls, there is an intricate, 3D network of interconnected void and capillary pores just nanometers in size. Viruses are thus filtered gradually and effectively, while proteins migrate outward with minimal adsorption and inactivation. Planova virus removal works on the principle of size exclusion, unaffected by physical or chemical effects such as adsorption. Therefore, even unknown viruses can be excluded as long as the virus size meets the exclusion specification of the filter. Planova 15N, 20N, and 35N filters are offered in 0.001, 0.01, 0.12, 0.3, 1.0, and 4.0 m² sizes. The 4.0 m² filter reduces the number of filters needed for a manufacturing cycle and shortens cumulative integrity test time. The polyvinylidene fluoride (PVDF) media Planova BioEX filter is offered in 0.001 and 1.0 m² sizes. Additional sizes, including 0.0003, 0.01, 0.1, and 4.0 m² are under development to extend the Planova BioEX line.

ChromaSorb membrane adsorber, an innovative, single-use, flow-through anion exchanger from Millipore (www.millipore.com), is designed to remove trace impurities—including HCP, DNA, endotoxins, and viruses. This device provides the greatest levels of impurity binding at the highest salt concentrations for MAbs and other protein purification steps. The ability to reliably perform at greater salt concentrations significantly reduces buffer volumes. Compared to traditional column-based anion exchange resins, ChromaSorb membrane adsorber reduces the validation requirements, capital equipment expenditures, time, and labor. The ChromaSorb membrane consists of uniform 0.65 μm pore structure, ultra-high molecular weight polyethylene (UPE) membrane—coated with a cationic primary amine ligand for high binding strength for negatively charged impurities.

Mobius FlexReady Solution for Virus Filtration from Millipore (www.millipore.com) provides the best combination of single-use assemblies (Flexware assemblies), innovative separation devices, and process-ready hardware specifically designed for virus filtration. It is pre-assembled and pretested, and integrates easily into any process. Designed for applications where feed volumes range between 1 and 200 L at protein concentrations from 5 to 10 g/L, the Mobius FlexReady Solution for Virus Filtration features Millipore's next generation virus clearance solution, Viresolve Pro Solution. Designed for applications where feed volumes range between 1 and 200 L at protein concentrations from 5 to 10 g/L, the Mobius FlexReady Solution for Virus Filtration features Millipore' s next generation virus clearance solution, Viresolve Pro Solution. The benefits include: unique low pulsation peristaltic pump, Constant pressure operation using pressure feedback and pump speed control, process end-point via percent flux decay, cumulative volume/weight or processing time, innovative low dead volume t-connectors, enabling the use of traditional pressure transducers, pre-sized sterilizing-grade filter and product collection assembly, ease of operation with an intuitive touch screen interface, and user-defined process and alarm set points.

Virus filtration with Virosart® CPV is an integral part of the orthogonal virus clearance technology platform at Sartorius Stedim Biotech (www.sartorius-stedim.com). This orthogonal technology platform features virus filtration, VI and virus adsorption. Virosart® CPV shows efficient removal of both small nonenveloped viruses (20 nm) and large enveloped viruses (>50 nm) from biopharmaceutical feed stream by size exclusion. The double layer 20 nm PESU membrane of Virosart® CPV features excellent flow rates and superior capacity. The filter offers highest viral safety over the entire flow decay profile up to 90%. Virosart® CPV filters are being tested for integrity using a water-based integrity test. All filters have been validated for 4 log10 removal of small nonenveloped viruses using bacteriophage PP7 as a model virus. Each individual Virosart® CPV filter is autoclaved and integrity tested during manufacturing assuring highest product reliability. Virosart® CPV provides highest viral safety to the biopharmaceutical product. This filter retains more than 4 log10 of small nonenveloped viruses (PPV or MVM) and more than 6 log10 of large enveloped viruses (e.g., MuLV). Based on the unique double layer 20 nm PESU membrane, Virosart® CPV provides excellent flow rates and superior capacity. This filter offers highest viral safety over the entire flow decay profile of up to 90%.

Scale-down work is being realized using the Virosart® CPV Minisart (5 cm² capsule) to enable filtration work for flow and capacity studies as well as for GLP virus spiking studies. Scale-up studies are being performed using this capsules size 9 with filter area of 2.000 cm² to reliably scale up into larger scale manufacturing. Typical batch sizes of products being subject to nanofiltration with this Virosart® CPV capsule size 9 are 5 to 50 L.

Pall (www.pall.com) offers Kleenpak Nova filters with either in-line or T-style configurations. The T-style configuration is ideal for manipulating multiple filters in series or in parallel configuration. Kleenpak Nova Capsule filters incorporate either a 10 in (254 mm), 20 in (508 mm), or 30 in (762 mm) length standard Pall cartridge filter, which have traditionally been installed in stainless-steel housings. In applications where a particular filter is already specified, the user can switch from a stainless-steel housing to a fully disposable assembly with minimal requalification. This means the extensive range of sterilizing-grade and virus filters currently available from Pall can easily be provided as a capsule filter, including: Low binding, high-flow Fluorodyne® II PVDF filters, Ultipor® N66 and positively-charged Posidyne® nylon 66 filters, Supor® polyethersulfone (PESu) filters, Ultipor VF DV20 and DV50 VR filters. Kleenpak Nova capsules are especially suited to pilot- and process-scale applications. They can be autoclaved or sterilized by gamma irradiation and can be supplied as part of pre-sterilized processing systems such as a filter/tubing/bag set. Additionally, the disposable Kleenpak sterile connector allows for the dry connection of two separate fluid pathways, while maintaining the sterile integrity of both. The connector consists of a male and a female connector, each covered by a vented peel away strip that protects the port and maintains the sterility of the sterile fluid pathway. Different connector options are available to allow for the connection of 15.8 mm (5/8 in), 13 mm (1/2 in), 9.6 mm (3/8 in), or 6 mm (1/4 in) nominal tubing. Kleenpak sterile connectors can either be autoclaved up to 130°C or gamma sterilized.

Viral clearance studies require viral spiking and many controls and validation protocols that might be difficult to conduct in-house. Several contract laboratories are available to do these studies and generally the author recommends outsourcing this phase of development.

- AppTec Laboratory Services, www.apptecls.com
- Bioreliance, Inc., www.bioreliance.com
- Charles River Laboratories, www.criver.com/products/biopharm/biosafety.html
- Inveresk Research Group, Inc., www.inveresk.com
- Microbix Biosystems, Inc., www.microbix.com
- Q-One Biotech, Ltd., www.q-one.com
- Texcell—Institut Pasteur, www.pasteur.fr/applications/dri/French/Texcell.html

11.11.4 Buffers

BP and storage requires large volume handling, generally about 10× the upstream media volume; some resins like Protein A require large buffer volumes. While there are several standard buffers, specific pH and electrolyte requirements make standardization of buffers difficult and these are often process-specific. While several development projects underway promise to reduce the volume of buffer needed, the current systems are likely to stay the same for some time. The main efforts in this regard include reducing the process steps.

The reduction in buffer volume is necessary because of the high cost of the water used in preparing buffers. While it is acceptable to use Purified Water USP to prepare buffers, many large manufacturing operations used instead WFI without choice because often this is the only choice available. Recently, a new manufacturing facility in Chicago (www. theraproteins.com) qualified a double reverse osmosis (RO) Edi water system for biological manufacturing saving almost 90% of the cost of water used, from about U.S. $ 3/L for WFI based on stainless-steel system to less than 5 cents/L.

Buffer storage was one of the first unit operations to transition to single-use systems. Recent analyses have confirmed that there is a clear economic advantage to this methodology over traditional hard-piped systems. Buffer mixing, however, continues to rely on more traditional technology. This is partially due to the scale of many BP processes and partially due to a reliance on existing infrastructure. However, as new facilities are commissioned and as new technologies are introduced that limit the volume of buffers required, SUMs are being chosen over traditional technologies. The shift to single use is driven by the needs to minimize capital investment, enable more rapid process setup, reduce downtime, and provide increased flexibility.

The largest disposable holding bags currently have a 3,000 L capacity (Sartorius Palletank), while mixing with disposables is limited to 5,000 L (Hynetics Disposable Mixing System) with more systems available at the 1,000 to 2,000 L scale. Preconfigured, disposable stand-alone systems for BP have been launched recently with 500 and 1,000 L capacities (e.g., Mobius). However, most of these packaged systems are very expensive and do not add any real value to the bioprocess since a simple system like a Dixie Poly Drum 330 gal Economy Tank with a PE liner would do the job as well (the cost of the entire system is less than U.S.$ 1,500); Class VI USP liners are readily available even in sterile state though that is not necessary. For company starting out, it is recommended that they develop their own configured system for storage of buffers and also use the same tanks for mixing purposes. Often a built-in system of a cage that will accommodate a liner is sufficient for the purpose.

As an example of integrated systems, for BP steps, GE Healthcare (www.gelifesciences.com) offers its WAVE™ Mixer. The WAVE Mixer provides efficient mixing in a sterile, sealed bag by an innovative method. Instead of using a pump or invasive impeller to induce circulation flow, it uses waves generated in the liquid by a precisely regulated rocking motion. The system has been optimized for extremely efficient mixing and dispersion. Wave motion moves large volumes of fluid and disperses solids. The WAVE Mixer eliminates the need for a mixing tank and conventional mixer. This also eliminates equipment cleaning, sterilization, and validation.

The WAVE Mixer system comprises two main components: a special rocking platform that induces a wave motion in the liquid without an impeller or other invasive mixer and the M*Bag™, which contains the ingredients to be mixed and dissolved. The unique M*Bag is made of a multilayer laminated clear plastic designed to provide high mechanical strength. A large screw cap port allows powders or other solids to be easily poured into the bag. Probes to measure pH and conductivity can be inserted. A large outlet port allows the M*Bag to be drained completely.

Standard systems are available for 20 and 50 L bags. These can be used to mix volumes from 1 to 35 L of liquid. Larger systems up to 500 L liquid volume are available. The WAVE Mixer principle has also been used for the mixing of materials in custom-shaped rigid containers.

Biological and particle contaminants present in buffers can have a large impact on process efficiencies and final product quality. Therefore, normal flow filtration is one of the first steps (after dissolution) in any BP process. Buffer filtration is key to protection of chromatography columns and ultrafiltration (UF) operations and to production of an endotoxin-free final product. Buffer filtration also aligns with the U.S. FDA guidelines on sterile drug products that advise to reduce and control bioburden across the process.

Buffer filters should be chosen based on the following characteristics:

- Validated retention of bacteria
- Broad chemical compatibility
- High permeability
- Physical robustness

For filtration of sterile and reduced-bioburden buffers, GE Healthcare offers ULTA™ Pure SG (for buffer sterilization) and ULTA Prime CG (for bioburden reduction). The ULTA family of filters uses membranes with industry-leading permeability that consistently outperforms competitive offerings. Both filter grades are constructed using PESu 0.2 μ membrane, which is physically robust and chemically resilient, so they perform reliably regardless of the buffer being prepared. Additionally, both filters employ a final membrane that is validated for bacterial retention using the ASTM F838-05 methodology. (LRV > 7 for ULTA Pure SG and LRV > 5 for ULTA Prime CG). ULTA filters are available in a wide variety of cartridge and capsule formats with surface areas ranging from 450 cm^2 to 1.5 m^2 in a single device.

11.11.5 Fluid Management

Once prepared, buffers are transferred to downstream processing stations, when using larger volumes, on carts or otherwise through a tubing system with the help of peristaltic pumps. In another chapter a review of the connectors, both aseptic and otherwise was presented.

ReadyCircuit assemblies comprise bags, tubing, and connectors. Together with ReadyToProcess filters and sensors, ReadyCircuit assemblies form self-contained bioprocessing modules that maintain an aseptic path and provide convenience by removing time-consuming process steps associated with conventional systems. Bags, tube sets, filters and related equipment can be secured in appropriate orientations for efficient operation using the ReadyKart mobile processing station. With an array of features, and optional accessories, the ReadyKart is designed to support a variety of process-specific, fluid-handling needs.

ReadyToProcess Konfigurator lets one design fluid-handling circuits with ease online. One enters the parameters to generate the design one needs; includes fast output of P&ID drawings and convenient Bill of Materials for simplified ordering.

ReadyMate connectors are genderless aseptic connectors that allow simple connection of components maintaining secure workflows and sterile integrity. Additional accessories such as tube fuser and sealer of thermoplastic tubing support secure aseptic connectivity throughout the manufacturing process.

ReadyToProcess filters are a range of preconditioned and ready to use cartridges and capsules for both cross-flow and normal-flow filtration operations. Factory prepared to WFI quality for endotoxins, TOC, and conductivity and sterilized via gamma radiation. They enable simpler and faster bioprocessing with maximum safety.

11.11.6 Bioseparation

Once the expression phase ends, the first step of bioseparation starts. In the case of bacterial expression, this would involve a continuous flow centrifuge (e.g., New Brunswick CEPA centrifuge, www.nbsc.com/cepa.aspx). Smaller volume can be processed in other standard centrifuges taking about 4–6 L in each run. At this point in the development, we do not have a disposable centrifuge option except the Centritech Cell II by Pneumatic Scale Angelus (www.pneumaticscale.com/) that can process up to 120 L/h. It will require running several centrifuges in parallel to process a typical 2,000–4,000 L run; this centrifuge however is capable of separation animal cells as well.

The next stage for handling the cell mass would be to use an enzyme method, a bead method, sonication, detergent, or solvent method. Homogenization using a French Press is most common for large-scale processing. At this time, there are no disposable mechanical systems available. And perhaps there is no need for it if the process can be isolated and more particularly if a single product is handled in a single facility.

11.11.7 Depth Filtration

Cell removal by filtration leaves media and its entire component in the same volume and this requires depth filtration. Depth filters are the variety of filters that use a porous filtration medium to retain particles throughout the medium, rather than just on the surface of the medium. These filters are commonly used when the fluid to be filtered contains a high load of particles because, relative to other types of filters, they can retain a large mass of particles before becoming clogged.

The performance of depth filters is largely dependent on the colloid content of the bioreactor offload and the cell debris removal capacity of the upstream centrifuge. Usually, depth filters are operated with a constant flow of 100 200 L/(m² h) and up to 150 L feed/m² of filter depending on the composition of the feed stream. The Millipore Millistak+ Pod system has a maximum capacity of 33 m² filter area, resulting in a batch capacity of 3–5,000 L. The Millipore Mobius FlexReady process equipment supports offers a larger 55 m²-filter area. Since the washing of these filters requires very large volumes of buffers, appropriate size holding tanks are required that can be lined with disposable PE liners.

11.11.8 Filtration

UF is a variety of membrane filtration in which hydrostatic pressure forces a liquid against a semipermeable membrane. Suspended solids and solutes of high molecular weight are retained, while water and low molecular weight solutes pass through the membrane. This separation process is used in industry and research for purifying and concentrating macromolecular (103–106 Da) solutions, especially protein solutions. UF is not fundamentally different from MF, nanofiltration or gas separation, except in terms of the size of the molecules it retains. UF is applied in cross-flow or dead-end mode and separation in UF undergoes concentration polarization.

Diafiltration is a membrane-based separation that is used to reduce, remove, or exchange salts and other small molecule contaminant from a process liquid or dispersion. In batch diafiltration, the process fluid is typically diluted by a factor of two using *clean* liquid, brought back to the original concentration by filtration, and the whole process repeated several times to achieve the required concentration contaminant. In continuous diafiltration the *clean* liquid is added at the same rate as the permeate flow.

Cross-flow filtration (also known as tangential flow filtration) is a type of filtration (a particular unit operation). Cross-flow filtration is different from dead-end filtration in which the feed is passed through a membrane or bed, the solids being trapped in the filter and the filtrate being released at the other end. Cross-flow filtration gets its name because the majority of the feed flow travels tangentially across the surface of the filter, rather than into the filter. The principal advantage of this is that the filter cake (which can blind the filter) is substantially washed away during the filtration process, increasing the length of time that a filter unit can be operational. It can be a continuous process, unlike batch-wise dead-end filtration. This type of filtration is typically selected for feeds containing a high proportion of small particle size solids (where the permeate is of most value) because solid material can quickly block (blind) the filter surface with dead-end filtration. Industrial examples of this include the extraction of soluble antibiotics from fermentation liquor.

UF and diafiltration steps are used to concentrate and change the buffer of a solution. During final formulation, UF/diafiltration is used to transfer the active pharmaceutical ingredient to a stabilizing environment and to achieve the correct concentration. Up to 300–5,000 L may need to be processed, depending on whether the column eluates can be fractionated. Membranes with a 30 kDa molecular weight cutoff are often used to retain antibodies, and the process intermediate is concentrated and washed with 5× volumes. Modules of up to 3 m^2 are available that can process 200 L/(h m^2). Several disposable systems are available (Scilog, Millipore) for a limited filter area (up to 2.5 m^2), but larger systems that might replace existing reusable systems with 14 m^2. Because there are already disposable modules and pumps available, its logical to carry the filtration steps in a closed system.

11.11.9 Integrated Systems

ÄKTA ready (www.gehealthcare.com) is a liquid chromatography system built for process scale up and production for early clinical phases. The system operates with ready-to-use, disposable flow paths and as a consequence, cleaning between products/batches and validation of cleaning procedures is not required. ÄKTA™ ready is a liquid chromatography system built for process scale up and production for early clinical phases. System meets GLP and cGMP requirements for Phase I III in drug development and full-scale production, provides improved economy and productivity due to simpler procedures, single use eliminates risk of cross-contamination between products/batches, easy connection to and operation with prepacked ReadyToProcess™ columns and other process columns, scalable processes using UNICORN™ software.

Studies conducted using the above ReadyToProcess system by GE to manufacture a MAb and comparing it with traditional system shows reduction in the total process time by half from almost 50 to 24 h. Most of the saving of time comes from obviating interim validation of equipment. The purity levels of the product obtained are generally comparable. However, in this particular example, the cost of materials is substantially higher when using the ReadyToProcess system; how much of it gets reduced by the time savings would depend on the cost of time to the individual processor (Table 11.7).

While the example above provide a very good view of the state of the art today, there remain many hurdles to providing a true cost-effective system. One way of achieving this goal would be to combine the upstream and downstream processes as suggested elsewhere in this book.

The above system however can be further modified by using Scilog's single-use UF system. The SciPure 200 (www.scilog.com) is a single-use bioprocessing platform for the automation, optimization, and documentation of TFF applications. The system has been designed to meet cGMP and 21 CFR Part 11 standards for data-collection and security as a standalone device with the ability to create and execute discrete or batch operations for filling, concentration, diafiltration, and normalized water permeability (NWP). User-selectable end points and alarms enable hands-free operation and ensure safe, consistent process performance. The patented proprietary technology enables the SciPure 200 system to respond to sensor feedback and thus maintain the user-defined flows and transmembrane pressure (TMP) simultaneously. All wetted flow-path manifold components of the SciPure 200 are considered Single-Use consumables.

SciLog (www.scilog.com) recently developed a fully automated, single-use purification platform that purportedly improves downstream processing efficiencies and may help cut costs. Other companies are developing disposable format expanded bed adsorption and high capacity monolith and membrane adsorbers to improve capacity during the capture.

MayaBio (www.mayabio.com) has recently developed a separative bioreactor where the binding resin is added directly to the bioreactor contained in a filter pouch with 30 μm size screen; once the protein in the media is absorbed onto resin or membrane, the bioreactor is

Table 11.7 Comparison between GE ReadyToProcess System and Traditional Systems Demonstrating the Time Savings Provided the GE ReadyToProcess System at Each Stage of Monoclonal Antibody Production

Step	ReadyToProcess	Traditional	% Time Saving
Upstream	Wave bioreactor	Stirred tank	0
Capture	ReadyToProcess Protein A	AxiChrom 70 column with Protein A	55
Buffer exchange, UF	ReadyToProcess hollow fiber cartridges	Kvick cassettes	55
Polishing	ReadyToProcess prepacked column, Capto	AxiCrom Capto	66
Formulation	ReadyToProcess hollow fiber cartridges	Kvick cassettes	30

drained out. The drain is closed and the resin/membrane is washed with buffers to remove debris and finally washed with an eluting buffer to a volume which is generally less than 5% of the original media volume. This process eliminates several steps: bioseparation, UF and buffer exchange. If the resin/membrane used to capture protein can be used in the column then this approach removes the lengthy procedure of column loading as well.

11.12 FILTRATION

Except for steel meshes in bulk manufacturing of nonsterile dosage forms, filters are rarely reused in the pharmaceutical industry. They take varied forms from muslin cloth to paper filters to membrane cartridges. Disposable filter devices in biological manufacturing were the earliest changes that went disposable mainly because of the problems with cleaning them; the cost of these parts have always been reasonable.

There are a multitude of filter designs and mechanisms utilized within the biopharmaceutical industry. Prefilters are commonly pleated or wound filter fleeces manufactured from melt-blown random fiber matrices. These filters are used to remove a high contaminant content within the fluid. Prefilters have a large band of retention ratings and can be optimized to all necessary applications. The most common application for prefilters is to protect membrane filters, which are tighter and more selective than prefilters. Membrane filters are used to polish or sterilize fluids. These filters need to be integrity testable to assess whether or not they meet the performance criteria. Cross-flow filtration can be utilized with micro or UF membranes. The fluid sweeps over the membrane layer and therefore keeps it unblocked. This mode of filtration also allows diafiltration or concentration of fluid streams. Nanofilters are commonly used as viral removal filters. The most common retention rating of these filters is 20 or 50 nm.

11.12.1 Dead-End Filtration

Dead-end filtration operates on the principle of passing a fluid feed stream through a filter device by means of a pressure drop, usually applied by either a pump or compressed gas pressure before the filter device. All contaminants larger in size than the pore size of the filter media are retained by the filter material and will finally cause a filter blockage by plugging its channels or pores. The dead-end filtration is one of the simplest modes of operation for filters and hence requires minimum accessories such as tubing/piping, tanks, controls, and footprint.

Dead-end filters described using microporous membranes manufactured out of synthetic polymers such as polyethersulfonate, PA, cyanoacrylate, and PVDF are used extensively for sterile processing. They are used for adding media to bioreactor, bioburden reduction in CH clarification, chromatography column protection, and final filtration of the purified bulk drug substance. These filters often come attached to disposable bags and are gamma sterilized.

The most common dead-end filtration devices are filter cartridges for reusable processes or capsules for fully disposable processes. They are used in wide-ranging applications as pre- and sterilizing-grade filters in upstream as well as downstream applications including media filtration; intermediate product pool filtrations; and in form, fill, and finish for the sterilization of drug substance. Dead-end filter devices are also used for sterilizing-grade air and vent filtration, for CIP and clarification, and, most recently, for viral clearance and membrane chromatography.

11.12.2 Cross-Flow Filtration

In chemical engineering, biochemical engineering, and protein purification, cross-flow filtration (also known as tangential flow filtration is a type of filtration, a particular unit operation). Cross-flow filtration is different from dead-end filtration in which the feed is passed through a membrane or bed, the solids being trapped in the filter and the filtrate being released at the other end. Cross-flow filtration gets its name because the majority of the feed flow travels tangentially across the surface of the filter, rather than into the filter. The principal advantage of this is that the filter cake (which can blind the filter) is substantially washed away during the filtration process, increasing the length of time that a filter unit can be operational. It can be a continuous process, unlike batch-wise dead-end filtration. This type of filtration is typically selected for feeds containing a high proportion of small particle size solids (where the permeate is of most value) because solid material can quickly block (blind) the filter surface with dead-end filtration. Industrial examples of this include the extraction of soluble antibiotics from fermentation liquors.

Since in cross-flow filtration the feed stream is led across or tangential to the filter material surface and is recycled continuously around the filter this requires more complex equipment and controls, but the retentate is allowed to pass through the filter device multiple times by recirculation. Thus, it is possible to perform concentration or buffer exchange processes. Additionally, the liquids with heavy load of suspended particles, the filter is kept from clogging as the turbulent flow of the feed across the filter removes deposited materials, something that is not possible in dead-end filtration.

11.12.3 Filtration Media

Filter media generally comprises layers of solid materials in a network or mesh with voids, pores, and channels that allow passage of liquid but retain larger particles, larger than the size of the openings, which may be in nanometers.

Depth filters use their entire depth to retain particulate on the basis of sieving compounded by adsorption effects unlike retentive filters where the filtered material is concentrated on the surface. The depth filter media dominate prefiltration and clarification applications because of the high solid mass that is generally required to be removed at this stage.

Sieving or size exclusion have more uniform pore sizes throughout the bed and are thus used to remove selective size of particles; these filters, mostly membrane types, are ideal as sterilizing filters for example, the commonly use 0.22 μm filter to sterilize liquid. While the main mechanism of their operation is sieving, the chemical nature of these membranes makes them a good base to adsorb organic substances.

Depth filter are made of fibers that are spread out on a substrate to make a mesh just like making paper; special additives such as activated carbon, ceramic fibers, and other such specific components are embedded with the help of a binder to form the filter.

Sheet filters are also made like paper using milled cellulose fibers and may contain diatomaceous earth or perlite along with a binder to strengthen the filter.

One of the world's largest suppliers of these filters in biopharmaceutical manufacturing is Pall (Table 11.8). Because of their thickness, the sheet filters provide a slow filtration option yet extensively used for prefiltration. Microglass fibers are also used filter media; these are nonwoven spun fibers of borosilicate glass whose web is strengthened by a binder allowing for a 3D structure of asymmetric voids as small as 0.2 μm to act as sterilizing filters.

Polypropylene and polyester fibers are also used by spinning from polymer melt and bonded by the polymer itself giving better chemical compatibility as no binder is added to them. These are always the preferred filters over PA and cellulose filters. The convention method of their manufacture leaves pore sizes 20–50 μm making them unsuitable for sterile filtration; special blown process is used to reduce the pore size in the range of 5–50 μm; further spinning is needed to reduce the size further to 1–10 μm range.

Table 11.8 Pall Filter Offering

Filter	Use	Type
Seitz® K–Series Depth Filter Sheets	Active pharmaceutical ingredients, clarification and prefiltration, plasma fractionation	Sheet filters and sheet filter modules
Seitz® K–Series Depth Filter Sheets	Beer, bottled water, dairy, food, soft drinks, spirits, wine	Sheet filters and sheet filter modules
Seitz® P-Series Depth Filter Sheets	Biotechnology, clarification and prefiltration, plasma fractionation	Sheet filters and sheet filter modules
Seitz® T-Series Depth Filter Sheets	Prefiltration, production	Sheet filters and sheet filter modules
Seitz® Z-Series Depth Filter Sheets	Active pharmaceutical ingredients, clarification and prefiltration	Sheet filters and sheet filter modules
Supracap™ 100 Depth Filter Capsules	Active pharmaceutical ingredients, biotechnology, cell separation, clarification and prefiltration, plasma fractionation, scale up/process development, vaccines	Capsules, sheet filters and sheet filter modules
SUPRAcap™ 200 Encapsulated Depth Filter Modules	Active pharmaceutical ingredients, biotechnology, cell separation, clarification and prefiltration, plasma fractionation, scale up/process development, vaccines	Capsules, sheet filters and sheet filter modules
Supracap™ 60 Depth Filter Capsules	Active pharmaceutical ingredients, biotechnology, cell separation, clarification and prefiltration, plasma fractionation, scale up/process development, vaccines	Capsules, sheet filters and sheet filter modules
SUPRAdisc™ Depth Filter Modules	Active pharmaceutical ingredients, biotechnology, cell separation, clarification and prefiltration, plasma fractionation, scale up/process development, vaccines	Sheet filters and sheet filter modules

(Continued)

413

Table 11.8 (Continued) Pall Filter Offering

Filter	Use	Type
SUPRAdisc™ Depth Filter Modules	Biofuels and biotechnology, chemicals	Sheet filters and sheet filter modules
SUPRAdisc™ HP Depth Filter Modules	Active pharmaceutical ingredients, biotechnology, cell separation, clarification and prefiltration, plasma fractionation, scale up/process development, vaccines	Sheet filters and sheet filter modules
SUPRAdisc™ II Depth Filter Modules	Beer, food, juice, spirits, wine	Sheet filters and sheet filter modules
SUPRAdisc™ II Modules	Active pharmaceutical ingredients, biotechnology, clarification and prefiltration, plasma fractionation, scale up/process development, vaccines	Sheet filters and sheet filter modules
SUPRApak™ Depth Filter Modules	Beer, spirits	Sheet filters and sheet filter modules
SUPRApak™ SW Series Modules	Beer, beer—corporate brewers, beer—microbreweries, food, soft drinks, spirits	Sheet filters and sheet filter modules
T-Series Depth Filter Sheets	Active pharmaceutical ingredients, biotechnology, cell separation, clarification and prefiltration, plasma fractionation, scale up/process development, vaccines	Sheet filters and sheet filter modules
T-Series Depth Filter Sheets	Biofuels and biotechnology, chemicals	Sheet filters and sheet filter modules
T-Series Membrane Cassettes	Active pharmaceutical ingredients, clarification and prefiltration	Sheet filters and sheet filter modules

Source: Pall Corporation, www.pall.com.

11.12.4 Polymer Membranes

The history of membrane filters goes back to hundreds of years.

Year	Important Development
1748	Abbe Nollet—water diffuses from dilute to concentrated solution
1846	The first synthetic (or semisynthetic) polymer studied by Schoenbein and produced commercially in 1869
1855	Fick employed cellulose nitrate membrane in his classic study *Ueber Diffusion*
1866	Fick, Traube, artificial membranes (nitrocellulose)
1907	Bechhold, pore size control, *ultrafiltration*
1927	Sartorius Company, membranes available commercially
1945	German scientists, methods for bacterial culturing
1957	USPH, officially accepts membrane procedure
1958	Sourirajan, first success in desalinating water

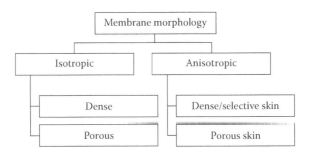

Figure 11.21 Basic membrane morphology.

The main advances in membrane technology (1960–1980) began in 1960 with the invention of the first asymmetric integrally skinned cellulose acetate (CA) RO membrane. This development simulated both commercial and academic interest, first in desalination by RO, and then in other membrane applications and processes. During this period, significant progress was made in virtually every phase of membrane technology: applications, research tools, membrane formation processes, chemical and physical structures, configurations and packaging.

Two basic morphology of hollow fiber membrane are *isotropic* and *anisotropic* (Figure 11.21). Membrane separation is achieved by using of these morphologies.

The anisotropic configuration is of special value. In the early 1960s, the development of anisotropic membranes exhibiting a dense, ultrathin skin on a porous structure provided a momentum to the progress of membrane separation technology. The semipermeability of the porous morphology is based essentially on the spatial cross section of the permeating species, that is, small molecules exhibit a higher permeability rate through the fiber wall. While the anisotropic morphology of the dense membrane, which exhibit the dense skin, is obtained through the solution-diffusion mechanism. The permeation species chemically interacts with the polymer matrix and selectively dissolves in it, resulting in diffusive mass transport along the chemical potential gradient, as what demonstrated in the pervaporation process.

Type of the membrane configuration are given in Figure 11.22 and are listed below.

Hollow fiber is one of the most popular membranes used in industries. It is because of its several beneficial features that make it attractive for those industries. Among them are

- *Modest energy requirement*: In hollow fiber filtration process, no phase change is involved. Consequently, it needs no latent heat. This makes the hollow fiber membrane have the potential to replace some unit operations which consume heat, such as distillation or evaporation columns.
- *No waste products*: Since the basic principal of hollow fiber is filtration, it does not create any waste from its operation except the unwanted component in the feed stream. This can help to decrease the cost of operation to handle the waste.

415

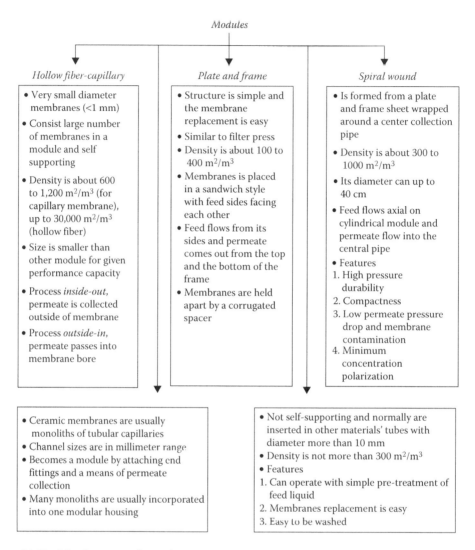

Figure 11.22 Membrane configuration.

- *Large surface per unit volume*: Hollow fiber has large membrane surface per module volume. Hence, the size of hollow fiber is smaller than other type of membrane but can give higher performance.
- *Flexible*: Hollow fiber is a flexible membrane, it can carry out the filtration by two ways, either is *inside-out* or *outside-in*.
- *Low operation cost*: Hollow fiber need low operational costs compare to other types of unit operation.

However, it also has some disadvantages which contribute to its application constraints. Among the disadvantages are

- *Membrane fouling*: Membrane fouling of hollow fiber is more frequent than other membrane due to is configuration. Contaminated feed will increase the rate of membrane fouling, especially for hollow fiber.
- *Expensive*: Hollow fiber is more expensive than other membrane which available in market. It is because of its fabrication method and expense is higher than other membranes.
- *Lack of research*: Hollow fiber is a new technology and, so far, there has been less research done on it compared to other types of membranes. Hence, more research will be done on it in the future.

Hollow fiber made of polymer cannot be used on corrosive substances and high temperature conditions. Various types of membrane processes can be found in almost all of the literature references.

There is considerable confusion in the open literature as to the distinction between few membrane separation processes, i.e., the MF, UF, and RO. Occasionally one will see it referred to by other names such as *hyperfiltration (HF)*. In order to distinguish these separation processes clearly that RO has the separation range of 0.0001 to 0.001 µm (i.e., 1 to 10 Å) or <300 mol wt. RO is a liquid-driven membrane process, with the RO membranes are capable of passing water while rejecting microsolutes, such as salts or low molecule weight organics (<1,000 Da). Pressure driving force (1 to 10 MPa) needed to overcome the force of osmosis that cause the water to flow from dilute permeate to concentrated feed. The principle use of this membrane process is desalination, which shows its great advantage over the conventional technique of desalination, that is, ion exchange.

The biotechnology industry, which originated in the late 1970s, has become one of the emerging industries that draws the attention of the world, especially with the emergence of the genetic engineering as a means of producing medically important proteins during the 1980s. Two of the major interest applications of membrane technology in the biotechnology industry will be the separation and purification of the biochemical product, as often known as downstream processing; and the membrane bioreactor, which developed for the transformation of certain substrates by enzymes (i.e., biological catalysts).

Since its introduction in the 1970s, the membrane bioreactor has gained a lot of attention over the other conventional production processes are the possibility of a high enzyme density and hence high space-time yields. Whereas downstream processing is usually based on discontinuously operated MF, membrane bioreactor are operated continuously and are equipped with UF membranes. Two types of bioreactor designs are possible: dissolved enzymes (as in used with the production of L-alanine from pyruvate), or immobilized enzymes membrane.

Membrane science began emerging as an independent technology only in the mid-1970s, and its engineering concepts still are being defined. Many developments that initially evolved from government-sponsored fundamental studies are now successfully gaining the interest of the industries as membrane separation has emerged as a feasible technology.

Today, membrane polymers used in pharmaceutical processes include PVDF; expanded polytetrafluorethylene (ePTFE); PESu; PA; CA; regenerated cellulose (RC); and mixed cellulose ester (MCE), a mixture of cellulose nitrate (CN) and CA. Membranes provide the highest retention efficiency or the smallest pore sizes; the MF membrane pore sizes range from 10 to 0.1 μm; the UF membranes have pore sizes from 0.1 μm to a few nanometers, making them even suitable for virus filtration. The nanofilters are in the range of 50 nm and smaller and rated for the molecular weight they can retain in kilodaltons. MF membranes are suitable for prefiltration, others for sterilization.

11.12.5 MF Cross-Flow

The traditional process for adopting cross-flow filtration involves the use of dense UF membranes for the purpose of performing a concentration and buffer exchange operation on the target molecule pre- and post-column chromatography. When the UF media is replaced with a microporous MF membrane, one has the option of performing a wide range of separations involving larger species, while usually operating in much lower pressures.

As in the case of the UF membrane applications, a suitable cross-flow MF process may involve the concentration and *washing* of a particulate material. For example, as an alternative to the use of centrifugation, one could aseptically recover cells from a cell culture process and proceed to concentrate and wash the cells to remove contaminating macrosolutes and replace the fluid with a solution suitable for freezing the cells. This same type of sequence could be used to aseptically process liposomes and other drug delivery emulsions.

A second widely practiced use of cross-flow MF is also an alternative to centrifugation or normal flow filtration for the clarification of the target molecule or virus from cells and cell debris. Highly permeable MF membranes allow a large target molecule to pass through the filter, while providing complete retention of the contaminating particulates in a single scaleable step.

The filter media needs a device to use; earlier devices were stainless-steel holders for flat discs; pleated inserts to provide larger surface area followed this and these were enclosed in plastic containers. While the stainless-steel devices could be autoclaved, the plastic components needed gamma radiation to sterilize.

Hollow fiber devices contain bundles of numerous hollow fiber membranes and they are placed coaxially into a pipe-like perforated cage and sealed using a resin in so that either one or both ends of the module are open to give access to the feed or allow exit to the filtrate or permeate. They can be operated from both sides, the tube or the shell side.

11.12.5.1 Hollow Fiber Devices Are Established, for Example, in Virus Clearance by Asahi Kasei Medical Planova®

Planova filters, the world's first filters designed specifically for VR, significantly enhance virus safety in biotherapeutic drug products, such as biopharmaceuticals and plasma derivatives. They exhibit unparalleled performance in removing viruses, ranging from HIV to parvovirus B19, while providing maximum product recovery.

11.12.5.2 BioOptimal MF-SL™
Designed specifically for use in cell culture clarification applications, BioOptimal MF-SL filters enable biopharmaceutical manufacturers to improve the efficiency and effectiveness of their protein harvest step.

11.12.5.3 TechniKrom™
Asahi Kasei Bioprocess, Inc. provides technologically advanced bioprocess equipment, products, and services to the biopharmaceutical, pharmaceutical, veterinary, and nutraceutical industries that permit the lowest cost of production and highest innate product quality, especially in cGMP-regulated environments. We help our clients implement true manufacturing science in their facilities to enable their achievement of these goals.

11.12.5.4 GE Healthcare
Process scale hollow fiber cartridges offered by GE Healthcare are provided in eight basic configurations covering a membrane area range of 0.92 to 28 m² (9.9 to 300 ft²) depending on the fiber internal diameter.

11.12.5.5 Spectrum
Spectrum disposable CellFlo hollow fiber membranes are specially designed for the gentle and efficient separation of whole cells in MF, bioreactor perfusion, and culture harvest applications. Much like GE's circulatory system, CellFlo combines the advantages of tangential flow MF (0.2 and 0.5 μm pore sizes) with larger hollow fiber flow channels (1 mm ID) to provide gentler efficacious micro-separations without the risk of cell lysis. Other cell separation technologies have a higher risk of lysis resulting in ruptured cells and culture harvests contaminated with intracellular macromolecules. Perfectly suited for continuous cell perfusion and bacterial fermentation, CellFlo membranes isolate secreted proteins while eliminating spent media containing metabolic wastes and drawing in fresh nutrient-rich media. Consequently, CellFlo enables cultures to grow to a higher cell density with higher viability providing as much as a ten-fold increase of daily production of secreted proteins.

Whether performing a cell perfusion or conducting a simple MF, disposable CellFlo modules can either be autoclaved or purchased irradiated (irr) for quick sterile assembly. Spectrum offers disposable CellFlo membrane modules in the full range of MiniKros and KrosFlo sizes and surface areas for processing volumes ranging from 500 mL to 1,000 L. All CellFlo membranes have a 1 mm fiber inner diameter, available in 0.2 and 0.5 μm pore sizes. Also to be considered are the MaxCell, Spectrum Laboratories CellFlo®, and KrosFlo®, module families.

Millipore has developed a derivative hollow fiber system, Pellicon and here is how it compares with standard hollow fiber filters (Table 11.9).

Flat sheets can be arranged in a stack in place of pleated or hollow fiber filter media. The sheets are sealed such that they leave channels open to allow feed to pass through.

Table 11.9 Comparison of the Millipore Pellicon Hollow Fiber Filter Relative to Traditional Hollow Fiber Filters

Hollow Fiber versus Pellicon 2—Summary		
Feature	Hollow Fiber	Pellicon 2
Robustness and reliability	Fibers are prone to stress failure	Very robust
Pressure capability	Low	High
Membrane choices	1. Polyethersulfone	1. Polyethersulfone 2. Regenerated cellulose 3. PVDF (for microfiltration)
Flow rate required to operate TFF processes	High flow rate resulting in • High energy consumption • Large piping • Compromised concentration ratio • Increased demand for floor space	Low flow rate resulting in • Low energy consumption • Small piping • High concentration ratio • Compact system size
Linear scale up	Compromised by differences in the length of the flow channel in laboratory versus process-scale cartridges	Identical length of flow channel length in all cartridge sizes to facilitate predictable scaling results
Consistency of retention relative to retentate channel design	Compromised consistency due to • Open flow channels. No internal mixing	High consistency due to • Build-in static mixer efficient internal mixing
Consistency of retention relative to the retentate flow channel length	Compromised consistency due to • Long flow channels	High consistency due to • Very short flow channels

11.12.6 Conclusion

From prefiltration to removing large sediments to harvesting bacterial cultures to removing viruses in the final stages of biological drug manufacturing, filters play one of the most important roles. There are dozens of companies specializing in specific filtration processes and giants dominate the market with their Millipore Pod® system, the Pall Stax® system, or Sartoclear® XL Drums from Sartorius Stedim. They also keep bringing newer filters, housings, arrangements, and recently in an integrated setup is their disposable factories concept. The manufacturer is highly advised to consult the current literature on the suitability of the type of filters used. More often than not, the suppliers are more than willing to understand the process and make recommendations. Obviously, cost is a serious concern but when it is realized that in a cGMP manufacturing environment having qualified a particular filter or a housing for a unit process, it is not easy to switch over to another type of filter or another supplier, the selection of these filters becomes a serious concern.

Questions

1. How is the manufacturing of some biologics going to change due to the expiration of patents coming soon?
2. Describe the three main categories of disposables.
   Answer:
   i.   Common disposables, petri dishes, flasks, pipets, PPE, test tubes.
   ii. Items for the line such as bags, connectors, tri-clamps, tubing, tank liners, valves.
   iii. Bioreactors, centrifuges, chromatography systems, pumps.
3. Since disposables make it easier to switch between production of different products and have been shown to reduce cost, name some of the perceived or real barriers to using disposables.
4. Describe the three classes of stabilizers used in polymers, their effect, and the major drawback of using a stabilizer.
   Answer: Melt processing aids that protect the polymer during extrusion and molding, thermal stabilizers that protect against heat in the final product, and light stabilizers that protect against UV. A major drawback is the introduction of new species that can be leached into the final product.
5. What benefit is derived from studying extractables in components for bioprocessing?
6. Describe some factors that may cause a leachable to not show up as an extractable.
   Answer: Products of reactions with the final drug formulation, different analytical methodologies.
7. In the USP 88 protocols, which of the six class classifications is the most stringent?
8. Why do many bag manufacturers recommend only partially filling the bags, especially if they are going to be used on a rocker?
   Answer: The pressure on the seals can cause them to burst.
9. Name some of the features that differentiate incubating containers from bioreactors.
10. When considering the selection of type of bioreactor, which design(s) might be selected to reduce the formation of foams in the culture media?

12

Upstream Processing

LEARNING OBJECTIVES

1. Identify the unique types of culture systems.
2. Recognize the advantages and disadvantages of each culture system.
3. Understand the challenges with scaling up cell culture systems.

12.1 INTRODUCTION

Upstream processing consists of a pure culture of the chosen organism, in sufficient quantity and in the correct physiological state; sterilized, properly formulated media, a seed bioreactor to develop inoculum to initiate the process in the main bioreactor; the production-scale bioreactor.

Downstream processing consists of equipment for drawing the culture medium in steady state, cell separation, collection of cell-free supernatant, product purification, and effluent treatment.

The upstream processing comprises production of target protein in a growth media in one of several forms: secretion to media, inclusion bodies in bacteria, and so on. Growing cells in supporting media under optimal conditions results in a wide range of products and process requires control of precise conditions to provide a commercially feasible yield of the target protein. The fermentation process (or bioprocess) is also used to generate biomass, various amino acids and vitamins, alcohol, or to modify compounds in addition to producing recombinant products, the focus of this book. Microorganisms (prokaryotic) and eukaryotic cell cultures are grown in volumes ranging from a few hundred mL to several thousand liters using a variety of cell growth methods and bioreactor designs. The large range of bioreactor sizes are needed because recombinant protein quantities needed vary widely, from hundreds of kilograms for albumin, hemoglobin, and insulin to perhaps a few grams for drugs like erythropoietins, interleukins, and so on. As a result, it is unlikely that the initial biogeneric therapeutic proteins will be of large volume type, due mainly to high initial investment required.

12.2 BIOREACTORS

A bioreactor is an equipment used to grow biological cells and organisms; historically, the word fermenter was used when microorganisms were grown and bioreactor when cells other than microorganisms are grown; however, these terms are now frequently used interchangeably, with preference for bioreactor in the recombinant production industry. A large variety of bioreactors are available such as shake flasks, roller bottles, spinner flasks, flexible cell culture flasks, wave bags, stirred tanks, and airlift reactors to support suspension, microcarrier, and cell encapsulation cultures. Many of these systems work at laboratory scale, yet a large array of them is used in the manufacturing operations if the required growth conditions are not reproduced in larger more efficient reactors. For biogeneric product manufacturer, another considerations must be made—to replicate the system of production used by the innovator and as approved by the regulatory authorities. At times, the biogeneric manufacturer may have to opt for a less efficient system merely to keep from introducing additional variable factors, like using cube system for cells that require stationary media vis-à-vis the use of roller bottles. The extent to which the biogeneric manufacturer will be able to modify the production technique will depend on the nature of validation required by the FDA in its comparability protocol guidelines for generic manufacturing; these guidelines are not yet released but are likely to be released in the coming months. The manufacturer may decide to forego the original method of production used and instead go for a more efficient and innovative system to obtain better yields even though this may require a larger investment upfront.

The wave technology offers, a newer addition, is a simple system up to 500 L culture with the advantage of using disposable materials. The technology is based on disposable plastic containers with ports to provide media and utility and monitoring probes; the bag rests on a plate that flips back and forth to create a wave motion inside the bag. The wave bioreactor is not free of shear forces and cell damage has been observed though improvement in the system are appearing rapidly and it is likely that this may turn out to be the premier system for mammalian cells and where contamination can be a problem, for example, using the same suite for multiple products.

The stirred tanks consist of stainless steel containers with rotating impellers of various configurations and devices that maintain constant agitation and control gas transfer, temperature, pH, and fluid level. Most stirred tanks use some form of sintered material or perforated tubing in order to sparge air or specific gas mixtures into the cell suspension. Figure 12.1 shows a typical (and perhaps one of the most popular) bioreactors.

Airlift bioreactors have no moving parts or mechanical seals and offers low hydrodynamic shear forces with a low power input per unit volume ($10–15$ W/m^3). This kind of bioreactors offers gentle gas circulation and good oxygen transfer. However, as the volume of the reactor increases, mixing becomes a limiting factor for the productivity (i.e., the amount of product formed per unit volume per unit time).

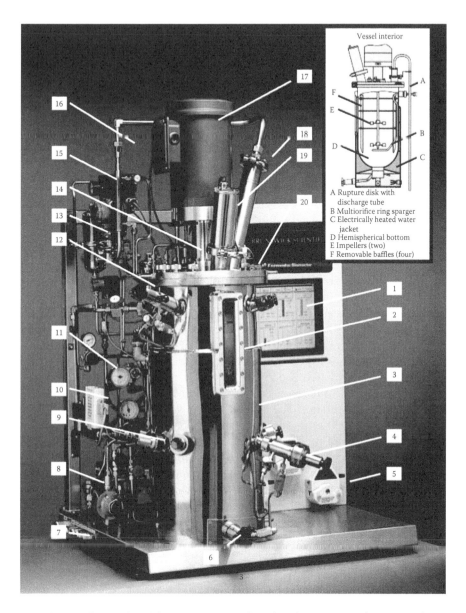

Figure 12.1 A typical stirred tank bioreactor. Reproduced with permission from manufacturer. Key: (1) controller with touch-screen interface; (2) viewing window; (3) sterilizer-in-place system; (4) resterilizable sample valve; (5) peristaltic pump; (6) resterilizable harvest/drain valve; (7) services, water, air, clean and house steam, water return and drain; (8) steam taps; (9) ports to allow addition of RTD, pH, DO, and other sensors; (10) thermal mass flow controller; (11) open frame piping to facilitate access for cleaning maintenance and servicing; (12) resterilizable inoculation/addition valves; (13) filters; (14) rupture disk to prevent overpressurization; (15) automatic back pressure regulator; (16) exhaust line with heat exchanger and view glass; (17) motor; (18) exhaust condenser; (19) combination light and fill port; (20) headplate ports for sampling and insertion of sensors and other devices.

425

12.3 BATCH CULTURE

A batch culture is a closed system with a fixed culture volume in which the cells grow until maximum cell density depending on medium nutrients, product toxicity, waste product toxicity, and other essential factors is reached. When a particular organism is introduced into a selected growth medium, the growth of the inoculum does not occur immediately, but takes a pause, the period of adaptation, called the lag phase. Following the lag phase, the rate of growth of the organism steadily increases, for a certain period, the period of logarithmic or exponential phase. After a certain time based on a variety of nutritional and cell characteristics, the rate of growth slows down, due to the continuously falling concentrations of nutrients and/or a continuously increasing (accumulating) concentration of toxic substances. This is called the deceleration phase. After the deceleration phase, growth ceases and the culture enters a stationary phase or a steady state. The biomass (or total quantity of cell mass) remains constant, except when certain accumulated chemicals in the culture begin to lyse the cells (chemolysis). Unless other microorganisms contaminate the culture, the chemical constitution remains unchanged. Mutation of the organism in the culture can also be a source of contamination, called internal contamination. If the desired product is produced in the log phase, it can be prolonged by manipulating the growth conditions but only for a very limited time, and if the desired amount is not produced that quickly, it will be reasonable to choose another culture method. At the onset of the stationary phase, the culture is disbanded for the recovery of its biomass (cells, organism) or the compounds (expressed proteins) that accumulated in the medium. This system of manufacturing is called batch processing or batch culture. A significant advantage of batch processing is the optimum levels of product recovery, control of growth conditions, and better regulatory compliance. The disadvantages are the wastage of unutilized nutrients, high labor costs, and the time lost in batch preparation. Batch cultivation however remains the simplest way to produce a recombinant protein. In batch cultivation, all the nutrients required for cell growth are supplied from the start, and the growth is initially unrestricted. However, the unrestricted growth commonly leads to unfavorable changes in the growth medium, such as oxygen limitation and pH changes. Also, certain metabolic pathways in the cell will be saturated, which potentially leads to the accumulation of inhibitory by-products in the medium. Therefore only moderate cell densities and production levels can normally be obtained with batch cultivations. To obtain high cell density and high protein production levels, fed-batch cultivation in a bioreactor is commonly used. Acetate is produced when the culture is growing in the presence of excess glucose or under oxygen-limiting conditions. A high concentration of acetate reduces growth rate, maximum obtainable cell density and the level of production of the recombinant protein. It is therefore important to maintain the acetate concentration below the inhibitory level. This can be achieved by controlling the cultivation in several ways: the growth rate could be controlled by limiting nutrients, such as sources of carbon or nitrogen; by using glycerol or fructose instead of glucose as the carbon/energy source; by addition of glycine and methionine or by lowering the cultivation temperature, or by metabolic engineering (http://www.babonline.org/bab/035/0091/bab0350091.htm—REF48#REF48). Other problems concerning growth to high cell densities are oxygen limitation, reduced mixing efficiency, heat generation, and high partial pressure of carbon dioxide.

12.4 CONTINUOUS CULTURE

In continuous processing the growth is limited by the availability of one or two components of the medium. As the initial quantity of a critical component is exhausted, growth ceases and a steady state is reached; growth is renewed by the addition of the limiting component. A certain amount of the whole culture medium can also be added periodically, after the steady state sets in. These additions increase the volume of the medium in the fermentation vessel, which is arranged such that the excess volume drains off as an overflow, which is collected and used for recovery of products. At each step of addition of the medium, the medium dilutes in the concentration of the biomass and the products. New growth, stimulated by the added medium increases the biomass and the products, till another steady state sets in; and another aliquot of medium reverses the process. It is called continuous culture or processing since the growth of the organism is controlled by the availability of growth-limiting chemical component of the medium, this system is called a chemostat. The rate at which aliquots are added or the dilution rate determines the growth rate.

Commercial adaptation of continuous processing is confined to biomass production, and to a limited extent to the production of potable and industrial alcohol. The production of growth-associated products like ethanol is more efficient in continuous processing, particularly for industrial use.

12.5 FED-BATCH CULTURE

In the fed-batch medium, a fresh aliquot of the medium is continuously or periodically added, without the removal of the culture fluid. The bioreactor is designed to accommodate the increasing volumes. The system is always at a quasi-steady state. Fed-batch processing requires greater degree of process and product control. A low but constantly replenished medium has the advantages of maintaining conditions in the culture within the aeration capacity of the bioreactor, removing the repressive effects of medium components such as rapidly used carbon and nitrogen sources and phosphate, avoiding the toxic effects of a medium component and providing limiting level of a required nutrient for an auxotrophic strain. Classically, the fed-batch culture is used in the production of baker's yeast, where biomass is the desired product. Diluting the culture with a batch of fresh medium prevents the production of ethanol, which affects the yield; in the production of yeast, the traces of ethanol were detected in the exhaust gas and the processing steps adjusted accordingly. Another classic fed-batch process product is penicillin, a secondary metabolite. Penicillin process has two stages: an initial growth phase followed by the production phase called the *iodophase*. The culture is maintained at low levels of biomass and phenyl acetic acid, the precursor of penicillin, is fed into the fermenter continuously, but at a low rate, as the precursor is toxic to the organism at higher concentrations.

In fed-batch cultivation, the carbon/energy source is added in proportion to the consumption rate. Thereby overflow metabolism and the accumulation of inhibitory by-products is minimized. Moreover, the growth rate can be balanced to achieve a maximal production level. The bioreactor should preferentially be equipped to maintain an optimal oxygen concentration, pH, and temperature. Defined media are generally used in fed-batch cultivation. As the concentrations of the nutrients are known and can be controlled during the cultivation, the cultivation is also more reproducible compared with the use of a complex growth medium. However, the addition of complex media, such as yeast extract, is sometimes necessary to obtain a high level of the desired recombinant protein.

In fed-batch process, neither cells nor medium are leaving the bioreactor keeping low the sugar levels for a long time and it is possible to switch from one substrate to another, thus rendering the use of inducible promoters possible. The process is usually performed at low growth rates adjusting the feed rate whose upper limit is dictated by the oxygen transfer limit and the cooling strategies available. The feed rate can be subjected to direct feedback control using substrate concentration and indirect feedback control parameters include cell concentration, culture fluorescence, carbon dioxide evolution rate, pDO, and pH-stat; constant, exponential, or increasing rate feeding are fixed and not subject to any feedback control as they are determined in the scale-up stage.

A variation of the classical fed-batch process is the semi-fed-batch process, where nutrients are added in dry form without changing the culture volume. In contrast to the batch mode, the operation of large-scale bioreactors in the fed-batch mode is subject to much variability. The substrate gradients formed may result in overflow metabolism locally in the bioreactor. The resulting product might be inhomogeneous as the cells produce variants of the target protein during different life cycle phases. Product stability might also be challenged by presence of proteolytic enzymes, as the product cannot be removed from the reactor before the end of production.

A mathematical model of a fed-batch reactor can be derived from a material balance across the reactor. Despite the apparent similarity between the fed-batch reactor model and the continuous culture model, they are very different. Whereas the chemostat equation for biomass accumulation is composed of a growth and a removal component:

$$\frac{dX}{dt} = \underset{\text{Biomass growth}}{\mu X} \cdot \underset{\text{Biomass removal}}{D X} \tag{12.1}$$

The fed-batch equation is composed of a growth and a dilution component (F/V):

$$\frac{dX}{dt} = \underset{\text{Growth}}{\mu X} \cdot \underset{\text{Dilution}}{\frac{F}{V} X} \tag{12.2}$$

The fed-batch reactor model contains an additional equation:

$$\frac{dV}{dt} = F \tag{12.3}$$

The concept of steady state cannot be as easily applied to a fed-batch reactor. The equations must therefore be solved numerically.

12.6 PERFUSION CULTURE

In perfusion batch cultivation, fresh media is added to the bioreactor and an equivalent amount is removed, with or without cells. A controlled perfusion bioreactor offers tight control of the growth conditions and cells can be kept in their productive phase for several

Table 12.1 Comparative Advantages and Disadvantages of Various Culture Systems

Culture	Advantages	Disadvantages
Batch	Well-tested technology, less contamination risk, less expensive	Limited cell density, downtime between batches, non-homogenous product, and variable quality between batches
Fed batch	High cell densities, longer culture periods using low medium viscosity	Non-homogenous product due to changing medium, large reactor size required, more susceptible to contamination, difficult to control, needs sophisticated monitoring systems
Perfusion	Long production phase, short down time, reducing cleaning and sterilization, waste removal, continuous expression, dilution of toxic medium, smaller reactor vessel	Susceptible to contamination due to frequent handling, difficult to control, requires sophisticated monitoring, nutrient gradients

months, if required. A significant risk in this process is contamination as the bioreactor is frequently handled in addition to accumulation of non-producing variants that can affect productivity. The advantages including short harvesting volumes, use of smaller bioreactor vessels, reducing initial capital costs despite lower yields obtained. Since the cells are maintained in the steady-state, the resulting product is often more homogeneous. The isolation of product can be controlled as the harvest can be selected from the steady-state production phase of the cell culture resulting in a more homogeneous product. The higher quality of product obtained from the steady-state culture in perfusion system makes downstream processing more efficient; there is also an option for batch processing of multiple harvests to reduce costs. These differences are often considered in making a choice for the perfusion system when considering the large media volume used in perfusion culture systems. Table 12.1 summarizes the advantages and disadvantages of the various types of culture processes used.

12.7 SUSPENSION CULTURE

A large variety of cells require adhesion to stationary surface to express proteins, for example, Chinese hamster ovary (CHO) cells in the production of erythropoietin. Classically, roller bottles are used to immobilize these cells whereby they secret the protein in the medium which is frequently harvested. These cells can also be immobilized onto the surface of microcarriers or to macroporous particles giving two advantages: easier control and high cell densities, for example, upward of 10^8 cells/ml. Microcarrier technology is used both in the batch and in the perfusion mode. See below for details on the use of microcarrier technology. Several bioreactor systems are based on immobilized cell technology (hollow fiber, ceramic matrix, packed-bed, and fluidized-bed reactors). Since suspension culture technology is relatively newer and the products approved by the FDA decades ago did not have the option of adopting them, many approved processes still rely on validated methods like the use of roller bottle. There are newer issues with suspension cultures such as cell aggregation and lack of system homogeneity when using hollow fiber systems. These remain to be resolved.

The absence of adventitious organisms in cell cultures is critical. In addition to demonstrating that bacteria, yeast, and molds are not present in cell cultures, the manufacturer must provide evidence for each culture that mycoplasmas and adventitious viruses are not present. It is important to recognize that certain hybridomas used for monoclonal antibody production may contain endogenous retroviruses. However, it must be demonstrated that any viruses present in the culture are removed from the final product. This requires the development of suitable analytical techniques to ensure the absence of contamination by mycoplasmas or human and animal adventitious viruses.

The degree and type of glycosylation may be important in the design of cell culture conditions for the production of glycosylated proteins. The degree of glycosylation present may affect the half-life of the product in vivo as well as its potency and antigenicity. Although the glycosylation status of a cell culture product is difficult to determine, it can be verified to be consistent if the culture conditions are highly reproducible.

Cell culture conditions are dependent upon the host system. Before performing a large-scale purification, it is important to check protein amplification in a small pilot experiment to establish optimum conditions for expression. The expression is monitored during growth and induction phase by retaining small samples at key steps in all procedures for analysis of the purification method. The yield of fusion proteins is highly variable and is affected by the nature of the fusion protein, the host cell, and the culture conditions.

12.8 MICROCARRIER SUPPORT

Microcarrier culture is a technique which makes possible the high yield culture of anchorage-dependent cells. By using macroporous microcarriers it is possible to immobilize semi-adherent and suspension cell lines, even in protein-free media. Growing cells on microcarriers can dramatically improve yield, reduce serum and media costs, decrease the risks of contamination and reduce the number of handling steps. The microcarrier surface supplies focal adhesion sites that support cellular traction, formation of the cytoskeleton, and orientation of organelles. Cells modify and lay down their own extracellular matrix on the microcarrier surface. Cells that form tight junctions can create a uniform cellular sheet around a microporous microcarrrier and generate a specific microenvironment inside the carrier. Cells in such sheets are polarized with typical apical and basolateral side. Microporous carriers allow cell-to-cell communication of low to medium molecular weight media components through the microcarrier. The volumetric cell densities in microcarriers allow use of serum or protein-free media, simplifying downstream processing. There is an additional protection of cells from the shear force stress due to aeration by sparging, spin filters and impellers. The use of microcarriers allow inoculation and growing one type of cells inside and another type outside where necessary such as in creating *artificial organs*. Compared to spin filters, immobilization of cells allows running perfusion cultures which allows use of serum-free media and switch from growth to production media; high density caused faster rate of exchange of nutrient minimizing retention times of secreted products, speeding harvesting of product at lower temperature—this can significantly improve product degradation profile and build up of toxic substances from the cells.

Amersham (Little Chalfont, UK) company was the first to produce these microporous microcarriers and offers several kinds such as Cytodex for use in animal cells; it is a transparent, hydrophilic and hydrated, cross-linked dextran for use in stirred cultures. Cytodex 1 is formed by cross-linking dextran matrix with positively charged DEAE groups making it more suitable for established cell lines for production from cultures of primary, and normal diploid cells. Cytodex 3 is formed by coupling a thin layer of denatured pig skin collagen type 1 to the cross-linked dextran matrix; this is more suitable for difficult to cultivate cells with an epithelial-type morphology. The collagen surface is susceptible to digestion by a variety of proteolytic enzymes which provides the opportunity to harvest cells from the microcarriers while maintaining maximum cell viability and membrane integrity.

Cytopore (http://www.amersham.com) is a transparent, hydrophilic and hydrated microporous cross-linked cellulose microcarrier with positively charged *N,N*-ethyl-aminoethyl groups; it is more rigid than Cytodex. Cytopores can also be used to immobilize insect cells, yeast and bacteria besides the CHO cells. Cytopore 1 is designed for use in suspension culture systems for growth of recombinant CHO cells with charge capacity of 1.00 meq/g; Cytopore 2 is optimized for anchorage-dependent cells where the optima charge density required is about 1.8 meq/g.

Cytoline (Amersham, http://www.amersham.com) is a range of weighted macroporous carriers for use in stirred tank, packed-bed, and fluidized-bed cultures; it is nontransparent and composed of medical quality polyethylene which is weighted by silica. Cytoline offers increased protection from shear forces, improves nutrition and aeration while reducing the need to use serum. Cytoline 1 is optimized for use in fluidized-bed cultures of CHO cells; its high sedimentation rate (120–220 cm/min) enables a high recirculation rate to allow better supply of oxygen. Cytoline 2 is a lower sedimentation rate 25–75 cm/min microcarrier for use in stirred cultures but mainly in the culture of hybridomas and other stress sensitive cells, in fluidized beds. Cytopilot Mini offered by Amersham is a laboratory-scale fluidized-bed reactor, designed specifically to exploit the potential of Cytoline.

Other suppliers of microporous microcarrier include Cultispher by Percell Biolytica AB (http://www.percell.se/). Hillex microcarriers by SoloHill (http://www.solohill.com/hillex.html).

Generally, microcarrier cultures can be contained in virtually any type of culture vessel. However, best results are obtained with equipment that gives even suspension of the microcarriers with gentle stirring. The most suitable vessels for general-purpose microcarrier culture are those with efficient gassing and mixing systems that do not generate high shear forces and provide a homogeneous culture environment. For really high cell densities a perfusion culture system is needed. However, when selecting a vessel for a perfusion culture some design criteria need consideration. The stirrer should never come into contact with the inside surface of the vessel during culture because it may damage the microcarriers. Similarly, spinner vessels with a bearing immersed in the culture medium are not suitable because the microcarriers can circulate through the bearing and get crushed. Alternatives to fermenters for perfusion culture exist for laboratory, pilot and production scale applications.*

The exact culture procedure depends on the type of cell and on the culture vessel. Macroporous microcarrier cultures normally contain 1–2 g Cytopore 1, and are usually inoculated with about 2×10^6 cells/ml. Perfused cultures may contain much higher microcarrier concentrations. In such instances the inoculum should be increased proportionally. Successful microcarrier culture depends on the state of the inoculum and correct operation during the initial stages. Conditions vary with cell type and the culture conditions. Anchorage-dependent cells cannot survive unattached in suspension for very long. The easy access to the interior of the carriers facilitates initiation of the culture at full culture volume, and enables continuous stirring at 30 rpm, from commencement of the culture.

For a stationary culture, cover the bottom of a bacteriological petri dish with microcarriers. The suggested starting concentration of microcarriers for a 60 mm of petri dish is approximately 2 mg/ml (about 0.1 cc/ml). For stirred cultures, the optimum concentration varies from cell to cell. The concentration for CHO cells is approximately 1–2 mg/ml. However, this very much depends on the feeding strategy for the culture. The high cell density experienced with macroporous carriers means that the culture rapidly consumes any available metabolites. A steady state should be maintained; toxic metabolites should not be allowed to accumulate and pH values should be maintained at the set level. Rapid changes in pH cause cell peeling and a reduction in the final cell yield. CO_2 should also be kept at the desired level. Cell growth can be monitored by glucose consumption and lactate build-up, CO_2 consumption, and cell counting.

12.9 ROLLER BOTTLE CULTURE SYSTEM

This is the most commonly used method for initial scale up of attached cells also known as anchorage-dependent cell lines. Roller bottles are cylindrical vessels that revolve slowly (between 5 and 60 revolutions per hour) which bathes the cells that are attached to the inner surface with medium. Roller bottles are available typically with surface areas of 1,050 cm². The size of some of the roller bottles presents problems since they are difficult to handle in the confined space of a microbiological safety cabinet. Recently roller bottles with expanded inner surfaces have become available which has made handling large surface area bottles more manageable, but repeated manipulations and subculture with roller bottles should be avoided if possible. A further problem with roller bottles is with the attachment of cells since as some cells lines do not attach evenly. This is a particular problem with epithelial cells. This may be partially overcome a little by optimizing the speed of rotation, generally by decreasing the speed, during the period of attachment for cells with low attachment efficiency.

---

* Glass culture vessels should be siliconized before use.

12.10 SPINNER FLASK CULTURE

This is the method of choice for suspension lines including hybridomas and attached lines that have been adapted to growth in suspension, for example, HeLa S3. Spinner flasks are either plastic or glass bottles with a central magnetic stirrer shaft and side arms for the addition and removal of cells and medium, and gassing with CO_2 enriched air. Inoculated spinner flasks are placed on a stirrer and incubated under the culture conditions appropriate for the cell line. Cultures should be stirred at 100–250 revolutions per minute. Spinner flask systems designed to handle culture volumes of 1–12 L are available from Techne (http://www.techne.com), Sigma (http://www.sigmaaldrich.com), and Bellco (http://www.bellcoglass.com/).

12.11 OTHER SCALE-UP OPTIONS

The next stage of scale up for both suspension and attached cell lines is the bioreactor that is used for large culture volumes (in the range 100–10,000 L). For suspension cell lines the cells are kept in suspension by either a propeller in the base of the chamber vessel or by air bubbling through the culture vessel. However both of these methods of agitation give rise to mechanical stresses. A further problem with suspension lines is that the density obtained is relatively low; in the order of 2×10^6 cells/ml.

For attached cell lines the cell densities obtained are increased by the addition of microcarrier beads. These small beads are 30–100 μm in diameter and can be made of dextran, cellulose, gelatin, glass or silica, and increase the surface area available for cell attachment considerably. The range of microcarriers available means that it is possible to grow most cell types in this system.

A recent advance has been the development of porous microcarriers which has increased the surface area available for cell attachment by a further 10–100 fold. The surface area on 2 g of beads is equivalent to 15 small roller bottles.

A newly introduced Roller Cell® system utilizes a rotary system of multiple bottles attached to a central collection duct avoiding labor costs associated with periodic harvesting of media. It can be used for a simple culture protocol with a *cell harvest* or multiharvest system (i.e., 10 × refeed/harvest). A comparison of the time taken to process the equivalent of 200 standard bottles manually, with a robotic automated system, and the RollerCell 40™ shows that for simple harvesting the total man hours are 15.5 in regular roller bottles, 5.7 h in robotic systems and only 1.5 h in RollerCell™ system. In multiple harvest system, if the manual hours are 37 in regular roller bottle system and 33.3 in robotic systems, it takes only 6.3 h. The RollerCell™ system (http://www.synthecon.com/Cellon/rc2.shtml) is certainly worth considering when scaling up production of suspension cell culture systems.

12.12 WAVE BIOREACTOR

This newer system of completely disposable bioreactor has many advantages including no cleaning, cross-contamination, or validation issues. Cells stay in contact with a disposable sterile biocompatible plastic which conforms to USP Class VI and ISO 10993. Bioreactors,

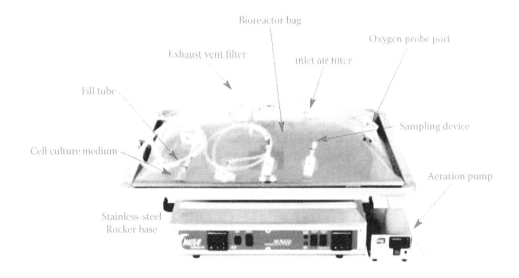

Figure 12.2 Essential features of wave bioreactor system.

including all fittings, and filters are delivered sterile and ready for use. These are ideal for cGMP applications and no biosafety cabinet is required in their use. These can be used in an incubator or on the bench with integral heater and optional CO_2/air mixing unit. For suspension, microcarrier or perfusion culture, spinners, roller bottles, and similar systems are not scalable due to inherently limited mass transfer surface area. The Wave Bioreactor® has no such limit and operation up to 580 L has been demonstrated, with cell densities over 6×10^7 cells/mL. Studies have shown excellent validation for CHO cells from 1–500 L capacity Wave Bioreactors (Figure 12.2) (http://www.wavebiotech.com).

The biogeneric recombinant protein manufacturers are advised to consider this system as their choice system to avoid many cGMP issues that are inevitable in any bioprocess scaling. The Wave Bioreactor system is an excellent option for suspension clones or attachment-dependent lines using microcarriers. It is not usually a good option for attachment-dependent cell lines that have hitherto been grown on rigid surfaces in roller bottles (e.g., currently available erythropoietin cell line). The surface of the bag is usually not designed for attachment. The Wave Bioreactor provides still too much disturbance during periodic harvesting that can cause a high degree of stress on the cells and probably cause them to slough off the surface and clump rather than maintain the confluent monolayer. Given below are some of the present applications of wave bioreactors:

Monoclonal antibodies: The wave bioreactor has been used extensively for monoclonal antibody production. Culture can be started at low volume and then fresh media is added whenever the cell count is sufficiently high. This enables inoculum scale up without transfers. In batches ranging from 100 mL to 580 L have been run with cell densities over 6×10^6 cells/mL, the productivity was comparable to stirred tank bioreactors. Dissolved oxygen concentrations were not limiting and remained above 50% saturation.

Insect cells/baculovirus: The high oxygen supply capability of the Wave Bioreactor makes it ideal for insect cell culture. Ten liter batch volumes are routine with cell densities over 9×10^6 cells/mL. Baculovirus yields are higher than with conventional bioreactors. The Wave Bioreactor system is extremely easy to operate and inoculum scale up and infection can be done inside the bioreactor, reducing the need for transfers.

Anchorage-dependent cells: Agitation in the wave bioreactor is powerful enough to mix and aerate the culture, yet it is gentle enough to cultivate anchorage-dependent cells on various microcarriers. Some reports indicate displacement and rupture of cells not specifically designed for the purpose.

Perfusion culture: Unique internal perfusion filter equipped Cellbags make perfusion culture easy. Bioreactors can be operated for weeks, and cell densities up to 6×10^7 cells/mL have been reported. Applications include high-density culture and patient-specific cell therapy. Wave bioreactors are in use in GMP applications producing inoculum for large conventional bioreactors, and also for clinical and commercial production of human therapeutics. Reduced cleaning and validation requirements make this an ideal system for GMP applications.

Other uses: The wave bioreactor has many other uses, for example keeping in-process inoculum pools agitated and aerated prior to use; bead-to-bead transfer; thawing, and mediamixing. Custom Cellbags can be provided for special applications.

12.13 CELL CUBE TECHNOLOGY

The CellCube® System offered by Corning (http://www.corning.com/lifesciences/news_center/press_releases/electronic_e-cube.asp) provides a fast, simple, and compact method for the mass culture of attachment-dependent cells. Disposable CellCube modules have a polystyrene tissue culture treated growth surface for cell attachment where the production can range from module with 8,500 cm² cell growth surface to one with 340,000 cm² using the same control package. The system continually perfuses the cells with fresh media for increased cell productivity. The CellCube System is comprised of four pieces of capital equipment—the system controller, oxygenator, circulation, and media pumps. The cell cubes consist of a series of parallel rigid plates designed for attached monolayers. One set of plates has the equivalent area to 200 roller bottles. The media is contained in a large reservoir which could be replaced on a daily basis (Figure 12.3).

12.14 ROTARY CULTURE SYSTEM

A newer entry to culture systems is the rotary cell culture system (e.g., Synthecon's RCCS™; http://www.synthecon.com), which is different from all other cell culture systems. The cylindrical culture vessel is filled with culture fluid and the cells or tissue particles are added. All air bubbles are removed from the culture vessel. The vessel is attached to the rotator base and rotated about the horizontal axis. Cells establish a fluid orbit within the culture medium in the horizontally rotating cylindrical vessel. They do not collide with the walls or any

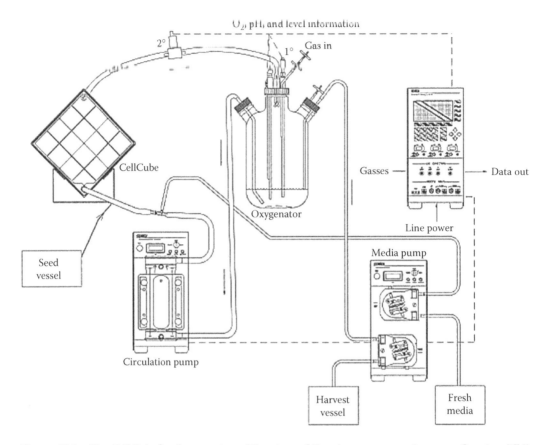

Figure 12.3 The CellCube® culture system. (Courtesy of Corning, www.corning.com, Corning, NY.)

other parts of the vessel and often appear as if embedded in gelatin. As cells grow in size the rotation speed is adjusted to compensate for the increased settling rates of the larger particles. The tissue particles do move enough within the fluid culture medium to exchange nutrients, wastes and dissolved gases, and make contact with other tissue particles. The cells and/or tissue particles often join to form larger tissue particles that continue the differentiation process.

Oxygen supply and carbon dioxide removal is achieved through a gas permeable silicone rubber membrane, which acts very much as lung membranes. Since The Rotary Cell Culture System™ has no impellers, airlifts, bubbles, or agitators, tissue damage from impact and turbulence is significantly decreased as compared to conventional bioreactors. Shear stress and damage is so low that it is essentially insignificant. Under these conditions, cells communicate and synthesize tissue as they would in the body rather than concentrate their energy on repair.

Unlike cell and tissue cultures grown in two-dimensional flat plate systems, cells grown in the Rotary Cell Culture System™ are functionally similar to tissues in the human body. You will be able to grow three-dimensional tissues in vitro that mimic the structure and function of the same tissue in vivo.

12.15 MEDIA

The integral component of upstream processing is the media used; its selection depends on the type of bioreactor used and type of culture system adopted. Whereas a large volume of data are available in the scientific literature on the selection of media, the best advice is available from the patent applications that described the original product as well as the information available from the media suppliers. Several environmental and regulatory considerations have changed the selection of media and the manufacturers are strongly advised to develop a good working relationship with media suppliers, who are more than cooperative in offering advice and frequently offer to run test batches to optimize the selection process. The search for media should begin with the following websites:

www.bd.com
www.cambrex.com
www.specialtymedia.com
www.hynetics.com
www.invitrogen.com
www.jrhbio.com
www.irvinesci.com
www.cellgro.com
www.pharma-ingredients.questint.com
www.serologicals.com
www.sial.com

The composition of the cell growth medium is very important as it significantly affects both the cells and the protein expression. For example, the translation of different mRNAs is differentially affected by temperature as well as changes in the culture medium. Nutrient composition and fermentation variables such as temperature, pH, and other parameters can affect proteolytic activity, secretion, and production levels. Specific manipulations of the culture medium have been shown to enhance protein release into the medium. Thus, supplementation of the growth medium with glycine enhances the release of periplasmic proteins into the medium without causing significant cell lysis. Similarly, growth of cells under osmotic stress in the presence of sorbitol and glycyl betaine causes more than a 400-fold increase in the production of soluble, active protein.

12.16 SCALING AND PRODUCTION COSTS

The upstream process is linked to downstream process and the selection of each step in the two phases is determined based on cost optimization considerations even though the expertise required in each of these steps is highly specialized. The downstream processing adds 80%–90% of the total cost of production; compare this with the cost of recovery in other biological fermentation productions: 5% for whole-cell yeast biomass, 10%–50% for bulk chemicals, 10% for extracellular enzymes, and 20%–50% for antibiotics. The high cost of recombinant DNA products arises from the low yields in aqueous fermentation broths and high purification regulatory requirements. As a result, it is not unusual to find market price for rDNA products in the range of $100,000 plus while the biomass and chemicals can be bought for pennies per kg.

Cost reduction in the manufacturing of recombinant products is an integrated approach wherein the upstream and downstream processing are developed to minimize waste, use of raw materials, capital, and energy. The large-scale process development for the upstream process takes into consideration several key factors such as

Organism selection, with regard to substrate versatility, by-product formation characteristics, robustness of the organism, for example, to process upsets, viability with regard to cell recycling, physiological characteristics (maximum growth rate, aeration requirements, etc.), and genetic accessibility.

Metabolic and cellular engineering to improve existing properties of the organism, to introduce novel functions, for example, by simplifying product recovery, expanding substrate and product ranges, and enabling fermentation to occur under nonstandard conditions.

Fermentation process development to achieve culture and media optimization (from complex to defined minimal media), optimization of cultivation parameters that take into account product recovery and purification (minimize by-product formation, minimize chemical inputs, and develop high-cell-density cultivation), and incorporation of cell retention/recycling. Several specific steps can be taken to minimize cost:

- Simplification of broth to remove whatever is nonessential, albeit at reduced efficiency, is a good general rule; inevitably, any added component burdens the downstream processing.
- Selecting alternate product form that is easier to separate in downstream processing.
- Reusing broth components, for example, recycling cells, although a technical challenge, holds promise for improving fermentation efficiency. The CHO cells show declining yield over 7-day period; however, adding fresh cells to already present cells may present a cost-reducing possibility. This cannot be done for processes where the drug is contained as inclusion body. Another strategy is reusing some or all of the broth after product separation. Often, optimum product synthesis and biomass growth take place when medium nutrients are present in excess. However, this results in nutrients being left over at the end of fermentation.
- Removing the product during fermentation improves the yield as the possible inhibitory effects of the product on production are reduced. Using continuous extraction, a side-stream can be routed out of the unit and the extracted broth returned to conserve broth as well. Further, two-phase fermentations have been developed to extract the product from a biomass-containing aqueous phase into an organic phase, which can then be removed on-line.

- Reducing the water content, which is typically as high as 90%, reduces downstream processing cost as well as the cost of purified water. This is accomplished by increasing the biomass concentration (i.e., high-cell-density [HCD] fermentation), engineering the organism to tolerate higher product concentrations, and removing inhibitory elements from the fermentation media composition.

Use of microcarriers in bioreactors for cells that requires stationary surface is an excellent approach to improve overall yield.

Introduction of downstream unit operations within a fermentation process reduce cost substantially, for example, extractive fermentation, electrodialysis, and in-line membrane separation technologies.

12.17 PROBLEM RESOLUTION IN FUSION PROTEIN EXPRESSION

A large expense should be budgeted for problem resolution during scale up of upstream processes. The inherent nature of cells, how they interact with media, the role of contamination, and so on, make it almost impossible to predict the fate of any scale-up batch. It is this knowledge and experience that the innovator companies purportedly adduce as the reason why a biological product cannot be produced as a generic equivalent. It is therefore imperative that the scale up should be fully validated. Following are some of the noted problems that may arise in the expression of fusion proteins and their solutions:

Too high a level of expression
Add 2% glucose to the growth medium. This will decrease the basal expression level associated with the upstream *lac* promoter but will not affect basal-level expression from the *tac* promoter. The presence of glucose should not significantly affect overall expression following induction with IPTG.

Basal-level expression (i.e., expression in the absence of an inducer, such as IPTG), present with most inducible promoters, can affect the outcome of cloning experiments for toxic inserts; it can select against inserts cloned in the proper orientation. Basal-level expression can be minimized by catabolite repression (e.g., growth in the presence of glucose). The *tac* promoter is not subject to catabolite repression. However, with the pGEX vector system there is a *lac* promoter located upstream between the 3′-end of the *lacIq* gene and the *tac* promoter. This *lac* promoter may contribute to the basal level of expression of inserts cloned into the pGEX multiple cloning site, and it is subject to catabolite repression.

No protein detected in bacterial sonicate.
Check DNA sequences. It is essential that protein-coding DNA sequences are cloned in the proper translation frame in the vectors. Cloning junctions should be sequenced to verify that inserts are in-frame.

Optimize culture conditions to improve yield. Investigate the effect of cell strain, medium composition, incubation temperature, and induction conditions. Exact conditions will vary for each fusion protein expressed.

Analyze a small aliquot of an overnight culture by SDS-PAGE. Generally, a highly expressed protein will be visible by Coomassie™ blue staining when 5–10 µL of an induced culture whose A600 is ~1.0 is loaded on the gel. Non-transformed host *E. coli* cells and cells transformed with the parental vector should be run in parallel as negative and positive controls, respectively. The presence of the fusion protein in this total cell preparation and its absence from a clarified sonicate may indicate the presence of inclusion bodies.

Check for expression by immunoblotting. Some fusion proteins may be masked on an SDS-polyacrylamide gel by a bacterial protein of approximately the same molecular weight. Immunoblotting can be used to identify fusion proteins in these cases. Run an SDS-polyacrylamide gel of induced cells and transfer the proteins to a nitrocellulose or PVDF membrane (such as Hybond™-C or Hybond-P). Detect fusion protein using anti-GST or anti-His antibody.

Most of the fusion protein is in the post-sonicate pellet

Check cell disruption procedure. Cell disruption is seen by partial clearing of the suspension or by microscopic examination. Addition of lysozyme (0.1 volume of a 10 mg/ml lysozyme solution in 25 mM Tris-HCl, pH 8.0) prior to sonication may improve results. Avoid frothing as this may denature the fusion protein.

Reduce sonication since oversonication can lead to co-purification of host proteins with the fusion protein.

Fusion protein may be produced as insoluble inclusion bodies. Try altering the growth conditions to slow the rate of translation, as suggested below. It may be necessary to combine these approaches. Exact conditions must be determined empirically for each fusion protein.

Lower the growth temperature (within the range of +20°C to +30°C) to improve solubility.

Decrease IPTG concentration to <0.1 mM to alter induction level.

Alter time of induction.

Induce for a shorter period of time.

Induce at a higher cell density for a short period of time.

Increase aeration. High oxygen transport can help prevent the formation of inclusion bodies. It may be necessary to combine the above approaches. Exact conditions must be determined empirically for each fusion protein.

Alter extraction conditions to improve solubilization of inclusion bodies.

Questions

1. Define fed-batch culture and the cell type for which it is best known
   Answer: Fresh media is continually or periodically added to attempt to obtain a quasi-steady state level of nutrients. It is best known for baker's yeast culture.
2. What types of cells are roller bottle systems best for?
   Answer: Adherent cells, which are attached along the walls of the roller bottle and gradually *washed* with media as the bottle rotates. Suspension cultures would see no benefit from a roller bottle relative to other culture systems.

3. What order of magnitude cell density can be expected by using microcarrier cell culture methods?

4. Aside from an increase in density, what benefits do microcarriers offer to the cell microenvironment?

5. Using microcarriers can sometimes reduce the need for serum in the media, what benefit does this have and what quality of the microcarrier is giving this effect?

6. What kind of modifications can be done to microcarriers to improve or tailor them to specific cell types?

   Answer: Coatings with extracellular matrix proteins, collagen, fibronectin, laminin, and so on.

7. Why can cost be reduced by in-stream extraction?

8. Define inclusion body (use outside source if necessary).

   Answer: Inclusion bodies are aggregates of a substance that shows up under staining. They can be a concern for bioprocessing especially as they can indicate bacterial contamination.

9. What is the culture method of choice for suspension cell cultures?

10. Considering that downstream processing often is a major cost in biological production, what reservation should a bioprocess planner or engineer have when considering the addition of a component to media?

    Answer: Removal of that component may make the downstream processing more costly.

13

Downstream Processing

LEARNING OBJECTIVES

1. Recognize the stages of downstream processing.
2. Understand the key considerations for selection of downstream processing techniques.
3. Identify the challenges presented by downstream processing techniques.

13.1 INTRODUCTION

Whereas upstream process generates the crude protein and much depends on the nature of gene construct and the conditions of upstream processing that determines the nature of protein, it is the downstream processing that defines the final product.

Downstream processing schemes include several stages (Figure 13.1), each serving a specific function; primarily this consists of Capture, Intermediate Purification and Polishing or final purification. Highest efficiency and cost reduction is achieved when the number of steps are reduced to a minimum, without appreciably affecting the final yield. The methods used in downstream processing are crucial to the safety of the product and as a result the processing area is required to be of the higher air quality standard than the upstream area (10,000 vs. 100,000). For recombinant proteins intended for use as human drugs, the purity must often exceed 99%, and some impurities, such as endotoxins and DNA, are limited to an upper level in the range of parts per million. Chromatographic methods available provide adequate purification and purity levels required and are easily scalable. The most frequently used chromatographic methods are ion-exchange chromatography, size-exclusion chromatography, hydrophobic-interaction chromatography, reversed-phase chromatography, and affinity chromatography.

A careful selection of the processes in any downstream processing begins with an understanding of the characteristics of the protein in question, its stability profile, and the factors that may alter its structure. The most important criteria the design of downstream process is the physical and chemical properties of the protein manufactured (Table 13.1).

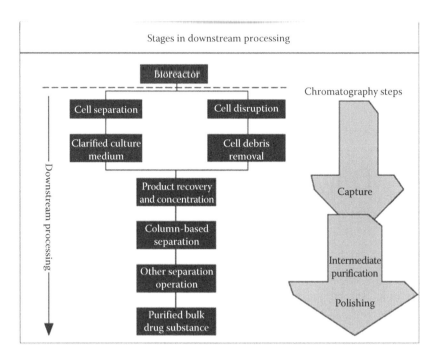

Figure 13.1 Downstream processing stages. (Data from Amersham Biotech Pharmacia, *Expanded Bed Adsorption Principles and Methods*, www.gelifesciences.com.)

Table 13.1 Protein Properties and Downstream Processing Systems

Property	Affects
Charge	Choice of purification methods, precipitation, crystallization, and chromatography.
Cofactors	Choice to add cofactors to stabilize proteins.
Co-solvents	Choice of co-solvents depends on function of pH, ionic strength, temperature, and redox potential on stability and solubility.
Detergent requirement	Choice and concentration of detergents depend on hydrophobicity of proteins during separation and purification.
Disulfide bonds	Control of redox potential; a shift of one pH unit results in a 60 mV change in redox potential (toward the reducing side when pH is raised); use of reducing agents such as dithiothreitol or cysteine to reduce the cysteine residues to cysteine conversion.
Free cysteines	Control of reducing agents and condition (mM amounts of reducing agents are added to the buffer to prevent air oxidation) to maintain free cysteine residues.

(Continued)

Table 13.1 (*Continued*)   Protein Properties and Downstream Processing Systems

Property	Affects
Hydrophobicity	Use of detergents to the buffers to prevent aggregation and binding to surfaces. Hydrophobic proteins are sticky and tend to bind to surfaces and to other proteins and hydrophobic co-solvents (detergents); choice of reverse phase chromatography depends on hydrophobicity.
Ionic strength	The solubility of the protein depends on the ionic strength of the solution.
Isoelectric point	pH adjustment to prevent unintended precipitation, particularly at low ionic concentration, during elution from chromatographic columns.
Metal ion sensitivity	Addition of EDTA to remove divalent metal ions.
Molecular weight	Selection of ultra- and microfiltration membranes and chromatographic columns.
Posttranslational modifications	Choice of methods including translation medium to control glycosylation and phosphorylation as essential properties for regulatory approvals.
Protease sensitivity	Storage of the harvest, or during downstream processing, to prevent protease activity.
Solubility	Conditions that cause unintended precipitation by electrostatic interaction at low ionic strength, especially at pH values close to the isoelectric point (isoelectric precipitation), hydrophobic interactions under conditions of high salt concentration (salting out) in the preparation of feedstock for hydrophobic interaction chromatography. (Precipitation of even small particles blocks filters, columns, and valves in preparative loadings to chromatographic columns.)
Stability	Control of pH, conductivity, temperature, redox potential, protein concentration, divalent metal ions, proteolytic enzymes, cofactors and presence of co-solvents to prevent degradation and aggregation. Biologic activity correlates with stability.

13.2 CAPTURE

Capture step may include a number of different unit operations such as cell harvesting, product release, feedstock clarification, concentration, and initial purification. Expanded bed adsorption technology is specifically designed to address the problems related to the beginning of the downstream sequence and may serve as the ultimate capture step since it combines clarification, concentration and initial purification into one single operation. Details of expanded bed operations are provided later in the chapter.

The overall purpose of the capture stage is to rapidly isolate the target molecule from critical contaminants such as proteases and glycosidases, remove particulate matter, concentrate, and transfer to an environment which conserves potency/activity. At this stage, high throughput (i.e., capacity and speed) and short process times are very important. Processing time is critical because the fermentation broths and crude cell homogenates contain proteases and glycosidases that reduce product recovery and produce degradation products that may be difficult to remove later. Adsorption of the target molecule on a solid adsorbent as done in expanded bed systems and adsorption chromatography decreases the likelihood of interaction between degradative enzymes and susceptible intramolecular bonds in the target molecule. The first step is a capturing step, where the product binds to the adsorbent while the impurities do not. The product is often eluted with a step gradient, giving a high concentration of the product but a moderate degree of purification. The main requirements of this first step are high capacity, high degree of product recovery, and high chemical and physical stability. Ion-exchange chromatography and, to some extent, hydrophobic-interaction chromatography are frequently used as the first chromatographic step.

13.2.1 Intermediate Purification

After the capturing step, the bulk of impurities, such as host-cell proteins, nucleic acids, and endotoxins, is typically removed with high-resolution techniques such as hydrophobic-interaction chromatography, ion-exchange chromatography, reversed-phase chromatography, or affinity chromatography. Lower flow rates, gradient elution, and matrices with particles of smaller size are used for enhanced resolution. After these steps, the product purity is typically at a level of 99%.

13.2.2 Polishing

The last step is a polishing step to remove any aggregates, degradation products, or target protein molecules that may have been modified during the purification procedure. It also serves to condition the purified product for its use or storage. Commonly used techniques for the final step are size-exclusion chromatography and reversed-phase chromatography.

13.3 SYSTEM SUITABILITY

The purification schemes should enable the eluted sample from one step to be applied directly on to the next step, avoiding buffer changes and concentration steps. It is also important to keep the number of steps as low as possible, since the total recovery decreases rapidly with the increasing number of steps. A convenient way to reduce the number of steps in the purification scheme without reducing the purity is to include a step with high selectivity, such as affinity chromatography, at each stage. Finally, the sanitization and cleanability of equipment is important. Cleaning chromatography columns is particularly challenging because of the inability to achieve the recommended linear velocities necessary to efficiently clean bioprocess equipment. Consequently, the mechanical design of the column plays a large role in its cleanability. The column's internal flow geometries and seal configurations must prevent dead flow areas that allow liquid to remain static during normal operation. All areas of the column must be swept with sufficient and consistent velocity to ensure effective cleaning and sanitization. The prospective manufacturer is advised to seek from manufacturers certification that the column is sanitizable and the regulatory authorities do accept this claim. Examples of sanitizable column include the QuikScale® biochromatography column, which is designed to distribute the solution evenly across the packed media bed to prevent any areas of stagnant liquid. This column can be easily and consistently sanitized and cleaned by FDA guidelines using typical sanitization protocols employing NaOH. As an example, the BioProcess™ HPLC columns from Amersham comprise a family of stainless steel, high-pressure chromatography columns with a wide range of bed heights and inner diameters and feature dynamic axial compression that uses solvent as the compression medium. In addition, dynamic axial piston pressure eliminates the formation of voids or channels in packed beds. Together with a specially designed flow distribution system fitted at both the piston and the bottom of the column, this ensures a uniform distribution of the mobile phase across the whole bed. These columns comply with the technical performance demands placed on equipment operated at pressures up to 100 bar in industrial bioprocessing. In addition, they withstand temperatures up to 50°C, which allows effective cleaning with warm water. Construction is in stainless steel AISI 316 L, and the sanitary design includes quick connections. Sealing materials are resistant to organic solvents and a leakage detection system is included.

13.4 DOWNSTREAM PROCESSING SYSTEMS

The choice of process equipment, the chemicals used, the columns selected, and the conditions under which processing is made are all critical. This section provides a general discussion of these elements. Details of processing can be found in the discussion of cell-specific processes described elsewhere in the book.

13.4.1 Buffers and Solvents

A large number of buffers and solvents are used in various unit operations associated with downstream processing. The largest range for buffers should normally be pKa ± 1. The solvents are selected based on their incompatibility with the proteins and the resins used. A list of most commonly used buffers and a list of most commonly used co-solvents along with the general conditions of their use are provided in Tables 13.2 and 13.3.

13.4.2 Sample Preparation

Each unit operation processes a prepared sample, which is generally a solution of target protein with variable levels of impurities and has specific chemical and physical properties suitable for the processing desired. Conditioning of samples includes such steps as centrifugation, filtration, microfiltration, ultrafiltration, desalting, and precipitation (Table 13.4).

An optimized sample preparation will include the least number of steps; for samples prepared for initial handling, use of expanded bed technology is advised

Table 13.2 Commonly Used Downstream Buffers and the Conditions of Their Use

Buffer	pKa	dpKa/dT	Comments
Acetic acid	4.76	−0.0002	Supplied as glacial acetic acid ($d = 0.1.058$ g/mL at 20°C). Acetic acid is corrosive and fumes irritant.
Ammonia	9.25	−31	Volatile. Fumes are harmful. Buffers are often prepared of ammonium hydrogen chloride or bicarbonate.
Boric acid	9.23	−0.008	Often used in combination with Tris and not so often as a stand-alone buffer.
Carbonic acid	6.35	−0.0055	CO_2 exchange with environment. Carbonate buffers
	10.33	−0.009	are commonly used in cell cultures to sustain CO_2 levels. Work above pH 7.5 to avoid release of CO_2.
Citric acid	3.14		Commonly used buffer in the pH range of 3–7.
	4.76		
	6.39		
Ethanolamine	9.50	−0.029	Smelly harmful liquid. Reacts with many amine-modifying agents.
Glycine	2.35	−0.002	Make sure the amino acid is not of animal origin.
	9.78	−0.025	It is a zwitterion with a reactive primary amine. Also used as a carbon and nitrogen source in cell cultures.
HEPES	7.66	−0.014	4-(2-hydroxyethyl)piperazine-I-ethanesulfonic acid. Low UV absorbance, commonly used in cell culture media.
Phosphoric acid	2.15	0.0044	Reacts with divalent metal ions. pH changes may
	7.20	−0.0028	occur if freezing samples stored in phosphate
	12.33		buffers.
Tris	8.06	−0.028	Tris(hydroxymethyl-aminomethane). High temperature sensitivity, reactive primary amine, influences pH measurements, undesirable effects on some biologic systems.

Source: Beynon, R.J., and Easterby, J.S., Properties of common buffers. In: *Buffer Solutions: The Basics.* Oxford University Press, Oxford, 1996, pp. 67–82.

(described later in the chapter). Any of these processes used can significantly affect sample stability (Table 13.5). Of greater importance is the physical stability of sample comprising of aggregation and precipitation that change in the secondary and tertiary structure of protein. Ideally, the protein should retain its biologically active form throughout the processing, though it is often not practical. The sample stability is monitored by the biological activity of sample (e.g., IU/mg) throughout the process development stages. A comprehensive stability assurance plan would include testing to study effects of overnight storage of sample, changes in pH (2–10), ionic strength (0.05–2.0 M), solvents, temperature (1°C–40°C), and sheer force. A factorial design is most optimal to evaluate these data.

Table 13.3 Commonly Used Downstream Solvents and the Conditions of Their Use

Co-solvent	Conditions for Use	Comments
Ammonium sulfate	1–3 M	Precipitating and stabilizing agent at concentrations above 0.5 mg/mL and to increase ionic strength in HIC.
Benzonase	9–90 U/ml	Enzyme used to degrade DNA and RNA.
Cysteine	1–100 mM	Reducing agent. Used in low mM concentrations in protein refolding, and in 50–100 mM concentrations in reduction of protein disulfide bonds. Relatively cheap.
Dextran sulfate	10%	Precipitates lipoproteins.
1,4-Dithiothreitol (DTT)	1–100 mM	Reducing agent. Used in low mM concentrations in protein refolding, and in 50–100 mM concentrations in reduction of protein disulfide bonds. Relatively expensive.
Ethylenediaminotetraacetic acid (EDTA)	1–10 mM	Binds strongly to divalent metal ions
EGTA	1–10 mM	Binds strongly to divalent metal ions
Dodecyl-β-D-maltoside	0.5%–1.0% v/v	Non-ionic detergent for membrane protein solubilization. May absorb at 280 nm. Expensive.
Glucose	20–50 mM	Protein stabilizer
Glycerol	5%–50% v/v	Protein stabilizer
Guanidinium hydrochloride	1–6 M	Protein denaturant used to dissolve inclusion bodies. Expensive.
Mannose	20–50 mM	Protein stabilizer
NaCl	0.1–1 M	Maintains ionic strength. Corrosive to stainless steel.
Nonidet P40	0.05%–2.0%	Non-ionic detergent. May absorb at 280 nm. Expensive.
Octyl-β-D-glucoside	0.05%–1.5%	Non-ionic detergent for membrane protein solubilization. May absorb at 280 nm. Expensive.
Polyethylene glycol	Up to 20% v/v	Precipitating agent with no denaturing effect. M_r usually less than 6000. Complete removal may be difficult, does not affect AC or IEC.
Polyethylene imine	0.1% v/v	Precipitates aggregated nucleoproteins.
1-propanol	0.05%–1.0%	Organic modifier
Protamine sulfate	1%	Precipitates aggregated nucleoproteins.
Sodium dodecyl sulfate (SDS)	0.1%–0.5%	Ionic detergent and denaturant. Expensive.
Sucrose	20–50 mM	Protein stabilizer
Tris	0.01–0.2 M	Maintains pH
Triton X-100	1%–2% v/v	Non-ionic denaturing detergent absorbing at 280 nm. Expensive.
Urea	1–8 M	Protein denaturant used to dissolve inclusion bodies. Cheap.

Table 13.4 Sample Conditioning Steps

Technique	Comments
Filtration	To clarify the sample, the sample must pass a 0.45 μm filter before being applied to the column. Filtration should be done just prior to chromatography as its composition may change with time due to precipitation or viscosity changes. These steps must be properly validated.
Ultrafiltration	For buffer exchange or to concentrate the sample. Sheer forces may result in protein destabilization.
Microfiltration	To remove cells or cell debris. Sheer forces may result in protein destabilization.
Centrifugation	To remove cells, cell debris or particulate matter.
Dilution	To reduce conductivity and/or viscosity when sample volume is not extremely large.
Removal of divalent metal ions	With EDTA or similar chelating agents.
Desalting	Chromatographic desalting is a very efficient buffer exchange method; used for removal of GuHCl or urea.
Hollow fiber dialysis	For buffer exchange.
Bio processing aids	Normally added batch-wise to crude protein solutions in order to remove particulate matter and hydrophobic compounds.
Benzonase	Enzyme used to degrade DNA and RNA.
Pre-column	Safety device to protect the main column.
Cyclodextrins	Bind strongly to detergents; used to remove detergents from protein surfaces.
Precipitation	Separation and concentration step; better to use other newer techniques allowing continuous operations.

M_r, relative molecular weight.

The stability of samples is further affected by the presence of co-solvents and other impurities (Table 13.6).

13.4.3 Protein Folding

When using *Escherichia coli*, the protein is retained in the inclusion bodies, which are brought into solution prior to downstream processing; at this stage the protein is likely to have incorrect disulfide pattern as *E. coli* does not carry out the intracellular folding of the cloned protein. The amino acid cysteine plays a dominant role in protein folding. Under oxidizing conditions, this amino acid will form a disulfide bridge to another cysteine residue making the redox potential of the solution an essential (but rarely measured) parameter in protein folding. It is a difficult task to re-establish the secondary and tertiary structure of proteins with disulfide bonds. Carefully designed folding buffers and fine-tuned parameter intervals (protein concentration, pH, conductivity,

Table 13.5 Sample Characteristics and Their Effect on Protein Stability

Parameter	Comments
Concentration	Very low protein concentration may limit the equilibrium capacity in adsorption chromatography.
Conductivity	The ionic strength of the solution affects protein solubility and binding to ion exchangers. Precipitation may occur slowly over time gradually transforming the clear solution to a filter blocking sample.
Holding times	The sample stability is function of time. Note that holding times in large-scale operations are much longer than in laboratory scale.
pH	The pH of the solution will affect the solubility of the protein, its ability to bind to ion exchangers and protein stability. pH will also influence the redox potential of the solution.
Redox potential	The redox potential of the solution influences disulfide bond stability. At reducing conditions, the disulfide bonds will open up resulting in free cysteinyl residues. The redox potential is a function of pH.
Temperature	The temperature influences pH, ionic strength, and the redox potential. The protein stability is a function of temperature. Proteolytic enzymes are less active at low temperatures.
Viscosity	Viscous samples are difficult to filter and apply to chromatographic columns.
Volume	When working with SEC or other isocratic techniques a large volume will call for a larger column to satisfy throughput.

Table 13.6 Co-solvents and Impurities That Can Affect Sample Stability

Co-solvent and Impurities	Comments
Cell debris	Increases column back pressure and blocks of filters.
Nucleic acids	Increase viscosity.
Enzymes	Proteolytic enzymes degrade the target protein.
Divalent metal ions	Bind to proteins and ion exchangers and affect in vitro renaturation. EDTA binds strongly to divalent metal ions.
Salts	Increase the conductivity (ionic strength) of the solution which may produce salting-in and salting-out effects; significantly affects affinity, ion exchange, and hydrophobic interaction chromatography, etc.
Non-ionic detergents	Affect affinity, hydrophobic interaction, reversed phase chromatography. Bind strongly to the protein.
Ionic detergents	Affect ion exchange, hydrophobic interaction, and reversed phase, and affinity chromatography. Bind strongly to the protein.
Zwitterionic detergents	Affect ion exchange, hydrophobic interaction, reversed phase, and affinity chromatography. Bind strongly to the protein.
Organic solvents	May cause precipitation. Affect hydrophobic and reversed phase chromatography. Large volumes require costly explosion proof facilities.

(Continued)

TABLE 18.8 (Continued) Co-solvents and Impurities That Can Affect Sample Stability

Co-solvent and Impurities	Comments
Poly-alcohols	May cause precipitation.
Anti-foam agents	Reduce formation of foam. These agents are hydrophobic in nature and bind to hydrophobic matrices.
Carbohydrates	Are present from the fermentation process. Rarely affect the subsequent purification step.
Lipids/lipoproteins	Hydrophobic in nature. May affect all forms of chromatography due to irreversible binding to the matrix.
Colored compounds	Very often bind irreversibly to chromatographic matrices.
Urea	Is present from *Escherichia coli* inclusion body extraction buffers. Does not affect ion exchange chromatography.
GuHCl	Is present from *E. coli* inclusion body extraction buffers. Does affect ion exchange chromatography.

temperature, and redox potential) are needed to assure even reasonable yields and to reduce the amount of incorrectly folded (scrambled) forms, which are often very difficult to separate from the native form.

During the renaturation process, proteins tend to aggregate either as a result of electrostatic and/or hydrophobic interactions or as a result of intermolecular disulfide formation. As the intramolecular folding reaction is of first order and the intermolecular aggregation reaction is of second order, it is often necessary to carry out the folding at low protein concentrations (0.05–0.2 mg/mL), resulting in large tank volumes, when folding takes place in an industrial environment. The composition of the buffer used to extract proteins produces first a denaturation (and reducing) and the buffer used to refold the protein (producing oxidation) is different. The final buffer used is the greatest importance. Final yields can be improved often by adding specific co-solvents; if detergent-assisted renaturation is used, the detergents can be removed by addition of cyclodextrins. The protein refolding generally takes place at alkaline pH (usually the interval 7.5–9.5 is used), as the deprotonated form of cysteine is required.

There are several methods for transfer from the initial denaturing or reducing buffer to the folding or oxidizing buffer. The dialysis in the bag is a common laboratory method, not suited for manufacturing scale production. Dilution is often used even in large sale but it required larger tanks and careful addition of denatured protein into the folding buffer to assure proper mixing to obtain low protein concentrations uniformly throughout the tank. Dilution folding can also be accomplished using a method of pulse renaturation where aliquots of the denatured protein are added at successive time intervals. Desalting assures a very efficient transfer to the folding buffer thus assuring well-defined folding conditions. If aggregation can be prevented by means of additional co-solvents, the method can be very efficient (moderate protein concentrations). The size exclusion chromatography allows high protein concentrations in the application sample as polymeric protein is removed from the folding zone due to size exclusion. The fast removal of aggregates will decrease the rate of the second-order aggregation reaction. Ultrafiltration is used for buffer exchange by using methods like hollow fiber dialysis which operates at low protein concentrations; the high capacity of hollow fiber devices makes this technique suited for industrial scale. The application sample is dialyzed against the folding buffer. In the technique of immobilized folding, the protein is immobilized to a chromatographic matrix in the presence of the initial buffer. Freedom for structure formation is facilitated by binding through N-terminal extensions (His-tags or cellulose tags), which are later removed by enzymatic cleavage. Folding is achieved by applying the renaturation buffer to the column. Aggregation is severely reduced and in situ purification can be achieved before eluting the protein.

The first buffer system used is for the purpose of denaturing a protein prior to renaturing. Commonly used denaturants are urea, guanidinium chloride, or detergents. Urea is cheap, but presence of cyanate will result in carbamylation of free amino groups. Therefore, cyanate must be removed (using a mixed anion exchange matrix) before the use of the urea solution. The temperature is often kept at 4°C–8°C during the operation to prevent formation of cyanate. A concentration of 7–8 M urea is recommended. Guanidinium chloride is a strong denaturant, but very expensive. A concentration of 4–6 M is recommended. Most detergents are also very efficient denaturants at 1%–2% solutions. They may bind strongly to the protein and certain chromatographic techniques cannot be carried out in presence of detergents. EDTA is often added to the buffer (to bind divalent metal ions) in order to prevent oxidative side reactions during folding. A concentration of 1–5 mM is recommended. Dithiothreitol (DTT) or cysteine is commonly used as the reducing agent. Cysteine is the cheaper of the two and does not smell. A concentration of 50–100 mM is recommended. A recommended buffer for denaturation includes 7 M urea or 6 M GuHCl or 0.1%–2.0% detergent, 1–5 mM EDTA, 50–100 mM reducing agent (dithiothreitol or cysteine), 50 mM buffer in the pH interval 7.5 to 9.5 (Tris or glycine). The buffer should have a pH range of 7.5–9.5; protein concentration 1–50 mg/mL; conductivity 10–50 mS/cm; temperature (urea) 4°C–8°C; temperature 4°C–25°C; redox potential −300 to −100 mV.

In the oxidation step or renaturation step, the typical conditions are low protein concentration, alkaline pH, low to medium denaturant concentration, presence of reducing or oxidizing disulfide agent, presence of EDTA, and often a specific co-solvent to facilitate folding. The folding is a slow process and up to 24 h reaction time should be expected for folding of proteins with disulfide bonds. Specific enzymes (protein disulfide isomerase) are rarely used in industrial scale. Refolding strategies depend on whether there is a concomitant disulfide bond formation or not. Where such bond is formed, the most common methods include air oxidation, the use of mixed disulfides and the use of low molecular weight thiols. The latter method is well suited for large-scale operations partly because of its simplicity and partly because of the few side reactions observed. The cysteinyl amino acid residue will form a disulfide bond with another cysteinyl residue at oxidizing conditions (some disulfide bonds form at a redox potential of −50 mV). The reagents used are 2-mercaptoethanol, glutathione, or cysteine, which are added to the reaction mixture. It may be useful to take advantage of the presence of oxygen (approximately 0.4 mM) in normal aqueous buffers and add instead the reduced mercapto reagents. Cysteine is a cheap, non-smelling, reagent well suited for large-scale operations (make sure the amino acid is of non-animal origin). It has been a common practice to make use of a specified ratio between the reduced and oxidized form of the mercapto reagent. However, in industrial application, it is strongly recommended to adjust the ratio between the reduced and oxidized form by controlling the redox potential of the solution. A typical folding buffer comprises 50–100 mM Tris or glycine, 0–3 M of denaturant, 1–5 mM EDTA, 2–5 mM mercapto reagent, and a co-solvent. The conditions of reaction should be at pH 9.0–9.5, protein concentration of 0.1–0.5 mg/mL (G25 or hollow fiber), 3–15 mg/mL (GPC), conductivity 10–30 mS/cm, temperature 4°C–25°C, and redox potential of −50 to +50 mV. Several co-solvents have been used to facilitate protein folding mainly by suppressing aggregation in the inhibition of intermolecular hydrophobic interactions. These include the following: acetamide; albumin; L-arginine hydrochloride; Brij 30, 35, and 58; carboxymethyl cellulose; cetyltrimethylammonium bromide (CTAB); CHAPS 3-(3-chloramidopropyl)dimethylammonia-1-propane sulfonate; CHAPSO; cyclodextrins, cyclohexanol; deoxycholate; dodecyl maltoside; dodecyltrimethyl ammonium bromide; ethanol; ethylurea; formamide; glycerol; n-hexanol; hexadecyldimethylethyl ammonium bromide; hexadecylpyridinium chloride monohydrate; laurylmaltoside; methylformamide; methylurea; myristyltrimethyl ammonium bromide; NP40, n-pentanol; POE(10)L ($CH_3(CH_2)_{11}(OCH_2CH_2)_{10}OH$); potassium sulfate; SB3-14 (N-tetradecyl-N,N-dimethyl-3-ammonio-1-propane sulfonate); SB12, sodium dodecyl sulfate; sodium sulfate; sorbitol; sulfobetaines; taurocholate; tetradecyl trimethyl ammonium bromide; Tris, Triton X-100; Tween 20, 40, 60, 80, and 81; and ZW3-14 ($CH_3(CH_2)_{13}(N(CH_3)_2CH_2CH_2SO_3)$).

Another co-solvent approach, called the dilution additive strategy, has been to employ small molecules to promote protein folding in which the interaction between the small molecule and the protein is transient. In another co-solvent approach, named artificial chaperone-assisted folding, aggregation is prevented by the formation of protein–detergent complexes. In the second step, the detergent is removed with cyclodextrins having a higher binding constant for the detergent than that of the protein. The stripping of the protein facilitates intramolecular folding. The naturally occurring chaperones GroEL and GroES are rarely used in industrial applications. Compounds used for chaperone-assisted refolding include cycloamylose, cyclodextrins, and linear dextrins.

In those instances where folding of proteins does not involve formation of disulfide bonds, a optimization for disulfide formation is omitted. Further those conditions that promote disulfide formation such as a correct redox potential is important. As most proteins comprise cysteinyl residues, it is a common practice to add from 1 to 10 mM reduced mercapto reagent to the folding mixture in order to prevent unintended disulfide bond formation.

Tables 13.7 and 13.8 show typical initial and final buffer conditions for two proteins, lysozyme and IGF-1:

Table 13.7 Buffer Conditions for Lysozyme

Parameter	Initial Conditions	Final Conditions
Protein concentration	50 mg/mL	0.2 mg/mL
Denaturant	6 M Guanidinium hydrochloride (GuHCl)	30 mM Guanidinium hydrochloride (GuHCl)
Buffer	0.1 M Tris-sulfate pH 8.5	0.1 M Tris-sulfate pH 8.5
EDTA		2 mM EDTA
Reducing agent	30 mM Dithiothreitol	
Oxidizing agent		4 mM Glutathione (GSH)/ Oxidized glutathione (GSSG)
Co-solvent		4 mM detergent
Cyclodextrin		16.5 mM methyl-beta-cyclodextrin

Table 13.8 Buffer Conditions for IGF-1

Parameter	Initial Conditions	Final Conditions
Protein concentration	1.5 mg/mL	
Denaturant	7 M urea	
Buffer	50–100 mM Tris	50 mM Tris
EDTA (ethylene diamino tetraacetic acid)	1–2 mM	2 mM EDTA
Reducing agent	50–100 mM cysteine	
Oxidizing agent		2 mM Cys/Cys-Cys
Co-solvent		25% v/v ethanol

13.4.4 Filtration

Filtration unit process is used for the following purposes:

- Harvesting, washing, or clarification of cell cultures, lysates, colloidal suspensions; microfiltration of cell cultures (prior to the capture operations) is an alternative to centrifugation or expanded bed technology.
- Removal of aggregates and precipitated proteins.
- Removal of particulate matter.
- Pre-chromatographic clarification to remove colloidal particles (chromatographic columns act as filters; a medium of particle size 50–100 μm is equivalent to a 0.45 μm filter); use a prefilter to columns to prolong their life.
- Buffer filtration.
- Sterile filtration and depyrogenation of small molecules.
- Specific virus removal.

- Buffer exchange; diafiltration can be used and tangential flow or hollow fibers are commonly used in parallel with chromatographic desalting procedures; force applied here can affect protein stability.
- Concentration, clarification, and desalting of proteins; ultrafiltration is used for sample concentration (e.g., prior to size exclusion chromatography or precipitation).

Alternates to filtration unit process are the techniques like expanded bed, precipitation, or desalting. The choice of filtration vis-à-vis other techniques is made by comparing the losses of target protein with the losses incurred in using other methods. The common losses during filtration consists of retention (0.4%–10%), adsorption (0.02%–2%), aggregation (0.1%–20%), and hold-up volumes (0.2%–10%). The wide range of losses are carefully optimized by choosing membranes with appropriate retention characteristics and adjusting various chemical and physical parameters such as pH and ionic strength. The adsorption depends on the membrane area, vis-à-vis the amount of protein present in the sample feed and the volume passed; generally, hydrophilic membranes will exhibit lower protein binding than hydrophobic membranes. Hold-up volumes can be reduced by careful piping design, optimization of membrane area, and flushing the system (and thereby diluting the filtrate or retentate). Aggregation in micro- and ultrafiltration affects protein stability by inducing aggregation.

Filtration is a pressure-driven separation process that uses membranes to separate components in a liquid solution or suspension based on their size and charge differences:

- Prefiltration (5 μm)
- Clarification (1 μm)
- Filtration (0.45 μm)
- Sterilization (0.22 μm)

In conventional flow, the fluid is pushed across the membrane; in tangential flow filtration, the fluid is pumped tangentially along the surface of the membrane such as microfiltration and ultrafiltration.

Microfiltration is usually used upstream in the recovery process to separate intact cells or cell debris from the harvest. Membrane pore size cutoff values are typically in the range from 0.05 to 1.0 μm. Ultrafiltration is used to separate protein from buffer components (buffer exchange), sample concentration or virus filtration. Depending on the protein to be retained, the nominal molecular weight limits are from 1 to 1,000 kD or even up to 0.05 μm (virus filtration). In tangential flow filtration, the liquid is divided into two streams, namely permeate and concentrate, the latter is too large to pass.

The ultrafiltration technique has traditionally been used to separate solutes that differ by more than 10-fold in size, making it ideal for buffer exchange and protein concentration. The low selectivity offered has mainly been attributed to the wide pore size distributions in commercial membranes, the presence of significant bulk mass transfer limitations, and membrane fouling phenomena. However, by proper selection of solute wall concentrations, in combination with the intrinsic sieving coefficients, the separation characteristics of the system can be altered toward better separation of the protein solute molecules.

The microfiltration technique is used early in the process to separate cells or cell debris from the harvest, in order to clarify the sample before the first chromatographic capture unit operation. Ultrafiltration may be used throughout the downstream process with the purpose of buffer exchange or protein concentration. However, the sheer forces applied to the target protein may affect its stability, and tangential flow operations should always be carefully controlled. It is a common practice to use ultrafiltration as the final downstream unit operation, in order to assure correct bulk buffer composition, but protein stability may be affected. Alternatively, desalting using size exclusion chromatography should be considered.

The most commonly used types of membranes are as follows:

- Flat membranes in a cartridge where the feed is applied tangential to the membrane. The incoming solution flows in the channels between the elements (filter surfaces), and the permeate filters through the elements. The channels can be open or equipped with a turbulent promoter (net). The concentrate, which is recycled, flows through the cartridge or modular elements. The system is easy to clean.
- Tubular membranes are used with a porous support assembly which is perforated inside and supports the tube. The input feed flows through the tube, and the permeate flows through the membrane outside the tube. It has a greater surface area than flat plate and high capital costs.
- Spiral membranes are rolled up flat sheets. Alternate layers of membrane, porous support, membrane, and a spacer are wound around a perforated tube. The surface is greater than tubular and flat plate. It may be difficult to clean deposited material on surface of the spacer.
- Hollow fiber filters are small porous fibers bundled together and sealed in a chamber. The feed is pumped through the fiber and the permeate flows through the tubing in the chamber. Hollow fiber filters have very large surface area; however, they cannot handle solids in the feed stream.

13.4.4.1 Filtration Optimization Considerations

The tangential flow filtration is controlled by adjusting the constant cross-flow rate to adjust changes in viscosity of sample, the pressure drop is maintained when cross-flow rates are adjusted, and the adjustment of retentate pressure and the transmembrane pressure are often kept constant. The process conditions that affect these adjustments include the following:

- Configuration of the membrane is important to obtain correct flux and pressure. The flux depends on the membrane configuration, where the energy input per membrane unit area may vary considerably. Typically, filtration is run at flux of 25–250 L/m^2 and pressure of 0.2–4 bar. The selection of the optimal membrane material/type is not straightforward and depends on fouling, membrane rejection, flux, pressure, time, energy consumption, and so on.
- Molecular weight cutoff of the membrane must match the need. A membrane with a higher molecular weight cutoff has a higher permeability and flux. Sometimes, the difference in rejection is not significant and there can be considerable economical advantages in optimizing the cutoff range.
- Intact cells/cell debris are retained on 0.05–1 μm membrane passing colloidal material, viruses, proteins, and salts.
- Viruses are retained on 100 kD–0.05 μm membrane passing proteins and salts.
- Proteins are retained on 10–300 kD or 1–1000 kD membrane passing other proteins including small peptides and salts.

Physicochemical characteristics are as follows:

- pH and ionic strength which affect protein solubility; precipitation of proteins reduces permeability of membrane.
- Temperature increases the diffusivity and decreases the viscosity. The effect is significant resulting in an increased flux. If the temperature is not adjusted, an increase in temperature should be expected as the filtration proceeds due to the energy input. Note that the protein stability might be affected by the temperature change.
- Protein concentration is a limiting factor for flux decreases with increasing protein concentration in the retentate; there is always a maximum concentration to which the feed can be concentrated.
- Diffusivity directly but not linearly determines process flux; higher diffusivity results in a higher flux, because solids are removed from the gel layer at a faster rate.
- Viscosity increased decrease flux.
- Transmembrane pressure increases compress the gel, lowering its permeability. At low protein concentrations, the flux is a function of the transmembrane pressure, while at high protein concentration, the flux becomes less dependent on transmembrane pressure. Membranes with relatively high water fluxes, such as polysulfones, are less pressure dependent than membranes that have low water fluxes (e.g., cellulose-based membranes).
- Fouling of membranes results from adsorption of solutes to the membrane surface or polymerization of solutes, which is an irreversible process leading to decreased flux.
- Cross-flow velocity (tangential flow) increases flux at equal transmembrane pressure but it can also affect protein stability.
- Filtrate velocity is normally uncontrolled (the operation depends on cross-flow velocity and transmembrane pressure); transmembrane pressure can be controlled by filtrate velocity.

13.4.5 Precipitation

It is often advantageous to precipitate the protein

- As an intermediary product for storage
- As final drug substance bulk material
- For buffer exchange and/or protein concentration

The advantages of protein precipitation include mainly the volume reduction, removal of specific impurities and enhanced stability when using certain co-solvents. The main drawbacks in using this unit process are that the precipitated protein may be difficult to re-dissolve, disposal of waste may create environmental issues, the high cost (large space, labor intensive, the use of explosion-proof environment when solvents are used, inefficiency at low protein concentration), and decreased protein stability when some solvents are used. A volume reduction remains the primary reason for using precipitation techniques.

Protein precipitation depends on the distribution of hydrophobic and charged patches on the surface and the properties of the surrounding aqueous phase. The most common technique of precipitation is salting out using high concentrations of salts, largely depending on the hydrophobicity of the protein (Table 13.9). The nature of the salt is of importance and salts, such as ammonium sulfate, that encourage hydration of polar regions and dehydration of the hydrophobic regions without interacting with the protein surface are favored. The salting-out effect of anions follows the Hofmeister series (phosphate > sulfate > acetate > chloride) and the most effective cations are ammonium > potassium > sodium. The heat of solution and change in solvent viscosity should be taken into account when choosing a precipitating salt as should be the presence of other contaminants in the salts that can also affect protein structure and stability (e.g., heavy metals in ammonium sulfate).

A globular protein will exhibit minimum solubility near its isoelectric point, as an overall charge close to zero minimizes the electrostatic repulsion between the solute molecules. This is called isoelectric precipitation, which is often carried out in the presence of polyalcohols in order to enhance the precipitation yield.

Addition of organic solvents (e.g., acetone, ethanol) to the aqueous phase reduces the water activity and decreases the dielectric constant of the solvent. It has been suggested that the precipitating forces are electrostatic in nature, much in the same way as under isoelectric precipitation, rather than through hydrophobic interaction. Larger proteins tend to precipitate at lower concentrations of organic solvent.

Table 13.9 Precipitation Agents in Downstream Processing

Precipitating Agent	Typical Conditions for Use	Comments
Acetone	0%–80% v/v at 2°C–8°C	Denatures irreversibly; explosion-proof area (10 L+) required; volume contraction calculations required.
Ammonium sulfate	1–3 M	May damage proteins; solid use produces uncontrolled precipitation locally; use saturated solution only; ideally protein concentration of 1 mg/mL is required to obtain acceptable yields.
Caprylic acid	Sample volume/15 g	Precipitates bulk of proteins from sera and ascites, leaving IgG in solution.
Dextran sulfate	0%–0.5% v/v	Precipitates lipoproteins.
Ethanol	0%–60% v/v	Denatures irreversibly; explosion-proof area (10 L+) required; volume contraction calculations required.
Polyethylene glycol (3000–20,000)	0–20 w/v	Rarely denatures; difficult to remove. The residual polymer will rarely interfere with the purification procedures used in industrial downstream processing.
Polyethylene imine	0%–0.1% w/v	Precipitates aggregated nucleoproteins.
Polyvinylpyrrolidine	0%–3% w/v	Precipitates lipoproteins. Alternative to dextran sulfate.
Protamine sulfate	0%–1% w/v	Precipitates aggregated nucleoproteins.

Polyethylene glycol of molecular weight 4000–20,000 is used to precipitate proteins (in concentrations up to 20% w/v). The mechanism is similar to that of organic solvents and PEG can be regarded as a polymerized organic solvent. It should be noted that PEG is not easy to remove from the protein, although its presence rarely affects chromatographic techniques.

13.4.6 Expanded Bed Adsorption System

The initial purification of the target molecule is traditionally treated with adsorption chromatography using a packed bed of adsorbent. However, this requires clarification of the crude feed before application to the chromatography column. The cells and/or cell debris are removed by centrifugation and/or microfiltration. Both of these traditional methods of separation have several disadvantages. For example, the efficiency of a centrifugation step depends on particle size, density difference between the particles and the surrounding liquid, and viscosity of the feedstock. When handling small cells, such as *E. coli*, or cell homogenates, small particle size and high viscosity reduce the feed capacity during centrifugation and sometimes make it difficult to obtain a completely particle-free liquid. To obtain a particle-free solution centrifugation is usually combined with microfiltration. Although microfiltration yields cell-free solutions, the disadvantages of this combination system include the following:

- Reduction in the flux of liquid per unit membrane area due to fouling of membrane
- Long process times
- Use of large units and thus large capital costs
- Recurrent cost of equipment maintenance
- Product loss due to degradation

The expanded bed adsorption (EBA) technology provides a fluidized adsorption resin; adsorption of the target molecule to an adsorbent in a fluidized bed also eliminates the need for particulate removal done by centrifugation and/or microfiltration. The properties of EBA make it the ultimate capture step for initial recovery of target proteins from crude feedstock. The process steps of clarification, concentration, and initial purification can be combined into one unit operation, providing increased process economy due to a decreased number of process steps, increased yield, shorter overall process time, reduced labor cost, and reduced running cost and capital expenditure. Successful processing by EBA has been reported in many commercial processes, for example, *E. coli* homogenate, lysate, inclusion bodies, and secreted products; yeast cell homogenate and secreted products; whole hybridoma fermentation broth; myeloma cell culture; whole mammalian cell culture broth; milk; and animal tissue extracts. The EBA technology has been pioneered by Amersham (GE Healthcare) through their Streamline® product line, which is fully scalable and widely used in the manufacturing of therapeutic proteins.

As the name describes, the adsorbent in the EBA system is expanded and equilibrated by applying an upward liquid flow to the column. A stable fluidized bed is formed when the adsorbent particles are suspended in equilibrium due to the balance between particle sedimentation velocity and upward liquid flow velocity. The column adaptor is positioned in the upper part of the column during this phase. Crude, unclarified feed is applied to the expanded bed with the same upward flow as used during expansion and equilibration. Target proteins are bound to the adsorbent while cell debris, cells, particulates and contaminants pass through unhindered. Weakly bound material, such as residual cells, cell debris, and other type of particulate material, is washed out from the expanded bed using upward liquid flow.

When all weakly retained material has been washed out from the bed, the liquid flow is stopped and the adsorbent particles quickly settle in the column. The column adaptor is then lowered to the surface of the sedimented bed. Flow is reversed and the captured proteins are eluted from the sedimented bed using suitable buffer conditions. The eluate contains the target protein, which is clarified and partly purified, ready for further purification by packed-bed chromatography. After elution, the bed is regenerated by washing it with downward flow in sedimented bed mode using buffers specific for the type of chromatographic principle applied. This regeneration removes the more strongly bound proteins which are not removed during the elution phase (Figure 13.2).

Finally a cleaning-in-place procedure is applied to remove non-specifically bound, precipitated, or denatured substances from the bed, and restore it to its original performance. During this phase, a moderate upward flow is used with the column adaptor positioned at approximately twice the sedimented bed height.

Tailoring the chromatographic characteristics of an adsorbent for use in expanded bed adsorption includes careful control of the sedimentation velocity of the adsorbent beads. The sedimentation velocity is proportional to the density difference between the adsorbent and the surrounding fluid multiplied by the square of the adsorbent particle diameter. To achieve the high throughput required in industrial applications of adsorption chromatography, flow velocities must be high throughout the complete purification cycle. Most EBA systems are based on adsorbent agarose, a material proven to work well for industrial-scale chromatography. The macroporous structure of the highly cross-linked agarose matrices combines good binding capacities for large molecules, such as proteins,

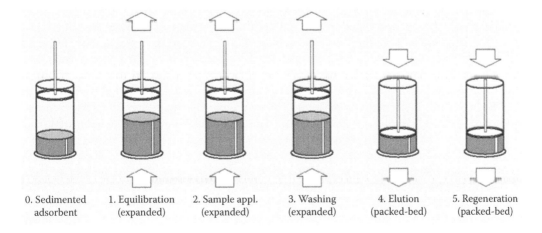

| 0. Sedimented adsorbent | 1. Equilibration (expanded) | 2. Sample appl. (expanded) | 3. Washing (expanded) | 4. Elution (packed-bed) | 5. Regeneration (packed-bed) |

Figure 13.2 Schematic presentation of the steps of expanded bed adsorption. (Data from Amersham Biotech Pharmacia, *Expanded Bed Adsorption Principles and Methods*, www.gelifesciences.com.)

with high chemical and mechanical stability. High mechanical stability is an important property of a matrix to be used in expanded bed mode to reduce the effects of attrition when particles are moving freely in the expanded bed. Agarose is also modified to make it less brittle to improve performance.

The column also has a significant impact on the formation of stable expanded beds. The columns are equipped with a specially designed liquid distribution system to allow the formation of a stable expanded bed. The need for a specially designed liquid distribution system for expanded beds derives from the low pressure drop over the expanded bed. Usually, the flow through a packed bed generates such a high pressure drop over the bed that it can assist the distributor in producing plug flow through the column. Since the pressure drop over an expanded bed is much smaller, the distributor in an expanded bed column must produce a plug flow itself. Consequently, it is necessary to build in an additional pressure drop into the distribution system. Besides generating a pressure drop, the distributor also has to direct the flow in a vertical direction only. Any flow in a radial direction inside the bed will cause turbulence that propagates through the column. Shear stress associated with flow constrictions also requires consideration when designing the liquid distributor. Shear stress should be kept to a minimum to reduce the risk of molecular degradation. Another function of the distribution system is to prevent the adsorbent from leaving the column. This is usually accomplished by a net mounted on that side of the distributor which is facing the adsorbent. The net must have a mesh size that allows particulate material to pass through and yet at the same time confine the adsorbent to the column. The distributor must also have a sanitary design, which means that it should be free from stagnant zones where cells/cell debris can accumulate.

Understanding the hydrodynamics of the expanded bed is critical for the performance of an expanded bed adsorption operation. The hydrodynamics of a stable expanded bed, run under well defined process conditions, are characterized by a high degree of reproducibility, which allows the use of simple and efficient test principles to verify the stability (i.e., functionality) of the expanded bed before the feed is applied to the column. The same type of test principles used to verify functionality of a packed chromatography column is used in expanded bed adsorption. The bed is stable when only small circulatory movements of the adsorbent beads are observed. Other movements may indicate turbulent flow or channeling, which leads to inefficient adsorption. Large circular movements of beads in the upper part of the bed usually indicate that the column is not in a vertical position. Channeling in the lower part of the bed usually indicates air under the distributor plate or a partially clogged distribution system. These visual patterns are illustrated in Figure 13.3.

Besides visual inspection, bed stability is evaluated by the degree of expansion and number of theoretical plates, before each run. The degree of expansion is determined from the ratio of expanded bed height to sedimented bed height, $H/H0$. If the degree of expansion differs from the expected value, it may indicate an unstable bed. Absolute values for the degree of expansion can only be compared if the buffer system (liquid density and viscosity) and temperature are constant between runs. A significant decrease in the degree of expansion may indicate poor stability or channeling due to trapped air under the distributor plate, infection or fouling of the adsorbent, the column not being in a vertical position, or a blocked distributor plate. The residence time distribution (RTD) test is a tracer stimulus method that can be used to assess the degree of longitudinal axial mixing (dispersion) in the expanded bed by defining the number of theoretical plates. A dilute acetone solution

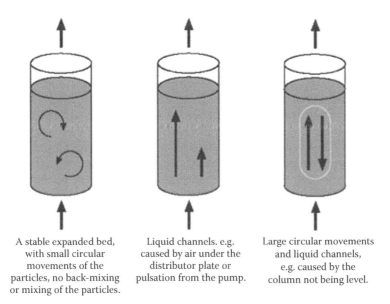

A stable expanded bed, with small circular movements of the particles, no back-mixing or mixing of the particles.

Liquid channels. e.g. caused by air under the distributor plate or pulsation from the pump.

Large circular movements and liquid channels, e.g. caused by the column not being level.

Figure 13.3 Visual patterns of movement of adsorbent beads in an expanded bed. (Data from Amersham Biotech Pharmacia, *Expanded Bed Adsorption Principles and Methods*, www.gelifesciences .com.)

is used as a tracer input into the fluid entering the column. The UV absorbance of the acetone is measured in the exit stream from the column. The number of theoretical plates is calculated from the mean residence time of the tracer in the column and the variance of the tracer output signal, representing the standard band broadening of a sample zone. The RTD test is a simple but efficient tool for function testing complete systems. If used to test systems before feed application, the risk of wasting valuable feed is reduced considerably. The test should be performed with the buffer and flow rate that are to be used during process operation. Note that when using a small tracer molecule (such as acetone) with a porous adsorbent the measurement of RTD is a function of tracer permeation in the matrix pores in addition to the actual dispersion in the liquid phase. Plate number of 170–200 N/m should be easily reached.

The critical parameters in expanded bed adsorption can be divided into chemical parameters, physical parameters, and the nature of feedstock.

Chemical parameters relate to the selectivity and capacity of the separation process and include pH, ionic strength, types of ions and buffers used. The influence on separation performance of these parameters is virtually the same in expanded bed adsorption as in traditional packed-bed chromatography. For example, high conductivity feedstock applied directly to an ion exchange adsorbent would reduce capacity requiring dilution prior to application. If conductivity is minimized at the end of the fermentation step, dilution is unnecessary. This results in less feed volume and shorter feed application time. In an intracellular system, conductivity of feedstock can be reduced by running the homogenization step in water or a dilute buffer. The pH range defined during method scouting should also be verified in expanded bed mode since reduced pH in some systems may cause aggregation of biomass. This aggregation can block the column distribution system causing poor flow distribution and an unstable bed.

Physical parameters relate to the hydrodynamics and stability of a homogeneous fluidization in the expanded bed. Some physical parameters are related to the broth composition, for example, cell density, biomass content, and viscosity. Others are related to operating conditions such as temperature, flow velocity, and bed height. Cell density and biomass content both affect viscosity, which may reduce the maximum operational flow rate by over-expanding the bed. Temperature also affects the viscosity and, hence, the operational flow rate in the system. Increased temperature can improve binding kinetics. Optimization experiments are usually carried out at room temperature but a broth taken directly from the fermenter may have a higher temperature. This difference in temperature must be considered when basing decisions on results from small-scale experiments.

Feedstock characteristics widely determine the application and efficiency of EBA systems (Table 13.10). Secretion systems generate dilute, low viscosity feedstock that contains rather low amounts of protein and intracellular contaminants, thus providing favorable conditions for downstream processing. Intracellular systems, on the other hand, generate feedstocks rich in intracellular contaminants and cell wall/cell membrane constituents. Along with the nutrient broth, these contaminants pose a greater challenge during the optimization phase of expanded bed adsorption. Much of the nutrient broth and associated contamination can be removed prior to cell lyses by thorough washing of the cells, but such steps introduce additional costs to the process. The main source of contaminants in feed where the target molecule is located within the host cell is the complex cell membrane that has to be disrupted to release the target molecule. Bacterial and yeast cell walls have a high polysaccharide content that can nucleate into larger structures that foul solid surfaces. Proteins and phospholipids are other integral parts of such cell walls that will be released upon cell disintegration. Bacterial cell walls are particularly rich in phospholipids, lipopolysaccharides, peptidoglycans, lipoproteins, and other types of large molecules that are associated with the outer membrane of a bacterial cell. These contaminants may complicate downstream processing by fouling the chromatographic adsorbent.

Contaminant may also be present as charged particulates that can act as ion exchangers and adsorb proteins, especially basic ones, if the ionic strength of the homogenate is low. This problem is, however, not specifically related to expanded bed adsorption and should be addressed when selecting conditions for cell disruption.

The main concern when processing a feed based on a secretion system would be to maintain intact cells, thereby avoiding the release of cell membrane components and intracellular contaminants such as DNA, lipids, and intracellular proteins that may foul the adsorbent or block the inlet distribution system of the column. Release of intracellular proteases is a further concern since it will have a negative impact on the recovery of biologically active material.

Animal cells lack a cell wall, which makes them more sensitive to shearing forces than microbial cells. The mammalian cell membrane is composed mainly of proteins and lipids. It is particularly rich in lipids, composing a central layer covered by protein layers and a thin mucopolysaccharide layer on the outside surface. Due to the high membrane content of mammalian cells, lysis can complicate the downstream process by causing extensive lipid fouling of the adsorbent. Another consequence of cell lysis is the release

Table 13.10 Characteristics of Feedstocks According to the Location of the Product in the Recombinant Organism

Escherichia coli	Yeast	Mammalian Cells
Secreted—Dilute, low viscosity feed containing low amounts of protein. Proteases, bacterial cells, and endotoxins are present. Cell lysis often occurs with handling and at low pH. DNA can be released and cause high viscosity.	Secreted—Dilute, low viscosity feed containing low amounts of protein. Proteases and yeast cells are present.	Secreted—Dilute, low viscosity feed containing low amounts of protein. Proteases and mammalian cells are present. Cell lyses often occur with handling and at low pH. DNA can be released and cause high viscosity. Cell lysis can also release significant amounts of lipids. Agglomeration of cells can occur.
Cytoplasmic—Cell debris, high content of protein. Lipid, DNA, and proteases are present. Very thick feedstock which needs dilution. Intact bacterial cells and endotoxins are present.	Cytoplasmic—Cell debris, high content of protein. Lipid, DNA, and proteases are present. Very thick feedstock which needs dilution. Intact yeast cells are present.	Cytoplasmic—Unusual location for product accumulation.
Periplasmic—Cell debris, high content of protein. Lipid and proteases are present. Thick feedstock which needs dilution. DNA is present if cytoplasmic membrane is pierced. Intact bacterial cells and endotoxin are present.	Periplasmic—Not applicable to yeast cells.	Periplasmic—Not applicable to mammalian cells.
Inclusion body—Cell debris, high content of protein. Lipid and proteases are present. Very diluted solutions after renaturation. Intact bacterial cells, DNA, and endotoxin are present. Precipitation of misfolded variants occurs in a time-dependent manner.	Inclusion body—Not applicable to yeast cells.	Inclusion body—Not applicable to mammalian cells.

of large fragments of nucleic acids, which can cause a significant increase in the viscosity of the feedstock or disturb the flow due to clogging the column inlet distribution system. Nucleic acids may also bind to cells and adsorbent causing aggregation in the expanded bed. These types of contamination also lead to problems in traditional processing where they cause severe fouling during microfiltration.

Hybridoma cells are generally considered to be particularly sensitive to shear forces resulting from vigorous agitation or sparging. In contrast, CHO cells have relatively high resistance to shear rates and a good tolerance to changes in osmotic pressure.

The use of expanded bed adsorption reduces the amount of cell lysis that occurs, as compared with traditional centrifugation and cross-flow filtration unit operations, since the cells are maintained in a freely flowing, low shear environment during the entire capture step. Nevertheless, it is important to actively prevent cell lysis during processing, for instance, by avoiding exposure to osmotic pressure shocks during dilution of the feedstock and by minimizing the sample application time.

Non-secreted products sometimes accumulate intracellularly as inclusion bodies, which are precipitated protein aggregates that result from overexpression of heterologous genes. Inclusion bodies are generally insoluble and recovery of the biologically active protein requires denaturation by exposure to high concentration of chaotropic salts such as guanidine hydrochloride or dissociants such as urea. The subsequent renaturation by dilution provides very large feedstock volumes. Expanded bed adsorption can be advantageous since precipitation of misfolded variants increases with time, which usually causes problems for traditional packed bed chromatography. Even after extensive centrifugation of the feed-stock, precipitation continues and may finally block a packed chromatography bed.

When a non-secreted product accumulates in the periplasmic compartment, it can be released by disrupting the outer membrane without disturbing the cytoplasmic membrane. Accumulation in the periplasmic space can thus reduce both the total volume of liquid to be processed and the amount of contamination from intracellular components. However, it is usually very difficult to release the product from the periplasmic space without piercing the cytoplasmic membrane and thereby releasing intracellular contaminants such as large fragments of nucleic acids, which may significantly increase the viscosity of the feedstock.

Method scouting, that is, defining the most suitable adsorbent and the optimal conditions for binding and elution, is performed at small scale using clarified feed in packed-bed mode. Selection of adsorbent is based on the same principles as in packed-bed chromatography. The medium showing strongest binding to the target protein while binding as few as possible of the contaminating proteins, that is, the medium with the highest selectivity and/or capacity for the protein of interest, will be the medium of choice. Regardless of the binding selectivity for the target protein, adsorbents are compatible with any type of feed material. The flow velocity during method scouting should be similar to the flow velocity to be used during the subsequent experiments in expanded mode. The nominal flow velocity for EBA is 300 cm/h. This may need adjustment during optimization, depending on the properties of the feedstock.

Elution can be performed step-wise or by applying a gradient. Linear gradients are applied in the initial experiments to reveal the relative binding of the target molecule versus the contaminants. This information can be used to optimize selectivity for the target molecule, that is, to avoid binding less strongly bound contaminants. It can also be used to define the step-wise elution to be used in the final expanded bed.

When selectivity has been optimized, the maximum dynamic binding capacity is determined by performing breakthrough capacity tests using the previously determined binding conditions. The breakthrough capacity determined at this stage will give a good indication of the breakthrough capacity in the final process in the expanded bed.

The purpose of the method optimization in expanded mode is to examine the effects of the crude feed on the stability of the expanded bed and on the chromatographic performance. If necessary, adjustments are made to achieve stable bed expansion with the highest possible recovery, purity, and throughput.

The principle for scale up is similar to that used in packed-bed chromatography. Scale up is performed by increasing the column diameter and maintaining the sedimented bed height, flow velocity, and expanded bed height. This preserves both the hydrodynamic and chromatographic properties of the system.

In any type of adsorption chromatography, the washing stage removes non-bound and weakly bound soluble contaminants from the chromatographic bed. In expanded bed adsorption, washing also removes remaining particulate material from the bed. Since expanded bed adsorption combines clarification, concentration, and initial purification, the particulate removal efficiency is a critical functional parameter for the optimal utilization of the technique. Washing may also be performed with a buffer containing a viscosity enhancer such as glycerol, which may reduce the number of bed volumes needed to clear the particulates from the bed. A viscous wash solution follows the feed-stock through the bed in a plug-like manner, increasing the efficiency of particulate removal. Even if the clarification efficiency of an expanded bed adsorption step is very high, some interaction between cell/cell debris material and adsorbent beads can be expected, which retain small amounts of cells and/or cell debris on the adsorbent. Such particulates may be removed from the bed during regeneration, for instance, when running a high salt buffer through an ion exchanger, or during cleaning between cycles using a well-defined CIP protocol.

Cells retained on the adsorbent may be subjected to lysis during the washing stage. Such cell lysis can be promoted by reduced ionic strength when wash buffer is introduced into the expanded bed. Nucleic acids released due to cell lysis can cause significant aggregation and clogging owing to the *glueing* effect of nucleic acids forming networks of cells and adsorbent beads. If not corrected during the washing stage, wash volume/time may increase due to channeling in the bed. Other problems may also arise during later phases of the purification cycle, such as high back pressure during elution in packed-bed mode and increased particulate content in the final product pool. If such effects are noted during washing, a modified wash procedure containing Benzonase (Merck, Nycomed Pharma A/S) can be applied to degrade and remove nucleic acids from the expanded bed.

Step-wise elution is often preferred to continuous gradients since it allows the target protein to be eluted in a more concentrated form, reduces buffer consumption, and gives shorter cycle times. Being a typical capture step, separation from impurities in expanded bed adsorption is usually achieved by selective binding of the product, which can simply be eluted from the column at high concentration with a single elution step.

The efficiency of the CIP protocol should be verified by running repetitive purification cycles and testing several functional parameters such as degree of expansion, number of theoretical plates in the expanded bed, and breakthrough capacity. If the nature of the coupled ligand allows it, an efficient CIP protocol would be based on 0.5–1.0 M NaOH as the main cleaning agent. If the medium to be cleaned is an ion exchange medium, the column should always be washed with a concentrated aqueous solution of a neutral salt, for example, 1–2 M NaCl, before cleaning with NaOH.

Occasionally, the presence of nucleic acids in the feed is the cause of fouling the adsorbent and in such a case, treating the adsorbent with a nuclease (e.g., Benzonase, Merck, Nycomed Pharma A/S) could restore performance. Benzonase can be pumped into the bed and be left standing for some hours before washing it out. Where the delicate nature of the attached ligand prevents, harsh chemicals such as NaOH, 6 M guanidine hydrochloride, 6 M urea, and 1 M acetic acid can be used.

13.4.7 Virus Inactivation and Removal

Mammalian cell cultures and monoclonal antibodies derived from hybridoma cell cultures pose an essential risk of contamination with retroviral particles or adventitious viruses. Despite the preventive actions (master cell bank characterization, use of raw materials of non-animal origin, end of production procedures), viral contamination remains a problem for all recombinant products as adventitious viruses can also be introduced during production (e.g., raw materials, cross contamination) with the risk of contaminating the final product. Virus inactivation and virus removal during protein purification are important steps, particularly in insect cells, mammalian cells, or transgenic animals. Though it is possible to inactivate the viruses without appreciably affecting the target protein, only prevention and partial inactivation techniques suitable for maintaining the purity of proteins are a viable choice. Besides inactivation, chromatographic and filtration procedures are used to clear viruses during downstream processing. The overall level of clearance is the ratio of the viral contamination per unit volume in the pretreatment suspension to the concentration per unit volume in the post treatment suspension. It is usually expressed in terms of the sum of the logarithm of the clearance found for individual steps possessing a significant reduction factor. Reduction of the virus titer of one $\log_{10}$ or less is considered negligible. Clearance should be demonstrated for viruses (or viruses of the same species) known to be present in the master cell bank (*relevant viruses*) or when a relevant virus is not available a *specific model virus* may be used as a substitute to challenge the samples and calculate clearance ratios. The choice of the viruses selected should be fully justified.

The accepted methods for virus clearance are: virus inactivation and virus removal; inactivation is the irreversible loss of any viral infectivity, while the virus removal is the physical reduction of viral particles in number achieved by such methods as depth and ultrafiltration and chromatography techniques exploiting electrostatic, hydrophobic and hydrophilic surface characteristics. Inactivation of virus is achieved by the following:

- *Radiation*: γ- and UV-irradiation destroy the virus genome; short wavelength UV treatment can course the formation of free radicals leading to protein damage. This can be minimized by the use of antioxidants or filters excluding the 185 nm wavelength).
- *Heat inactivation*: It contributes significantly to the inactivation of viruses. The introduction of high temperature short time (HTST) heat treatment offers substantial inactivation of small non-enveloped viruses while fully maintaining the integrity of the protein product. This method features the unique opportunity to spike and re-collect a virus sample of a volume as low as 20–30 mL into the fluid pathway using a designed sample applicator under operational conditions for the manufacturing process (flow rate 35–80/Lh, peak temperature 60°C–165°C) at full scale. The complete pathway is disposable, hence offering an extraordinary validation opportunity as well as a multi-product use and avoiding any potential cross-contamination
- *pH*: Acid treatment results in destruction in the nucleocapsid and genome. Acid treatment works well with larger virus particles. Particles <40 nm may require a

combination of pH < 3 and 3 M urea. Acid treatment at pH > 3 does not inactivate non-enveloped viruses. Enveloped viruses are not inactivated in a reliable manner

- *Pressure*: High pressure procedures at near-zero temperatures may be useful in inactivation of viruses.
- *Co-solvents*: Organic solvents dissolve the virus envelope and/or disintegrate the nucleocapsid.
- *Detergents*: Detergents dissolve the virus envelope and/or disintegrate the nucleocapsid. The method is very efficient for lipid-enveloped viruses, but is ineffective against non-enveloped viruses.
- *Denaturation*: The method selected for inactivation depends to a great degree on the nature of virus, results in disintegration of the nucleocapsid. Urea treatment does not inactivate small non-enveloped viruses. Large enveloped viruses are inactivated to some extent. Urea treatment works well with larger virus particles. Particles < 40 nm may require a combination of pH < 3 and 3 M urea. Chaotropic agents dissolve the virus envelope and/or disintegrate the nucleocapsid.
- *Fatty acids*: Treatment with caprylate is a useful approach to remove the risk of lipid-enveloped viruses from protein pharmaceuticals.
- β-*propiolactone*: This is an effective virucidal agent; 3.5–5 log reduction of viral infectivity is observed but it is toxic and removal must be assured by analytical testing validation.
- *Inactine*: The technology is based on disruption of nucleic acid replication while preserving the integrity of lipids and protein.
- *Biosurfactants*: Surfactin, a cyclic lipopeptide antibioic with a molecular weight of 1036, possessing antiviral effect (enveloped RNA and DNA viruses) and anti-mycoplasma properties. The activity decreases with increasing protein concentration and the reagent is not effective in solutions of high protein concentration. The in vivo toxicity is low.
- *Imines*: 0.05% v/v N-acetylethylenimine (AEI) inactivates infectious units of polio-virus and foot-and-mouth disease virus at 4°C or 37°C without damaging a variety of proteins tested.
- *Quaternary ammonium chloride*: 3-(trimethyloxysilyl)-propyldimethyloctadecylammonium chloride (Si-QAC) covalently binds to alginate and removes viruses from protein solutions.

Because of the differences in the nature of viruses and their in vitro reactivity, it is difficult to adopt general methods for their clearance, for example, solvent-detergent treatment is highly effective for inactivation of enveloped viruses, but has no or little effect on non-enveloped viruses. Low pH is effective in mammalian cell systems but has little effect on parvoviruses. It is important to include at least one virus inactivation step in the downstream process scheme. The process should be properly validated keeping in mind that the inactivation is a biphasic process. The sample is ordinarily spiked with virus in small amounts so as not to change the sample characteristics (e.g., buffer composition, protein concentration, conductivity). Parallel control assays should be included to assess loss of infectivity due to dilution, concentration, or storage. Buffers and products should be evaluated independently for toxicity or interference in assays used to determine the virus filter, as these components may adversely affect the indicator cells. Virus escaping a first inactivation step may be more resistant to subsequent steps (e.g., virus aggregates).

Most downstream processes include at least three different chromatographic procedures that also help remove adventitious agents. The virus capsid is a shell consisting of different proteins and the virus particle might behave as any other protein present in the sample to be purified. Also the envelope of enveloped viruses contains a variety of proteins. Given the diversity in the nature of viruses, these methods cannot be relied upon to definitely remove viruses. Generally, anion exchange chromatography at basic pH and low conductivity proves most useful.

Filtration work through two mechanisms: size exclusion and absorptive retention of particulates. Size exclusion, which occurs due to geometric or spatial constraint, provides a predictable method of particle removal, as it is not directly influenced by process and filtration conditions. In contrast, a number of process-dependent factors (e.g., charge, hydrophobicity, pH, ionic strength) influence the absorption of particulates in a much less controlled manner. Size exclusion and adsorptive filtration are not mutually exclusive. Depth filters with anion exchanging characteristics are very efficient virus removers.

The viruses of interest, such as retroviruses (100–140 nm) and small viruses (about 30 nm) can be removed by use of nanofiltration or by ultrafiltration. Nanofilters featuring pore sizes in the range of 20–70 nm utilize the classical depth structures, which are typical for commercial microfiltration membranes. Tighter pore sizes results in high back-pressure (>0.3 Mpa). Nanofilters are inexpensive in practical use and can be used anywhere in the downstream process as long as the load solution is 0.1 μm prefiltered. A significant feature of nanofilters is the possibility of measuring their integrity. Complete clearance (to the limits of detection) was demonstrated in the removal of viruses above 35 nm from human globulin by 35 nm nanofiltration.

Ultrafiltration offers the possibility to operate at much smaller pore sizes (>1 kDa cutoff) more or less depending on the stokes radius of the protein. A cutoff of 200 kDa allows for the passage of IgG-type antibodies (Mw around 150 kDa) resulting in excellent clearance factors for virus particles >40 nm. Depending on process parameters, even a 100 kDa filter may be used successfully with significant retention of particles <40 nm[3].

Membrane filtration is an effective, reliable, and controllable technique to remove viruses. In many cases large viruses could be removed to the detection limit of the assay used. Small viruses (e.g., parvoviruses) may require filtration through special membranes that have limited protein transmission. cGMP facilities are typically divided into an area where viruses are expected to be present (harvest and capture) and non-virus areas potentially free of viruses. An early virus filtration step is therefore of advantage, but is challenged by the composition (viscosity, particulates) of the sample material in early downstream processing. Virus filtration should also be used whenever cell culture media or buffers are believed to include a virus contamination risk.

13.5 PROCESS FLOW

The entire downstream process is presented in a process flow diagram that specifies the details of processes in a logical order, properly sized to meet the requirements of each operation. The process flow for the manufacturing of erythropoietin is provided in Table 13.11.

Table 13.11 Process Flow for the Manufacturing of Erythropoietin

Equipments Used	Process and Material	Process Description
• XX L S.S. vessel • Sartorius membrane filter 2.0 and 0.45 μm	Growing media preparation: Using fetal bovine serum, gentamicin, DMEM, high glucose ↓	• Add X L of DMEM, high glucose in XX L vessel. • Add X L fetal bovine serum and X g gentamicin, mix till dissolve. • QS to XX L with high glucose. • Filter the solution and keep at X°C for XX h
• X L sterile S.S. vessel • Sartorius membrane filter 2.0 and 0.45 μm	Harvesting media preparation using human insulin gentamicin, DMEM, high glucose ↓	• Add X L of DMEM, high glucose in XX L sterile vessel. • Add XX mg human insulin and X g Gentamicin, mix for XX min. • QS to XX L with high glucose. • Filter the solution and keep at X°C for XX h.
• Water Bath • Centrifuge • CO_2 incubator • Rolling bottle apparatus	Cell sub-culture for XX frozen vials of CHO EPO ↓	• Thaw the vials at X°C in water bath, wash vials with X% ethanol, transfer the contents of each vial into XX mL centrifuge tube. • Wash the cell by centrifugation at XX rpm for X min. with x-y mL growing media for X times. • Disperse the cellular pellets in X mL of growing media in X mL flask and divide the dispersion into X flasks and complete the volume to X mL with growing media. • Repeat the above steps for all vials. • Incubate all flasks at X°C for X days. • Split the contents of each flask into X flasks and complete the volume to X mL with growing media. • Incubate all flasks at X°C for X days. • Split the contents of each flask into X roller bottles and complete the volume to X mL with growing media.
• Centrifuge • Sartorius membrane filter 2.0 and 0.45 μm	Harvesting for X days ↓	• Transfer the contents of each bottle to a centrifuge flask and wash the cell by centrifugation two times with PBS 15–20 mL. • Inoculate the cell dispersion of each flask with harvesting medium into roller bottles. • Media containing EPO collected every 24 h, filtered through 2.0 and 0.45 μm. • Collected medium replaced with new medium for X days.
• Column blue sepharose XK	Purification: Affinity chromatography ↓	• Filtered cellular supernatant rh-EPO is purified through a affinity column. • Filtered collected media is loaded in the column equilibrated in PBS.

(Continued)

471

Table 13.11 (Continued)   Process Flow for the Manufacturing of Erythropoietin

Equipments Used	Process and Material	Process Description
		• The column is then washed with X column volumes with PBS and elute the bounded protein with PBS-1.4 M NaCL (X g of NaCl/L of PBS). The sample obtained are stored at −4°C. • After the EPO elution the column is washed first with X mL of NaOH 0.1 M and later with 2 column volume of PBS-X M NaCl. Finally, the column is equilibrated in PBS for the next day.
• Column Sephadex Fine	Desalting	• The rh-EPO recovered from previous step is desalted using column. • The column is equilibrated in X mM Tris-HCl pH X with an increasing flow going from X mL/min. to XmL/min with a limit pressure of X MPa. The maximum volume loaded is around X mL. • The elution of the protein is controlled at X nm and the salts concentration is followed by the conductimeter in line. • The column is cleaned with X column volumes of X M NaOH and re-equilibrated with X mM Tris-HCl pH X for the next day.
• Column Hi Trap Q Sepharose	Anion exchange ↓	• The desalted fraction containing the rh-EPO is purified using a Hi Trap Q Sepharose. • The column is equilibrated with X volumes of XmM Tris-HCl pH X and later with X volumes of 50 mM Tris-HCl pH X—X mM NaCl (X% Buffer B, X mM Tris—HCl pH X—NaCl X M).
• Column Hi Prep	Desalting ↓	• The rh-EPO recovered from previous step is desalted using column Hi Prep. • The column is equilibrated in X mM NaAC pH X at X mL/min. The maximum volume loaded in the column is X mL. • The solution is monitored at X nm controlling the elution of the protein and of the salt with the conductimeter line. The flow through is collected and the salt is left to complete its elution. • The column is cleaned with X volumes of X M NaOH and re-equilibrated with X mM NaAC pH 6.0 for the next day.
• Column Hi Trap SP Sepharose	Cation exchange ↓	• The rh-EPO containing fractions eluted from the Q-Sepharose column and desalted is loaded in a Hi Trap SP-Sepharose column.

(Continued)

472

Table 13.11 (*Continued*)   Process Flow for the Manufacturing of Erythropoietin

Equipments Used	Process and Material	Process Description
		• This SP-column retains isoforms of incomplete glycosylation enriching the specific activity and another high molecular weight contaminant products.
		• The fraction containing the EPO molecules with high glycosylation elute with the flow through (FT) of the column using X mM NaAC, pH X.
		• The column is first equilibrated with 10 volumes of X mM NaAC pH X.
		• The fraction containing the rh-EPO is loaded in the column at X mL/min.
		• Measure the optical density with a spectrophotometer to determine the quantity of protein present in the sample.
		• Measure the volume obtained.
		• Filter the flow through in a Millipore Stericup 0.22 μ.
		• Store the product obtained at 2°C–8°C.
		• The column is then washed with X volumes of Xm M NaAC, pH X-XM NaCl and re-equilibrated in Xm M NaAC, pH X.
• Gel filtration column, Superose	Gel formation ↓	• The final polishing of the purified rh-EPO is performed using a gel filtration column.
		• The fraction is loaded at X mL/min. following the spectrum at X nm, collecting the peak containing the purified rh-EPO.
• Polyethylene storage container	Final product	• Erythropoietin concentrated solution has a concentration of X mg/mL to X mg/mL and potency of not less than 100,000 international units (IU) per milligram of active substance determined.

Questions

1. Describe the broad stages in downstream processing.
   Answer: Cell separation from media or cell disruption and cell debris removal, product recovery and concentration, column based separation, other separation operations, purified bulk drug substances.
2. What is the major consideration in choosing the downstream processing technique?
   Answer: The physical and chemical properties of the manufactured protein.
3. Why is the solubility of the protein is an important consideration?
   Answer: Particles of precipitate can clog chromatography parts, filters, and so on.

4. Even though the capture step does not often increase the purity of the substance, what are the main requirements of these steps?
   Answer: High degrees of capacity, product recovery, chemical and physical stability.
   Questions 5 through 8 are focused on expanded bed chromatography.

5. Although whole cells can be added to the column, what can be expected from having the cells there and should be kept in mind although it may not prevent the use of this technique.
   Answer: Interaction of the product with the cells or cell fragments will occur, but the risk to the product may not prevent it from being a good technique.

6. Why does it work to put particles into this type of column?
   Answer: When loading there is expanded area for particles to pass through the chromatography media.

7. Will it work if the desired product has no affinity for the bed?
   Answer: No.

8. Why is it important to monitor the degree of expansion?
   Answer: A variance in the degree of expansion can indicate problems with the manifold, and infection, or fouling of the column.

9. Describe ways to inactivate viruses.
   Answer: Heat inactivation, pressure, co-solvents, pH, fatty acids, quaternary ammonium chloride, and radiation.

10. What is a limitation of pH treatment when considering inactivation of viruses?
    Answer: Enveloped viruses are not reliably inactivated by pH treatment.

14

Purification

LEARNING OBJECTIVES

1. Understand the role that protein chemistry plays in purification.
2. Recognize the differences in chromatography methods.
3. Identify chromatography techniques that are appropriate for the desired product and the challenges with scaling up the selected chromatography technique.

14.1 INTRODUCTION

The downstream purification steps comprise the most important part of the manufacturing of therapeutic proteins. The upstream process accumulates a large number of impurities including viruses, electrolytes, and other uncharged degradation products and structurally related molecules. Cleaning out these unwanted components to a level where it can comply with compendial requirements where available is accomplished in the purification steps. The chromatography techniques used can add contaminants of their own, cause protein degradation or modification of protein structure. Additionally, the yield obtained through the purification process is critical in making the system commercially feasible. Establishing optimal separation on a cost-effective basis requires a good understanding of the physicochemical nature of the target protein, particularly its physical and chemical stability profile. The first part of this chapter deals with the properties of protein that can have significant effect on its separation potential; this is followed by a description of the most commonly used chromatography techniques.

14.2 PROTEIN PROPERTIES

All proteins are made up of amino acids and may contain other molecules as well. Amino acid contain amino group (NH_2), a carboxyl group (COOH), and an R group with a general formula, R-CH(NH_2)-COOH. The R group differs among various amino acids. In a protein, the R group is also called a side chain. There are over 300 naturally occurring amino acids, those of interest to humans are 20, the type of R attached determines if they would at neutral pH retain a negative charge (acidic; aspartic and glutamic acid), positive charge (basic; lysine, arginine, and histidine), or are aromatic in nature (tyrosine, tryptophan, and phenylalanine), contain sulfur (cysteine and methio nine), are uncharged hydrophilic (serine, threonine, asparagine and glutamine), inactive hydrophobic (glycine, alanine, valine, leucine, and isoleucine), or have special structures (proline, where amino acid groups are not directly connected and thus appear at the end of the peptide chain). These classifications are important in imparting certain prop erties to proteins, besides the charge, that should be evaluated in the selection of an appropriate separation procedure. For example, interaction between positive and nega tive R groups may form a salt bridge, which is an important stabilizing force in pro teins. The disulfide bond formed between two cysteine residues provides a strong force for stabilizing the globular structure. A unique feature about methionine is that the synthesis of all peptide chains starts from methionine. Hydrophilic groups can form hydrogen bonds. The inactive hydrophobic amino acids are found inside the protein interior and do not form hydrogen bonds and rarely interact.

The amino acids are designated specific symbols to represent them in a complex struc ture. One of the most significant property of proteins derives from their hydrophobicity imparted by the component amino acids. Table 14.1 lists the hydrophobicity indices of the 20 amino acids found in proteins. The hydrophobicity index, as given below, tells the rela tive hydrophobicity among amino acids. A higher value means higher hydrophobicity, the likely to be found in the protein interior. Table 14.1 arranges amino acids in the increasing order of hydrophobicity except for proline.

14.3 AFFINITY CHROMATOGRAPHY

Molecules are separated in affinity chromatography (AC) through structure-specific inter actions with ligand. AC is preferably used for capture operations, where high selectivity assures good separation between the protein and cell culture components and impuri ties. The advantages of AC include its high specificity and mild elution conditions; the disadvantages include its inability to separate derivatives from target protein, inability to use sodium hydroxide for cleaning and the overall cost of operation. In the elution stage, the adsorption is carried out using a specific substrate ion in combination with one of the above mentioned principles. To be effective, the dissociation constant must be in a range of 10^{-5}–10^{-7} M to allow efficient elution of the protein generally accomplished by changing pH, ionic strength, polarity or by addition of specific co-solvents. The commonly available affinity interactions used are as follows: antibody–antigen, enzyme–substrate, inhibitor– enzyme, lectin–polysaccharide, hormone–receptor, protein A–IgG, triazine–protein, pep tide–protein, metal ion–protein, and glutathione–glutathione-S-transferase. As a result, this chromatographic technique is highly selective but offers poor resolution of related derivative products making it an ideal unit operation for initial capture of product where the pass through volumes may be very large and where step-elution of target protein is made after washing away impurities.

Table 14.1 Structure and Hydrophobicity of Amino Acids

Name	Symbol		R group	Terminal group	Hydro-phobicity
	3 Lett.	1 Lett.			
Aspartate	Asp	D			−3.5
Glutamate	Glu	E			−3.5
Lysine	Lys	K			−3.9
Arginine	Arg	R			−4.5
Histidine	His	H			−3.2
Tyrosine	Tyr	Y			−1.3
Tryptophan	Trp	W			−0.9

(*Continued*)

477

Table 14.1 (*Continued*)   Structure and Hydrophobicity of Amino Acids

Name	Symbol		R group	Terminal group	Hydro-phobicity
	3 Lett.	1 Lett.			
Phenylalanine	Phe	F	$\bigcirc$–CH$_2$–C(H)(NH$_3^+$)–COO$^-$		2.8
Cysteine	Cys	C	HS–CH$_2$–C(H)(NH$_3^+$)–COO$^-$		2.5
Methionine	Met	M	CH$_3$–S–CH$_2$–CH$_2$–C(H)(NH$_3^+$)–COO$^-$		1.9
Serine	Ser	S	HO–CH$_2$–C(H)(NH$_3^+$)–COO$^-$		−0.8
Threonine	Thr	T	CH$_3$–CH(OH)–C(H)(NH$_3^+$)–COO$^-$		−0.7
Asparagine	Asn	N	NH$_2$–C(=O)–CH$_2$–C(H)(NH$_3^+$)–COO$^-$		−3.5
Glutamine	Gln	Q	NH$_2$–C(=O)–CH$_2$–CH$_2$–C(H)(NH$_3^+$)–COO$^-$		−3.5

(*Continued*)

Table 14.1 (*Continued*)   Structure and Hydrophobicity of Amino Acids

Name	Symbol		R group	Terminal group	Hydro-phobicity
	3 Lett.	1 Lett.			
Glycine	Gly	G		H—C($\cdot$COO$^-$)(H)(NH$_3^+$)	−0.4
Alanine	Ala	A		CH$_3$—C(H)(COO$^-$)(NH$_3^+$)	1.8
Valine	Val	V	(CH$_3$)$_2$CH—	C(H)(COO$^-$)(NH$_3^+$)	4.2
Leucine	Leu	L	(CH$_3$)$_2$CH—CH$_2$—	C(H)(COO$^-$)(NH$_3^+$)	3.8
Isoleucine	Ile	I	CH$_3$—CH$_2$—CH(CH$_3$)—	C(H)(COO$^-$)(NH$_3^+$)	4.5
Proline	Pro	P	(CH$_2$)$_3$ ring	C(H)(COO$^-$)(N—H)	−1.6

The advantage of using AC in large-scale capture operations has resulted in the availability of several generic options based on ligand screening technology such as the use of

Small organic triazine-based ligands, which are identified by screening against the target protein, which is immobilized to a matrix and optimized in a column mode. Aminimide molecules as molecular recognition agents.

Ligands protein A and protein G for antibody purification or from the cell culture harvest. Protein A binds effectively to the human IgG subclasses IgG_1, IgG_2, IgG_4, and protein G binds effectively to the human IgG subclasses IgG_{1-4}.

Fusion protein capture. Ligands are chosen to take into account their toxicity and environmental impact, if these are not already in wide use. Commonly used ligands are antibodies, antigens, cofactors, protein A, metal chelators, miomimetic triazine compounds, and structural peptides. Both expanded bed and packed-bed technology are used for capture operations.

The elution techniques used in AC include the following:

Isocratic elution (not very practical in large-scale productions).

Stepwise elution of several isocratic elution to remove bound impurities by passing 1–2 bed volumes at each step. This process is more robust than gradient operations.

Gradient elution where the concentration of the eluting buffer is increased continuously by mixing starting and final buffer so that the percentage of final buffer pumped into the column is gradually increased.

Gel filtration should be evaluated during elution. If used, the non-binding solutes will be fractioned according to size as in size exclusion chromatography and some molecules may be affected (delayed elution) by the pore size of the particles. The sample molecules cannot migrate ahead of the eluting buffer since they encounter conditions which favor their re-binding to the matrix.

The column size is usually not a critical parameter and determined by the capacity of the adsorbent. Short bed heights (10–30 cm) and wide columns will allow for high throughput of the often large volumes handled during capture. Some of the common media used that comply with cGMP purification qualification include: Blue Sepharose 6 FF, Chelating Sepharose FF, Heparin Sepharose 6 FF, Streamline Heparin, Protein A Sepharose 4 FF. Protein A Sepharose 6 FF, Streamline rProtein A, rProtein A Sepharose FF, rmp Protein A Sepharose FF, MabSelect, Protein G Sepharose 4 FF, Chelating Sepharose FF, and Streamline Chelating all from Amersham.

The operating conditions are optimizing through adjustment of pH where variations affect the affinity between the protein and the ligand due to a change of surface charge properties of the protein. An increase in pH will mostly result in enhanced binding and thus the elution is done at lower pH values though high pH may be necessary in some instances. The ionic strength is adjusted by adding salt (typically 0.15 M) to the buffer to suppress non-specific electrostatic interactions. This may be unnecessary in situations where the ligand interacts predominantly by electrostatic forces where higher ionic strength (1–3 M) is used such as in the binding to dye resins. When the binding is dominated by hydrophobic interactions, high salt concentrations enhance binding (e.g., binding of IgG to Protein A resins). The binding capacity should not be exceeded to avoid precipitation; for example, the theoretical binding capacity of a protein with M_r 60,000 is approximately 80 mg/mL on a 4% agarose-based affinity matrix. The polarity is important where binding is a result of hydrophobicity where elution is not easily achieved through changes in pH or ionic strength; this requires reduction of polarity or inclusion of a chaotropic salt, denaturing agent, or detergent in the eluting buffer. Useful detergents are Lubrol, Nonidet P-40, octylglycosides, and Triton X-100 (note that it causes high UV-absorption) at concentrations below the critical micelle concentration. Chaotropic salts, such as KSCN and KI (1–3 M), are typical. Polarity reducing agents such as ethylene glycol and dioxan often promote desorption at concentrations of 20%–40% (v/v) and 10% (v/v), respectively. Denaturants such as GuHCl or urea, used at moderate concentrations, affect the structure of the protein and thereby the ability to bind to the ligand. Other displacers include monomeric (e.g., imidazole) and polymeric displacers (e.g., vinyl imidazole and vinyl caprolactam). The common buffers used in elution in AC on A and G resins depend on the target proteins. For example, for most IgGs, the starting buffer would be sodium phosphate at pH7 but the elution buffer can be glycine-HCl, ammonium acetate, sodium citrate, or sodium phosphate.

14.4 IMMOBILIZED METAL AC

The immobilized metal ion AC (IMAC) is a special type of AC where the target protein is captured based on its affinity to for metal ions complexed with a chelating group (e.g., iminodiacetic acid). Since the strength of binding is highly dependent on the protein structure IMAC provides a high selectivity. To be bound to metal ions, the protein must exhibit certain amino acid residues such as histidine, cysteine, or tryptophan; since histidine tagged proteins are widely expressed in *Escherichia coli*, the use of IMAC is common. The binding potential remains viable even when proteins are denatured such as by using 7–8 M urea or 6 M GuHCl; ionic adsorption is obviated using high ionic strength buffers. The binding is influenced by pH, where low pH often leads to desorption. Clearance of viruses is often in some instances; however, this must be thoroughly validated.

Briefly, the main advantages of IMAC are high selectivity, mild elution conditions, effective in the presence of denaturants, detergents, glycol and ethanol, and binding at high ionic strength is possible. The main disadvantages are that it cannot separate derivatives from the protein of interest, and there is a potential leakage of metal ions. IMAC is preferably used for capture or first intermediary purification operations, where good separation between the protein, cell culture components, and impurities is needed.

IMAC is highly useful for purification of IgGs as they bind to metal chelating columns at neutral to alkaline pH, the binding being relatively independent of salt concentration, presence of non-ionic detergents and of urea in low concentrations. As a result, the cell culture medium can be applied to the column with no required conditioning. Elution is performed by decreasing pH in the range of 8–4, mainly reflecting titration of histidyl residues or, by using competitive elution with imidazole, providing a more gentle technique in case the target molecule shows limited stability at low pH. Since the leakage of metal ions is inevitable, further purification is needed in subsequent steps.

The capture feature of IMAC are highly desirable because there is little or no adjustment of the large volume of cell culture application sample required, the majority of contaminants pass through the column at loading conditions and the divalent metal ions can be readily removed in simple additional steps. The elution techniques in the use of IMAC are similar to those described above for AC. Same holds true for column dimensions. The most common media used in IMAC are Chelating Sepharose FF and Streamline Chelating from Amersham Biosciences. The most optimal binding conditions obtained are a neutral to slightly alkaline pH, and pH variation is a good tool to discriminate binding to histidyl residues. A decrease in pH will generally lead to desorption of the protein. Most proteins elute between pH 6.0 and 4.2. High concentrations of salt in the buffer do not appreciably affect the adsorption of protein and as a result it is common to include sodium chloride (0.1–1.0 M) in buffers used in IMAC in order to suppress ion exchange effects as well as formation of electrostatic complexes between the contaminants and target protein. Loading considerations are similar to those observed for AC. The choice of metal ion depends on the relative stability of complexes formed with iminodiacetic acid and for divalent metal ions it is in the following order: $Cu^{2+} > Ni^{2+} > Zn^{2+} > Co^{2+} > Ca^{2+}, Mg^{2+}$. Some proteins bind only to Cu^{2+}; the use weakly binding Zn^{2+} is often made to enhance selectivity. When using Ni^{2+}, generally for polyhistidine tagged proteins, the choice must be balanced with the possibility that remnants of nickel may produce allergic reactions. Additives that alter polarity have only minor effect. And denaturants only slightly affect the performance of IMAC. Most suitable elution solvents are ammonium chloride, glycine, histamine, histidine, tris or imidazole, EDTA with affinity for the chelated metal at high ionic strength as they strip the metal ions from the column. A milder elution system comprises solutes such as ammonium chloride and glycine for competitive elution from the column. EDTA is used to recover very tightly bound proteins but it also strips metal ions. Buffers used in IMAC are phosphate, borate, or acetate for initial screening as they do not interfere with binding. If the protein:metal affinity is high, a buffer that tends to reduce the binding strength can be used (e.g., Tris-HCl). However, amine-based buffers may affect both metal leakage and binding capacity. Most commonly used starter buffers are Tris-HCl, Tris, sodium borate, sodium acetate and phosphate, and the common elution buffers are likely to be the starting buffer with histidine, sodium acetate with sodium chloride, phosphate-acetic acid, EDTA, sodium acetate, imidazole, histidine, or phosphate.

14.5 ANION EXCHANGE CHROMATOGRAPHY

The most widely used purification technique in the manufacturing of therapeutic proteins is ion exchange chromatography because of the system robustness, excellent scalability, high-resolution power, and capacity. These are widely for capture, intermediary purification, and polishing; high resolution possible only surpassed by RPC; organic solvents, urea, and detergents do not affect the efficiency, it is highly flexible, and low protein concentration samples can be applied directly without significant loss. The disadvantages of AEC include poor binding at medium to high ionic strength, high ionic strength in eluted fractions when salt desorption is used, localized pH extremes during elution that can affect protein stability, uncontrolled pH during elution that may cause precipitation in the column, and that some glycoproteins may exhibit a very complex purification pattern.

While the science behind the binding of protein to charged surfaces is not well understood, the use of protein characteristics like pI, and M_r, the charge, the matrix used, and the pH and conductivity of solvent provide good predictability of separation. Anion exchangers are basic ion exchangers containing positive ligands binding negatively charged proteins (or counterions, anions). They are traditionally divided into two groups, weak and strong anion exchangers based on the pKa of the charged group. The trend goes toward use of the strong anion exchangers (quaternary amines) capable of binding proteins in the pH range of 2–12 depending on the pI of the protein (a protein of pI 3.1 is expected to bind at pH 4.1, while a protein of pI 6.1 is expected to bind at pH 7.1). A pH change in the interval of 2–12 will consequently not affect the net charge of a strong anion exchanger. The corresponding pH interval for a weak anion exchanger is 2–9.

Seven out of 20 amino acid residues contain charged groups affecting binding to ion exchangers. The simplest model will assume the protein net charge to be the dominant binding force (the more highly charged a protein is, the more strongly it binds), but local charge distributions on the protein surface should be taken into consideration. It is the chromatographic contact region of the protein surface that determines the chromatographic behavior illustrated in binding of proteins at their pI to ion exchangers. The number of charged sites of the protein interacting with the ion exchanger is called the Z value. An increase in Z indicates stronger and stronger binding. The Z value depends on pH, protein conformation, solvent, amount of protein bound, and ion exchanger properties. There is little relation between the protein net charge and the Z value.

Most proteins have an isoelectric point at pH below 7 expanding the range in which anion exchange chromatography can be used. A rule of thumb says that the protein will bind to the ion exchanger one pH unit from the isoelectric point, which should be the starting point before going into experimental design (a protein with pI of 5.5 is expected to bind at pH 6.5 and over).

As a rule, a negatively charged protein will bind to the anion exchanger making adsorption strongly pH dependent. At pH values far from the isoelectric point, proteins bind strongly. Near the isoelectric point, weaker binding may be expected and, at the isoelectric point, local charge distributions may occur even if the net charge is neutral. The pH of the solution is therefore a very essential parameter in ion exchange chromatography and a decrease in pH may be used to elute the protein.

Negatively charged ions (chloride, acetate, citrate, phosphate) are used as counterions to replace the protein during elution. The protein competes with those ions for binding to the ion exchanger. To assure high binding capacity, low buffer concentrations are used during column equilibrium and sample application (0.01–0.05 M), which makes it important to use buffers with a pKa close to the pH working range (±0.5 units) to assure sufficient buffer capacity. Note that pKa varies with temperature. The effect of ions on chromatographic behavior has been studied extensively, but safety, economy, robustness, and large scale considerations very often restrict industrial applications to a few well-characterized buffer systems such as acetate, citrate, phosphate, carbonate, and ammonia. Generally, the steric factors only affect the separation of charged solutes as a result of their influence on the available capacity for each substrate.

There are several different elution techniques utilized. In isocratic elution, which is rarely used, the solvent composition is constant and all components move simultaneously. A stepwise elution is a serial application of several isocratic elutions. At each step, typically 1–2 bed volumes of eluant are passed through the column. Column wash procedures are often step elutions used to remove bound impurities. Stepwise elution of the target protein is often a good alternative to gradient elution as it provides a more robust system. In gradient elution, the concentration of the eluting buffer is increased continuously by mixing starting and final buffer so that the percentage of final buffer pumped into the column is gradually increased. The elution process depends on the stage at which AEC is applied; in the capture stage, the ionic strength may be too high requiring an additional ultrafiltration step which will increase process volume; though one can use high-resolution procedures (gradients) at capture, it is recommended to make use of simple elution techniques (on/off) and use the column in a similar way to affinity columns. At the intermediate stage, an ion exchanger may be used where sample conductivity is low (e.g., after a HIC step) to keep sample handling to a minimum. In the polishing stage, the use of such high separation media as the monodispersed small particle (15 and 30 μ) ion exchangers (e.g., Source 30Q) helps to separate even the closely related compounds (e.g., des-amido forms and oxidized forms and target protein).

In the capture mode, the column dimensions may be defined to obtain maximum throughput of the broth. If ion exchange is used for intermediary purification or polishing, the bed height is a critical parameter. The normal range is between 10 and 30 cm bed height. Columns used for isocratic elution should have a larger bed height than columns used for gradient elution. Some of the most popular media used include the following: ANX Sepharose 4 FF, DEAE Sepharose FF, Q Sepharose FF, Q Sepharose Big Beads, Q, Sepharose High Performance, Q Sepharose XL, Source 15Q, Source 30Q, Streamline DEAE, Streamline Q XL from Amersham Biosciences. Only marginal gains are made from choosing a weak ion exchanger over a strong ion exchanger. The more important considerations include the size of particle; larger proteins require media with large pore sizes and it must be assure that the protein is not excluded from the inner part of the particle due to a pore size being too small. This will considerably lower the capacity. The pore size of the particles is an important consideration as size exclusion effects may occur following elution. To protect media, sample should be filtered with a 0.45 μm filter prior to application, which may result in increased back pressure. Filtration is not necessary if expanded bed technology is used.

Typically the pH of the application sample should be at least one pH unit above the isoelectric point of the target molecule. A pH farther away from the isoelectric point will increase the net charge of the target molecule inducing stronger binding but also increased capacity. The choice of optimal pH will always be a balance between binding capacity and selectivity, and this must be defined by experimental work. An increase in pH will result in desorption from the column as pH becomes closer to pI. Electrophoretic titration curves allow optimization of the charge-pH relationship and are particularly useful way of predicting suitable conditions for an ion exchange separation.

As a rule, the ionic strength of the sample and the mobile phase should be low to assure firm binding of the target molecule. Typical buffer concentration should be within 0.01–0.05 M (resulting in an ionic strength of around 5 mS/cm) in order to assure maximum binding capacity. Increasing the ionic strength of the solution will lead to desorption of the protein. It is possible to influence both resolution and the elution pattern by changing the nature of counterions, as proteins behave differently to the said changes (in a non-predictable way). Commonly used anions are acetate, citrate, sulfate, and phosphate. Chloride may also be used, but due to its corrosive effect on stainless steel, chlorides are often exchanged with acetate counterions in large scale. There is also a concern due to the buffering effect of some of the counterions (e.g., acetate). Polyvalent anions are better displacers (less retention) of small molecules from an anion exchanger than monovalent ions (compared at the same ionic strength). The elution strength of different anions is acetate < formate < chloride < bromide < sulfate < citrate.

The reason why temperature is important in ion exchange chromatography is not because of its effect on ion behavior but for the change in pKa brought about by changes in temperature, particularly as samples are subjected to wide range of transition from cold room to work areas.

Though the capacity of ion exchange matrices is generally high, precipitation can occur inside the column during elution at high local protein concentration.

Polarity of solvents due to the presence of non-ionic detergents and organic solvents (such as ethanol, ethylene glycol) does not affect the protein binding significantly; zwitterions, such as betaine and taurine, decrease aggregate formation and strength of binding to the ion exchanger, thus increasing the resolution. PEG, a neutral polymer, increases the interaction with the ion exchanger resulting in increased resolution.

The chaotropic effect of anions increase in the order sulfate, phosphate, acetate, carbonate, and chloride. Presence of chaotropic salts (e.g., thiocyanate) or denaturing agents (e.g., urea) increases the solubility of the protein; urea does not influence the binding of protein to the ion exchanger.

Example of common and elution buffers used in AEC include ammonium acetate, sodium phosphate, and Tris (for elution Tris will contain additional sodium chloride). It is important to assure optimal buffer capacity (pKa $\pm$ pH unit) in sufficient concentration (usually in the interval of 25–50 mM). The charged form of the buffer species should be of the same sign as the ligand on the adsorbent (e.g., NH_4^+, Htris$^+$) to prevent these ion from becoming part of the ion exchange process and inducing localized pH changes.

14.6 CATION EXCHANGE CHROMATOGRAPHY

The advantages and disadvantages of selecting and using CEC are similar to those described above for AEC and are not repeated in this section. Cation exchangers are acidic ion exchangers containing negative ligands binding positively charged proteins (or counterions, cations) that can be weak or strong based on the pKa of the charged group. The stronger cation exchangers are more popular such as sulfopropyl, or methyl sulfonate, which can bind proteins in the pH range of 4 13, depending on the pI of the protein. Weak cation exchangers will work to a lower pH of 6. Most proteins have an isoelectric point at a pH below 7, restricting the range in which cation exchange chromatography can be used, for example, a protein with a pI of 5.5 is expected to bind at pH 4.5 and under that might exclude strong cation exchangers. Positively charged ions (sodium, ammonium, potassium) are used as counterions to replace the protein during elution. The protein competes with those ions for binding to the ion exchanger. To assure high binding capacity, low buffer concentrations are used during column equilibrium and sample application (0.01–0.05 M), which makes it important to use buffers with a pKa close to the pH working range ($\pm$0.5 units) in order to assure enough buffer capacity.

The media commonly used in CEC include the following: CM Sepharose FF, SP Sepharose FF, SP Sepharose BigBeads, SP Sepharose XL, SP Sepharose High Performance, Source 15S, Source 30S, Streamline SP, Streamline SP XL.

As a general rule, the ionic strength of the sample and the mobile phase should be low to assure firm binding of the target molecule. Typical buffer concentration should be within 0.01–0.05 M (resulting in an ionic strength of around 5 mS/cm) in order to assure maximum binding capacity.

Increasing the ionic strength of the solution will lead to desorption of the protein. It is possible to influence both resolution and the elution pattern by changing the nature of counterions, as proteins behave differently to the said changes (in an unpredictable way). Commonly used anions are acetate, citrate, sulfate, and phosphate. Chloride may also be used, but due to its corrosive effect on stainless steel, chlorides are often exchanged with acetate counterions in large scale. One should be aware of the buffering effect of some of the counterions (e.g., acetate). The elution strength of different anions is acetate < formate < chloride < bromide < sulfate < citrate. Examples of common starting and elution buffers are ammonium acetate and water (for starting buffer).

14.7 SIZE EXCLUSION CHROMATOGRAPHY

SEC (gel filtration, gel permeation chromatography, molecular sieving chromatography) is a high-resolution separation process used to separate molecules based on the difference in molecular size (e.g., poly- and dimeric compounds), to desalt, where low molecular compounds are exchanged, for group separations (e.g., removal of low molecular weight impurities, and to facilitate refolding of denatured proteins). The main advantages of SEC are the effective removal of di- and polymers (highly desirable in finishing or polishing operations), fast method development, does not affect protein stability, and that the buffer can be exchanged independent of the chromatographic technique. The disadvantages include its low capacity (the application sample volume should not exceed more than 5% v/v of the column volume; as a result, SEC is rarely used in capture and intermediary operations), high cost of columns, long cycle times due to long beds. and low flow velocities and the dilution of sample (or increase in volume).

The solute molecules are separated on the basis of the pore volume of media. Large molecules, which cannot enter the intraparticle volume are not retained, while small molecules, able to enter the particles and diffuse into a larger volume, are retained. The elution volume of a non-retained solute is equal to the inter particle volume (the void volume, V_0). The ratio between the intraparticle volume (V_i) and V_0 is called the permeability of the chromatographic medium (Figure 14.1).

As the sample moves down the bed of media under elution medium, the small molecules, which diffuse into the bed (including the buffer components of the sample), are delayed compared with the large molecules, which cannot diffuse (or only partly diffuse) into the gel particles. The result is a separation according to molecular size (or approximately molecular weight) (Figure 14.2).

The resolution is determined by the size difference between the solutes and the selectivity of the gel and parameters such as load, flow rate, particle size, and column dimensions. The application sample should be highly concentrated in order to reduce its volume. Ultra-filtration is a commonly used technique to achieve concentrated samples. The capacity can be improved by concentrating the sample prior to application. This may cause an

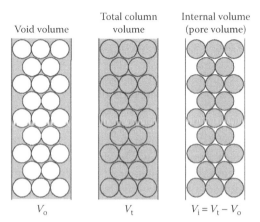

Figure 14.1 Description of volume parameters in gel chromatography. (Data from GE Healthcare, *Gel Filtration Principles and Methods*, www.gelifesciences.com.)

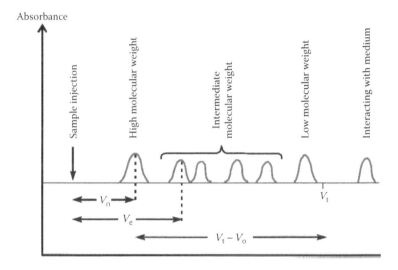

Figure 14.2 Isocratic elution in gel filtration. (Data from GE Healthcare, *Gel Filtration Principles and Methods*, www.gelifesciences.com.)

increase in viscosity and may lead to precipitation. The costs included in introducing an extra step should be balanced against the increased capacity.

Gel filtration separates mixtures of biomolecules according to size. Large molecules elute either in the void volume or early in a chromatographic separation. Smaller molecules elute later, depending on their degree of penetration of the pores of the matrix. Gel filtration is a simple and mild technique which complements ion exchange, hydrophobic interaction, and AC. In process-scale chromatography, gel filtration is principally used for desalting the product, for buffer exchange, for rapid removal of reagents to terminate a reaction, or for specific removal of contaminants with molecular weights above or below that of the desired product. Typically, molecules must differ in size by 2-fold to yield a good separation, although other adsorptive effects can augment some separations where molecules are similar in size. Gel filtration is useful for at the polishing stage where volumes are much lower than at the capture or intermediate stages and there is a need to remove dimers or aggregates. Gel filtration separates mixtures of biomolecules according to size. Large molecules elute either in the void volume or early in a chromatographic separation. Smaller molecules elute later, depending on their degree of penetration of the pores of the matrix. Gel filtration is a simple and mild technique which complements ion exchange, hydrophobic interaction, and AC. In process-scale chromatography, gel filtration is principally used for desalting the product, for buffer exchange, for rapid removal of reagents to terminate a reaction, or for specific removal of contaminants with molecular weights above or below that of the desired product. Typically, molecules must differ in size by twofold to yield a good separation, although other adsorptive effects can augment some separations where molecules are similar in size. Gel filtration is useful for at the polishing stage where volumes are much lower than at the capture or intermediate stages and there is a need to remove dimers or aggregates. Gel filtration has successfully been employed for size based separations of macromolecules since the late 1950s. Gel filtration, or size exclusion chromatography, may be performed in three principally different modes, depending on the size differences of the solutes to be separated: (1) group separation, (2) fractionation, and (3) determination of molecular mass (distributions). When the size difference is large, that is, a factor of more than 10, we talk about group separation (e.g., desalting, buffer exchange) and when the size difference is small, that is a factor of 2 to 5, we talk about fractionation. The third mode is analytical gel filtration, for example, determination of molecular mass distributions, where an array of molecular masses is to be separated. These different modes put different requirements on the equipment and media used and will yield widely different productivity in terms of information or material processed. Desalting and buffer exchange of protein samples are two examples of group separation. The large size difference between the protein and the low molecular solute makes it possible to select a gel filtration medium that will exclude the protein from the porous network while allowing full permeation of the low molecular weight solute. This is the most productive mode of preparative gel filtration (in terms of mass of product per volume medium and unit time) and will, as we shall see below, allow large freedom for choosing experimental conditions that otherwise would be detrimental to the separation of more closely sized molecules. In gel filtration the separation takes place due to the, for steric reasons, different access to the pore volume of molecules of different sizes. The separation thus takes place over a volume equal to the pore volume. In desalting (used for describing group separation) the gel filtration medium is used to selectively exclude the large molecular weight solute, for example, protein or DNA from entering the porous gel phase. Thus, a rational choice of matrix will allow the protein to be eluted in the void or interstitial, volume of the column. As a result the protein zone will be diluted to a minimum, as caused by eddy dispersion only (e.g., non-equilibrium effects are eliminated). This also means that the zone broadening, or dilution of the protein zone, is rather insensitive to fluid velocity and high velocities (e.g., exceeding 500 cm/h) may be employed for fast desalting (since the zone broadening of low molecular weight solutes is also generally small unless extreme velocities are used). Low molecular weight impurities, for example, salt, will permeate the pore volume and will have a retention volume equal to the total liquid volume of the column (if provided the size of the molecule is small as compared to the pore size of the gel filtration medium). If the impurities have an intermediate size they will only permeate part of the pore volume giving a less favorable situation. From the principles of group separation we may conclude that the following characteristics of the gel filtration medium are important: (1) pore size, (2) pore volume, (3) particle size, and (4) matrix rigidity. The pore size is chosen such that the large molecular weight solute is excluded from the gel matrix. However, the pore size must not be too small since the low molecular weight impurities will then not elute at the total volume and this will limit the applicable sample volume. The pore volume is a very important characteristic of the gel filtration medium and will directly influence the sample volume that is applicable. Therefore the matrix volume of a desalting gel filtration medium used for preparative use should be kept as low as possible. However, this is contradictory to the demand of high matrix rigidity which generally is increased with increased matrix volume. A small pore volume may of course be compensated for by using a larger bed volume but this will be at the expense of lower productivity. The particle size will influence the sample dispersion in the bed. However, since the large molecular mass solute will not enter the porous phase, the main cause of zone broadening in gel filtration (i.e., due to non-equilibrium) is not present and only eddy dispersion contributes. This effect may be small compared to dispersion from sample application and column dead volumes (e.g., at inlet and outlet). It may be concluded that the influence of particle size in the range of 50 to 300 µm on the bed dispersion is rather small for column lengths above 15 cm. However, for shorter columns bed dispersion reduces the sample volume that can be applicable, especially for media of large particle size. In addition to the effect from the dispersion of the bed, a contribution from column dead volumes may be anticipated, the extent being dependent upon the column design. This will reduce the relative influence of the particle size to some degree. The effect will be largest for small particles since these yield lower dispersion than larger particles. If the sample volume is very small a column of small size is recommended. If dilution of the sample must be kept to a minimum a small particle size gel filtration medium should be selected. The particle size has a large influence on the pressure drop over the packed bed. In principle the pressure drop is inversely proportional to the particle size squared. This is due to that smaller intraparticle channels are formed by smaller particles. The higher liquid velocities in these smaller channels will result in higher friction forces acting on the particles yielding higher pressure drops but also leading to higher stress which may result in compaction of the bead. The reduced size of the flow channels with lower particle size will also lead to a higher sensitivity to viscous fingering effects, that is, the distortion of highly concentrated sample zones due to hydrodynamic instability of the rear part of the zone. A high matrix rigidity will allow high flow rates to be employed for fast desalting but this may be at the expense of the maximum sample volume that can be applied and these factors need to be considered simultaneously. If large sample volumes are to be quickly desalted it may be better to use a larger particle of low matrix volume. The productivity is expressed as the amount of product purified per unit time and unit bed volume. The amount of purified product is equal to the concentration times the sample volume times the yield. The yield for desalting (and gel filtration in general) is very high and may be set to 100%. The maximum concentration of proteins that may be applied is restricted by the relative viscosity of the sample compared to eluant and a sample concentration of 50 mg/mL of a protein having a molecular mass of 50,000 seems to be the upper limit in simple aqueous eluants. The productivity decreases with increasing column length. Thus it is advantageous to use *short and fat* columns as long as the column construction minimizes column dead volumes. In order to utilize the entire pore volume for desalting it is important that the pore size is not too small since this will lead to low molecular weight impurities being eluted too early. A gel filtration medium of larger pore size which still excludes the protein of interest should be used, or the sample volume must be reduced to allow for separation (the sample volume may not exceed the difference in elution volume of the impurity and the void volume). Gel filtration can offer a very robust purification for initial buffer exchange of raw plasma in a large-scale albumin fractionation plant. HiPrep™ 26/10 Desalting offers a quick, easy, and convenient way for group separation of high and low molecular weight substances. Since proteins and other biomolecules differ greatly in size from salts and other small molecules, gel filtration is particularly efficient for many everyday laboratory operations. *Group separation* separates the components of a sample into two groups, for example, high molecular weight substances, which are excluded from the gel and thus elute first, from low molecular weight substances that enter the pores freely and thus elute later. Buffer exchange and desalting are common operations in any laboratory engaged in sample purification and analysis. It is often necessary to change the buffer composition of a sample between chromatography steps or to satisfy special requirements of an assay. Desalting of a sample is a prerequisite for mass spectroscopy analysis, lyophilization, and after certain procedures such as ion exchange chromatography. Although both procedures can be accomplished by dialysis, this is a time-consuming process, and samples sensitive to degradation may be at risk. Because of its high speed and high volume capacity, HiPrep 26/10 Desalting is an excellent alternative to dialysis, especially when larger sample volumes are used or when samples need to be processed rapidly to avoid degradation. The most critical parameter affecting resolution in desalting applications is the sample-to-gel volume ratio. To minimize dilution and still retain good separation, sample volumes up to approximately 30% of the total bed volume are recommended. Desalting can be done at high flow rates as flow rate has a minor impact on resolution.

Gel filtration is used for several different purposes. For example, it is used for fractionation as last *polishing* step where process volume has been reduced by previous step(s), to remove aggregates; in the desalting step anywhere in the process for easy conditioning. The stationary phase or media generally comprises inert chemically stable uniform spheres with a defined particle and pore size distribution. The pore size is chosen according to optimal separation between the target protein and impurities. The optimal condition is to exclude the target protein from the intraparticle volume to avoid zone broadening. If the size difference between the target protein and the impurities is small, a pore size from which the target molecule is eluted at roughly half a column volume is optimal. It should be noted that most gel permeation chromatography media contain small amounts of ionic groups; the ionic interaction between charged solutes and the matrix is prevented by the addition of 25–150 mM salt. Larger proteins require media with large pore sizes. Verify that your protein is not excluded from the inner part of the particle due to a pore size being too small. This will considerably lower the capacity.

The mobile phase is selected based on desired outcome. Preparative SEC includes buffer exchange and fractionation. Buffer exchange or desalting is the exchange of low molecular components of the sample (typically salt molecules) with another buffering substance. In fractionation, the solute is separated from other solutes according to their molecular size, typically separation of poly- and dimers from the monomeric target protein.

Commonly used SEC media are Sephadex (based on cross-linked dextran), Superdex (based on highly cross-linked agarose), Superose (based on highly cross-linked agarose), and Sepharose (based on cross-linked agarose) from Amersham. The SEC media are not inert and can induce electrostatic, hydrophobic, hydrogen bonding and biospecific interactions. The resolution is proportional to the square root of the bed height. The effective column length may be increased by adding columns in series (column stacking). The sample volume is the single parameter having the greatest impact on resolution. The sample volume should not exceed 5% v/v of the column volume. (Even smaller loads are often necessary in order to obtain the desired resolution.) In desalting mode, up to 30% v/v of the total bed volume may be applied without disrupting the separation effect.

The sample concentration is restricted by the protein precipitation and the viscosity of the sample plug compared to that of the mobile phase. The general rule is that the viscosity of the sample should be less than 1.5. This corresponds to a sample concentration of 70 mg/mL of a globular protein such as albumin. At lower temperature the viscosity increased by a large factor, often doubling the back pressure and slowing the diffusion rate of the solute molecules. The resolution decreases with increasing flow velocity relative to the viscosity of the eluant. Typical flow velocities at large scale are in the range of 30–50 cm/h. In desalting mode (e.g., Sephadex G-25), it can be as high as 200 cm/h depending on the bed diameter and height. An increase in bed height increases the resolution. The increase in resolution relates directly to the square root of the increase in bed height. The application sample should be filtered with a 0.45 μm filter prior to application in order to protect the column against particles, aggregates, and so on, which may result in increased back pressure.

The common buffers used include ammonium acetate and sodium phosphate (alone or in combination with ammonium sulfate). To avoid precipitation due to change of pH, ionic strength, presence of co-solvent or changes in temperature, assure that the application sample complies with the equilibration buffer.

The problems of later or earlier elution are readily solved by adjusting a large number of parameters available.

When elution is later than expected, it can be caused by the following:

- Ionic adsorption due to negatively charged groups on the support (carboxyl-, sulfate) and positively charged groups on sample molecules. It is resolved by including 150 mM NaCl (or other salt) in buffer.
- Hydrophobic adsorption. It is resolved by adding 10%–20% ethanol or other organic solvents to buffer or decrease salt concentration in high ionic strength buffer.
- More compact shape of the sample molecule due to hydrogen bridge bonds. It is resolved by including 8 M urea or 6 M guanidine hydrochloride in buffer.
- Digestion by proteases. It is resolved by adding protease inhibitors to buffer.

When elution is earlier than desired, its causes and remediation are as follows:

- Ionic aggregates and complexes due to carbohydrate chains (glycoproteins). It is changed by including 150 mM NaCl or up to 10% betaine in buffer.
- Complexes associated via SH groups. It is resolved by adding reducing agent (e.g., DTT) to buffer.
- Hydrophobic aggregates are removed by adding 10%–20% ethanol or other organic solvents to buffer.
- Gel filtration of micelles/protein aggregates is resolved by decreasing buffer detergent concentration until below CMC or use a different detergent (stay below its CMC).
- Exclusion of molecules due to ionic repulsion of negatively charged groups on sample and support is resolved by including 150 mM NaCl or 0.1% TFA in buffers.

14.8 REVERSED PHASE CHROMATOGRAPHY

This is one of the most widely used chromatography method in the downstream processing as well as in the analytical testing of therapeutic proteins. Whereas other methods rely on the size of molecule, RPC is governed by the hydrophobic interaction between the solute molecules (in the mobile phase) and the ligand (in the stationary phase). This should not be confused with HIC (hydrophobic interaction chromatography), where the ligands interact individually with the solutes; in the RPC, the stationary phase is a continuous hydrophobic phase with the solute molecules partitioning between the mobile phase and the stationary phase. The separation occurs by a reversible dynamic absorption/desorption onto a matrix of hydrophobic ligand, which are chemically attached to a porous, insoluble matrix generally composed of silica or a synthetic organic polymer, such as polystyrene. The unattached silanol groups on silica (when used) interact with the solute molecules (an undesirable situation reduced by blocking the groups with alkyl silane reagents—end-capping) as well making the media support an important element. Whereas silica-based matrices are chemically stable at acidic pH, synthetic organic polymers are stable throughout the pH range from 1 to 12. The unattached surface of polymers is also strongly hydrophobic, in contract to the unattached ends on silica. The selectivity in separation is determined by the type of ligand attached to the medium, such as n-alkyl hydrocarbon or aryl hydrocarbon compounds; if solute is highly hydrophobic, the ligands must be less hydrophobic (or else they will elute). Proteins bind C4–C8 columns. If impurities present are charged they can bind to ligand which can be reduced by a proper selection of the mobile phase. The mobile phase is generally a mixture of water, organic modifier (e.g., water-ethanol), and a buffering substance to assure that the solutes are uncharged during separation. The organic modifier or more than modifier is often present in concentrations from 0% to 60% v/v such as 2-propanol, acetonitrile, methanol, and ethanol (listed in decreasing elution strength order). (The use of organic solvents in large-scale operations requires explosion proof equipment and facilities.) The concentration of modifier is important and often a gradient system is used to improve separation where the initial binding conditions are designed to favor adsorption of the solute from the mobile phase (aqueous solution with little or no organic modifier present). In this case, adsorption is considered the extreme equilibrium state where the distribution of solute molecules is essentially 100% in the stationary phase. This is followed by desorption where the solute is essentially 100% distributed in the mobile phase achieved by decreasing the polarity (increasing the concentration of organic modifier). Several elution techniques are used with RPC, isocratic, stepwise, gradient, affinity elution, gel filtration, etc. Common media include Source 15RPC or Source 30RPC from Amersham.

The primary advantages of RPC are its very high resolution even with closely related molecules and the use of high ionic strength solutions; RPC is a perfect polishing technique, but rarely used in intermediary purification and not in the capture mode. Presence of organic solvent in the eluted fractions makes it often necessary to introduce a subsequent buffer exchange step. The disadvantages in using RPC include the mandatory use of organic solvents which often denature the target or affect their solubility, the ligand may also denature the proteins; RPC is also not suitable for proteins with molecular weight above 25 kD.

The common mobile phase solvents include HCl, phosphoric acid, trifluoroacetic acid, triethylammonium phosphate, and ammonium acetate. The PRC matrix is stable at wide pH ranges (silica unstable at alkaline pH). At low pH the silanol groups of silica-based matrices will be uncharged reducing binding of ionic impurities. When using low pH, basic proteins shows a tail when eluted; this can be obviated by increasing pH. The competition between carboxyl and basic groups is eliminated at low pH, where the carboxyl group ionization and the amino groups are essentially fully protonated. Generally, higher selectivity is seen when running below the pI of the protein (the mechanism is not well explained). In the absence of ions that stabilize secondary and tertiary structure, lowering of pH results in loss of resolution; since ionic strength does not have any significant direct effect, RPC offers great flexibility; however, where ion pairing agents is involved, it results in increased hydrophobicity of the solute molecules and thus its resolution on the columns; examples of ion pairing agents include TFA, PFPA, HFBA, ammonium acetate, phosphoric acid, tetramethylammonium chloride, tetrabutylammonium chloride, and triethylamine. Before any of these agents can be used, their toxicity must be considered. Presence of denaturing agents does not affect the capacity of the column.

Elevated temperatures expedite mass transfer of the solutes, more rapid unfolding/refolding, and interactions with ions and solvents, all improving efficiency of system; however, protein denaturation at high temperature should be the controlling factor.

Whereas much higher loading can be done compared to ion exchange chromatography, generally more than 30% of maximum capacity would lead to losses in resolution and chemical deterioration as irreversible adsorption, denaturation, or conformational alterations. When the samples are very dilute, losses are minimal.

14.9 HYDROXYAPATITE CHROMATOGRAPHY

Hydroxyapatite matrix (poly-calcium phosphate $[Ca_{10}(PO_4)_6(OH)_2]$) is both the support and ligand where positively charged pairs of crystal calcium ions and clusters of six negatively charged oxygen atoms associated with triplets of crystal phosphates bind proteins through nonspecific and by specific complexing of protein carboxyls with calcium loci on the mineral. At low pH (5 or below) or in the presence of chelating agents, the crystal structure and efficiency is lost; however, hydroxyapatite media are resistant to sodium hydroxide, detergents, organic solvents, and denaturing agents. The major advantages in the use of HAC are its applicability during capture, intermediary purification, and polishing stages, often offering unique separation of even between closely related compounds, effective with different buffers and organic solvents and allowing mixed mode purification. HAC is applicable to all antibodies, providing good fractionation regardless of the production medium, species, class, or subclass. The disadvantage relates to stability of matrix at low pH and in the presence of chelating agents; matrix can degrade due to microbial secretion of acidic contaminants (this can be obviated using 50%–60% methanol, though it represents a hazardous situation). The availability of different size uniform stable particles in the range from 10 to 100 µm is suitable for intermediate purification and polishing operations, as an alternate to IMAC, IEC, HIC, and RPC.

Proteins are eluted either as a result of the nonspecific ion screening of charges or by specific displacement of protein groups from the sites of the column with which they have complexed. The good results obtained using HAC are surprising in absence of a solid theory how it works. It is particularly useful for the purification of medium to large size proteins with a well-defined tertiary structure; low molecular weight solutes and denatured proteins show lower affinity to hydroxyapatite. The adsorption depends on pH and ionic strength. The elution behavior is a function of the isoelectric point of the protein; basic proteins elute at moderate concentrations of phosphate, fluoride, chloride, or thiocyanate (0.1–0.3 M), alternately low concentrations (<0.003 M) of Ca^{2+} or Mg^{2+}; acidic proteins elute at equal moderate concentrations of phosphate and fluoride but do not elute with Ca^{2+} and usually not with chloride; neutral proteins elute with phosphate, fluoride, and chloride and not with Ca^{2+} or thiocyanate.

The elution techniques used are isocratic, stepwise, gradient, gel filtration, and so on. The common media are the Macro-prep Ceramic Hydroxyapatite I and II from BioRad. Generally, an increase in pH would result in decreased binding capacity at a given ionic strength and the matrix is unstable below pH 5. In general, low ionic strength favors protein adsorption and moderate to high salt concentrations may be workable depending on protein and salt. However, increasing phosphate concentration (even at low concentration) results in desorption of the protein. All proteins elute at moderate phosphate ion concentrations. Basic proteins elute at less than 3 mM Ca^{++} or Mg^{++} and with moderate Cl^-. Neutral proteins do not elute with Ca^{++} or other divalent metal ions. Acidic proteins do not elute with Ca^{++} or other divalent metal ions and do not usually elute with chloride. 0.005 M $MgCl_2$ or 1 M NaCl/KCl is recommended to elute basic proteins, 1.0 M $MgCl_2$ to elute protein with pI between 5.5 and 8.0 and 0.3 M phosphate to elute acidic proteins. The load capacity of HAC is high but there remains a possibility of localized precipitation of target protein at high local concentration. Organic solvents (such as ethanol, ethylene glycol) do not affect the protein binding significantly and are even desired to keep hydrophobic proteins in solution or to keep the protein in its monomeric form. Proteins usually do not bind in presence of detergents or denaturing agents, such as urea. As only native proteins bind to hydroxyapatite, binding of weakly interacting basic proteins can be strengthened by inclusion of 1 mM phosphate in the buffer.

The common starting buffers are potassium phosphate, sodium phosphate, sodium chloride and magnesium chloride; the elution buffers are mainly phosphates.

14.10 HYDROPHOBIC INTERACTION CHROMATOGRAPHY

HIC is based on interaction between hydrophobic patches on the protein surface and hydrophobic ligands of the matrix and is a result of the solvophobic effect, solute avoiding solvent. As a result, the high ionic strength of the solvent favors binding or the presence of salts that imparts the solution higher surface tension. (Balance this with risk of salting out of proteins.) Unlike the RPC where the absorbent was a continuous phase, the ligands interact individually with the solutes in HIC, which is a much stronger chromatographic method with lesser risk of protein denaturation compared to RPC. The factors of importance are the type of ligand and base matrix, the solvent properties, temperature, and type and concentration of salt. Retention is proportional to the length of the alkyl ligand chain (hydrophobic character); ligands containing 4 to 10 carbon atoms are suited for most purposes. Aryl ligands, showing both aromatic and hydrophobic interactions, offer a mixed mode. Solvent additives (alcohols, detergents, chaotropic salts) that decrease the surface tension of water weaken the hydrophobic interaction leading to desorption of the bound protein. Different salts give rise to differences in hydrophobic interaction and combinations of strong ligand–weak salt, medium ligand–medium salt, and weak ligand–strong salt can be used in the unit operation optimization. In summary, the HIC shows advantage of using high and low salt concentrations, giving high recovery with high binding capacity and makes an excellent complementary technique to IEC. The conductivity of fermentation samples is often relatively high (10–30 mS/cm), making HIC an excellent capture step for hydrophobic proteins. Additionally, the binding capacity often decreases in the presence of anti-foam agents added during fermentation. The disadvantage includes protein precipitation at high salt concentrations and the environment risk considerations in large-scale operations (high salt consumption and disposal). (If used in intermediate purification, it is an excellent step following ion exchange chromatography, where high salt concentrations have been used to elute the target protein.) HIC is used in the polishing mode, but the resolution cannot be compared to that of IEC and RPC.

In the capture mode, the column dimensions are generally short (heights from 5 to 20 cm). The common media used are Butyl Sepharose 4 FF, Octyl Sepharose 4 FF, Phenyl Sepharose6 FF (high sub), Phenyl Sepharose FF (low sub), Phenyl Sepharose High Performance, Source 15ETH, Source 15SO, Source15PHE from Amersham. Since there is a correlation between increase in pH and weakened hydrophobic interaction, binding capacity must be tested at various pH values. Adsorption of proteins to HIC columns is favored by high salt concentrations (typically from 0.5 to 3 M concentrations are used). The strength of interaction depends on the salt used following the series (Hofmeister) ammonium sulfate > ammonium chloride > sodium sulfate > sodium chloride > sodium bromide > sodium thiocyanate, with ammonium sulfate as one of the most utilized salts. The concentration of salt needed for protein binding may vary considerably from protein to protein. The HIC medium of choice should bind the protein of interest at relatively low salt concentration (<1 M). The effect of salts in HIC can be accounted for by reference to the Hofmeister series for the precipitation of proteins or for their positive influence in increasing the molal surface tension of water. Elution is carried out with salt free buffers of low ionic strength. Less hydrophobic matrix is used if non-polar solvents are needed for elution. Elution is achieved by a linear or stepwise decrease in the concentration of salt in the mobile phase. Temperature significantly affects HIC, lower temperature reducing interaction. Presence of polarity-decreasing solvents (low levels of alcohols, detergents, ethylene glycol) decreases the binding of the target protein; these can be added after the salt has been removed from the column. Presence of chaotropic ions (e.g., Gu^{2+}, SCN^-) or urea decreases the binding of the target protein with risk for protein denaturation. Charged molecules containing short alkyl and/or aryl groups can be used as displacers in HIC.

The common starting buffers are potassium phosphate, sodium phosphate with aluminum sulfate, Tris with ammonium sulfate, Tris with EDTA and ammonium sulfate, sodium phosphate with sodium chloride, sodium succinate with ammonium sulfate, glycine, and sodium acetate with ammonium sulfate. The elution buffers include potassium phosphate, sodium phosphate, Tris with EDTA, sodium phosphate with sodium chloride, sodium succinate with ammonium sulfate, glycine, and ethylene glycol.

14.11 SCALE UP AND OPTIMIZATION

Scale up requires an in-depth understanding of parameters prior to establishing a scale-up plan. These parameters include the following:

- Chromatography medium type
- Sample concentration
- Protein load/mL gel (adsorption techniques)
- Sample volume/mL gel (gel filtration)
- Linear flow rate
- Productivity (g/h/liter of gel)
- Column bed height
- Back pressure
- Buffer type and allowed variations in pH and conductivity
- Feedstock and buffer storage stability
- Acceptable materials in contact with liquid
- Protein sensitivity to shear forces
- Recovery based on a well-defined product quality assay
- Washing procedures
- Gel life length
- Buffer consumption
- Product volumes
- Number of product fractions to be collected
- Monitoring parameters

There are several approaches to scale up; for example, we can maintain bed height, linear flow rate, gradient volume: media volume, sample concentration and composition, sample volume: media volume. Another choice will be to increase column diameter, volumetric flow rate, sample volume proportionally, gradient volume proportionally. In scale up of adsorption techniques, the diameter is increased but the bed height is maintained. When using gel filtration we can increase diameter, maintain bed height and additionally use columns in series. Most parameters that can be changed hover around the column used wherein the wall support and wall effects determine the choice of which parameter to change and which one to keep constant. The wall support affects distribution system, handling/packability, chemical resistance, pressure rating, and hygienic design (referring to cGMP compliance). The wall effects include pressure/flow curves in columns with different diameters; the system considerations include extra column zone spreading, accuracy (flow rate, gradient), chemical resistance, pressure rating, and hygienic design. The non-chromatographic factors that may affect performance upon scale up include changes in sample composition, changes in sample concentration, longer holding times, buffer preparation. In fine tuning the adjustments generally include adjustment of gradient volume, adjustment of flow rate, adjustment of equilibration volume, modification of fractionation, modification of CIP-routines. Scale up from 10- to 500-fold are routinely made; however, a stepwise approach is suggested to take into account unexpected nonlinearities particularly with reference to the column characteristics that may arise. One of the premier sources of support is obviously the column and media supplier such as Amersham, who are more than likely to walk you through the entire process of scale up. When projects of large dimension are installed, many suppliers would even offer to run your process to assure you are making the right selection. Chromatography media is one of the most expensive component of the entire process and every effort should be made to make this as optimal as possible for long-term cost savings.

The primary objective of optimization is to reach the specified purity at highest possible yield, at lowest possible cost and in the shortest possible time. There are two parallel activities, the optimization of each chromatographic step and the optimization of the process.

The method optimization using process chromatography operates on a different principle than does analytical chromatography; in process chromatography, the resolution is adjusted to increase sample loading (productivity) and increased yield through less peak cutting within a defined purity Rs; in analytical chromatography, resolution concerns maximum number of peaks, identity, purity, and quantification. Similarly, in process chromatography the size of sample is as large as possible while opposite holds true for analytical chromatography. The speed is measure in g/mL gel/h in process and in cycles/h in analytical chromatography. The optimization parameters related to chromatography and process are given in Table 14.2.

Bed height optimization techniques depend on the required selectivity. For high selectivity techniques where efficiency less important, chemistry is used to improve RS and adsorption techniques such as IEC, HIC, AC are used with typical bed height of 5–20 cm. In low selectivity techniques where efficiency is more important, isocratic techniques such as SEC are used with typical bed heights: 60–90 cm.

Table 14.2 Optimization Parameters in Chromatography and Process

Chromatographic	Process
Column length and diameter	Stability
Bead size	Working temperature
Flow rates	Viscosity
Sample capacity (volume/mass), conditioning, application	Concentration/dilution
Buffers and salts	Batch size
Gradient volumes and shape	Logistics of handling liquids and consumables
Regeneration/re-equilibration	Cooperation between research/development and production

Particle size is important; for purification, the bead size ranges from 15 to 90 mm and for polishing, 10–34 mm. Bead size greater than 90 mm causes fouling, pressure drop, flow rate, and higher costs.

Flow rate adjustment requires equilibration, adsorption, wash, desorption, regeneration consideration.

Gradient optimization starts with a simple linear gradient wherein slopes and shapes are varied to improve Rs; in step gradients often artifacts are discovered.

Sample loading optimization depends on the technique used. For adsorption techniques where very high selectivity or capture is desired, complete bed volume is used for sample binding. In adsorption chromatography used for purification, only first past of bed volume is used for sample binding; in isocratic techniques, the sample volume is limiting.

Steps in the process inversely affect the yield regardless of the step yield proportion; therefore, keeping steps to minimum is probably the most effective optimization for cost, yield, and productivity.

Buffer systems are modified by setting range of buffer conditions, avoiding expensive buffers and instead using the standard phosphate, acetate, or citrate buffers.

Temperature increase increases throughput and is a good parameter to adjust if stability of target protein, of media, and resultant interactions would allow.

Gel filtration is optimized taking into account, the matrix, selectivity, rigidity, chemical stability, bead size distribution, bed height, column packing, flow rate, sample volume, and viscosity.

Ion exchange is optimized by binding pH and ionic strength, sample load (mass), flow rate (equilibration, adsorption, desorption, wash), gradient volume, and shape. The elution strength of different ions in anion exchange chromatography is: Acetate < formate < chloride < bromide < sulfate < citrate; in cation exchange chromatography: lithium < sodium < ammonium < potassium < magnesium < calcium.

AC critical parameters include the type of ligand and ligand density, binding conditions, dynamic capacity, elution conditions. The binding of hIgG is increased due to coupling of the legend. The elution is affected often by denaturing conditions (low pH, chaotropic salts, urea, guanidine-HCL), in AF attempts should be made to immediately neutralize or remove eluting agents and remove aggregates simultaneously using gel filtration.

Hydrophobic interaction chromatography optimization parameters include sample load, sample application, flow rate, gradient volume and shape, temperature dependence, hydrophobicity of ligand and additives. Increased ligand density gives increased strength of interaction and increased capacity; increased temperature gives increased strength of hydrophobic interaction; however, one must be cognizant of temperature-dependent alteration of protein structure; lower pH shows increased hydrophobic interaction. The productivity is improved by optimizing starting conditions like type of salt, concentration and application mode, by optimizing the dynamic loading capacity and by tuning the gradient, flow rate, and sample relationship similar to what is normally done for ion exchange chromatography.

Questions

1. List some advantages and disadvantages of affinity chromatography.
   Answer: Adv: high specificity, mild elution conditions; Disadv: hard to distinguish target from derivatives.
2. When selecting elution buffers in an affinity chromatography setup, list some factors that need to be considered.
   Answer: Polarity, pH, ionic strength.
3. What kind of production system is often used for IMAC?
4. List some of the pros and cons of AEC, the most used chromatography method.
   Answer: Pro: scalability, high resolution, Con: usually high ionic strength in elution buffer.
5. If a protein has a pI of 6.75 what pH would be a good starting point in AEC?
6. Should the ionic strength of the solution be low or high for binding on an AEC column?
7. For gel permeation chromatography, what is the maximum recommended percentage of the total bed volume that a sample should be?
8. When the process requirements indicate that the solution or mobile phase should be acidic, which chromatographic technique may be useful?
   Answer: Reverse phase chromatography
9. Which method can be used to distinguish relatively similar compounds, or even denatured verses native conformations?
10. Describe the parameters that are useful to consider when designing the transition between lab scale and production scale, or scale up.
    Answer: Chromatography medium type, protein load, sample volumes/concentrations, protein sensitivity to shear forces, washing procedures, gel life length, buffer consumption, and so on.

15

Manufacturing Systems

LEARNING OBJECTIVES

1. Identify the four types of expression systems that can be used for protein production.
2. Understand the advantages and challenges present with each manufacturing system for protein production.
3. Recognize the engineering similarities between the manufacturing systems.

15.1 BACTERIAL EXPRESSION SYSTEMS

The typical protein to be expressed in gram-negative bacteria comprises 100–300 amino acids, has no posttranslational modifications, and possesses a restricted number of cysteine residues to make in vitro refolding possible. Whereas this chapter pertains mainly to gram-negative bacteria, a discussion of how the gram-positive bacteria are viewed with great interest should be made. The problems of methionine blocking the N-terminus and the intracellular formation of inclusion bodies which add host cell impurities in the use of gram-negative bacteria can be resolved by using gram-positive bacteria such as *Bacillus subtilis* and *Lactococcus lactis*. Also, the presence of endotoxin is of little concern in gram-positive bacteria. On the negative side, while using *Bacillus*, endogenous proteolytic degradation can be significant, a drawback not found in *Lactococcus*. The extracellular expression of the folded target protein in the use of gram-positive bacteria additionally eliminates significant problems in the use of *Escherichia coli* expression system: the requirements of in vitro folding and performing cleavage of the N-terminal tag. This results in simpler process design comprising of harvest, capture, intermediate purification, polishing, concentration, and finishing as described below for gram-negative bacteria. The rest of the chapter refers to expression system comprising gram-negative bacteria, particularly *E. coli*.

Although bacteria cannot be used to express some large, complex proteins (with eukaryotic posttranslational modifications including glycosylation, acetylation, and amidation), other proteins such as interferons, interleukins, colony stimulating factors, growth hormones, growth factors, and human serum albumin have been successfully produced.

Marketed products produced include human growth hormone; human insulin; α, β, and γ-interferon; and interleukin 2. This chapter deals with the upstream and downstream processing for the manufacturing of therapeutic proteins using bacteria, particularly the gram-negative bacteria such as *E. coli*. This system is most popular because of its low fermentation cost and high expression yields. The most common form of bacterial expression is cytoplasmatic or intracellular expression where inclusion bodies contain the target protein, which is in an inactive form and thus harmful to bacteria; the yield is generally high and the system requires simpler plasmid construct. The disadvantages include need for in vitro folding, expression of Met-protein and complex purification steps needed. The cell disruption to recover inclusion bodies releases a large volume of host cell proteins, nucleic acids, and proteolyitc enzymes that can damage target protein. Measures to reduce this proteolysis include use of thioredoxin-deficient strains, processing at low temperatures, and co-expression of chaperones, co-expression of protein disulfide-isomerase, and fusion partners; unfortunately, none of the methods have been developed far enough to be useful in commercial processing operations. Cytosolic expression in *E. coli* also produces methionine blocking of the N-terminus requiring a specific enzymatic cleavage step to produce the native molecule. To eliminate expression of Met-protein, N-terminally extended protein constructs are expressed followed by an enzymatic cleavage step in which the extension is cleaved with an endopeptidase or removed step by step with an exopeptidase. Typical extensions are fusion proteins, histidine tags, or, if proline is the second amino acid in the protein, a few amino acids. These disadvantages, particularly the inability of gram-negative organisms to express folded proteins to the periplasm or to the medium has resulted in attempts to use other forms of expression, namely, periplasmic and secretion. Attention has been focused on gram-positive bacteria, for example, *Bacillus* species, which naturally secretes large amounts of protein to the medium, but endogenous proteolytic degradation is of general concern. *Lactococcus*, traditionally used in the dairy industry, has no detectable extracellular proteases or toxins and also offers direct expression to the medium. The periplasmic expression has the advantage of producing native protein with correct N-terminal structure, requiring simpler purification and less extensive incidence of proteolysis. The disadvantages include inefficient translocation through the inner membrane and the fact that inclusion bodies may still form. The extracellular secretion system would be idea for it results in least extensive proteolysis, provides for simpler purification, and corrects N-terminus situation; however, there is little secretion that results in very low yields; one exception being the expression of β-glucanase.

15.2 GENETICALLY MODIFIED BACTERIA

The genetically modified bacteria are prepared by introducing a recombinant gene into the bacteria on a plasmid, modified to optimize heterologous protein expression comprising complete genetic elements to enhance transcription and translation and to stabilize mRNA. A plasmid is a double stranded circular DNA, small 2–25 Kbp (some bigger), bacterial artificial chromosome that has the characteristics of autonomous replication. Plasmid vectors are very useful as a quick way to introduce genes to the cell and are much more easy to manipulate than the chromosome. Components of a gene include promoter, operator, ribosome binding sites (RBSs), coding sequence, start, and stop codon. All vectors comprise an origin of replication (Ori) that determines the vector copy number. The stability of the expression cassette has a high impact on productivity. Loss of the cassette during the course of the fermentation (the cell tends to minimize the stress by getting rid of the plasmid) results in formation of nonproductive, plasmid-free cells, which usually outgrow plasmid-carrying cells in fermentation unless selective pressure can be effectively employed. Plasmid stability is increased by using vectors that confer an antibiotic resistance (e.g., ampicillin) to the host or complement some auxotrophic feature of the host strain. If periplasmic or extracellular expression is desired, the vector must also include a signal sequence for the transport of the protein.

Great advances have been made in the availability of commercial systems that help resolve some of the problem related to expressed protein harming the host, formation of inclusion bodies, target proteins appearing translationally, and complex purification procedures. The popular commercial systems provide supporting materials and reagents in kit to cone, express, and purify recombinant proteins with a fair amount of ease. These support systems are broadly classified as promoters; stabilizing and optimizing elements; RBSs; and transcriptional and translational termination sequences.

15.2.1 Promoters

Promoters are DNA sequences to which the endogenous bacterial RNA polymerase will bind to initiate transcription. The promoter has an important function in that it determines the polarity of the transcript by specifying which strand will be transcribed. More important, how tightly regulated a promoter/operator is will greatly affect the ability to express proteins. Most bacterial promoters used in expression vectors consist of two elements located (−35) and (−10) from the actual transcriptional start. These elements comprise the consensus sequences that are bound by a specific transcription factor and the RNA polymerase. One of the most commonly encountered promoters is the trc promoter.

DNA sequences that act in conjunction with promoters and bind repressor molecules regulate the induction of transcription. One of the most commonly used in *E. coli* is the lacO/*lacIq* repressor system. In this system, transcription is virtually shut off until the promoter is derepressed by the addition of IPTG. At this point, the promoter is freed (i.e., the repressor no longer physically blocks transcription) and transcription is turned on. Inducible elements provide the ability to keep expression of the target gene off, should it produce a product that might be toxic to the host strain. There are a number of different methods of regulation that are available in commercial expression systems. While most are capable of inducing tremendous levels of expression, even slightly leaky expression during culture expansion can limit final product yield.

15.2.2 Terminators

In prokaryotic systems, anti-termination elements are incorporated into vectors to stabilize the RNA polymerase on the DNA template. These elements help ensure optimal transcript elongation during message synthesis. Transcription terminators are used to signal the active RNA polymerase to release the DNA template and halt transcription of the newly transcribed RNA. These terminators are ordinarily positioned downstream of the multicloning site and act to prevent pausing, prevent premature termination, and limit read-through of transcription, which adversely affects plasmid replication. Use of transcription terminators such as rrnB T1 and T2 from *E. coli* 5S rRNA is especially important for use with strong promoters.

15.2.3 Ribosome Binding Sites

RBSs are small, open reading frames upstream of the coding sequence of interest engineered to encourage ribosomes to bind and translate the sequence of interest. An RBS (Shine–Dalgarno sequence) is required just upstream of the translational start to provide the context for efficient translation initiation. RBS sequences are engineered into vectors to enhance and stabilize ribosome binding. Often RBS elements may be *borrowed* from different sources or are the native RBSs for the fusion species. Frequently used RBS elements are obtained from either the *lacZ* gene or the gene 10 of the bacteriophage T7.

Several commercial systems are now available with more appearing on the scene regularly; what used to be a great deal of science and art has been practically reduced to a kit approach with remarkable consistency and proven results. Given below are some of these systems, the Novogen pET system remains one of the best systems that we have used:

Arabinose-regulated promoter (Invitrogen pBAD Vector): This system generates very low levels of uninduced expression through glucose-catabolite-dependent repression. The pBAD promoter is induced by arabinose. Adding arabinose into the medium in increasing concentrations induces transcription in a dose-dependent manner.

T7 expression systems (Novagen, Promega, Stratagene): The pET-based vectors utilize the T7 RNA polymerase-based expression vector of Moffat and Studier (1986) to achieve very high levels of protein expression. The power of the pET system is that the T7 RNA polymerase is specific for its own promoter, which is found only on the expression plasmid. During growth and culture expansion, the T7 promoter is under the tight control of the *lacIq* gene, repressing any expression that might adversely affect bacterial growth. When induced with IPTG, rather than directly inducing the T7 promoter 5′ to the target gene, a T7 RNA polymerase is expressed in host *E. coli*, allowing transcription from the T7 promoter. Transcription and translation can be accomplished in only a few hours, with the expressed protein often comprising the most abundant cellular component. It is important to know that some of these commercial systems are sold under intellectual property rights that may require royalty agreements. For example, the Invitrogen's pET system is licensed from Brookhaven Institute that has no fee when used for development in the laboratory, $5,000 if used to test products in humans and a royalty of 1% if the product derived from using the T7 pET system results in a commercial product used in humans in the United States. The licensing agreement is signed directly with Brookhaven and requires that the manufacturer carry a liability insurance.

Trc/Tac promoter systems (Clontech, Invitrogen, Kodak, Life Technologies, MBI Fermentas, New England BioLabs, Amersham Biotech, Promega): Trc promoters are IPTG-inducible hybrid promoters. The Trc promoter is a trp/lac fusion, where the (−35) position is derived from trp and the (−10) position is obtained from lacUV5 promoter elements. While extremely strong, some low-level expression of the recombinant protein may occur during growth.

P_L *promoters (Invitrogen pLEX and pTrxFus Vectors):* P_L-based systems place the protein of interest under the tight transcriptional control of the lambda cI repressor protein. The repressor protein must be engineered into the *E. coli* host or be incorporated into the vector itself. The repressor protein is placed under the control of an inducible promoter. Expression of the cI repressor binds to the operator of the P_L promoter to prevent transcription of the recombinant gene. Induction occurs with the addition of tryptophan, which prevents expression of the repressor, allowing transcription for the P_L promoter.

Lambda PR promoter (Amersham pRIT2T Vector): The PR promoter of the bacteriophage lambda provides for thermo-inducible expression of proteins when temperatures are shifted during growth from 37°C to 42°C. Induction is accomplished in 90 min.

Phage T5 promoter (Qiagen): The phage T5 promoter provides a strong recognition site for *E. coli* RNA polymerase and can direct the expression of targets to levels up to 50% of total cellular protein. The promoter is regulated by two lactose operator elements.

tetA promoter (Biometra pASK75 Vector): The tetA promoter is induced by the addition of anhydrotetracycline in concentrations that are not antibiotically effective. This promoter is not regulated by any endogenous cellular mechanisms and therefore is not influenced by catabolic repression.

15.2.4 Fusion Proteins and Tags

One-step purification of the recombinant protein by high-affinity binding can be accomplished in some situations using vectors engineered with DNA sequences encoding a specific peptide fused to the expressed protein. One of the most popular systems is the 6xHis system in which six histidine residues enable the tagged-recombinant protein to be purified by a nickel-chelating resin. Often, an endopeptidase recognition sequence is also engineered between the affinity tag and the protein of interest to allow subsequent removal of the leader sequence, peptide tag, or fusion sequences by enzymatic digestion.

Tags serve several function providing purification and stabilization of the expressed protein; fusion may act as tag with the generation of antibodies.

Calmodulin-binding peptide (CBP) tag (Stratagene pCAL Vectors): pCAL expression vectors contain a sequence encoding a CBP. The CBP tag allows the hybrid recombinant protein to bind to a calmodulin resin in the presence of low concentrations of calcium. Elution is accomplished in the presence of 2 mM EGTA and neutral pH. The conditions are milder than in other tag systems. The CAP tag is one of the smaller tags, encoding a 4 kDa tag. Smaller tags have potentially less impact on the protein of interest than larger tags.

Glutathione S-transferase (GST) tag (Amersham pGEX Vectors): Vectors containing the GST-fusion tag allow encoded proteins to be efficiently purified from bacterial lysates utilizing an affinity matrix containing glutathione. Elution of the purified protein is accomplished under mild, nondenaturing conditions. The GST fusion adds a 26 kDa tag to the recombinant protein, which can be removed when an endopeptidase cleavage site sequence is incorporated between the tag and the protein.

6xHIS tag (Invitrogen, Kodak, Life Technologies, New England BioLab, Pierce, Amersham [GE], Promega, Qiagen, Novagen): 6xHis-tagging vectors fuse a six-histidine peptide to the recombinant protein. This small addition rarely affects protein structure to a significant degree and therefore usually does not require removal following purification of the protein. The 6-His residues impart a remarkable affinity for matrices containing nickel. The fact that binding can occur under native as well as under denaturing conditions distinguishes this affinity purification method from the others. Recombinant proteins, frequently encountered in inclusion bodies in bacterial expression systems, can be solubilized under denaturing conditions using urea or guanidine hydrochloride. The solubilized 6xHis-tagged proteins can then be purified by binding to nickel ions on the matrix. The strong affinity of the 6xHis tag tolerates denaturing conditions that facilitate the removal of non-specific contaminants often associated with recombinant proteins expressed in bacteria. Elution is accomplished under mild conditions by either reducing the pH or adding imidazole as a competitor. With great advances taking place in the field of commercial kits and systems, the reader is referred to market leaders to obtain information on a system suitable for their use.

Dihydrofolate reductase (QIAGEN): Short peptide sequences from the murine dihydro-folate reductase (DHFR) are fused to target proteins to increase stability of the target protein, as well as enhance its antigenicity. Thioredoxin fusion sequences (Invitrogen, pTrxFUS and pThioHis Vectors, Novagen pET-32 Vectors): Designed to maximize the accumulation of fusion proteins in the soluble fraction, a number of additional advantages are imparted when recombinant proteins are fused with sequences encoding thioredoxin. Fusion with thioredoxin helps overcome insolubility encountered with some bacterial systems. Additionally, in *E. coli*, thio-redoxin accumulates in adhesion zones, which can be selectively released by rapid osmotic shock. The temperature stability of thioredoxin also allows temperatures as high as 80°C to be tolerated during purification. These features can be exploited to simplify purification of expressed fusion proteins. Finally, thioredoxin pos-sesses a unique active dithiol, which directs high-affinity binding to phenylarsine oxide, allowing rapid purification of expressed proteins.

Protein A (Amersham pEZZ 18 and pRIT2T): The ability of Protein A to bind to IgG immunoglobulins continues to be a workhorse in biotechnology. pEZZ 18 con-tains two synthetic Z domains of the *B* IgG binding domains of Protein A and pRIT2T contains the natural IgG binding domains of protein A. Fusion proteins are easily purified using IgG Sepharose resins. The two Z domains add a 14-kDa peptide to the recombinant protein.

Biotinylation (Promega PinPoint™ Vector): Biotinylation-based epitopes encode pep-tide sequences that become biotinylated in vivo during expression. Relying on the strong affinity of streptavidin for biotin, the biotinylated peptide acts as a purification tag for the fusion protein. Promega provides a unique monomeric avidin that allows elution of the fused proteins under mild non-denaturing conditions (5 mM biotin), not possible with native avidin.

Cellulose-binding domain (CBD) (Novagen, pET CBD Vectors): CBDs allow for the purification of expressed proteins with cellulose or chitin matrices. These materials are generally very low cost and quite stable and may be found in a variety of forms including beads, powders, fibers, membranes, filters, and sheets. Additionally, the CDD fusion often increases thermostability of the recombinant protein, which may be useful in purification strategies or in simply increasing the stability of expressed proteins.

Maltose-binding protein (MBP) (New England BioLabs, pMAL Vectors): The malE gene encodes the MBP, which has the capability to bind tightly to amylose. The MBP is separated from the desired expressed sequence by a polylinker encoding 10 asparagine residues. The linker is designed to assure the MBP can adequately bind amylose, which is immobilized on resin. In addition to aiding in expression and purification, the MBP fusion partner also helps keep proteins soluble and provides a choice of folding pathways.

S-Peptide tag (Novagen, selected pET Vectors): The 15 amino acid peptide (S-Tag) encoded by these vectors is a small, hydrophilic tag that has a strong affinity (Kd = 109 M) for a 104 amino acid protein (S-protein) derived from pancreatic ribonuclease A. When associated, the S-protein:S-peptide complex possesses ribonuclease activity (ribonuclease S). This strong association and activity have been exploited to measure S-Tag fusion protein (ribonuclease assay, which can detect as little as 5 fmol target) and can be used with reagents and resins for detection and purification purposes. For example, the S-protein itself can be directly conjugated to alkaline phosphatase or horseradish peroxidase and used as a probe to detect S-Tag fusion protein by Western blot.

Strep-tag (Biometra pASK75 Vector): A C-terminal fusion tag, the strep-tag encodes a 10 amino acid sequence, which binds streptavidin. Affinity of the tag for streptavidin allows purification of recombinant proteins under mild conditions. Along with affinity-purification applications, the strep-tag can be utilized to directly detect recombinant proteins by Western blot or ELISA assays using streptavidin-enzyme (alkaline phosphatase) conjugates.

Intein-mediated purification with affinity chitin-binding tag (New England BioLabs, pCYB Vectors/IMPACT System): This chimeric system produces a C-terminally tagged protein in which a small 5-kDa chitin-binding domain (ChBD) from *Bacillus circulans* is physically separated from the target protein by the protein splicing element derived from the *Saccharomyces cerevisiae* VMA gene 1. The splicing element, or intein, has been modified such that it undergoes a self-cleavage reaction at its N-terminus at low temperatures in the presence of thiols. The fusion protein is purified by passing extracts through a chitin column; the purified protein is then induced to undergo the intein-mediated self-cleavage on the column by overnight incubation at 4°C in the presence of dithiothreitol or β-mercaptoethanol. The target protein without additional residues is released while the chitin-binding fusion domain remains adhered to the resin.

immunoreactive epitopes (Invitrogen, Novagen, Kodak). While many vectors utilize fusion or epitope tags for multifunctional purposes, some vectors encode fragments that are essentially immunoreactive epitopes. Immunoreactive tags provide a rapid means of detecting tag-hybrid proteins with high specificity and affinity without needing to generate specific antisera to each protein of interest. The monoclonal anti-myc antibody detects recombinant proteins containing the myc epitope (GluGlnLysLeuIleSerGluGluAspLeuAsn). An alternative is the 11 amino acid epitope tag (GlnProGluLeuAlaProGluAspProGluAsp) derived from herpes simplex virus (HSV) glycoprotein D, which can be recognized by an anti-HSV monoclonal antibody.

Kinase sequences for in vitro labeling (Stratagene, Amersham): To enable rapid in vitro labeling of proteins with 32P, some vectors incorporate the recognition sequence for the catalytic subunit of cAMP-dependent protein kinase as a fusion epitope. The site encoding the sequence (ArgArgAlaSerVal) is usually located between a primary fusion sequence and the sequence for the gene of interest. Expressed proteins can be directly labeled using protein kinase and [gamma 32P]-ATP (Kaelin et al., 1992).

Protein A signal sequence (Amersham pEZZ18): The protein A signal sequence of this vector results in the secretion of the expressed protein into the aqueous culture.

ompT and ompA leader signal peptides (Biometra, New England BioLabs, Kodak): The ompT and ompA leader sequence directs secretion of proteins into the periplasmic space. This periplasmic localization can simplify recovery of expressed proteins since osmotic shock treatments can enrich for proteins localized within the periplasm.

malE signal sequence (New England BioLabs pMAL-p2): The normal malE signal sequence contains residues that direct the expressed fusion protein through the cytoplasmic membrane to the periplasm. This provides an alternate folding pathway that particularly helps in the formation of disulfide bonds.

T7 gene 10 leader peptide (Novagen, Stratagene, Promega, Invitrogen): An 11 amino acid leader peptide (MetAlaSerMetThrGlyGlyGlnGlnMetGly) derived from the T7 major capsid protein (gene 10) is incorporated into vectors to provide an ATG source for fused proteins. This leader peptide is often used in T7 expression systems. Antibodies generated against this epitope can be used to detect the production of expressed protein in Western or immunoprecipitation assays.

15.2.5 Fusion and Tagged Protein Cleavage Systems

Whereas the use of tagged or fusion proteins allows for rapid quantitation and purification of recombinant proteins, this requires an addition to the vector-derived epitope to provide a cleavage system. While some epitopes such as the 6XHis tag are small and may be inconsequential, others are significantly larger and may affect the downstream use of the recombinant protein. By incorporating site-specific protease cleavage sites between the epitope/fusion and the target protein, these sequences can be removed. One complication arises when the recombinant protein has proteolytic cleavage site within its own sequence making it difficult for the protease to recognize its target site intended. Using a protease to mediate cleavage eventually requires that the protease itself must be removed following the reaction, in order to obtain a truly purified recombinant protein. To address this issue, some manufacturers have incorporated novel methods of releasing the target protein from the fusion product while simultaneously including a strategy of immobilizing the protease on a resin through use of an engineered tag on a recombinant endopeptidase. The PreScission Protease from Amersham is a genetically engineered fusion protein consisting of the 3C protease of the human rhinovirus type 14 and glutathione S-tranferase. This protease can be used either following purification of the recombinant protein, or while the target protein is bound to glutathione Sepharose. Since the protease itself contains a GST tag, it remains bound to the Sepharose matrix allowing rapid purification of the target away from the protease. New England BioLabs has recently introduced a vector that relies on intein-mediated self-cleavage rather than proteolytic cleavage of the fusion. The intein sequence mediates self-cleavage between the tag epitope and the target sequence and liberates the target protein from the fusion species without the introduction of additional proteins. The affinity tag can remain immobilized, and purification of the target is relatively easy.

Some commonly encountered protease/cleavage sites are as follows:

- Thrombin (KeyValProArg/GlySer)
- Factor Xa Protease (IleGluGlyArg)
- Enterokinase (AspAspAspAspLys)
- Rtev (GluAsnLeuTyrPheGln/Gly): rTEV is a recombinant endopeptidase from the tobacco etch virus
- Intein-mediated self-cleavage (New England BioLabs)
- 3C Human rhinovirus protease (Amersham Biotech) (LeuGluValLeuPhe Gln/GlyPro)

Polylinkers or MCSs are synthetic DNA sequences encoding a series of restriction endonuclease recognition sites that are engineered for convenient cloning of DNA into a vector at a specific position. MCSs can range in size from two restriction sites and up. To accommodate reading frame differences with translational start sequences, many vectors are offered in an *A, B, C* format, meaning there is a single base shift between each vector, allowing easy cloning into each of the three reading frames. Additionally, some vectors are provided where the MCSs are in opposite orientations. For sequences where the aminoterminus has not been precisely defined, Kodak has developed a FLAG-Shift vector. These vectors contain a *shift* sequence that allows expression of an open reading frame without regard to the reading frame in which it was originally cloned. This shift is facilitated by ribosomal slippage caused by a run of A/Ts.

LIC vectors (ligation-independent cloning, Novagen, Stratagene) allow directional cloning of PCR products without restriction digestion or ligation reactions of the amplified products. LIC vectors rely on sequence complimentarity between the primer used for amplification and the ends of the vector. These overhangs, following treatment with T4 polymerase, allow specific and efficient annealing and subsequent transformation directly into bacteria. Primers for the overhang can also be engineered to accomplish additional tasks. Novagen, for example, uses primers that encode the recognition site for enterokinase. All vectors must contain a DNA sequence that directs binding of DNA polymerase and associated factors in order to maintain copies of the vector. Most vectors utilize elements from pBR322. Many vectors also provide an M13 origin of DNA replication (f1) allowing the production of single-stranded DNA for sequencing and mutagenesis.

15.2.6 Selection Pressure

All vectors contain sequences that provide a means to select only those cells containing a vector. As a selection pressure, an antibiotic is usually added to the medium. The following markers function by either conveying drug resistance on the host or enabling the host to compensate for the absence of an essential component in the media (auxotrophic markers):

Ampicillin: It interferes with a terminal reaction in bacterial cell wall synthesis. The resistance gene (bla) encoding beta-lactamase cleaves the beta-lactam ring of ampicillin. Ampicillin is rapidly degraded by the extracellular enzyme β-lactamase secreted by the plasmid-carrying cells. This can be a major problem decreasing yields significantly due to the outgrowing of plasmid-carrying cells by non-carrying ones. This problem has been addressed adding ampicillin during the fermentation or using carbenicillin, which is more stable but expensive.

Tetracycline: It prevents bacterial protein synthesis by binding to the 30S ribosomal subunit. The resistance gene (tet) specifies a protein that modifies the bacterial membrane and prevents transport of the antibiotic into the cell.

Kanamycin: It binds to the 70S ribosomes and causes misreading of messenger RNA. The resistant gene (Km) modifies the antibiotic and prevents interaction with the ribosome.

With the ever-increasing rate of discovering new genes comes the equal challenge of understanding how the products of these genes are used and regulated, when they appear, and how they interact within cells. While much attention has been given to high-throughput PCR and sequencing, numerous advancements have been made in lower profile areas such as developing tools to rapidly express and purify proteins.

15.2.7 Process Optimization

Commercial success of a bacterial cell production system depends on a large number of factors, from the cell density to type of media to the conditions of process; optimization remains a trial and error based through some basic principles that help us avoid obvious pitfalls.

15.2.7.1 Cell Density and Viability

As most proteins are intracellular accumulated in *E. coli*, productivity is proportional to the final cell density and the specific productivity, that is, the amount of product formed per unit cell mass per unit time. High cell densities require sufficient oxygen supply to avoid formation of acetate, lactate, or pyruvate when *E. coli* is grown under anaerobic or oxygen-limiting conditions (mixed acid fermentation). A further complication of *E. coli* growth on glucose under aerobic conditions is incomplete glucose oxidation resulting in accumulation of acetate, sometimes referred to as the bacterial *Crab tree* effect; therefore, excess glucose in the medium should be avoided.

Proteolysis is often a major problem especially when the microorganism is stressed, where a high proteolytic protein turnover can be expected. Variations between shake flasks and large-scale bioreactors have been observed challenging the scale up and limiting the value of down-scale studies.

Higher cell densities are also obtained when using *E. coli* by separating growth and production phases taking advantage of regulated promoters to achieve high cell densities in the first phase (promoter off) and high rate of target protein expression in the second phase (promoter on). Inducers such as 3,β-indolacrylic acid (IAA), isopropyl-β-D-thiogalactoside (IPTG), and lactose are used to turn the promoter on (trp and Lac promoters, respectively).

High cell density growth is inevitably faced with problems of oxygen supply, formation of toxic products, high carbon dioxide, and heat generation; one way to resolve this would be to switch to modes other than batch mode since merely increasing the concentration of nutrients is not advised. For example, the maximum concentration of glucose in media should not exceed 50 g/L; ammonia by 3 g/L, iron(II) by 1.15 g/L; magnesium by 8.7 g/L; manganese by 68 mg/L; phosphate by 10 g/L; zinc by 0.038 g/L; molybdenum by 0.8 g/L; boron by 44 mg/L; and cobalt by 0.5 mg/L. Even in fed-batch mode and in some situations perfusion mode, the longevity of continuous culturing causes accumulation of non-producing variants of the microbial cells resulting in decreasing productivity.

Cell density is calculated from OD_{470} on the basis of a calibration curve or by laser turbidimetry and expressed as unit g/L. The viscosity of culture broth increases sharply when the cell concentration exceeds 200 g/L, which is regarded as the maximum attainable cell density of *E. coli*. The cell dry weight is calculated from OD_{470} or OD_{500} on the basis of a calibration curve or by centrifugation and weight of the pellet. Viable cells can be identified by spread out of the cell suspension on nutrient agar plates with or without kanamycin or like selection markers. Cell lysis can be measured from the DNA content in the supernatant following centrifugation. Plasmid instability influences the productivity. Instability may result from defective partitioning during cell division (loss) or undesired modifications (insertion, deletion, rearrangement of DNA). Most plasmids of industrial interest are lost at frequencies of 10^{-2} to 10^{-5} per cell generation. The plasmid-free cells will have a higher specific growth rate and they will, over time, reach a higher concentration. Plasmid instability is influenced by plasmid construction, plasmid copy number, cultivation conditions, and the bioreactor configuration. The stability can be estimated by replica plating to ampicillin, kanamycin or like selection marker agar plates. The method sensitivity is 1%. The number of plasmid molecules per genome in a single cell. Plasmid copy number (PCN) is a criterion for the strength of the expression system on the DNA level. The production of target protein depends on the PCN. The PCN is calculated from measurement of the total DNA content and the plasmid DNA content of the biomass by quantitative DNA assays (e.g., agarose slab gel electrophoresis, capillary electrophoresis) after cell disintegration.

15.2.7.2 Media
The common media include

Complex systems containing chemically undefined nutrients such as yeast extract, peptone, tryptone, and casamino acids; it typically comprises tryptone, yeast extract, mineral salts (e.g., sodium choride, potassiumhydrogen phosphate, magnesium sulfate), glucose, and an antibiotic (e.g., kanamycin, ampicillin, chloramphenicol).

Defined media comprising solely defined nutrients, it typically comprises mineral salts including ammonium sulfate, trace elements, foam controlling agents, glucose, and eventually additional components such as thiamine and ampicillin.

Semi-complex media which are a combination of the above two types.

15.2.7.3 Control Parameters

The in process control parameters have well-defined lower and upper parameter limits and measurement of a variety of output parameters (responses):

pH is typically set at 6.9; repeated sterilization of probe may delay response time.

Dissolved oxygen must exceed 20%; because of low solubility in media (approx 7.6 mg/L), the oxygen transfer rate is a limiting factor when scaling up bacterial cultures. The dissolved oxygen is measured by a polarographic oxygen electrode.

Temperature lowering to 26°C–30°C reduces nutrient uptake and growth rate as well as inclusion bodies but also reduces toxic by-product formation. Heat generation during culture in large-scale fermenters requires cooling.

Agitation rate is adjusted to keep dissolved oxygen above critical value; generally, 300–1,000 rpm are maintained.

Aeration rate of 1 vvm at 30–70 kPa proves optimal.

Ammonia feed is maintained to keep ammonium concentrations below 170 mM; ammonia is determined by Kjeldahl analysis.

Glucose feed is adjusted not exceed optimal glucose levels using feedback mechanisms. The levels of glucose are measured by HPLC, RI, or commercial kits.

Acetate forms in complex and defined media when the specific growth rate exceeds 0.2 and 0.35/h, respectively; $pCO_2 > 0.3$ atm decreases growth rate and stimulates acetate formation, which is reduced by using glycerol as a carbon source instead of glucose and by using the exponential feeding method. A concentration of less than 20 mM of acetate maintains an exponential growth. Acetate concentration is monitored by gas chromatography or with an acetate kit.

Foam level should be minimized by adding anti-foam agents.

By-products are routinely monitored; ethanol detected by gas chromatography (flame ionization detector) or ethanol sensor; propionate and lactate detected by gas chromatography (flame ionization detector); amino acids detected by HPLC and the product by specific assay (see BP, EP, or USP for assay methods).

15.2.8 Downstream Processing

The downstream process comprises harvest, capture, in vitro refolding, intermediary purification, enzymatic cleavage, and polishing after the step of generating starting material from fermentation and extraction. The most commonly used techniques used in downstream processing include chromatography, filtration, microfiltration, ultrafiltration, active filtration, centrifugation, precipitation, and crystallization. The downstream process is designed for effective and efficient removal of cell debris, host cell proteins, nucleic acids, and endotoxins that arise from the disruption of the cells. It is also important to remove the closely related target protein derivates such as cleaved forms, deamidated forms, oxidized forms, and scrambled forms as much as possible. As a result of these considerations, a minimum of three different chromatographic steps are generally required. In most instances, the last step would be size exclusion chromatography (and thus four steps). Virus removal is required (in instances where animal-derived raw materials are used), this would add an additional step to the total processing scheme.

The biogeneric manufacturing client should make a thorough search of the intellectual property infringement in using any technique since a large number of patents often protect the innovator's molecules (see Chapter 17).

15.2.8.1 Harvest

Harvesting step generally uses techniques like centrifugation, filtration, microfiltration, or ultrafiltration. The purpose of the harvest step is to isolate the inclusion bodies from cell culture impurities such as cell debris and to condition the sample for the following chromatographic capture step. Generally, centrifugation separates the cells from media; the cells are washed and their disruption is a mechanical (e.g., french press), chemical (e.g., urea and cysteine), or enzymatic nature (e.g., lysozyme) process to release host cell proteins (and therefore also proteolytic enzymes) to the medium. If the cells are exposed directly to the extraction buffer, cell debris is removed by centrifugation. It is recommended to use urea (7–8 M) as the denaturing agent and cysteine (50–100 mM, of non-animal origin) as the reducing agent. Note that urea solution must be free of cyanate to prevent carbamylation of primary amino groups (for further information see the carbamylation document). Ethylenediaminetetraacetic acid (EDTA) is often added to the extraction buffer in 1–2 mM concentrations in order to inhibit metalloproteases. The typical result of the harvest and extraction procedure is a viscous sample at 4C with high levels of target protein, host cell proteins, DNA, and endotoxins in a 7–8 M urea, 50–100 mM cysteine, 1–2 mM EDTA buffer at pH 7.5–9.0. The use of expanded bed adsorption technique recovers proteins directly from preparations of broken cells, saving one or several centrifugation and/or filtration steps. Since during cell lysis and extraction, the recombinant product is exposed to a variety of proteolytic enzymes, enzyme inhibitors should not be used at this stage. The enzymatic activity can be reduced by using protease negative mutant hosts, low temperatures, and fast procedures. Inevitably, the presence of denaturing agents leads to the formation of minor amounts of cleaved products, such as split and truncated forms

15.2.8.2 Capture

Capture step follows the harvesting and generally uses chromatographic techniques like affinity chromatography (AC), ion exchange chromatography (IEC), IMAC; expanded bed; packed-bed. The purpose of the capture step is to remove cell culture and process-related impurities and to prepare for in vitro folding. The nature of the capture step depends on the protein construct expressed. For example, histidine tags are exceptional, binding to metal chelating matrices under denaturing conditions. AC can be used for fusion proteins if in vitro refolding has been carried out prior to the capture step. For non-tagged proteins with short N-terminal extensions IEC can be used under denaturing conditions provided urea is used as denaturant. The particle size of media should be in the range of 100–300 nm. It may be an advantage to use expanded bed technology. The typical result of the capture procedure is a purified sample comprising the target protein (1–5 mg/mL) and low to medium levels of impurities in 7–8 M urea, 50–100 mM cysteine, 1–2 mM EDTA buffer at pH 7.5–9.0.

15.2.8.3 In Vitro Refolding

As mentioned above, inclusion bodies do not produce target protein in its natural form requiring refolding that is often chaotrope mediated, co-solvent assisted, requires dilution, desalting, use of hollow fiber, size exclusion chromatography (SEC), or immobilized protein. In some instance, prior to refolding of the proteins, some purification can be made by means of dilution, SEC, dialysis or immobilization techniques ahead of addition of refolding buffer. The purpose of the in vitro folding step is to bring the denatured target protein into its native biological active form. From a regulatory point, it is important to keep this procedure as a separate unit operation as random in vitro refolding is very difficult to control and impossible to document. Note that whereas the inclusion bodies from different sub-batches can be pooled, refolding step requires use of single container and uniform conditions. The in vitro refolding comprises transfer from the initial denaturation buffer (e.g., in 7–8 M urea, 50–100 mM cysteine, 1–2 mM EDTA buffer at pH 7.5–9.0) by means of dilution, desalting, dialysis, size exclusion chromatography or immobilization technologies to the renaturation buffer (e.g., 1–5 mM cysteine, 1–2 mM EDTA, co-solvent, buffer pH 7–9.5), which is also the composition of the sample for intermediary purification. The sample should be directly taken to intermediate purification column avoiding excessive handling to prevent aggregation of the newly folded target protein.

The refolding is always carried out at low protein concentration (0.1–0.5 mg/mL) to prevent protein aggregation; as a result, the volume of buffer used at this stage is large. Additionally, this may require use of co-solvents added to the folding buffer, typically salts, sugars, detergents, sulfobetaines, or short chain alcohols. The most difficult refolding, formation of disulfide bonds between cysteine residues, is managed by adjusting the redox potential, pH, temperature, conductivity, and protein concentration. Whereas refolding is often spontaneous when the environment is more oxidizing, a validated system is needed to reduce the losses of proteins at this stage. It is not uncommon to lose 50% of protein at this stage and therefore to make a commercial yield possible, this step must be most carefully monitored.

15.2.8.4 Enzymatic Cleavage

The purpose of the cleavage procedure is to remove the N-terminal extension. The enzyme used to remove the tag must be of non-animal origin. The enzyme may be immobilized in order to reduce its amount in the final product. If immobilized folding is being used, the cleavage enzyme may be added after refolding thus combining the two operations. A specific immobilized refolding method using the FXa cleavage site has been described and used in small scale. The folded protein is eluted from the column by means of FXa leaving the tag immobilized to the column. The composition of the sample for polishing depends on the cleavage procedure used. Typical tags are fusion proteins or repeated histidine sequences. If the second amino acid (N-terminally) is proline, this amino acid will act as a stop codon for specific di-amino acid exopeptidases and the tag can be removed without the enzymatic cleavage site insert. There are several types of cleavage sites, for example, where there is an enzymatic cleavage site insert between a fusion protein or tag and the mature protein, and thus, the cleavage is performed with an endopeptidase, such as Factor Xa (FXa), which recognizes the sequence -Ile-Glu-Gly-Arg- resulting in a correct N-terminal sequence of the mature protein as FXa cleaves after the arginine residue. More than 10 eukaryotic proteins have been expressed by this method. Another construct type makes use of the exopeptidase, dipeptidyl amino peptidase I (DPPI), which cleaves every second peptide bond from the N-terminal end of the molecule except for the amino acid residues Glu or Pro acting as terminators for proteolytic degradation. The Glu stop terminator is used in constructs where the second amino acid residue is not proline. The N-terminal extension, be it a fusion protein, a His-tag or a few selected amino acids, must be removed using specific bioprocess grade enzymes of recombinant origin. Well-characterized bioprocess enzymes for this purpose are rare (an exception is DPPI), limiting the number of protein constructs to be used in biopharmaceutical processes.

15.2.8.5 Intermediary Purification

This step utilized techniques like IEC, IMAC, HAC, hydrophobic interaction chromatography (HIC), or packed-bed to remove cell culture and process-derived impurities and to prepare the sample for polishing. Anion exchange, cation exchange, or hydroxyapatite chromatography will apply for the purification step following in vitro folding. Chromatography based on hydrophobic interaction should be avoided, as the renatured protein tends to aggregate during such procedures. The particle size of media should be in the range of 50–120 nm. An important part of the process design is to assure a smooth transfer between unit operations making use of the ability of ion exchangers to bind proteins at low salt concentrations and hydrophobic interaction media to bind proteins at high salt concentrations. However, in certain cases buffer exchange or sample concentration is required. It is recommended to use chromatographic desalting as the buffer exchange principle (no shear forces) and ultrafiltration (or precipitation) for sample concentration. Note that variations in the composition of eluted samples (e.g., protein concentration, conductivity, pH) may influence the proceeding sample application and thus interfere with process robustness.

15.2.8.6 Polishing

This step typically used techniques like reversed phase chromatography (RPC), IEC, or packed-bed. This is the most refined step in purification to remove host cell, process and product related impurities. Powerful chromatographic methods (high-performance reverse phased chromatography [HP-RPC] or high-performance ion exchange chromatography [HP-IEC]) should be used to separate the protein from its derivatives (enzymatic cleaved forms, des-amido forms, oxidized forms, scrambled forms, etc.). To obtain optimal resolution, the particle size of media should be in the range of 15–60 nm.

15.2.8.7 Concentration

In most instances, the eluant from the polishing step would provide the final product in a concentrated form. However, in some instances, reduction of volume may be required. This can be accomplished by ultrafiltration (see comments under intermediate purification relating to buffer exchange).

15.2.8.8 Finishing

This is generally the final step using SEC, desalting, or packed-bed. SEC (packed-bed) removes di- and polymer forms and small molecules (e.g., endotoxins, co-solvents, and leachables) and prepares the drug substance for formulation into drug product. Whereas the host cell proteins are removed all along wherein DNA is removed by means of anion exchange or hydroxyapatite chromatography (DNA binds strongly to both types), endo-toxins are removed by binding to anion exchange matrices, polymyxin, Sepharose or histamine-Sepharose; additionally, endotoxins are removed by ultrafiltration, gel filtration, or phase separation with the detergent Triton X114, the final step of finishing assure that the drug substance is ready to be used in the drug product formulation.

15.3 MAMMALIAN CELLS MANUFACTURING SYSTEMS

The main disadvantage in the *de novo* synthesis of recombinant eukaryotic proteins in a prokaryotic system is the improper protein folding and assembly, and the lack of post-translational modification, principally glycosylation and phosphorylation. This leads to utilization of eukaryotic cells wherein viruses are used as vectors. Eukaryotic expression systems fall into four distinct classes based upon host type: yeast, drosophila, insect (nondrosophila), and mammalian. This chapter highlights the use of mammalian eukaryotic cells.

15.3.1 Genetically Modified Cell Lines

Mammalian cell culture systems offer the distinct advantages of extracellular expression in native form including complex posttranslational-modified proteins; the expression vectors are commercially available with large-scale production batches (2 to 5,000 L) and the track record for FDA and other regulatory body approvals has been very good. On the negative side, mammalian cells take longer time (4–6 months) to develop from introduction of gene to protein production; they grow slowly with density not exceeding beyond 100 million cells/mL; the culture media used are expensive, provide low yields (generally less than 100 mg/L; recently, systems have begun to yield gram quantities per liter), and may contain bovine products and allergens; the ICH requirements for characterization are elaborate and extensive as there is a possibility of carrying virus contamination; the process is subject to sheer stress and thus difficult to use as suspension culture or even in wave bioreactors; cell lines are also sensitive to osmolarity changes and finally there are safety issues in the management of cell lines.

The most popular cell lines used include Chinese hamster ovary (CHO), human cervix (HeLa), African green monkey kidney (COS), baby hamster kidney (BHK) cells, and hybridomas. Well-characterized cell lines can be obtained from the American Type Culture Collection (ATCC) and the European Collection of Cell Cultures (ECACC). These continuous cell lines have the potential of an infinite life span and can usually be culti-vated as perfusion cultures. A cell bank system comprising the master cell bank (MCB) and the working cell bank (WCB) provides the means for production of well-characterized and standardized cells.

The establishment of cell banks for newly developed cell lines is critical to the successful development of many biological products. The cell bank system assures that the cell line is preserved, its integrity is maintained, and a sufficient supply is readily available. A well-characterized cell bank is the consistent source of production cells throughout the life of the product. Worldwide regulatory authorities require screening cell cultures for the presence of contaminating agents by testing for adventitious viral or microbial agents using both in vivo and in vitro methodologies. The cGMP compliant preparation of MCBs and MWCBs is performed in a class 100 environment with in-phase testing for mycoplasma and sterility. Cell banks are stored in validated and continuously monitored liquid nitrogen dewars.

Given below are suggested for testing MCBs and end of production cells:

Microbial contamination: Sterility (USP 24) determines the presence of aerobic and anaerobic bacteria and fungi, mycoplasma (1993 PTC CBER/FDA).

Cell line authenticity: Karyology and isoenzyme analysis determines the species of origin of the cell line.

Transmission electron microscopy (TEM): TEM determines cellular morphology, presence of microbial contaminants, and enumeration of retroviral and retrovirus-like particles.

Endogenous retroviruses: Reverse transcriptase assays and retroviral infectivity assays detect the presence of retroviruses.

In vitro and in vivo adventitious virus testing.

Mouse, rat & hamster antibody production assays (MAP, RAP, & HAP): They detect species-specific viruses in rodent cell lines.

Bovine and porcine virus assays (9 CFR).

Human viruses: HIV-I & HIV-II, HTLV-I & HTLV-II, HAV, HBV, HCV, CMV, EBV, HSV-2, HHV-6, AAV-2, and B-19.

Primate viruses: SIV, STLV, foamy agent, and SMRV.

The following tests are required for the WCBs:

Microbial contamination: Sterility (USP 24) determines the presence of aerobic and anaerobic bacteria and fungi, mycoplasma (1993 PTC CBER/FDA).

In vitro adventitious virus testing.

Eukaryotic expression vectors are of two basic types: virion or virion–plasmid hybrids. Virion-type vectors are most commonly used for the delivery of foreign genes, or a replacement for a defective host gene, into mammalian cell hosts. The virion–plasmid hybrid vectors are used to facilitate the overexpression of protein in native form. Additionally, the availability of authentic pure protein has hastened the development of structure-dependent epitope-specific antibodies to native proteins, the crystallization and subsequent X-ray/NMR analysis of proteins in their native, correctly folded, posttranslationally modified state, the characterization of gene products for genes whose phenotype may or may not be known, and the isolation of proteins whose native form is in such low abundance that they are very difficult to purify from the original natural organism or tissue. The main features of eukaryotic expression vectors include various sequence elements that explicitly define the level of expression, the transcriptional start and stop points, postprocessing (transcript splicing, poly-adenylation, etc.) transport, selectable markers, and in some cases, a peptide tag to facil itate isolation and purification of the gene product. The earliest expression vectors, pSV2, is a composite of sequence elements from the papovavirus, Simian virus 40 and the prokaryotic cloning vector, pBR322. SV40 sequence provided transcriptional enhancers, promoter (early region), splicing signal (small t-antigen gene), and the polyadenylation signal element, and pBR322 provided the origin of replication (ori) element. The presence of a selectable marker, pBR322 AmpR gene, completes this model eukaryotic expression vector. Practically, all modern eukaryotic expression vectors possess one or more of these elements. Other viruses used include cytomegalovirus (CMV), murine sarcoma virus (MSV), Rous sarcoma virus (RSV), mouse mammary tumor virus (MMTV), and Semliki forest virus (SFV).

Generally, recombinant proteins are expressed in a constitutive manner in most eukaryotic expression systems and frequently with inducible promoters heat shock protein, metallothionien, and human and mouse growth hormone, MMTV-LTR, and inducible enhancer elements ecdysone, muristerone A, and tetracycline/doxycycline.

Two principal strategies have been employed to increase cell productivity: gene regulation and gene amplification. Gene regulation aims to increase the number of times a single gene is transcribed and then translated into product. Gene amplification aims to increase the number of genes that are available for transcription to produce the product (e.g., use of BPV virus, use of DNA amplifying drugs such as methotrexate).

Commercial systems that incorporate the entire gene sequences to support the expression of desired proteins are available from Clontech, Invitrogen, Novagen, Life Technologies, Promega, Pharmacia Biotech (GE), Strategene, Quantum Biotech, and many more. Selectable markers generally are either recessive or dominant; the recessive markers are usually genes that encode products that are not produced in the host cells (cells that lack the *marker* product or function). Marker genes for thymidine kinase (TK), dihydrofolate reductase DHFR, adenine phosphoribosyl transferase (APRT), and hypoxanthine-guanine phosphoribosyl transferase (HGPRT) are in this category. Dominant markers include genes that encode products that confer resistance to growth-suppressing compounds (antibiotics, drugs) and/or permit growth of the host cells in metabolically restrictive environments. Commonly used markers within this category include a mutant DHFR gene that confers resistance to methotrexate; the gpt gene for xanthine-guanine phosphoribosyl transferase, which permits host cell growth in mycophenolic acid/xanthine containing media; and the neo gene for aminoglycoside 3'-phosphotransferase, which can confer resistance to G418, gentamycin, kanamycin, and neomycin. Practically, all eukaryotic expression vectors used today possess at least one marker from either or both of these categories, although dominant markers are the most common.

Host-range specificity for virion vectors is determined primarily by the presence of recognizable host cell surface receptors, whereas for virion–plasmid hybrid vectors, the determinant is the degree to which the host's cellular machinery recognizes the transcriptional control signals of the hybrid vector. Transcriptional enhancers appear to be the primary determinants of cell-type specificity.

After the target gene has been engineered into the appropriate cloning vector, the vector will need to be introduced into the host cell. Given the infectious nature of the viruses from which most eukaryotic expression vectors are derived, it would seem that the introduction of the vector into the host would be rather straightforward. Unfortunately, this process can be complicated.

The introduction of the vector into mammalian cells can be effected by microinjection, electroporation, and calcium phosphate-, DEAE-dextran-, polybrene-, DMSO-, or cationic lipid-mediated transfection. Although the method of choice usually depends on the cell type and cloning application, cationic lipids or liposome-mediated transfection protocols generally yield the highest and most consistent transfection efficiencies in mammalian cell systems. Thus, many corporate suppliers of expression systems recommend a lipid-based transfection protocol, with many providing proprietary liposome reagents (e.g., Clonetech's Clonfectin Transfection Reagent, Novogen's GeneJuice, Invitrogen's PerFect Transfection Kit, Promega's Transfectin and Tfx-50 reagents, or Life Technologies Lipofectin Reagent).

15.3.2 Monoclonal Antibodies Production

Monoclonal antibodies are expressed in mammalian cells and also in mouse ascites. This section refers to special considerations involved in the production of monoclonal antibodies using mammalian cells. The typical expression level of the target protein is from 50 to 1,000 mg/L. The protein purification strategy takes into consideration the poor stability at pH below 4.5 and irreversible structural changes that may result in loss of immunoactivity. This consideration is different from the manufacturing of other classes of therapeutic proteins where the goal is keep the protein as non-immunogenic as possible through structural modifications. IgM tends to precipitate at low conductivity where the protein is in its pentameric form. Generally, IgMs are less stable than IgGs. Most IgGs are stable and soluble at medium to high pH and low conductivity, a condition often used in application samples for chromatographic procedures. However, some mAbs (up to 20% of IgMs) are cryoglobulins with reduced solubility below 37°C. mAbs being highly basic, form stable ionic complexes with polyvalent anions (phosphate, citrate, sulfate, borate). The complexes easily aggregate. mAbs also form complexes with nucleic acids; the reaction can be reversed in presence of 0.3–1.0 M NaCl. mAbs strongly bind to divalent metal ions; the resulting change in the net charge of the molecule leads to destabilization. Table 15.1 lists the principles used to remove adventitious agents in the manufacturing of human monoclonal antibodies. Many of these principles apply to removal of adventitious agents in general as well.

15.3.3 Upstream Process Optimization

Commercial-scale manufacturing is carried out in closed reactors with no or limited supply of medium (batch or rarely fed-batch mode) or in bioreactors allowing media throughput with cell retention (perfusion systems). Immobilized cells can be utilized in both modes resulting in cell densities from 10^6 cells/mL (suspension cultures) to 10^8 cells/mL (immobilized cells). The productivity of batch cultures is often relatively high (up to 2 g/L for antibodies), but product stability, toxicity and bioreactor volume reduction make perfusion bioreactors fairly competitive. The total process yield following downstream processing may be better using the perfusion mode (less purification problems due to higher quality of the starting material), despite the slightly lower productivity.

519

Table 15.1 Removal of Adventitious Agents

Principle	Endotoxins	Nucleic Acids	Viruses	Note
Anion exchange	++	+++	+++	Strongly basic IgGs and IgMs form stable complexes with DNA, especially at low conductivity reducing clearance.
Cation exchange	+	+++	++	Nucleic acids do not bind to cation exchangers.
HIC	+	+++	++	Nucleic acids do not bind to HIC media. Antibody–nucleic acid complexes are dissociated at high salt concentrations. Endotoxins may form micelles or higher secondary structures in aqueous solutions, especially at high salt concentrations and thus get excluded from the matrix.
Hydroxyapatite	+	+	+	Nucleic acid clearance is variable in phosphate gradients.
IMAC	++	++	+++	Assuming similar purification properties as for Protein A.
Protein A	++	++	+++	Complexes between monoclonal antibodies and nucleic acids are dissociated at high salt concentrations tolerated in the Protein A application.
Size exclusion	+	+	+	Nucleic acids form complexes with monoclonal antibodies at low conductivity resulting in a reduced clearance factor. The endotoxin clearance factor is less for IgM.

There are two types of media used, one as growth media to support multiplication of cells and production media to maintain cells in the most productive phase. The culture media used for establishing MCBs still uses serum; but the fact that MCB is extensively characterized, the use of serum is justified. However, the rest of the media used should be free of adventitious agents (e.g., viruses, prions), which restricts use of fetal calf serum, peptones of animal origin, and porcine trypsin. Several commercial supplier these types of media and the claims made regarding their suitability should be evaluated vis-à-vis the process requirements. The serum-free media consist of salts, vitamins, amino acids, and carbohydrates supplemented with specific growth and attachment factors such as insulin, IGF-1, transferrin, epidermal growth factor, somatostatin, fibronectin, and collagen. In addition cells often need steroid-type hormones such as dexamethasone, testosterone, progesterone, and hydrocortisone and lipid-based factors including phospholipids, cholesterol, and sphingomyelin. Protein additives (e.g., albumin, transferrin, growth factors, peptones) are often of recombinant or plant origin. Albumin, which is the most important protein of all animal sera, is included in many serum free media. It exhibits a number of functions (transport, detoxification, buffering, mechanical protection against sheer forces). However, the growth stimulatory effect seems to be associated with a factor not present in the recombinant form indicating that recombinant albumin can only partially replace the natural source. Transferrin, which transports Fe-ions to the cells, is used in almost any serum free medium or is replaced with iron-complexes (e.g., ferri-sulfate, iminodiacetic acid complexes, ferri-sulfate-glycine-glycine-complexes, ferri-citrate, ferri-tropolone, phosphate compounds). Peptones are often produced from Soya by enzymatic degradation. Typical concentrations of additives are 5 mg/L of insulin, 5–35 mg/L of transferring, 20 μM of ethanolamine, and 5 μg of selenium. Sometimes, sodium carboxymethyl cellulose (0.1%) is added to prevent mechanical damage to cells. Pluronic F68 (0.1%) is used to reduce foaming and to protect cells from bubble sheer forces in sparged cultures.

Cell detachment has been achieved by the use of trypsin or trypsin/EDTA derived from porcine or bovine pancreas. Serum-free media are devoid of the anti-trypsin activity of serum and trypsin has been sought replaced by dispase I/II, papain or pronase or by use of thermo-responsive polymer surfaces.

N-linked glycosylation is a posttranslational modification commonly performed on proteins by eukaryotic cells and it can significantly alter the efficacy of a human therapeutic protein. The use of mammalian cells, such as CHO cells, for the commercial production of recombinant human proteins is often attributed to their ability to impart desired glycosylation features on proteins. An essential step in N-linked glycosylation is the transfer of oligosaccharide from a lipid in the endoplasmic reticulum membrane to an asparagine residue within a specific amino acid consensus sequence on a nascent polypeptide. In cultured cells, this reaction does not occur at every identical potential glycosylation site on different molecules of the same protein. The resulting variation in the extent of glycosylation for a given protein is known as site occupancy heterogeneity. Although current regulatory practice permits product heterogeneity, demonstration of specific and reproducible glycosylation is required. Hence heterogeneity in protein glycosylation presents special challenges to the development and production of a candidate therapeutic with consistent properties. In view of the inevitable occurrence and significance of glycosylation heterogeneity in protein therapeutics derived from mammalian cells, much research has been directed toward understanding factors that influence glycosylation heterogeneity during a bioprocess. When using CHO cells, there occurs a gradual decline in glycosylation site occupancy over the course of batch and fed-batch cultures of recombinant CHO cells: the proportion of fully glycosylated molecule can decrease by 9%–25% during the exponential growth phase]. This deterioration in glycosylation does not arise from extracellular degradation of product, nor could it be overcome by supplementation of the cultures with extra nutrients, such as

521

nucleotide sugars, glucose, and glutamine. Certain lipid supplements can minimize the glycosylation changes; since lipid-linked oligosaccharides (LLOs) are the oligosaccharide donors in N-linked glycosylation, their availability may be a key regulatory mechanism for controlling the extent of protein glycosylation. Inadequate formation or excessive degradation of LLOs can result in LLO shortages and consequently limit cellular glycosylation capacity. Under subsaturating LLO levels, a gradual decrease in the intracellular pool of LLOs would lead to a corresponding decrease in protein glycosylation. The CHO cells glycosylate their proteins to a gradually increasing extent as culture progresses, until the onset of massive cell death (15%–25%). The glycosylation site occupancy of different proteins may undergo distinct changes over the length of culture even though the net glycosylation efficiency in CHO cells improves with cultivation time. The glycosylation pattern of each individual glycoprotein product needs to be tracked over the course of culture because different proteins may exhibit different glycosylation variations with time, even when the same culture method is used.

Process parameters of importance in optimizing mammalian cell yields include:

pH, which is optimal at 6.8 to 7.2; lower pH inhibits growth; since CO_2 is generated, control of pH throughout fermentation may be needed due to formation of lactic acid. pH must be controlled to compensate lactic acid formation by adjusting supply of CO_2. The problems associated with deterioration of pH measuring devices as described in bacterial cell culture applies here as well

Redox potential optimal value is +75 mV, which equals a pO_2 of 8%–10%, which is approximately 50% of air saturation. The redox potential depends on the concentration of reducing and oxidizing agents, the temperature and the pH of the solution. The redox potential falls under logarithmic growth and is at its lowest 24 h before the onset of stationary phase

Dissolved oxygen should be in the range of 0.06–0.3 µmol oxygen/10^6 cells/h. As oxygen solubility in aqueous solutions is very low (7.6 µg/mL) the oxygen transfer rate (OTR) is a main limiting factor when scaling up cell cultures

Temperature The optimal temperature range is from 33°C to 38°C. The relative low level of metabolic activity makes it easier to control temperature in animal cell bioreactors

Osmolality in culture medium used with lepidoteran cell lines is 345–380 mOsm/kg

Agitation rate ranging from 50 to 200 rpm are common but need optimization depending on the size of equipment

Ammonia production rate (mmol/10^6 cells/h) is an indicator of metabolic rate and should be continuously measured and kept under control. The specific ammonia production rate (mmol/10^6 cells/h) is an indicator of metabolic rate. Analysis of ammonia can be performed using a BioProfile 100 analyzer or similar instrument. Ammonia may also be determined using an enzyme based assay kit

Glucose levels should be analyzed to monitor glucose utilization (mmol/10^6 cells/h) is an indicator of metabolic rate

Glutamine, an essential amino acid for cell growth, should not be used as an energy source. The metabolic product, ammonia, which is toxic to the cells, should be controlled. The glutamine concentration should be kept in the range of 2–8 mM

Lactate is formed by conversion of glucose—a balance between glycolysis and oxidation of glucose is maintained

PCO_2 is used to adjust the CO_2 flow to regulate the pH of the cell culture, and the flow is maintained only as long as the pH is above the set point. In late stage cultures, the CO_2-HCO_3 buffer system is no longer sufficient to maintain pH and sodium hydrogen carbonate or NaOH is used instead

Foam level is controlled by addition of anti-foam agents

Growth rates are measured in terms of cell density (using a hematocytometer); cell viability is tested using trypan blue, erythrosine staining, or electronic counting (e.g., Coulter counter); and specific production rates are monitored using a cell-hour approach which expresses the relationship between protein productivity and cell population dynamics. LDH activity reflects the extent of cell lyses, since LDH is not secreted by mammalian cells. The concentration of the reduced form of nicotinamide adenine dinucleotide or its phosphorylated form correlates with cell mass during the lag phase and exponential growth phase and provides information of the physiological state of the culture. The reduced form fluoresce at 460 nm when irradiated with light at 340 nm, while the oxidized form do not fluoresce. Various amino acids can be analyzed by HP-RPC after derivatization with o-pthalaldehyde, 3-mercaptopropionic acid, and 9-fluorenylmethylchloroformate using a fluorescence detector. Glutamine can be analyzed using a BioProfile 100 analyzer or similar instrument.

Adventitious agents are tested at the end of the cell culture in the unprocessed bulk and where multiple harvest pools are prepared at different times, the culture is tested at the time of the collection of each pool. The test program should include test for bacteria, fungi, mycoplasma and viruses. Test for adventitious viruses in continuous cell line cultures used for expression of recombinant proteins should include inoculation onto monolayer cultures of the same species and tissue type as that used for production, of human diploid cell line, of another cell line from a different species. If appropriate, a PCR test or another suitable method may be used. When cells are readily accessible (e.g., hollow fiber), the unprocessed bulk would constitute harvest from the fermenter.

15.3.4 Downstream Process Optimization

Since the target protein is typically expressed directly to the medium, the typical procedures of harvest capture, intermediary purification and polishing are used, in addition to viral clearance steps where required (when used, it is advisable to clear virus as early as possible despite the difficulties in handling early samples of media due to their viscosity etc.) Since mammalian cell lines are subject to shear, milder bioreactor conditions are used; roller bottles are still widely used despite the high cost; similarly the downstream processes chosen should be of such nature as to maintain the structural integrity of protein. For example, the use of chromatographic desalting as the buffer exchange principle (no shear forces) and ultrafiltration (or precipitation) for sample concentration is recommended. The process design should assure a smooth transfer between unit operations making use of the ability of ion exchangers to bind proteins at low salt concentrations and hydrophobic interaction media to bind proteins at high salt concentrations fully coordinated.

15.3.4.1 Harvest

This stage conditions the sample for the capture step. Cells and cell debris are typically removed by means of centrifugation, microfiltration or expanded bed technology. The expanded bed technology may prove impractical due to cell aggregation. Several new membrane technologies obviate the problems of cell aggregation and improve the efficiency of tangential flow filtration. Mammalian cell cultures are sometimes carried out as continuous cultures running over several weeks (typically from 4 to 8 weeks). The harvest is collected into sub-batches at regular intervals and sometimes even processed further before pooling. It should be emphasized that each sub-batch must undergo testing before being added to the pool of batches in order to demonstrate process control.

15.3.4.2 Capture

This step removes cell culture and process-derived impurities and prepares the sample for intermediary purification. Both packed-bed and expanded bed technology are used. The typical chromatographic capture procedure used are ion exchange chromatography, although AC or HIC work for some proteins. Presence of anti-foam agents in the harvest may eliminate use of HIC due to their relative high hydrophobicity. The particle size of chromatographic media is ideally in the range of 100–300 nm.

Several purification principles are suited for capture purification of IgG. Protein A affinity chromatography has been used in a number of cases, but the less common Protein G or IMAC technology should offer advantage as well as many monoclonal antibodies bind strongly to metal affinity matrices. Note that monoclonal antibodies bind to nucleic acids and divalent metal ions. Protein A binds to all subclasses of human IgG (except for IgG class 3) in the Fc region at neutral to alkaline pH with low to high conductivity. Generally, only slight adjustment of the culture medium is needed for application and binding, although high ionic strength increases the binding capacity of the column. The binding is unaffected by the nature and variations of the glycosylation pattern. The mAb is eluted by decreasing pH, but the instability at low pH must seriously be taken into consideration. Addition of co-solvents, such as 30%–60% ethylene glycol or 1–2 M urea to the buffer is sometimes used to elute the protein at a higher pH. Further, a stabilizing effect is obtained if the mAb is eluted into a neutral pH buffer. If fetal calf serum has been added to the culture medium, bovine IgG may amount up to 50% of the IgG eluted. Several IgMs bind to protein A, but elution often requires lower pH than 4.5, which seriously challenges the protein stability. Leakage of the protein A ligand is a serious drawback and specific analytical assays must be introduced to prove efficient removal. IMAC is a very attractive capture purification principle for IgG's, which binds to metal chelating columns at neutral to alkaline pH (buffers containing chelating agents, free ammonium ions, free amino acids, amines or aminated zwitterion should not be used). The binding is relatively independent of salt concentration, presence of non-ionic detergents and of urea in low concentrations. The cell culture medium can therefore be applied to the column with little or no conditioning. Elution is performed by decreasing pH in the range of 8–4, mainly reflecting titration of histidyl residues or with chelating agents such as EDTA displacing the metal from the column. Leakage of Ni^{++} or similar metal ions must be expected and thus further purification is needed in subsequent steps. Although IMAC can be used virtually anywhere in the downstream process with only minor adjustment of the application sample, the capture features dominate because there is little or no adjustment of the large volume of cell culture application sample required, the majority of contaminants pass through the column at loading conditions and that metal ions can be removed in later steps. IMAC binds IgG from more species and subclasses than do Protein A and it operates under far milder conditions. It is less expensive and does not leach cytotoxic biological material into the product. IMAC will selectively recover intact IgG from supernatants in which the light chain is in surplus. It should be emphasized that the expanded bed technology offers the advantages of very gentle isolation of the expressed mAb, saving at least one centrifugation or filtration step.

15.3.4.3 Virus Inactivation
Inactivation is typically (but not necessarily) performed after the capture step, where the sample volume has been severely reduced. The virus inactivation program should be linked to the infectious viruses used for transfection of the cells.

15.3.4.4 Intermediary Purification
This step removes cell culture and process-derived impurities and prepares the sample for polishing. The intermediary purification step offers a wide range of chromatographic principles (IMAC, HIC, IEC, HAC). The particle size of chromatographic media should be in the range of 50–120 nm. Both cation and anion exchange chromatography (IEC) are suited purification principles for all mAbs, although the former is restricted in that very few mAbs are soluble at low pH and low conductivity. Binding conditions and choice of ion exchanger depends on the pI of the antibody and thus some IgG class 3 mAb may be too basic to support high binding capacities on anion exchangers. HIC is applicable to all mAbs. Application in highly concentrated salt solutions and elution in low conductivity buffers may result in precipitation of the antibody and care should therefore be taken to investigate the stability of the mAb under these conditions. Mixed mode ion exchangers, such as hydroxyapatite, is a suited purification principle, also for IgM. However, chelating agents cannot be tolerated in the application buffer and the matrix does not withstand acidic pH buffers.

15.3.4.5 Virus Filtration
The techniques used include pH modification, addition of detergents, and use of micro-wave heating. Membrane filtration can contribute to the overall virus reduction in a reliable and controlled manner without damaging the target protein. In many cases, large viruses could be removed to the detection limit of the assay used. Small viruses (e.g., parvoviruses) may require filtration through special membranes that have limited protein transmission. cGMP facilities are typically divided into an area where viruses are expected to be present (harvest and capture) and non-virus areas potentially free of viruses. An early virus filtration step is recommended if the viscosity and particulates levels would allow an effective process (Table 15.1).

15.3.4.6 Polishing
This step removes host cell, process and product related impurities. Powerful chromatographic methods (HP-IEC) should be used to separate the protein from its derivatives

(enzymatic cleaved forms, des-amido forms, oxidized forms, scrambled forms, etc.). The polishing step makes use of the most highly developed purification methods to obtain optimal resolution. The particle size of chromatographic media should be in the range of 15–60 nm.

15.3.4.7 Finishing

This step removes di- and polymer forms and small molecules (e.g., endotoxins, co-solvents, leachables) and allows for easy reformulation of the drug substance. Techniques used include SEC, desalting; packed-bed. The high molecular weight of IgM at 900 KDa makes SEC a powerful purification tool for IgM antibodies.

15.4 YEAST CELL EXPRESSION SYSTEM

The use of nonmammalian hosts has a distinct generic advantage that these hosts are generally regarded as safe since they are not pathogenic to humans. Yeasts are particularly attractive as they can be rapidly grown on minimal (inexpensive) media. Recombinants can be easily selected by complementation, using any one of a number of selectable (complementation) markers. Expressed proteins can be specifically engineered for cytoplasmic localization or for extracellular export. And finally yeasts are exceedingly well suited for large-scale fermentation to produce large quantities of heterologous protein. Classical studies in yeast genetics have generated a wide array of potential cloning vectors and, in the process, defined which plasmid and host genomic sequences are important in expression technology.

In a summary, the yeast culture system has many significant advantages such as it is easy and cheap to grow in large scale, has good regulatory track record, the genetics of yeast is well understood, allows some posttranslational modifications, short doubling time, high cell densities and yield is achievable, no endotoxin release from host cell organism, extracellular expression to low viscosity medium is possible, minor secretion of host cell proteins, no specialized bioreactor required and it is safer than working with mammalian tissue or cell lines.

The disadvantages of yeast system include problems with correct glycosylation, over-glycosylation can ruin protein bioactivity, glycosylation is not identical to mammalian glycosylation, extensive proteolysis of target protein, non-native proteins are not always correctly folded, fewer cloning vectors are available, gene expression less easy to control, *S. cerevisiae* is unable to excise introns in gene transcripts of higher eukaryotes.

The use of yeast expression systems involves an entirely different set of techniques and principles than those used for other eukaryotic or prokaryotic systems. Commonly used yeast hosts are *Saccharomyces cerevisiae*, *Schizosaccharomyces pombe*, *Pichia pastoris*, *Hansela polymorpha*, *Kluyveromyces lactis*, and *Yarrowia lipolytica*. Newer research tools like lithium acetate and electroporation-mediated transformation of intact yeast cells and the creation of 2 µ yeast episomal plasmids have helped yeast rise to the most favorite list of expression systems.

Wild-type yeasts are prototrophic, that is, they are nutritionally self-sufficient, capable of growing on minimal media. Classical genetic studies have created auxotrophic strains—those that require specific nutritional supplements to grow in minimal media. The nutritional requirements of the auxotrophic strains are the basis for selection of successfully transformed strains. By including a gene in the plasmid expression cassette that complements one or more defective genes in the host auxotroph, one can easily select recombinants on minimal media. Hence, strains requiring leucine will grow on minimal media if they harbor a plasmid expressing the LEU2 gene. The most commonly used selectable markers found in yeast are for leucine, uracil, histidine, and tryptophan deficiencies.

While the number and variety of *S. cerevisiae* and *S. pombe* strains possessing nutrition selectable markers make these yeasts attractive hosts, their limitations include hyperglycosylation; weak, poorly regulated promoters; and biomass fermentation. Many of these and other problems are circumvented using, *P. pastoris, K. lactis,* and *Y. lipolytica* that have been extensively utilized in the industrial-scale production of metabolites and native proteins (e.g., β-galactosidase). Vector-host genetic incompatibilities and a relatively undefined biology have limited their use as heterologous expression hosts.

The methylotrophic yeast, *H. polymorpha*, and to a greater extent *P. pastoris*—unique in that they will grow using methanol as the sole carbon source—are becoming a favorite expression host alternative for many researchers. *Pichia pastoris* has produced some of the highest heterologous protein yields to date (12 g/L fermentation culture), 10- to 100-fold higher than in *S. cerevisiae*. In *P. pastoris*, growth in methanol is mediated by alcohol oxidase, an enzyme whose de novo synthesis is tightly regulated by the alcohol oxidase promoter. The enzyme has a very low specific activity. To compensate for this, it is over-produced, accounting for more than 30% of total soluble protein in methanol-induced cells. Thus, by engineering a heterologous protein gene downstream of the genomic AOX1 promoter, one can induce its overproduction. This is the basis for the *P. pastoris* expression system. *Hansela polymorpha* produces the methanol oxidase (MOX) protein under control of the MOX1 promoter. A complete *P. pastoris* expression system is available from Invitrogen.

Most yeast vectors for protein expression contain one or more of these basic elements: the *S. cerevisiae* 2 μ plasmid origin of replication, a ColE1 element, a antibiotic resistance *marker* gene to aid development and screening of plasmid constructs in *E. coli*, a heterologous (constitutive or inducible) promoter, a termination signal, signal sequence (encoding secretion leader peptides), and occasionally fusion protein genes (to facilitate purification).

Constitutive gene expression by the yeast plasmid cassette is commonly mediated (in *S. cerevisiae* and *S. pombe*) by the promoters for genes to the glycolytic enzymes: glyceraldehyde-3-phosphate dehydrogenase (TDH3), triose phosphate isomerase (TPI1), or phosphoglycerate isomerase (PGK1). Protein expression can also be regulated (induced) using the alcohol dehydrogenase isozyme II (ADH2) gene promoter (glucose-repressed), glucocorticoid responsive elements (GREs, induced with deoxycorticosterone), GAL1 and GAL10 promoters (to control galactose utilization pathway enzymes, which are glucose-repressed and galactose induced), the metallothionein promoter from the CUP1 gene (induced by copper sulfate), and the PHO5 promoter (induced by phosphate limitation). Most native yeast gene termination signals, when included in the plasmid expression cassette, will provide proper termination of RNA transcripts. The most commonly used are terminator signals for the MF-alpha-1, TPI1, CYC1, and PGK1 genes.

Complete packaged system for quickly developing yeast expression systems is available from Clontech, Invitrogen, or Stratagene and others. For example, Invitrogen sells an expression vector for *S. cerevisiae* and a complete system for *P. pastoris* expression cloning. The Easy Select Pichia Expression Kit includes vectors (pPICZ series), *P. pastoris* strains, reagents for transformation, sequencing primers, media, and a comprehensive manual. Researchers can clone their protein gene into any reading frame contained in each of three different vectors, select recombinants by zeocin resistance, induce protein expression with methanol (sole carbon source), and identify expression using antibody to a C-terminal c-myc peptide tag. These vectors also harbor an *S. cerevisiae* alpha-factor secretion gene and polyHIS-encoding element, thus expressed protein is easily recovered from culture extract supernatant and purified using metal-chelate chromatography (e.g., ProBond resin packaged in Invitrogen's Xpress Purification System).

The yeast species *S. cerevisiae* and *P. pastoris* are the most widely used species for therapeutic protein manufacturing as they offer high efficiency, lower cost and large yields (10G+/L). The development time from introduced gene to protein is about 14 days (in comparison, *E. coli* is 5 days and mammalian cells from 4 to 5 months). In contrast to *E. coli*, yeast can express correctly folded proteins directly to the medium, which greatly facilitates purification (low level of host cell proteins, non-viscous solution, low DNA level). The rigid cell wall renders the use of all sorts of bioreactors possible regardless of stirring and shaking mechanisms. Yeast cell cultures have been widely used for the production of biopharmaceuticals such as insulin, streptokinase, hirudin, interferons, tissue necrosis factor, tissue plasminogen activator, hepatitis B vaccine, and epidermal growth factor.

Large-scale operations are associated with a number of restrictions related to host strain physiology and fermentation technology. Many promoter systems that work well in small scale cannot be implemented in production processes demanding a substantial number of generations. Use of low-expression cassettes reduces the loss of plasmid to some extent, but a profound effect on productivity may be observed due to lack of stability. Expression systems characterized by a high specific rate of product formation at low specific growth rates are highly favorable for large-scale operations. Oxygen demand and temperature control are key factors in controlling yeast fermentations, which are mainly carried out as fed-batch cultivations. Proteolysis of the target protein can be a major problem.

15.4.1 Cell Substrates

15.4.1.1 *Saccharomyces cerevisiae*

The baker's yeast *S. cerevisiae* is the most extensively studied yeast strain. Its genetics are well known and it has obtained a generally regarded as safe (GRAS) status. Protease deficient strains, such as BT150, deficient in proteases A and B, carboxypeptidase Y, and carboxypeptidase S, are available. *Saccharomyces cerevisiae* exhibits alcoholic fermentation under aerobic conditions, unless the sugar supply rate is low. This response occurs at glucose concentrations of 0.15 g/L, hence the demand for low sugar supply rate (which is growth limiting). To prevent this, the use of non-repressing substrates such as raffinose or continuous culture is employed. It is common practice to measure the ethanol concentration or the respiratory quotient (RQ). An indirect feedback control of RQ data has been applied to assure effective production (RQ < 1.3), but it must be kept in mind that the low growth rate may affect target protein expression.

A commonly employed strategy when expressing recombinant proteins in yeast is to put the gene of interest under the control of an inducible promoter. The use of inducible promoters (e.g., GAL1 induced by galactose) provides for the separation of growth and recombinant protein production. There is no strong inducible promoter available in *S. cerevisiae*, and the expression of recombinant protein will only amount to about 1%–5% of total cellular protein, as compared to 35% in *P. pastoris*. An example is the expression of recombinant hirudin, a thrombin inhibitor and therapeutic for cardiovascular diseases. If separation of growth and production is not desired (e.g., if protein expression is growth associated), the use of a constitutive promoter such as PHO5 can be employed.

The stability of the expression cassette has a high impact on productivity. Loss of the cassette during the course of the fermentation results in formation of nonproductive, plasmid free cells, which usually outgrow plasmid carrying cells in fermentation unless selective pressure can be effectively employed. More than 30 generations are required from stock culture to the final stage, and if the expression cassette is lost during the process, this will result in loss of productivity.

To target the recombinant protein for secretion, a signal sequence is needed. This can be derived directly from the protein of interest if it is recognized and correctly processed in yeast. If not, the signal sequence of the *S. cerevisiae* α-mating pre-pro leader sequence or invertase may be used. This signal directs the recombinant protein to the endoplasmatic reticulum for further processing and secretion.

While *S. cerevisiae* has been fermented in several different ways, the fermentation protocol of *Pichia pastoris* cultures is, broadly speaking, nearly always the same. This fermentation process is carried out by generating biomass by growing on excess glycerol then inducing protein production with methanol. It is a three-stage combination of batch and fed-batch modes. The first stage is a 24 h glycerol batch usually conducted with 4% v/v glycerol. The end of this stage is indicated by a sharp rise in dissolved oxygen (DO) after which a glycerol fed-batch phase is started, typically with a 50% v/v glycerol solution at a feed rate of 15 ml/L. This phase de-represses the AOX1 promoter and must last for at least one hour. Examples of glycerol fed-batch stages lasting all the way up to 32 h have been employed. The third stage, a methanol fed-batch, is initiated either with a 100% methanol feed when the last batch of glycerol is exhausted or by slowly adapting the cells to growing on methanol typically on 5% v/v methanol while still feeding glycerol. This induction phase triggers the production of heterologous protein and usually lasts about 80–90 h. Tight control of the methanol concentration is obtained by regularly performing *spike tests* to make sure the methanol is present at limiting amounts. The rapid proliferation of *P. pastoris* cells set high demands to oxygen supply and cooling.

The nutritional needs of yeast are simple and depend on the yeast species, strain and growth conditions. The main culture media components are a carbon source (which also functions as the energy source), salts, trace elements, nitrogen, and growth factors.

For *S. cerevisiae* fermentations, glucose is often chosen as the carbon source because of its inexpensiveness and relative high solubility, whereas for *P. pastoris* (see below) fermentations glycerol and methanol are used. The growth factor requirements vary in a case-to-case manner. *Saccharomyces cerevisiae* has in some cases a requirement for inositol, pantothenate, pyridoxine, thiamine, nicotinic acid, and biotin, whereas *P. pastoris* has been reported to require biotin.

15.4.1.2 *Pichia pastoris*

Pichia pastoris is a methylotrophic yeast, which means that it can grow on methanol as the only carbon source. The knowledge of this yeast's genetics stems from the extensive research on the production of single-cell protein (SCP). It is characterized as glucose insensitive yeast. *Pichia pastoris* has a high oxygen demand and as so the fermentation of this yeast generates considerable amounts of heat. It has the advantage of a very strong inducible promoter, the AOX1 promoter. The AOX1 gene encodes one of two alcohol oxidases expressed in the presence of methanol. When growing on glucose, transcription from the AOX1 promoter is completely repressed even in the presence of methanol. Growth on glycerol allows for induction with methanol, but the total effect of glycerol is not completely understood. It has become evident, that glycerol even at low levels also inhibits expression from the AOX1 promoter, though not as pronounced as glucose. The availability of the strong AOX1 has provided for protein expression levels as high as 22 g/L for intracellular expressed proteins and 11 g/L for secreted ones. In contrast to *S. cerevisiae* this species exhibits relatively short glycosylation chain length, and the major problem is enzymic deglycosylation and varying glycosylation patterns.

15.4.2 Cell Cultures

Yeast can grow both anaerobically and aerobically. In anaerobic growth, most of the carbon substrate is metabolized into inorganic substances like ethanol and carbon dioxide, making this growth less desirable for protein production. The preferred large-scale aerobic fermentation yields more biomass. However, the presence of high levels of readily metabolically available sugars (e.g., glucose) represses aerobic respiration (the Crab tree effect) in certain yeast species (e.g., *S. cerevisiae*) and it can be difficult in practice to completely suppress the anaerobic growth. The use of a non-repressing substrates (e.g., raffinose) or continuous culture are often employed to overcome this problem.

Basically, the fermentation of yeast can be divided into two modes: batch systems with its different variants and continuous systems. The classical batch systems offer minor risks, relative inexpensiveness and well-tested procedures. The crab tree effect of *S. cerevisiae* and other limiting factors of batch fermentations have led to the development of fed-batch systems and this is now the most commonly employed fermentation strategy. Continuous modes offer the possibility of prolonged fermentation, high productivity, and greater flexibility than do batch modes. However, the higher risk of contamination and greater expense make it less amenable. When choosing fermentation mode, the volumetric productivity, final product concentration, stability and reproducibility must be considered in a case-to-case manner.

15.4.3 Batch Culture

This is a closed system with a definite amount of nutrients and one single harvest. The cells follow classic kinetics with a log phase of rapid proliferation where some products are produced and a stationary phase where the amount of cells does not change and where other products are produced. If the desired product is produced in the log phase, it can be prolonged by manipulating the growth conditions but only for a very limited time.

If the desired amount is not produced that quickly, it will be reasonable to choose another culture method. When fermenting *S. cerevisiae,* the cells will start by producing ethanol due to the crab tree effect and will not enter the log phase of aerobic respiration until the sugar level is low enough. The osmotic sensitivity of yeast cells puts another constraint on the initial sugar concentration. In addition to these disadvantages, batch culture does not allow for control of the growth rate and the culture becomes rapidly limited by oxygen. All together these factors restrict the duration of batch fermentations. Higher yield of biomass can be achieved in batch fermentations by keeping the sugar level low, using a glucose insensitive yeast like *Candida* or replacing glucose with a non-repressive substrate such as acetate, galactose, or glycerol.

15.4.4 Fed-Batch Culture

Another solution to the problems with the crab tree effect and osmotic sensitivity is to conduct the fermentation in a fed-batch mode. Medium is added in fixed volumes throughout the process thus increasing the volume of the cell culture with time. Neither cells nor medium are leaving the bioreactor. In this way, the sugar levels can be kept low for a long time, and it is possible to switch from one substrate to another thus rendering the use of inducible promoters possible. The process is usually performed at low growth rates the key control parameter being the feed rate whose upper limit is dictated by the oxygen transfer limit and cooling strategies available. The feed rate is often subjected to feedback control strategies using for instance measurement of the RQ, biomass production, or heat generation. In *S. cerevisiae*, this feedback includes on-line analysis of glucose and ethanol, whereas *P. pastoris* fermentations often are controlled by either direct on-line measurement of methanol but more frequently by *spike tests.* (The *spike tests* confirm that the compound in question [e.g., methanol, glycerol, glucose] is the rate-limiting factor.) Variants of the classical fed-batch strategy such as semi-fed batch where nutrients and vitamins are added in dry form not changing the culture volume have also been employed with success.

15.4.5 Perfusion Culture

An alternative approach to batch cultivation is to continuously add fresh medium to the bioreactor and to remove equivalent amounts of medium with cells. Continuous cultures are performed at low dilution rates usually up to 0.3/h. It has been reported that higher dilution rates causes washout even though successful fermentation has been performed with dilution rates up to 0.6/h after a time of adaptation. Low dilution rates usually promote a high yield of biomass and a RQ of about 1. In *S. cerevisiae* fermentations, high dilution rates promote a switch to anaerobic fermentation because of too much accessible sugar. Continuous cultures are conducted in chemostats having all the sophisticated monitoring and control apparatus necessary to maintain a successful continuous culture. In the chemostat, the cell density will not be as high as in batch fermenters resulting in a lower productivity, but the long-term continuous expression of product will in many cases be advantageous to the batch mode. In contrast to batch cultures, a steady state is reached, where the cell density, the substrate concentration, and the product concentration are constant. The disadvantages of continuous cultures are high risk of contamination with faster growing organisms and demand for very complex and expensive apparatus. The longevity of continuous culturing can cause accumulation of non-producing variants of the yeast cells resulting in decreasing productivity.

15.4.6 Cell Immobilization Strategies

It has been shown that immobilizing cells increases the achievable cell density and plasmid stability enabling longer cultivation time and higher productivity. The reason for this is not yet clear. Conventional immobilizing methods such as chemical cross-linking or entrapment of cells in a gel matrix can alter cell physiology, increase contamination risks, and decrease efficiency, reasons for why these methods have not become very widespread. However, it has been reported that immobilization of *S. cerevisiae* strain XV2181 cells in a fibrous bed bioreactor promoted a stable long-term production of GM-CSF with a relatively high volumetric productivity (0.98 mg/L/h) performed for 4 weeks without any contamination or cell physiology alteration. The specific protein production and total product yield were, however, much lower than the control batch fermentation with cells in suspension.

15.4.7 Media

Media can be divided into two categories: complex and defined. The complex media are rich broths comprising yeast extract or yeast nitrogen base along with the carbon source and can be supplemented with biotin and peptone. They can be buffered with potassium phosphate. Typical concentrations are 1% yeast extract, 2% peptone, and 0.00004% biotin and the carbon source can be 2% glucose, 1% glycerol, or 0,5% methanol. The defined media comprise salts, trace elements, and optionally amino acids. Often the trace elements are added after sterilization along with the carbon substrate and the required vitamins. Commonly used additives are casein hydrolysates that can prevent proteolytic degradation of the final product by inhibiting extracellular proteases and anti-foam agents.

15.4.7.1 In Process Control

In process control is becoming an increasingly important part of the safety measurements taken in biopharmaceutical development and manufacture. The control program comprises strict parameter control using defined lower and upper parameter limits and measurement of a variety of output parameters (responses). Critical parameters and interactions should be identified from the data collected. The aim is to assure a robust and reproducible process. Below is listed a number of important parameters and responses related to bacterial cell cultures (Table 15.2).

The responses monitored during yeast culture are listed in Table 15.3. The regulatory issues relating to yeast systems are relatively simpler. The risk related directly to the cells fall into three categories: viruses and other transmissible agents, cellular DNA, and host

Table 15.2 Important Parameters in Yeast Cultures

Parameter	Comments
Aeration rate	The aeration rate is commonly set to a fixed value or to increase as the biomass increases. Typical values are 1–2 vvm (liter oxygen per liter of culture per min).
Agitation rate	The stirrer speed is either fixed on a value known to be sufficient to keep the DO above the critical 20% (common values are 500–600 rpm) or established empirically in response to the DO9.
Dissolved oxygen	The dissolved oxygen must exceed 20% and is most commonly set to 30%. Since oxygen solubility in aqueous solution is very low (7.6 µg/mL) the oxygen transfer rate (OTR) is a main limiting factor when scaling up yeast cultures. The oxygen level can be controlled via the aeration rate, vessel top pressure and agitation rate. The DO is a valuable tool for analyzing the actual culture composition via the *spike test*. The *spike tests* confirm that the compound in question (e.g., methanol, glycerol, glucose) is the rate-limiting factor. The feeding of the said compound is stopped and the DO is measured. If the response time is long (1–2 min) or the rise in DO is small (~10%), the fermentation is not limited by the compound. A typical rate limited culture will have spike times of 15–30 s.
Foam level	The foam level is controlled by addition of anti-foam agents.
Glucose and glycerol feed	These carbon substrates can be determined on-line with a near infrared analyzer or off-line with HPLC. Glucose is often determined off-line using an enzymatic analytical kit. Spike tests are used to see if these substrates are present at limiting amounts.
Methanol and ethanol	Since high levels (2%–3%) of methanol are toxic to the cells, it is important to keep strict control with the concentration in the cell culture and adjust the feed rate often. Traditionally the culture is kept methanol limited by performing spike tests regularly. Since a limiting concentration of methanol may not be optimal, it can be advantageous to perform on-line control with an alcohol sensor in the exhaust gas or a near infrared analyzer. Alternatively, the alcohol content can be analyzed off-line with gas chromatography. It has been reported, that a methanol concentration of 1% is optimal for *P. pastoris* fermentations. The same analytical methods apply to ethanol measurement in *S. cerevisiae* fermentations.
pCO_2	It is not certain that pCO_2 have any effect on yeast cultures, but a negative effect on cell growth has been observed at pressures above 350 mbar1. pCO_2 is used to calculate the respiration quotient (RQ), an important parameter, as described below.
pH	Yeast grow well at pH 5–6, although it has been reported that lowering pH to 4 has no effect on the growth of *S. cerevisiae*. A pH decrease to 3 has been employed to reduce the action of proteases. pH 4 has been reported to increase plasmid stability and thereby protein production and has been employed to lower the risk of bacterial contamination. The metabolism of actively growing yeast will result in a decrease in pH; this is opposed by the automatic addition of ammonia hydroxide which can also be a nitrogen

(Continued)

Table 15.2 (Continued) Important Parameters in Yeast Cultures

Parameter	Comments
	source. pH is measured with permanently sealed gel filled glass combination electrodes or with pressurized electrodes. They are standardized against commercially available standard solutions. Repeated sterilization over a prolonged period of time depletes the outer gel layer of the glass membrane increasing the response time. Pilot scale and larger vessels are sterilized with steam in situ. NaOH or HCl is often used to adjust pH. Care should be taken to avoid locally high pH during addition. It is recommended to use less concentrated NaOH solutions (0.1 M).
RQ	The RQ is defined as the ratio of CO_2 production to oxygen consumption. It is a valuable guide to the metabolic state of the yeast cell culture. Aerobic growth yields RQ values above one, whereas values below one indicates a switch to anaerobic fermentation with the concomitant decrease in biomass. For *S. cerevisiae* BT150, an RQ of 1 is optimal for biomass production. The optimal value for protein production must be determined from case to case.
Temperature	The optimal temperature is 30°C. Temperature is sometimes shifted to 28°C or lower to prevent overheating. Respiration generates heat and especially *P. pastoris* fermentations, demanding high amounts of oxygen, generate substantial heat.

Table 15.3 Important Responses in Yeast Cultures

Response	Comments
Amino acids	Detected by HPLC.
Ammonia	Can be determined by Kjeldahl analysis.
Biomass and cell density	The biomass states the amount of wet cell weight (WCW) that can be converted to the dry cell weight (DCW). DCW can be measured gravimetrically. DCW has a linear relationship with the absorbance at a given wavelength (A_{590}–A_{660}) over a certain range, a relationship that must be established on case-by-case, since it varies with size and shape of the cells. For a typical diploid strain $A_{660} = 2$ equals 10^7 cells and for a typical haploid strain $A_{660} = 2$ equals 2×10^7 cells. The linear range is often very short (usually within 0.1–0.3 absorbance units at 660 nm). The actual cell number can be calculated electronically (Coulter counter) or visually by coupling a hemocytometer to a light microscope. The normal convention with budding yeast cells is to consider a daughter cell only an individual cell when completely separated from the mother cell. A brief sonification of the cells before counting will separate cells that have completed cytokinesis. Cell aggregations should not be a frequently encountered problem since the yeast strains used in the industry usually aggregate only when contaminated with bacteria or fungi. In addition, indirect methods measuring the metabolic activities such as glucose or oxygen consumption, RQ and increase in product formation can be applied.

(Continued)

Table 15.3 (*Continued*)   Important Responses in Yeast Cultures

Response	Comments
Cell viability	A wide variety of marker genes is currently available. Use of marker genes that encode resistance against antibiotics is generally recommended.
Methanol and ethanol	Since high levels (2%–3%) of methanol are toxic to the cells, it is important to keep strict control with the concentration in the cell culture and adjust the feed rate often. Traditionally, the culture is kept methanol limited by performing spike tests regularly. Since a limiting concentration of methanol may not be optimal, it can be advantageous to perform on-line control with an alcohol sensor in the exhaust gas or a near infrared analyzer. Alternatively the alcohol content can be analyzed off-line with gas chromatography. It has been reported, that a methanol concentration of 1% is optimal for *P. pastoris* fermentations. The same analytical methods apply to ethanol measurement in *S. cerevisiae* fermentations.
Product	Specific assay.

cell proteins (e.g., growth factors). The potential introduction of adventitious agents such as fungi, bacteria, viruses, and prions in cell culture media is of major concern and has let the biotech community to constantly search for safe media and raw materials. Thus, raw materials possessing high contamination risk (e.g., hydrolysates and peptones produced from animals or by means of animal derived enzymes) should be avoided. Use of antibiotics is discouraged. Yeast is generally regarded as a safe expression system (GRAS status). Its use is not associated with release of endotoxins and adventitious agents such as viruses or prions are not present. The major concern is the presence of DNA and host cell proteins in the final product.

15.4.8 Downstream Processing

In contrast to the bacterial expression systems, yeast does express proteins with the correct N terminal amino acid residue. Consequently, use of tagged proteins is rarely observed with this expression system. The protein is normally expressed to the medium in its native form, although disulfide rearrangement or reduction may appear due to the low redox potential of the fermentation broth. Proteins are often expressed in yields ranging from 50 to 300 mg/L. Besides being regarded as generally safe to use, the yeast expression system does not raise any concerns related to endotoxin release from cell walls and possible virus infections. The cell wall is rigid and separation of cells from the medium is relatively easy using centrifugation or expanded bed technology.

The purification techniques generally used are similar to those used for bacterial expression systems except there is no refolding and cleavage steps involved. There are no specific purification methods for removal of host cell proteins, but use of three to four different chromatographic methods during downstream processing will, in most cases, result in an acceptable level. Unintended glycosylation products may be co-expressed together

Table 15.4 Steps in Yeast-Derived Systems

Harvest (centrifugation, filtration, microfiltration, ultrafiltration)	The purpose of the harvest step is to condition the sample for the capture step. Cells and cell debris are typically removed by means of centrifugation or expanded bed technology. The latter may in some cases prove difficult to operate due to cell aggregation. Several new membrane technologies have been developed to improve the efficiency of tangential flow filtration. The redox potential of the solution may be close to reducing conditions (<100 mV) resulting in cleavage of the disulfide bonds. This parameter should therefore be closely monitored during operation.
Capture (AC, IEC, IMAC; expanded bed packed bed)	The purpose of the capture step is to remove cell culture and process derived impurities and to prepare the sample for intermediary purification. Both packed-bed and expanded bed technology will apply. The typical chromatographic capture procedure is ion exchange chromatography, although AC or HIC may apply for some proteins. Presence of anti-foam agents in the harvest may eliminate use of HIC due to their relative high hydrophobicity. The particle size of chromatographic media should be in the range of 100–300 nm. The sample composition depends on the chromatographic principle used.
Intermediary purification (IEC, IMAC, HAC, HIC; packed bed)	The purpose of the intermediary purification step is to remove cell culture and process derived impurities and to prepare the sample for polishing. The intermediary purification step offers a wide range of chromatographic principles (IMAC, HIC, IEC, HAC). The choice of media not only includes the protein purification ability, but also the ability to *receive* pooled fraction from the capture step and to *deliver* a suitable application sample to the polishing step. The particle size of chromatographic media should be in the range of 50–120 nm. The nature of the sample for polishing depends on the chromatographic principle used.
Polishing (RPC, IEC, HIC; packed bed)	The purpose of the polishing step is to remove host cell, process and product-related impurities. Powerful chromatographic methods (high performance HP-RPC or HP-IEC) should be used to separate the protein from its derivatives (enzymatic cleaved forms, des-amido forms, oxidized forms, scrambled forms, etc.). The polishing part of the process makes use of the most highly developed purification methods to obtain optimal resolution. Minor amounts of glycosylated products may be present from the fermentation broth and specific care should be taken to remove these products during polishing. The particle size of chromatographic media should be in the range of 15–60 nm.
Concentration (ultrafiltration)	This step may be required to concentrate the output to meet the product formulation requirements.
Finish (SEC, desalting; packed bed)	The purpose of the SEC step is to remove di- and polymer forms and small molecules (e.g., endotoxins, co-solvents, leachables) and to allow for easy reformulation of the drug substance.

with the target protein (e.g., mono- and di-glycosylated forms). They can be difficult to separate from the target molecule even during polishing. The major steps in the downstream processing of yeast-derived proteins are provided in Table 15.4.

15.5 INSECT CELLS SYSTEMS

The nonmammalian hosts like insect cells have several advantages:

- The protein is secreted to the medium in its native form.
- They express posttranslational modified proteins including glycosylation, phosphorylation, palmitoylation, myristoylation, and glycosyl-phosphatidylinositol anchors.
- Expression vectors are commercially available.
- The system is suited for expression of cell toxic products since the cells can be grown in a healthy state before infection.
- The baculovirus vectors are harmless to humans.
- They are safer to handle.
- They provide high yields (1–600 mg/L).
- They are easy to develop (taking about a month to prepare and purify a recombinant virus, compared to more than 6 months for mammalian cells).
- They are less expensive to operate.

The main drawbacks include the following:

- Minimal regulatory track record; FDA is yet to approve the first product.
- Semi-expensive culture media.
- Cell line stability.
- Cells are killed during infection releasing intracellular proteins (*Lepidopteran* species).
- Inactivation of the secretory pathway results in low expression yields due to aeration requirements not met.
- Presence of immunogenic host cell proteins due torelease of proteolytic enzymes upon cell disruption.
- Inability to produce eukaryotic glycoproteins with complex N-linked glycans.
- Inability to proper processing of proteins that are initially synthesized as larger inactive precursor proteins (e.g., peptide hormones, neuropeptides, growth factors, matrix metalloproteases).
- Risk of infection with mammalian viruses.
- Sensitive to sheer forces.
- Difficulties in scale up.

The classical strategy for production of proteins in insect cells involves the distinct stages of growing insect cells (*Lepidopteran* species) to mid-exponential growth phase, infecting the cells with the vector, *Autographa californica* nuclear polyhedrosis virus (AcNPV) or *Bombyx mori* nuclear polyhedrosis virus (BmNPV), containing the gene cloning for the target protein and finally harvest and purification of the expressed protein. The reason for using the AcNPV infection step is the ability of baculovirus to replicate in established insect cell lines, where the polyhedrin gene is replaced with a gene of choice (under the control of the strong polyhedrin promoter). The result is high-level expression of the gene insert and the accumulation of the target protein. In contrast to other microbial or mammalian cell expression systems, the host cells are killed during each infection cycle.

Eukaryotic expression systems employing insect cell hosts are based upon one of two vector types: plasmid or plasmid–virion hybrids. Although the latter is the most commonly used, plasmid-based systems offer methodological advantages. The typical insect host is the common fruit fly, *Drosophila melanogaster*. Other insect hosts include mosquito (*Aedes albopictus*), fall army worm (*Spodoptera frugiperda*), cabbage looper (*Trichoplusia ni*), salt marsh caterpillar (*Estigmene acrea*), and silkworm (*Bombyx mori*). In most all cases, heterologous protein overexpression occurs in suspension cell cultures. The exception, and one of the advantages of plasmid–virion systems, is that the recombinant virus may also be injected into larval host hemocel or literally fed to the mature host. Three basic options are available for protein expression in insect cells: vectors that enable high level transient expression; vectors that enable continuous expression from stably transfected cells; and the lytic baculovirus system.

15.5.1 Transient Expression Systems

Transient expression is the most rapid method requiring simple transfection of insect cell expression vectors containing appropriate promoters (e.g., ie1 and gp64 promoters) in the absence of selection. Expression when optimized peaks between 24 and 48 h after transfection. Novogen's InsectDirect® System (http://www.novogen.com) is a complete system based on several vectors featuring an enhanced ie1 promoter. The plasmid-based vector systems provide a mechanism for both transient and long-term expression of recombinant protein. This expression system is exemplified by the Drosophila Expression System (DES) available from Invitrogen. The transfection of competent *D. melanogaster* cells with engineered plasmid will mediate the transient (2–7 days) expression of heterologous protein.

15.5.2 Continuous Expression Systems

Continuous expression using stably transfected insect cells lines is useful for the study of glycoproteins, secreted proteins, and membrane proteins such as receptors. An alternative to the discontinuous insect cell system (cells are killed by the bacoluvirus infection, see below) is continuous culture of permanently transfected cells. Cell cultures of the fruit fly, *D. melanogaster*, grown to cell densities of 5.7×10^7 cells/ml in a low-cost media makes this system a promising candidate for future recombinant protein expression.

The gene of interest is cloned into a vector that utilizes a promoter recognized by the insect cell transcription machinery (e.g., baculovirus ie1 or gp64 promoters). The majority of resistant cells will express the target protein at various intervals. Such cell lines maintain stable expression for many passages (more than 50), enabling long-term culture for the accumulation and study of expressed protein. Establishing transformed cells that will express protein for longer time periods requires that the host cells be cotransfected with a *selection* vector, which results in the stable integration of the expression cassette into the host genome. This system offers two advantages over plasmid–virion systems: methodological simplicity, saving the researcher time, effort, and materials; and a choice of expression regimes, constitutive or inducible. Constitutive expression is mediated using the Ac5 Drosophila promoter, whereas a metallothionein promoter guides copper-inducible expression. The DES vectors are designed with multiple cloning sites for insertion of the heterologous protein gene in any of three reading frames. A choice of vectors also provides for the expression of a variety of C-terminal fusion tags: V5 epitope for identification of expressed protein with V5 epitope antibody, polyhistidine peptide for simplified purification with metal chelate affinity resin, and the BiP secretion leader peptide. The DES system also includes media for maintenance of the host cell line and expression of protein, as well as reagents to facilitate transfection. The commonly used stable cell lines include *Aedes aegypti*, *Aedes albopictus,* and *Anopheles gambia*; in addition, the following lines can be stable cell lines or used with baculovirus system (see below): *D. melanogaster* (Schneider S2 and S3), *S. frugiperda* (Sf9), *S. frugiperda* (Sf21), *T. ni* (High Five), and *T. ni* (BTI-TN-5B1-4).

15.5.3 Baculovirus Expression Systems

The baculovirus expression cassette contains all the genetic information needed for propagation of progeny virus, so no helper virus is needed in the transfection process. The biology of the virus provides a simple means, using plaque morphology, to identify transformed host cells. The virus does not appear to be transmissible to vertebrate species; therefore, this virus-based system is safe for human handlers. Since with many virus vectors, heterologous protein genes are under the control of the late-stage baculovirus p10 and polyhedrin promoters, recombinant protein is, in most cases, the sole product produced. Hence, cells harboring the baculovirus expression cassette integrated in their genomes can produce relatively high amounts of heterologous protein. Most of this protein is easily extracted from the cytoplasm (no inclusion bodies characteristic of prokaryotic systems) or harvested from extracellular culture filtrate (when the expression cassette includes a secretory leader fusion peptide engineered to the recombinant protein). However, the cell machinery may be starting to shut down late in infection, which can impact, in particular, proteins requiring processing. Hence, some companies have introduced viral vectors with hybrid early/late promoters that permits the still functioning cell to process glycosylated or secreted proteins. The commonly used cell lines are *Drosophila melanogaster* (Schneider S2 and S3), *S. frugiperda* (Sf9), *S. frugiperda* (Sf21), *T. ni* (High Five), *T. ni* (BTI-TN-5B1-4; HighFive™).

Baculovirus expression system provides one of the highest levels of target protein expression using baculovirus expression vector system such as BacVector offered by Novogen. In this system, insect cells are infected with a recombinant baculovirus bearing the gene of interest. The infected cells undergo a burst of protein expression, after which the cells die and may lyse. High-level expression is obtained by the of very late baculovirus promoters (e.g., polh and p10 promoters), which are only active during the final stages of the infection cycle. Expression at earlier times can be advantageous to allow more complete protein modification such as glycoprotein processing and is obtained by using alternative baculoviral promoters, for example, iel and gp64 promoters. The process of creating and expressing heterologous protein with the plasmid–virion system is rather straightforward, in theory, but does require a bit of technical finesse and close attention to detail. The process begins with the engineering of the heterologous protein gene into a *transfer plasmid*. This plasmid contains all the elements for autonomous replication in *E. coli*, a bacterial selection marker (usually an ampicillin resistance gene), and elements of the baculovirus genome. The heterologous protein gene is inserted in a specific orientation and location into the plasmid so it is flanked by elements of the baculovirus genome. Successfully engineered plasmids are then cotransfected with viral expression vector (essentially wild-type baculovirus DNA with p10 and/or polyhedrin genes removed) into permissive host cells. Cell-mediated double recombination between viral sequences flanking the heterologous protein gene and the corresponding sequences of the viral expression vector results in the incorporation of the heterologous protein gene into the viral genome. Hence, recombinant progeny viruses will produce heterologous protein late in their life cycle. Novagen's pIE vectors are based on the baculovirus immediate early promoter iel. These plasmids can be used with G418 selection to generate stable cell lines from Sf0 or Sf21 cell lines. Other suppliers of vectors and complete Baculovirus systems are Clontech, Invitrogen, Life Technologies, Novagen, Pharmingen, Quantum Biotechnologies, and Stratagene. (Check out the vendors offering as these are upgraded frequently.)

The baculovirus system has several drawbacks:

The cyclic killing and lysis of the host cell releases intracellular proteins to the medium adversely affecting the purification of the target protein.

The production can only be achieved in batches or at best, semi-continuously.

The expression yield is often much lower than expected due to inactivation of the secretory pathway during the late phase of infection.

Inactivation of secretory path affects posttranslational events such as glycosylation (the sugar chain will end in a mannose and not contain galactose or terminal sialic acid) rendering the expressed protein unsuitable for in vivo applications.

Baculovirus infected cells do not efficiently excise introns from expressed genomic DNA, thus limiting foreign protein expression from cDNAs.

Recent developments to obviate these disadvantages novel expression vectors have been used to transform *Lepidopteran* insect cells into high-level expression systems using both the Bm5 and the HighFive™ transfected cell lines to achieve high yield and complex glycosylation under the control of the enhanced actin promoter system; a yield of 27 mg/L has been possible using this system for GM-CSF in suspension cultures. Though currently not significant, insect cell technology is likely to produce many dramatic advances in the near future.

15.5.4 Process Optimization

Large-scale insect cell cultures are processed in a batch or fed-batch suspension culture grown in a serum-free medium to a cell density of 1–3×10^6 cells/ml before the viral infection is conducted at early or middle exponential phase. Late exponential phase infection can be done if cells are re-suspended in fresh medium leading since production is limited either by depletion of nutrients or by accumulation of toxic compounds.

Suspension cultures are the preferred choice for large-scale insect cell processes although in some cases relative higher yields have been reported in static cultures.

Growing the culture to higher cell densities in spinner flasks ($2–3 \times 10^6$ cells/mL in uninfected cells) often results in decreased target protein expression due to an unusually high oxygen demand; as a result, culture volumes above 500 mL requires additional oxygen sparging that can damage the shear-sensitive insect cells. As a result, airlift fermenters are recommended that provide good agitation at low shear. Polymers (e.g., 0.1% w/v Pluronic polyol F-68) are added to reduce foam formation and thus provide protection of the cells. Typical doubling times are 20–40 h.

If the fed-batch mode is used, addition of nutrients such as yeastolate ultrafiltrate, lipids, amino acids, vitamins, trace elements, and glucose is done under controlled conditions.

The recombinant baculovirus is generated by homologous recombination to stock solution of a titer of 1×10^7 to 1×10^8 pfu/ml, which is used to infect the insect cells around day 40–47. Protein expression usually takes place shortly after infection. The product yield decreases sharply when cultures are infected later than an optimal time of infection (TOI), which is in the early or mid-exponential phase of a culture.

Replacement of growth media prior to infection and feeding with glucose, glutamine, and yestolate in later stages of the infection improves yield.

Addition of human nerve growth factor also improves yield if the cells are grown in the fed-batch mode feeding with a mixture of glutamine, yestolate, and lipids.

Use of efficient medium like YPR for *sf9* and HighFive™ cells.

Assure that all components, oxygen, glucose and glutamine feeding are available in ample supply during protein synthesis and also viral replication stages.

Use of microemulsions to introduce lipids to culture to avoid presence of insoluble lipid droplets in the culture medium.

Where serum-free media cannot be used, assure that it is free of TSE; serum-free media may contain discrete proteins or bulk protein fractions but not of animal origin; also there should be no components of unknown origin.

pH range of 6.0–6.4 is optimal for most *Lepidopteran* cell lines.

Dissolved oxygen (DO) corresponding to 10%–50% of air saturation is needed in large-scale bioreactors. Supply of pure oxygen may be needed for high-density cell cultures. A standard oxygen probe (e.g., Ingold) is used for oxygen measurements.

Temperature range is from 25°C to 30°C for optimal operations; lower temperatures (20°C) are useful for keeping the cells as a slower growing stock.

Osmolality is optimally maintained at 345–380 mOsm/kg for culture medium used with lepidoteran cell lines.

Agitation rates are determined empirically; range of 50 to 200 rpm are most common.

Ammonia production rate ($mmol/10^6$ cells/h) is an indicator of metabolic rate.

Glucose utilization ($mmol/10^6$ cells/h) is an indicator of metabolic rate.

pCO_2 is monitored through pH changes; the CO_2 flow is used to regulate the pH of the cell culture, and the flow is maintained only as long as the pH is above the set point. In late stage cultures the CO_2-HCO_3 buffer system is no longer sufficient to maintain pH and sodium hydrogen carbonate or NaOH is used instead.

Lactate dehydrogenase activity reflects the extent of cell lysis, since LDH is not secreted by insect cells.

MOI has a limited effect on the maximum achievable yield, it is generally in the interval between 0.1 and 1.0 pfu/cell for most efficient operation; lower MOI are used for fed-batch production.

TOI is typically initiated at cell densities of $1-3 \times 10^6$ cells/ml.

Adventitious agent contamination is best detected is at the end of the cell culture in the unprocessed bulk (if multiple harvest pools are prepared at different times, the culture shall be tested at the time of the collection of each pool). The test program should include test for bacteria, fungi, mycoplasma and viruses.

15.5.5 Downstream Processing

The use of the standard *baculovirus* system requires cyclic killing and lysis of the host cell that releases intracellular proteins to the medium complicates the purification of the target protein; as a result, alternate systems like transfection with appropriate plasmids are often preferred. The typical expression level of the target protein is from 50 to 500 mg/L and tags are not necessary. Insect cells are sensitive to shear forces, a factor that is not relevant when using baculovirus systems. Since there is a release of proteolytic enzymes, harvesting and capturing should is done under conditions, where the enzymatic activity is decreased (low temperature and fast procedures) without using any enzyme inhibitors. The standard procedures of harvesting, capturing, intermediate purification, and polishing apply to insect cells as well as they to other systems described above and additionally a step of virus decontamination is introduced. It is recommended to use this virus inactivation step early in the purification process despite the difficulties in the filtration in the early stages of processing.

15.5.5.1 Harvest
Most insect cell cultures are run as batch or fed-batch cultures; hollow fiber modules prove useful.

15.5.5.2 Capture
The typical chromatographic capture procedure is ion exchange chromatography, although AC or HIC may apply for some proteins. Presence of anti-foam agents in the harvest may eliminate use of HIC due to their relative high hydrophobicity. The particle size of chromatographic media should be in the range of 100–300 nm.

15.5.5.3 Virus Inactivation
Since pathogenic or infectious viruses are not used to transform, it is difficult to define a suitable inactivation program. Generic inactivation methods (e.g., microwave) may be considered, but it may be enough to highlight inactivation measures taken as part of the downstream process (e.g., low pH, presence of co-solvents).

15.5.5.4 Intermediary Purification
The intermediary purification step offers a wide range of chromatographic principles (IMAC, HIC, IEC, HAC).

15.5.5.5 Virus Filtration

Small viruses (e.g., parvoviruses) may require filtration through special membranes that have limited protein transmission. Harvest and capture are the areas where viruses can be expected, use early viral filtration where possible taking into account viscosity and particulate load.

15.5.5.6 Polishing

Chromatographic methods (high performance HP-RPC or HP-IEC) are used to separate the protein from its derivatives (enzymatic cleaved forms, des-amido forms, oxidized forms, scrambled forms, etc.).

15.5.5.7 Finishing

SEC removes di- and polymer forms, small molecules (e.g., endotoxins, co-solvents, leach-ables). DNA is removed by means of anion exchange or hydroxyapatite chromatography (DNA binds strongly to both types).

15.6 TRANSGENIC ANIMAL SYSTEMS

A transgenic animal is one that carries a foreign gene that has been deliberately inserted into its genome. The foreign gene is constructed using recombinant DNA methodology. In addition to a structural gene, the DNA usually includes other sequences to enable it to be incorporated into the DNA of the host and to be expressed correctly by the cells of the host. Transgenic sheep and goats have been produced that express foreign proteins in their milk. Transgenic chickens are now able to synthesize human proteins in the *white* of the eggs. These animals should eventually prove to be valuable sources of proteins for human therapy. In July 2000, researchers from the team that produced Dolly reported success in producing transgenic lambs in which the transgene had been inserted at a specific site in the genome and functioned well. Transgenic mice have provided the tools for exploring many biological questions.

Until recently, the transgenes introduced into sheep inserted randomly in the genome and often worked poorly. However, in July 2000, success at inserting a transgene into a specific gene locus was reported. The gene was the human gene for alpha 1-antitrypsin, and two of the animals expressed large quantities of the human protein in their milk. The method used to create transgenic sheep is as follows. Sheep fibroblasts (connective tissue cells) growing in tissue culture are treated with a vector that contained the seg-ments of DNA: 2 regions homologous to the sheep *COL1A1* gene. This gene encodes Type 1 collagen. This locus is chosen because fibroblasts secrete large amounts of collagen and thus one would expect the gene to be easily accessible in the chromatin. Also inserted is a neomycin-resistance gene to aid in isolating those cells that successfully incorporates the vector and the human gene encoding alpha1-antitrypsin. The vector further contains promoter sites from beta lactoglobulin gene to promote hormone-driven gene expression milk producing cells and also binding sites for ribosomes for efficient translation of the mRNAs. Successfully transformed cells are then fused with enucleated sheep eggs and implanted in the uterus of a ewe (female sheep). The off spring secrete milk containing large amounts of alpha-1-antitrypsin (650 µg/mL; 50 times higher than previous results using random insertion of the transgene). This project has now been abandoned because of its high cost despite remarkable success.

Chickens grow faster than sheep and large numbers can be grown in close quarters; synthesize several grams of protein in the *white* of their eggs. Two methods have succeeded in producing chickens carrying and expressing foreign genes: infecting embryos with a viral vector carrying the human gene for a therapeutic protein, and the promoter sequences that will respond to the signals for making proteins such as lysozyme in egg white. This is followed by transforming rooster sperm with a human gene and the appropriate promoters and checking for any transgenic offspring. Initial results from both methods indicate that it may be possible for chickens to produce as much as 0.1 g of human protein in each egg that they lay and these proteins are likely to have correct sugars to glycosylate proteins, something not possible when using *E. coli*.

Transgenic pigs have also been produced by fertilizing normal eggs with sperm cells that have incorporated foreign DNA. This procedure, called *sperm-mediated gene transfer* (SMGT), may someday be able to produce transgenic pigs that can serve as a source of transplanted organs for humans. Progress is being made on several fronts to introduce new traits into plants using recombinant DNA. The genetic manipulation of plants has been going on since the dawn of agriculture, but until recently this has required the slow and tedious process of cross-breeding varieties. Genetic engineering promises to speed the process and broaden the scope of what can be done. There are several methods for introducing genes into plants, including infecting plant cells with plasmids as vectors carrying the desired gene and shooting microscopic pellets containing the gene directly into the cell. In contrast to animals, there is no real distinction between somatic cells and germline cells. Somatic tissues of plants, for example, root cells grown in culture can be transformed in the laboratory with the desired gene and grown into mature plants with flowers. Therapeutic protein genes can be inserted into plants and expressed by them with glycosylation, reduced dangers inherent in tissue culture techniques and offer simple purification potential. Corn is the most popular plant for these purposes, but tobacco, tomatoes, potatoes, and rice are also being used. Some of the proteins that are being produced by transgenic crop plants: human growth hormone with the gene inserted into the chloroplast DNA of tobacco plants, humanized antibodies against such infectious agents as HIV, respiratory syncytial virus (RSV), sperm (a possible contraceptive), HSV, the cause of *cold sores*; protein antigens to be used in vaccines and other useful proteins like lysozymes and trypsin.

Transgenic animals are one of the most promising recombinant protein expression systems making it possible to produce plasma proteins, human antibodies and other proteins not easily derived from other sources; however, the development process is long as it takes 18–33 months from introduction of gene to production at usable levels. The FDA is about to approve first transgenic product, a human antibiotic expressed in milk.

The target protein is usually expressed in the mammary gland, often at high protein concentrations (50 mg/mL), resulting in a yearly production of 10–100 kg per animal (cows). The animal husbandry and milking procedures are known technologies upgraded to good agricultural practices (GAP). The whey fraction can be processed by known chromatographic procedures, resulting in high quality pathogen free drug substance bulk materials— a prerequisite for preclinical and clinical trials. For large-scale production (>100 kg/yr), the costs of raw products are approximately 10 times lower for transgenic animals compared to mammalian cell cultures, mainly because of reduction in capital investment.

Examples of major products undergoing clinical trials are alpha-1 antitrypsin (cystic fibrosis), alpha-glucosidase (Pompe's disease), and antithrombin III (coronary artery bypass grafting).

The considerations in the use of transgenic animals are different from those of cell culture techniques:

Need to redefine the MCB/WCB concept.

Consider the variation of milk composition with lactation period.

Control of sick animals and use of medications.

Presence of pathogenic agents in the expressed proteins.

Virus inactivation and documented clearance is required. There is a link between bovine spongiform encephalopathy (BSE) and Creutzfeldt-Jakob disease (CJD). Both types of CJD and other forms of transmissible spongiform encephalopathy (TSE) are probably caused by aberrant protein agents, named prions. Prions are notoriously difficult to inactivate without denaturing the protein product, but specific filters are entering the market. Prions have not been found in milk from bovine spongiform encephalopathy (BSE) infected cows, and use of good breeding practice and pathogen free purification facilities should reduce the risk of infections to a minimum.

Strategic methodologies such as milking pigs and rabbits can be very arduous besides other problems of herd control.

Coexpression of the animal protein in milk, often possessing close physical and chemical properties with the target protein (bovine serum albumin has, e.g., 76% homology with serum albumin); process design should include powerful purification procedures for removal of the co-expressed protein.

Regulatory controls are poorly defined.

High bioburden (levels up to 10,000 cfu/mL are common) can affect stability; raw milk cannot be stored for more than 12 h and some expressed proteins may not tolerate pasteurization; freezing and low temperature storage is therefore required.

15.6.1 Downstream Processing

Assuming the starting material is raw milk, it is normally converted to skim milk by centrifugation using techniques common in the dairy industry. After removal of casein the capture, intermediary purification, polishing concept can be applied using the same purification principles as for cell culture harvests. Special attention should be paid to proteases and to separation of the target protein from its animal counterpart co-expressed in milk.

15.6.1.1 Harvest

This step consists of removing fat micelles and casein; centrifugation, filtration, microfiltration, and possibly use of expanded bed. Variations in the starting material composition is associated with the lactation cycle, presence of sub-clinical infections, and so on, requiring testing after each milking to establish conditions of separation of therapeutic proteins. The most dominant proteins present in cow or sheep milk is α- and β-lactoglobulin, immunoglobulin, and serum albumin, but a number of plasma proteins may also be found. Skimming removes 95%–98% of lipid, still enough fat to affect the useful life of chromatographic capture column and to block filters used.

15.6.1.2 Capture

This step removes cell culture and process-derived impurities and to prepare the sample for intermediary purification. The shear bulk of casein (40 g/L) can be removed by precipitation at pH 4.5 or by adding precipitating agents such as polyethylene glycol. Use of low pH should be avoided as many proteins lose their biological activity such as glycoproteins may loose sialic acid residues. The casein micelles are solubilized by chelation of the calcium with EDTA or citrate prior to chromatography. Ceramic and organic membranes are used to remove casein micelles by micro- or ultrafiltration. Finally, clarification of skim milk using EDTA followed by addition calcium phosphate based particles has been used to reform casein micelles away from the target protein. Many proteins such as protein C bind to the casein micelles, and if the micelles are not dissolved, the protein C can be lost. The process is suitable for expanded bed or big bead technology in the capture step assuming that the protein does not bind to casein micelles. In a simple two-step procedure (de-creaming and capture), the protein solution is made ready for virus inactivation and purification. The typical chromatographic capture procedure is ion exchange chromatography, although AC or HIC may apply for some proteins. The particle size of chromatographic media should be in the range of 100–300 nm.

15.6.1.3 Virus Inactivation

Inactivation is typically (but not necessarily) performed after the capture step, where the sample volume has been severely reduced. Details provided for virus inactivation in other chapters on cell cultures apply here as well.

15.6.1.4 Intermediary Purification

This step removes cell culture and process derived impurities and to prepare the sample for polishing. The intermediary purification step offers a wide range of chromatographic principles (IMAC, HIC, IEC, HAC).

15.6.1.5 Virus Filtration

Membrane filtration can contribute to the overall virus reduction in a reliable and controlled manner without damaging the target protein.

15.6.1.6 Polishing

This step removes host cells, process and product related impurities. Powerful chromatographic methods (HP-IEC) are used to separate the protein from its derivatives (enzymatic cleaved forms, des-amido forms, oxidized forms, scrambled forms, etc.). RPC is probably not an option taking the type of molecules expressed in transgenic animals into consideration (monoclonal antibodies, complex proteins). The particle size of chromatographic media should be in the range of 15–60 nm.

15.6.1.7 Finishing

The use of SEC removes di- and polymer forms, small molecules (e.g., endotoxins, co-solvents, leachables). The co-expressed animal target protein must be efficiently removed.

Questions

1. While *E. coli* produce proteins efficiently, the most common use for *E. coli* is for the production of circular DNA. What additional step is often required to ensure that the protein will have the correct tertiary structure?
   Answer: An in vitro folding step is required since *E. coli* lacks the necessary chaperon proteins.
2. Name some of the benefits of using mammalian cells as the expression system.
3. If using a mammalian cell what validations of the cell bank are required?
   Answer: Absence of microbial contamination, absence of mycoplasma, absence of viruses and viral particles of species that it is raised in or will be used in.
4. Define the difference between gene regulation and amplification as used for increasing production in mammalian cells.
5. List the various ways a gene can be introduced into mammalian cells. Which is the most common?
   Answer: Microinjection, electroporation, calcium phosphate, DEAE-dextran, DMSO, polybrene, cationic lipid-mediated transfection. Lipid-based transfection is very common and available in many commercial kits.
6. What problems can using serum free media avoid?
7. If complexation with nucleic acids during the production of monoclonal antibodies is suspected, what can be done to reverse this process.
8. When a process designer is considering the use of yeast as the expression system, what are some of the possible problems that should be taken into account?
9. Why can yeast be used in many types of bioreactors?
   Answer: The hard cell wall makes them more resistant to damage from the mechanical parts of the bioreactors.
10. Which two purification steps can often be avoided with yeast as compared to bacterial expression systems?
11. While animal systems can offer high yield, what are some of the challenges in this field?
    Answer: What would be the analogous regulation in an animal system to the cell bank for mammalian cellular systems? How are diseases controlled in the animals? What steps need to be taken to prevent the presence of pathogens in the product?

16

Quality Consideration

LEARNING OBJECTIVES

1. Understand the roles of quality control and quality assurance in bioprocess design.
2. Recognize the key regulatory agencies in the United States and abroad.
3. Identity the key steps involved in product validation and how they relate to overall quality assurance.

16.1 INTRODUCTION

The overarching philosophy articulated in both the cGMP regulations and robust modern quality systems is that "Quality should be built into the product, and testing alone cannot be relied on to ensure product quality." Several key concepts are critical for any discussion of modern quality systems. Every pharmaceutical product has established identity, strength, purity, and other quality characteristics designed to ensure the required levels of safety and effectiveness. *Quality by design* means designing and developing manufacturing processes *during the product development* stage to consistently ensure a predefined quality at the end of the manufacturing process. A quality system provides a sound framework for the transfer of process knowledge from the development to commercial manufacturing processes and for postdevelopmental changes and optimization. Corrective and preventive action is a well-known cGMP regulatory concept that focuses on investigating and correcting discrepancies and attempting to prevent recurrence.

Change control is another well-known cGMP regulatory concept that focuses on managing change to prevent unintended consequences. The major implementation of change control in the cGMP regulations is through the assigned responsibilities of the quality control unit. Certain manufacturing changes (e.g., changes that alter specifications, a critical product attribute, or bioavailability) require regulatory filings and prior regulatory approval. A quality system also contains change control activities, including quality planning and control of revisions to specifications, process parameters, and procedures. In this guidance, *change* is discussed in terms of creating a regulatory environment that encourages change toward continuous improvement. This means a manufacturer is empowered to make changes based on the variability of materials used in manufacturing and optimization of the process from learning over time.

Many of the modern quality systems correlate very closely with the cGMP regulations. Current industry practice generally divides the responsibilities of the quality control unit (QCU), as defined in the cGMP regulations, between quality control (QC) and quality assurance (QA) functions.

QC usually consists of the testing of selected in-process materials and finished products to evaluate the performance of the manufacturing process and to ensure adherence to proper specifications and limits.

QA primarily includes the review and approval of all procedures related to production, maintenance, and review of associated records, auditing, and performing trend analyses.

The concept *quality unit* is consistent with modern quality systems in ensuring that the various operations associated with all systems are appropriately conducted, approved, and monitored. The cGMP regulations specifically assign the quality unit the authority to create, monitor, and implement the quality system. However, the quality unit is not meant to take on the responsibilities of other units of a manufacturer's organization, such as the responsibilities handled by manufacturing personnel, engineers, and development scientists.

The following are the other cGMP-assigned responsibilities of the quality unit are consistent with a modern quality system approach:

- Ensuring that controls are implemented and completed satisfactorily during manufacturing operations
- Ensuring that developed procedures and specifications are appropriate and followed, including those used by a firm under contract to the manufacturer
- Approving or rejecting in-process materials and drug products—although such activities do not substitute for, or preclude, the daily responsibility of manufacturing personnel to build quality into the product
- Reviewing production records and investigating any unexplained discrepancies

Under a robust quality system, the manufacturing units and the quality unit can remain independent but still be included in the total concept of producing quality products. In very small operations, a single individual can function as the quality unit. That person is still accountable for implementing all the controls and reviewing results of manufacture to ensure that product quality standards have been met.

Figure 16.1 shows the relationship among the six systems: one quality system and five manufacturing systems. The quality system provides the foundation for the manufacturing systems that are linked and function within it. The quality system model described in this guidance does not treat the five manufacturing systems as discrete entities but instead integrates them into appropriate sections of the model. Those familiar with the six-system inspection approach will see organizational differences in this guidance; however, the interrelationship should be readily apparent. One of the important themes of the systems-based inspection compliance program is to be able to assess whether each of the systems is in a state of control. The quality system model presented in this guidance will

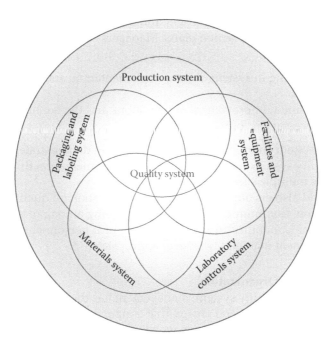

Figure 16.1 Six-way quality system.

also serve to help firms achieve the desired state of control. The model is organized into the following four major sections:

- Management responsibilities
- Resources
- Manufacturing operations
- Evaluation activities

16.2 MANAGEMENT RESPONSIBILITIES

Robust modern quality system models call for management to play a key role in the design, implementation, and management of the quality system. For example, management is responsible for establishing the quality system structure appropriate for a specific organization. Management has ultimate responsibility to provide the leadership needed for the successful functioning of the quality system.

16.2.1 Provide Leadership

In a robust modern quality system, senior management demonstrates commitment to developing and maintaining their quality system. Leadership is demonstrated by aligning quality system plans with the manufacturer's strategic plans to ensure that the quality system supports the manufacturer's mission and strategies. Senior managers set implementation priorities and develop action plans. Managers can provide support of the quality system by

- Actively participating in system design, implementation, and monitoring, including system review
- Advocating continual improvement of operations and the quality system
- Committing necessary resources

In a robust quality system environment, managers should demonstrate strong and visible support for the quality system and ensure its global implementation throughout the organization (e.g., across multiple sites).

Managers should also encourage internal communication on quality issues at all levels in the organization. Communication should be ongoing among research and development, regulatory affairs, manufacturing, and quality unit personnel on issues that affect quality, with management included whenever appropriate.

16.2.1.1 Structure of the Organization

When designing a robust quality system, management has the responsibility to determine the structure of the organization and ensure that assigned authorities and responsibilities support the production, quality, and management activities needed to produce quality products. Senior managers have the responsibility to ensure that the organization's structure is documented.

Managers have the responsibility to communicate employee roles, responsibilities, and authorities within the system and ensure that interactions are defined and understood.

An organization also has the responsibility to give the individual who is appointed to manage the quality system the authority to detect problems and effect solutions. Usually, a senior manager administers the quality system and can, thus, ensure that the organization receives prompt feedback on quality issues.

16.2.2 Build Your Quality System to Meet Requirements

Implementing a robust quality system can help ensure compliance with regulations related to safety, identity, strength, quality, and purity as long as the quality system addresses the minimum requirements of cGMP regulations as well as the needs of the manufacturer. Under the quality system model, the agency recommends that senior managers should ensure that the quality system they design and implement provides clear organizational guidance and facilitates systematic evaluation of issues. For example, according to the model, when documenting a quality system, the following should be included

- Scope of the quality system, including any outsourcing
- Standard of quality that will be used
- Manufacturer's policies to implement the quality system criteria and the supporting objectives
- Procedures needed to establish and maintain the quality system

It is recommended under a modern quality system approach that a formal process be established to submit change requests to directives. It is also recommended that, when operating under a quality system, manufacturers develop and document record control procedures to complete, secure, protect, and archive records, including data, which act as evidence of operational and quality system activities. This approach is consistent with the cGMP regulations, which require manufacturers to develop and document controls for specifications, plans, and procedures that direct operational and quality system activities and to ensure that these directives are accurate, appropriately reviewed and approved, and available for use.

16.2.3 Establish Policies, Objectives, and Plans

Under a modern quality system, policies, objectives, and plans provide the means by which senior managers articulate their vision of quality to all levels of the organization.

It is expected that under a quality system senior management would incorporate a strong commitment to quality into the organizational mission. Senior managers are expected to develop an organizational quality policy that aligns with this mission; commit to meeting requirements and improving the quality system; and propose objectives to fulfill the quality policy. Under a quality system, to make the policy relevant, it must be communicated to, and understood by, personnel and contractors (as applicable) and revised as needed.

Managers operating within a quality system are expected to define the quality objectives needed to implement the quality policy. Senior management is expected to ensure that the quality objectives are created at the top level of the organization (and other levels as needed) through a formal quality planning process. Objectives are typically aligned with the manufacturer's strategic plans. A quality system seeks to ensure that managers support the objectives with necessary resources and have measurable goals that are monitored regularly.

Under a quality system, managers would be expected to use quality planning to identify resources and define methods to achieve the quality objectives. It is recommended that quality plans be documented and communicated to personnel to ensure awareness of how their operational activities are aligned with strategic and quality goals.

16.2.4 Review the System

System review is a key component in any robust quality system to ensure its continuing suitability, adequacy, and effectiveness. Under a quality system, senior managers are expected to conduct reviews of the whole quality system according to a planned schedule. Such a review typically includes both an assessment of the product and customer needs (in this section, *customer* is defined as the recipient of the product and the product is the goods or services being provided). Under a quality system, the review should consider at least the following:

- Appropriateness of the quality policy and objectives
- Results of audits and other assessments

- Customer feedback, including complaints
- Analysis of data trending results
- Status of actions to prevent a potential problem or a recurrence
- Any follow-up actions from previous management reviews
- Any changes in business practices or environment that may affect the quality system (such as the volume or type of operations)
- Product characteristics that meet the customer's needs

When developing and implementing new quality systems, reviews should take place more frequently than when the system has matured. Outside of scheduled reviews, the quality system is typically included as a standing agenda item in general management meetings.

Review outcomes typically include

- Improvements to the quality system and related quality processes
- Improvements to manufacturing processes and products
- Realignment of resources

Under a quality system, the results of a management review are expected to be recorded. Planned actions should be implemented using effective corrective and preventive action and change control procedures.

Table 16.1 shows how the cGMP regulations correlate to specific elements in the quality system model for this section. Manufacturers should always refer to specific regulations to ensure that they are complying with all regulations.

Table 16.1 CFR cGMP Regulations Related to Management Responsibilities

Quality System Element	Regulatory Citations
1. Leadership	–
2. Structure	Establish quality function: §211.22(a) (see definition §210.3[b][15])
	Notification: §211.180(f)
3. Build quality system	QU procedures: §211.22(d)
	QU procedures, specifications: §211.22(c), with reinforcement in §§211.100(a), 211.160(a)
	QU control steps: §211.22(a), with reinforcement in §§211.42(c), 211.84(a), 211.87, 211.101(c)(1), 211.110(c), 211.115(b), 211.142, 211.165(d), 211.192
	QU quality assurance; review/investigate: §211.22(a), 211.100(a–b), 211.180(f), 211.192, 211.198(a)
	Record control: §211.180(a–d), 211.180(c), 211.180(d), 211.180(e), 211.186, 211.192, 211.194, 211.198(b)
4. Establish policies, objectives, and plans	Procedures: §211.22(c–d), 211.100(a)
5. System review	Record review: §211.180(e), 211.192, 211.198(b)(2)

16.3 RESOURCES

An appropriate allocation of resources is key to creating a robust quality system and to complying with the cGMP regulations.

16.3.1 General Arrangements

Under a robust quality system, there should be sufficient allocation of resources for quality system and operational activities. Under the model, senior management, or a designee, is responsible for providing adequate resources for the following:

- To supply and maintain the appropriate facilities and equipment to consistently manufacture a quality product
- To acquire and receive materials that are suitable for their intended purpose
- For processing the materials to produce the finished drug product
- For laboratory analysis of the finished drug product, including collection, storage, and examination of in-process, stability, and reserve samples

16.3.2 Develop Personnel

Under a quality system, senior management is expected to support a problem-solving and communicative organizational culture. Managers are expected to encourage communication by creating an environment that values employee suggestions and acts on suggestions for improvement. Management is also expected to develop cross-cutting groups to share ideas to improve procedures and processes.

In the quality system, it is recommended that personnel be qualified to do the operations that are assigned to them in accordance with the nature of, and potential risk to quality presented by, their operational activities. Under a quality system, managers are expected to define appropriate qualifications for each position to help ensure individuals are assigned appropriate responsibilities. Personnel should also understand the impact of their activities on the product and the customer (this quality system parameter is also found in the cGMP regulations, which identify specific qualifications—that is, education, training, and experience or any combination thereof).

Under a quality system, continued training is critical to ensure that the employees remain proficient in their operational functions and understanding of cGMP regulations. Typical quality system training would address the policies, processes, procedures, and written instructions related to operational activities, the product/service, the quality system, and the desired work culture (e.g., team building, communication, change, behavior). Under a quality system (and the cGMP regulations), training is expected to focus on both the employees' specific job functions and the related cGMP regulatory requirements.

Under a quality system, managers are expected to establish training programs that include the following:

- Evaluation of training needs
- Provision of training to satisfy these needs
- Evaluation of effectiveness of training
- Documentation of training and/or re-training

555

When operating in a robust quality system environment, it is important that supervisory managers ensure that skills gained from training be incorporated into day-to-day performance.

16.3.3 Facilities and Equipment

Under a quality system, technical experts (e.g., engineers, development scientists), who have an understanding of pharmaceutical science, risk factors, and manufacturing processes related to the product, are responsible for specific facility and equipment requirements.

According to cGMP regulations, the QCU has the responsibility of reviewing and approving all initial design criteria and procedures pertaining to facilities and equipment and any subsequent changes (see §211.22[c]). The Food and Drug Administration (FDA) can, as resources permit, provide a preoperational review of manufacturing facilities.

According to the cGMP regulations, equipment must be qualified, calibrated, cleaned, and maintained to prevent contamination and mix-ups. Note that the cGMP regulations require a higher standard for calibration and maintenance than most generic quality system models. The cGMP regulations place as much emphasis on process equipment as on testing equipment, while most quality systems focus only on testing equipment.

16.3.4 Control Outsourced Operations

When outsourcing, a second party is hired under a contract to perform the operational processes that are part of a manufacturer's inherent responsibilities. For example, a manufacturer may hire another firm to package and label or to perform cGMP regulation training. Quality systems call for contracts (quality agreements) that clearly describe the materials or service, quality specification responsibilities, and communication mechanisms.

Under a quality system, the manufacturer ensures that the contract firm is qualified. The firm's personnel should be adequately trained and monitored for performance according to their quality system, and the contract firm's and contracting manufacturer's quality standards should not conflict. It is critical in a quality system to ensure that the contracting manufacturer's officers are familiar with specific requirements of the contract. However, under the cGMP requirements, the QCU is responsible for approving or rejecting products or services provided under contract.

As Table 16.2 illustrates, the cGMP regulations are consistent with the elements of a quality system in many areas in this section. However, manufacturers should always refer to specific regulations to ensure that they are complying with all regulations.

16.4 MANUFACTURING OPERATIONS

There is a significant overlap between the elements of a quality system and the cGMP regulation requirements for manufacturing operations. It is important to emphasize again that FDA's enforcement programs and inspectional coverage remain based on the cGMP regulations.

Table 16.2 CFR cGMP Regulations Related to Resources

Quality System Element	Regulatory Citations
1. General arrangements	–
2. Develop personnel	Qualifications: §211.25(a)
	Staff number: §211.25(c)
	Staff training: §211.25(a–b)
3. Facilities and equipment	Buildings and facilities: §§211.22(b), 211.28(c), 211.42–211.50, 211.173
	Equipment: §211.63–211.72, 211.105, 211.160(b)(4), 211.182
	Lab facilities: §211.22(b)
4. Control outsourced operations	Consultants: §211.34
	Outsourcing: §211.22(a)

16.4.1 Design and Develop Product and Processes

In a modern quality system manufacturing environment, the significant characteristics of the product being manufactured should be defined, from design to delivery, and control should be exercised over all changes. Quality and manufacturing processes and procedures—and changes to them—should be defined, approved, and controlled. It is important to establish responsibility for designing or changing products. Documenting associated processes will ensure that critical variables are identified.

This documentation includes

- Resources and facilities needed
- Procedures to carry out the process
- Identification of the process owner who will maintain and update the process as needed
- Identification and control of critical variables
- QC measures, necessary data collection, monitoring, and appropriate controls for the product and process
- Any validation activities, including operating ranges and acceptance criteria
- Effects on related process, functions, or personnel

Management calls for managers to ensure that product specifications and process parameters are determined by appropriate technical experts (e.g., engineers, development scientists). In the pharmaceutical environment, experts would have an understanding of pharmaceutical science, risk factors, and manufacturing processes as well as how variations in materials and processes can ultimately affect the finished product.

16.4.2 Monitor Packaging and Labeling Processes

Packaging and labeling controls, critical stages in the pharmaceutical manufacturing process, are not specifically addressed in quality system models. Therefore, the FDA recommends that manufacturers always refer to the packaging and labeling control regulations at 21 CFR 211 subpart G.

In modern quality system environments, when new or reengineered processes are developed, it is expected that they will be designed in a controlled manner. A design plan would include authorities and responsibilities; design and development stages; and appropriate review, verification, and validation. If different groups are involved in design and development, the model recommends that responsibilities of different groups be documented to avoid omission of key duties and ensure that the groups communicate effectively. Plans should be updated when needed during the design process. Prior to implementation of processes (or shipment of a product), a robust quality system will ensure that the process and product will perform as intended. Change controls should be maintained throughout the design process.

16.4.3 Examine Inputs

In modern quality system models, the term *input* refers to any material that goes into a final product, no matter whether the material is purchased by the manufacturer or produced by the manufacturer for the purpose of processing. *Materials* can include items such as components (e.g., ingredients, process water, and gas), containers, and closures. A robust quality system will ensure that all inputs to the manufacturing process are reliable because QCs will be established for the receipt, production, storage, and use of all inputs.

The quality system model calls for the verification of components and services provided by suppliers and contractors; however, the model offers a method for implementing verification that is different from those in the cGMP regulations.

The cGMP regulations require either testing or using certificate of analysis (COA) plus an identity analysis. The preamble to cGMP states that reliability can be validated by conducting tests or examinations and comparing the results to the supplier's COA. Sufficient initial tests must be done to establish reliability and to determine a schedule for periodic rechecking. As an essential element of purchasing controls, it is recommended that data for acceptance and rejection of materials be analyzed for information on supplier performance.

The quality system approach also calls for the auditing of suppliers on a periodic basis. During the audit, the manufacturer can observe the testing or examinations conducted by the supplier to help determine the reliability of the supplier's COA. An audit should also include a systematic examination of the supplier's quality system to ensure that reliability is maintained. The FDA recommends that a combination approach be used (i.e., verifying the suppliers' COA through analysis and audits of the supplier). If full analytical testing is not done, the audit should cover the supplier's analysis; however, a specific identity test is still required.

Under a quality system approach, there should be procedures to verify that materials are from approved sources (for application and licensed products, certain sources are specified in the submissions). Procedures should also be established to encompass the acceptance, use, or rejection and disposition of materials produced by the facility (e.g., purified water). Systems that produce these in-house materials should be designed, maintained, qualified, and validated where appropriate to ensure that the materials meet their acceptance criteria.

In addition, we recommend that changes to materials (e.g., specification, supplier, or material handling) be implemented through a change control system (certain changes require review and approval by the QCU). It is also important to have a system in place to respond to changes in materials from suppliers so that necessary adjustments to the process can be made and unintended consequences prevented.

16.4.4 Perform and Monitor Operations

The core purpose of implementing a quality system approach is to enable a manufacturer to more efficiently and effectively perform and monitor operations. The goal of establishing, adhering to, measuring, and documenting specifications and process parameters is to objectively assess whether an operation is meeting its design (and product performance) objectives. In a robust quality system, production and process controls should be designed to ensure that the finished products have the identity, strength, quality, and purity they purport or are represented to possess.

In a modern quality system, a design concept established during product development typically matures into a commercial design after process experimentation and progressive modification. Areas of process weakness should be identified, and factors that are influential on critical quality attributes should receive increased scrutiny. The FDA recommends that scale-up studies be used to help demonstrate that a fundamentally sound *design* has been fully realized. A sufficiently robust manufacturing process should be in place prior to commercial production. With proper design, and reliable mechanisms to transfer process knowledge from development to commercial production, a manufacturer should be able to validate the manufacturing process. In a quality system, process validation provides initial proof, through commercial batch manufacture, that the design of the process produces the intended product quality. Sufficient testing data will provide essential information on performance of the new process, as well as a mechanism for continuous improvement. Modern equipment with the potential for continuous monitoring and control can further enhance this knowledge base. Although initial commercial batches can provide evidence to support the validity and consistency of the process, the *entire life cycle* should be addressed by the establishment of continuous improvement mechanisms in the quality system. Thus, in accordance with the quality system approach, process validation is not a onetime event but an activity that continues.

As experience is gained in commercial production, opportunities for process improvements may become evident. cGMP regulations require the review and evaluation of records to determine the need for any change. These records contain data and information from production that provide insights into the product's state of control. Change control systems should provide for a dependable mechanism for prompt implementation of technically sound manufacturing improvements.

Under a quality system, written procedures are followed, and deviations from them are justified and documented to ensure that the manufacturer can trace the history of the product, as appropriate, concerning personnel, materials, equipment, and chronology and that processes for product release are complete and recorded.

Both the cGMP regulations and quality system models call for the monitoring of critical process parameters during production.

- Process steps should be verified using a validated computer system or a second person. Batch production records should be prepared contemporaneously with each phase of production. Although time limits can be established when they are important to the quality of the finished product, this does not preclude the ability to establish production controls based on in-process parameters that can be based on desired process endpoints measured using real time testing or monitoring apparatus (e.g., blend until mixed vs. blend for 10 min).
- Procedures should be in place to prevent objectionable microorganisms in finished product that is not required to be sterile and to prevent microbial contamination of finished products purported to be sterile. Sterilization processes should be validated.

Pharmaceutical products must meet their specifications, and manufacturing processes must consistently meet their parameters. Under a quality system, selected data are used to evaluate the quality of a process or product. In addition, data collection can provide a means to encourage and analyze potential suggestions for improvement. A quality system approach calls for the manufacturer to develop procedures that monitor, measure, and analyze the operations (including analytical methods and/or statistical techniques). Knowledge continues to accumulate from development through the entire commercial life of the product. Significant unanticipated variables should be detected by a well-managed quality system and adjustments implemented. Procedures should be revisited as needed to refine operational design based on new knowledge. Process understanding increases with experience and helps identify the need for change toward continuous improvement. When implementing data collection procedures, consider the following:

- Are collection methods documented?
- Will the data be collected when in the product life cycle?
- How and to whom will measurement and monitoring activities be assigned?
- When should analysis and evaluation (e.g., trending) of laboratory data be performed?
- What records are needed?

A modern quality system approach indicates that change control is warranted when data analysis or other information reveals an area needing improvement. Changes to an established process should be controlled and documented to ensure that desired attributes for the finished product will be met.

Change control with regard to pharmaceuticals is addressed in more detail in the cGMP regulations. When developing a process change, it is important to keep the process design and scientific knowledge of the product in mind. When major design issues are encountered through process experience, a firm may need to revisit the adequacy of the design of the manufacturing facility, the design of the manufacturing equipment, the design of the production and control procedures, or the design of laboratory controls. When implementing a change, determining its effect should be based on monitoring and evaluating those specific elements that may be affected based on understanding of the process. This allows the steps taken to implement a change and the effects of the change on the process to be considered systematically. Evaluating the effects of a change can entail additional tests or examinations of subsequent batches (e.g., additional in-process testing or additional stability studies).

The quality system elements identified in this guidance, if implemented, will help a manufacturer manage change and implement continuous improvement in manufacturing.

Under a quality system, procedures should be in place to ensure the accuracy of test results. Test results that are out of specification may be due to testing problems or manufacturing problems and should be investigated. Invalidation of test results should be scientifically and statistically sound and justified.

The agency recommends that, upon the completion of manufacturing and maintaining quality, the manufacturer should consider shipment requirements to meet special handling needs (in the case of pharmaceuticals, one example might be refrigeration).

Under a quality system, trends should be continually identified and evaluated. One way of accomplishing this is the use of statistical process control. The information from trend analyses can be used to continually monitor quality, identify potential variances before they become problems, bolster data already collected for the annual review, and facilitate improvement throughout the product life cycle. Process capability assessment can serve as a basis for determining the need for changes that can result in process improvements and efficiency.

16.4.5 Address Nonconformities

A key component in any quality system is handling nonconformities and/or deviations. The investigation, conclusion, and follow-up should be documented. To ensure that a product conforms to requirements and expectations, it is important to measure process and product attributes (e.g., specified control parameters strength) as planned. Discrepancies may be detected during any stage of the process by an employee or during QC activities. Not all discrepancies will result in product defects; however, it is important to document and handle them appropriately. A discrepancy investigation process is critical when a discrepancy is found that affects product quality.

In a quality system, it is critical to develop and document procedures to define responsibilities for halting and resuming operations, recording the nonconformity, investigating the discrepancy, and taking remedial action. The corrected product or process should also be reexamined for conformance and assessed for the significance of nonconformity. If the nonconformity is significant, based on consequences to process efficiency, product quality, safety, and availability, it is important to evaluate how to prevent recurrence.

Under a quality system, if a product or process does not meet requirements and has not been released for use, it is essential to identify or segregate it so that it is not distributed to the customer by accident. Remedial action may include correcting the nonconformity, allowing the product to proceed with proper authorization and the problem documented, using the product for another application, or rejecting the product. If an individual product that does not meet requirements has been released, the product can be recalled. Customer complaints should be handled as discrepancies and investigated.

Table 16.3 shows how the cGMP regulations correlate to specific elements in the quality system model. Manufacturers should always refer to specific regulations to ensure that they are complying with all regulations.

Table 16.3   CFR cGMP Regulations Related to Manufacturing Operations

Quality System Element	Regulatory Citations
1. Design and Develop Product and Processes	Production: §211.100(a)
2. Examine Inputs	Materials: §§210.3(b), 211.80–211.94, 211.101, 211.122, 211.125
3. Perform and Monitor Operations	Production: §§211.100, 211.103, 211.110, 211.111, 211.113
	QC criteria: §§211.22(a–c), 211.115(b), 211.160(a), 211.165(d)
	QC checkpoints: §§211.22(a), 211.84(a), 211.87, 211.110(c)
4. Address Nonconformities	Discrepancy investigation: §§211.22(a), 211.115, 211.192, 211.198
	Recalls: 21 CFR Part 7

16.5 EVALUATION ACTIVITIES

As in the previous section, the elements of a quality system correlate closely with the requirements in the cGMP regulations. See Table 16.4 for specifics.

16.5.1 Analyze Data for Trends

Quality systems call for continually monitoring trends and improving systems. This can be achieved by monitoring data and information, identifying and resolving problems, and anticipating and preventing problems.

Quality system procedures involve collecting data from monitoring, measurement, complaint handling, or other activities and tracking this data over time, as appropriate. Analysis of data can provide indications that controls are losing effectiveness. The information generated will be essential to achieving problem resolution or problem prevention.

Although the annual review required in the cGMP regulations call for review of representative batches on an annual basis, quality systems call for trending on a regular basis. Trending enables the detection of potential problems as early as possible to plan corrective

Table 16.4   CFR cGMP Regulations Related to Evaluation Activities

Quality System Element	Regulatory Citations
1. Analyze Data for Trends	Annual review: §211.180(e)
2. Conduct Internal Audits	Annual review: §211.180(e)
3. Risk Assessment	–
4. Corrective Action	Discrepancy investigation: §211.22(a), 211.192
5. Preventive Action	–
6. Promote Improvement	–

and preventive actions. Another important concept of modern quality systems is the use of trending to examine processes as a whole; this is consistent with the annual review approach. These trending analyses can help focus internal audits.

16.5.2 Conduct Internal Audits

A quality system approach calls for audits to be conducted at planned intervals to evaluate effective implementation and maintenance of the quality system and to determine if processes and products meet established parameters and specifications. As with other procedures, audit procedures should be developed and documented to ensure that the planned audit schedule takes into account the relative risks of the various quality system activities, the results of previous audits and corrective actions, and the need to audit the entire system at least annually. Quality systems recommend that procedures describe how auditors are trained in objective evidence gathering, their responsibilities, and auditing procedures. Procedures should also define auditing activities such as the scope and methodology of the audit, selection of auditors, and audit conduct (audit plans, opening meetings, interviews, closing meeting, and reports). It is critical to maintain records of audit findings and assign responsibility for follow-up to prevent problems from recurring.

The quality system model calls for managers who are responsible for the areas audited to take timely action to resolve audit findings and ensure that follow-up actions are completed, verified, and recorded.

16.5.3 Risk Assessment

Effective decision-making in a quality system environment is based on an informed understanding of quality issues. Elements of risk should be considered relative to intended use, and in the case of pharmaceuticals, patient safety and ensuring availability of medically necessary drug products. Management should assign priorities to activities or actions based on the consequences of action or inaction—otherwise known as *risk assessment*. It is important to engage appropriate parties in assessing the consequences. Such parties include customers, appropriate manufacturing personnel, and other stakeholders. Assessing consequences includes using the manufacturer's risk assessment model to address risks, developing a strategy by deciding which options to implement, taking actions to implement the strategy, and evaluating the results. As risk assessment is a reiterative process, the assessment should be repeated if new information is developed that changes the need for, or nature of, risk management.

In a manufacturing quality system environment, risk assessment is used as a tool in the development of product specifications and critical process parameters. Used in conjunction with process understanding, risk assessment helps manage and control change.

16.5.4 Corrective Action

Corrective action is a reactive tool for system improvement to ensure that significant problems do not recur. Both quality systems and the cGMP regulations emphasize corrective actions. Quality system approaches call for procedures to be developed and documented

563

to ensure that the need for action is evaluated relevant to the possible consequences, the root cause of the problem is investigated, possible actions are determined, a selected action is taken within a defined timeframe, and the effectiveness of the action taken is evaluated. It is essential to maintain records of corrective actions taken.

It is essential to determine what actions are needed to prevent problem recurrence using information from sources such as

- Nonconformance reports and rejections
- Complaints
- Internal and external audits
- Data and risk analyses related to operations and quality system processes
- Management review decisions

16.5.5 Preventive Action

Being proactive is an essential tool in quality system management. Tasks can include succession planning, training, capturing institutional knowledge, and planning for personnel, policy, and process changes.

A preventive action procedure will help ensure that potential problems and root causes are identified, possible consequences assessed, and actions considered. The selected preventative action should be evaluated and recorded, and the system should be monitored for the effectiveness of the action. Problems can be anticipated and their occurrence prevented using information from reviews of data and risk analyses associated with operational and quality system processes, and by keeping abreast of changes in scientific and regulatory requirements.

16.5.6 Promote Improvement

The effectiveness and efficiency of the quality system can be improved through the quality activities described in this guidance. Management may choose to use other improvement activities, as appropriate. It is critical that senior management be involved in the evaluation of this improvement process.

Table 16.4 shows how the cGMP regulations correlate to specific elements in the quality systems model for this section. Manufacturers should always refer to specific regulations to ensure that they are complying with all regulations.

16.5.7 Conclusion

Implementation of a *comprehensive quality system model for* human and veterinary pharmaceutical products, including biological products, will facilitate compliance with 21 CFR 210 and 211. The central goal of a quality system is to ensure consistent production of safe and effective products and that these activities are sustainable. Quality professionals are aware that good intentions alone will not ensure good products. A robust quality system will promote process consistency by integrating effective knowledge-building mechanisms into daily operational decisions. Specifically, successful quality systems share the following characteristics, each of which have been discussed in detail earlier:

- Science-based approaches
- Decisions based on an understanding of the intended use of a product
- Proper identification and control of areas of potential process weakness
- Responsive deviation and investigation systems that lead to timely remediation
- Sound methods for assessing risk
- Well-defined processes and products, starting from development and extending throughout the product life cycle
- Systems for careful analyses of product quality
- Supportive management (philosophically and financially)

Both good manufacturing practice and good business practice require a robust quality system. When fully developed and effectively managed, a quality system will lead to consistent, predictable processes that ensure that pharmaceuticals are safe, effective, and available for the consumer.

16.6 QA SYSTEMS

QA systems are established to assure that every batch produced has similar characteristics. Whereas the role of in-process controls, standard operating procedures, and extensive documentation control are the keys to good QA practices, the specific process requirements in recombinant manufacturing and the inherent variability of biological systems make the QA systems more complicated; the need for stringent controls is evident in light of reported incidents in the use of biological products where the most common incidents involve incomplete virus inactivation, endogenous viral contamination, adventitious viral contamination, or entry of other infectious agents such as prions. It is important to realize that the QA systems are supposed to prevent manufacturing of out-of-specification product and not to prevent side effects or lack of efficacy if that is built into the process. For example, the most recent reporting of pure red-cell aplasia (PRCA) in the use of epoetin formulation in Europe was not a QA issue but a design issue; when albumin was removed and replaced with polysorbate, an aggregation that could not be predicted resulted in several PRCA cases. Such incidences are less frequent than the issues related to products being out of specification. The regulatory guidelines from ICH, FDA, European Medicines Evaluation Agency (EMEA), and Japan are very detailed in how the specifications are to be laid out and the tolerance allowed for each test. However, the manufacturers inevitably develop their in-house specifications and limits and QA procedures that are generally more stringent; in some instances, manufacturers add tests that are neither required nor reported to the regulatory agencies. This is one of the strongest claim made by innovator companies as they defend their position that there can never be a biogeneric product.

When new products are developed, whether generic or innovative, the planning for regulatory controls and compliance starts very early in the process; despite this well established practice, most delays in the approval of drug products occur because of poor early planning relating to QA issues. Some of these issues are listed as follows:

- Companies should arrange meetings with FDA as early as possible; the Division of Therapeutic Proteins is now a well-defined section under the Center for Drug Evaluation and Research (CDER) that is fully staffed to attend to all enquiries. The well-established system of filing for pre-IND conferences should be used extensively.
- The timelines should be made realistic; however, marketing pressures often cause the regulatory staff to squeeze the timelines. The same holds for adequate resources, both manpower and financial set aside, to develop the chemistry manufacturing and controls CMC sections.
- The problems related to product definition area readily solved in a generic situation, but when faced with a new product, the final product composition and definition often changes during development, making the regulatory filings more difficult and time consuming.
- The choice of cell line is critical; for example, growth hormone is produced using different types of cell lines; the choice of one over the other will depend on a large number of factors, not necessarily the financial ones; the safety of product and ease of production should be the prime considerations. Cell lines must be optimized and characterized in accordance with the ICH guidelines. The cells must come from certified traceable sources.
- The process design for cGMP manufacturing should be robust and scalable; though the FDA allows for process change through comparability protocols, these are expensive to run and should be highly discouraged; all factors should be studied prior to finalizing the process as little changes are made to it later.
- The availability of raw materials can often be a major problem, such as when securing albumin from a reliable source; all materials should be manufactured under cGMP compliance.
- In-process controls often prove inadequate when the process is scaled up; provisions should be made for this as well as for assuring that the documentation is as comprehensive as possible. Analytical procedures should be adequately validated, the assays rugged, and sufficient testing included. Parameters should be stated in intervals with a set point. Product specification and acceptance criteria should be well defined.

16.7 VALIDATION MASTER PLAN

The U.S. FDA defines process validation as "Establishing documented evidence which provides a high degree of assurance that a specific process will consistently produce a product meeting its pre-determined specifications and quality characteristics." The validation of pharmaceutical production is a general requirement of cGMP for finished pharmaceuticals (21 CFR 210 and 211). The validation procedure is often separated into a production facility qualification and a process validation, considering all features of a new product and its manufacture. Validation ensures that safe and efficacious products are manufactured, and this requires controlling not just the finished product but the manufacturing process itself. Process validation starts early; however, a full validation is not required until phase III cGMP manufacture.

The process validation program comprises acceptance criteria of raw materials, process rationale and strategy, a flow sheet, defining parameter intervals, defining critical parameters, column cleaning, column lifetime, filter cleaning, filter lifetime, and process performance qualification and addresses removal of process- and product-related impurities. However, each product is unique and requires a dedicated listing of important elements of validation.

The validation master plan (VMP) is a document that contains many components of QA systems; it begins with the process development and is updated throughout the process. An appropriate validation plan reduces the risk of missing out essential components in the CMC section, assuring batch compliance. The process validation is a major component of the VMP and includes elements such as

- Acceptance criteria for every analysis of in-process materials, active pharmaceutical ingredient (API), and drug product (DP).
- Identification of all analytical methods used including plans for qualification and validation.
- Characterization of cells used for propagation into cell cultures. The program comprises cell line history, substrate and raw material characterization, and test for microbial agents, fungi, mycoplasma, viruses, and prions. The ICH guideline on cell characterization is usually followed.
- Identification of critical parameters for each unit operation. Statistical factorial design is used to identify critical parameters.
- Stability studies, both short and long term:
  - For the product
  - For intermediary products stored for a certain amount of time. Product stability under the given storage conditions must be assured throughout the storage period.
- Process robustness testing results include specified parameter intervals, identification of critical parameters by statistical analysis, recoveries, yields, batch data, column and filter performances, and column and filter lifetimes.
- Flow sheets describing every unit operation.
- Identification and clearance methods for impurities:
  - Host cell–related impurities come from the host organism (e.g., endotoxins from *Escherichia coli*; viruses from insect cells, animal cells or transgenic animals, host cell proteins [HCPs], host cell DNA). Process steps, which are especially powerful in removing a specific impurity, should be identified and a clearance factor calculated, if possible.
  - Process-related impurities are substrates and reagents required by the process (viruses, prions, chemical compounds, enzymes, leachable from chromatographic resins). Process steps, which are especially suitable for removing a specific impurity, should be identified and a clearance factor calculated, if possible.
  - Product-related impurities are derivatives or isoforms of the target protein (e.g., di- and polymers, des-amido forms, oxidized forms, split products, scrambled forms, carbamylated forms). These impurities are normally removed at the polishing step(s).

- Protocols for every validation study conducted; these include statement of experimental objective, definition of what is to be qualified or validated, experimental plan, sampling plans, test plans with acceptance criteria to be met or established, and description of statistical analyses to be applied.
- Parameter intervals should be established for every unit operation and include: proven acceptable range (PAR), regulatory range, control range, and operating range.
- Identity, safety, process criticality, release procedures, and COAs must be addressed. ISO 9000-9004 standards are often used.
- References to
  - Analytical methods used: descriptions, method qualification, and validation
  - Pilot and manufacturing protocols and batch documentation
  - Relevant development documentation, direct or indirect (development report)
  - Summary reports, unit operation descriptions, protocols, and batch records
  - Stability reports, short and long term
- Sampling and testing plans to include sampling for end-of-production test, in-process control, QC, target protein characterization, holding times, and stability studies.
- Specifications include the analytical test program for API and DP.
- Validation task reports include product development summary, lot summary report, process performance report, in-process control report, and validation protocol completion report.

Validation studies depend on the type of protein, but mostly these comprise the following:

- Column lifetime is crucial and requires cleaning validation, sanitization, and test for leachables and assessment of column performance.
- Critical parameters are determined by statistical methods (e.g., fractional factorial design is common practice).
- Filter lifetime requires cleaning validation, sanitization, and test for filter extractables.
- Process robustness requires manufacturing of 3–5 continuous batches in small or pilot scale to meet specified acceptance criteria. The measurement of unit operation are recoveries and total yield.
- Raw materials require identification of critical raw materials, and identity, purity, suitability, and traceability are included.
- Removal of impurities comprises control of host cell–, process-, and product-related impurities.
- Virus validation requires assurance of virus removal from the target protein.

In regulatory filings, the requirement of validation studies depends on the phase of study:

Phase I: Virus validation with one or two model viruses; sterility and mycoplasma tests; critical analytical methods; removal of impurities of biological origin; generic assays for HCP, DNA, and endotoxins; product impurity profile; and API and DP to meet specified acceptance criteria. Process validation is not required.

Phase II: Critical analytical methods, others qualified; product impurity profile; and API and DP to meet acceptance criteria. No virus validation studies and no specific process validation are required, unless changes are made.

Phase III: Extensive virus validation; process validation on three or more consecutive batches; all analyses; specific assay for HCP; cleaning validation and lifetime studies for chromatographic columns; clearance studies for removal of HCP, DNA, and specific impurities; product-related impurities characterized if present in amounts of >0.1%; API and DP to meet specified acceptance criteria; critical process parameters and operating ranges defined; and worst-case scenario addressed.

16.8 RAW MATERIALS

Both biological and chemical raw materials are used such as cell culture nutrients, serum components, and inorganic salts, detergents, antifoam agents, enzymes, reagents, organic compounds, organic solvents, cleaning agents, growth factors, and chromatographic media. These should be manufactured under cGMP; pay closer attention to materials such as chromatographic media where the supplier should certify its cGMP status. Some raw materials such as chromatographic media require substantial testing before release for clinical production (a test period of one year or more should be expected). Some vendors have overcome this hurdle by providing regulatory support files for media to be used in biopharmaceutical processes. The qualification of raw materials is an ongoing process starting during process development. It is recommended to draft the master plan prior to entering production of material for phase I clinical studies and to establish specifications and standard operation procedures for all materials used. Critical materials should be identified and supplier data obtained. During phase II production, the master plan is updated, critical raw material assays are in put place, and the test for noncritical materials should be initiated. Stability assays should be established, where relevant.

The basic quality concepts include assurance of the identity, purity, suitability, and traceability of all the raw materials used to meet standards appropriate for their intended use. Raw materials must be quarantined, identified, and released by an authorized person and their identity proven by specific assays (often available from the vendor). COAs should be received for each lot of raw material. Each vendor must undergo a vendor qualification program (audit) such as described by the Parenteral Drug Association.

16.9 COLUMN LIFE

A typical chromatographic unit operation comprises application of sample, cleaning buffer removes impurities tightly bound to the matrix, elution buffer releases the target protein from the column, and equilibration brings column to its initial condition. The column is washed in one to several volumes of a specific wash buffer intended to remove impurities. If the process is run in campaigns, storage of the column(s) is an integrated part of the procedure requiring to define storage time and conditions. Each one of these unit operation steps is characterized by a set of parameter ranges (e.g., pH, conductivity, temperature, flow) and the buffer components used. Changes may take place within the specified intervals, but it is strongly recommended not to introduce changes outside the tested ranges as unforeseen responses may result. Thus, the entire chromatographic unit operation is an interlinked set of events, which in most cases are repeated several times before the matrix is replaced. Even use of strong cleaning agents such as NaOH, NaCl, or detergents cannot guarantee total removal of impurities, making each run a new event in which the outcome cannot be predicted. It is therefore necessary carefully to investigate the lifetime of the column by repeated runs. Such studies are for economical reasons and usually carried out in small-scale test columns operating under identical conditions except for the column diameter and load (prospective validation). Another approach is to correlate column performance with readily measurable attributes (e.g., recovery, clearance of specific impurities, back pressure, total organic carbon [TOC]) with specified acceptance criteria (concurrent validation). The advantage of the latter procedure is that it can be carried out in full scale during manufacture. However, demands to fast and reliable analytical methods and the risk of failed batches due to column failure should be taken into consideration.

The cleaning procedure is obviously a very important part of the chromatographic unit operation. The lifetime of a column may be several hundred cycles and build up of impurities that may severely affect the column performance (e.g., reduced capacity) and even result in leakage of tightly bound impurities into the product. Therefore, critical factors such as type and concentration of cleaning agent, contact time, flow rate, and temperature should already be investigated during process development. Typically, analytical methods such as enzyme-linked immunosorbent assay (ELISA), high performance liquid chromatography (HPLC), TOC, total protein, and visual inspection are used to measure the outcome. The final cleaning validation must be carried out in full scale.

The cleaning procedure should also be tested (challenge studies) for its ability to sanitize the column with respect to microorganisms, fungi, and spores. Examples of sanitizing agents are NaOH or hibitane (0.5%) in 20% ethanol or 20% ethanol with Hibitane.

Virus validation is an integrated part of the program if the target protein has been expressed in insect cells, mammalian cells, or transgenic animals. The first virus validation study is carried out before or during manufacture for phase I clinical material. Although column lifetime usually comprises a few cycles at this stage, the issue should be a part of the overall strategy. A more comprehensive virus validation study is carried out usually prior to phase III manufacture. The ICH guideline on viral safety states that "over time and after repeated use, the ability of chromatographic columns and other devices used in the purification scheme to clear virus may vary." Thus, a repeated virus validation study may be needed at the end of the column lifetime study.

The integrity of the column bed needs to be measured to confirm the quality and consistency of the chromatographic operation. Commonly used measures are the number of theoretical plates (N), the height equivalent to theoretical plate (HETP), the tailing factor (T), and the asymmetry (As). A high HETP indicates inefficient column packing, whereas a low HETP indicates that the probe molecule is retained on the column. The typical range of As is from 0.8 to 1.4. Values lower than 0.8 indicate column over packing, packing a too high pressure, or bed cracking. A value over 1.4 indicates that the column is not packed tight enough, and air pockets in column hardware void spaces or poor injection technique.

16.10 PROCESS

The process rationale is stated based on input on the target protein, expression system used, and specific demands to posttranslational modifications such as glycosylation, acylation, phosphorylation, or PEGylation. The process strategy should include the considerations related to product safety, process robustness, scale up, cGMP manufacture, and economy. The strategy should allow VMP revisions as the process "changes" from a phase I to a mature phase III. A flow sheet showing all process unit operation with indication of where critical raw materials or adventitious agents are entering the process and at which steps they are removed is provided. This includes removal of host cell–, product–, and process-related impurities.

16.10.1 Parameters and Responses

Robustness is introduced by controlling each step, and this requires developing critical process parameters. In fermentation/cell culture and downstream processing, the parameter intervals are identified; the operational parameters (factors) are linked to performance parameters (responses) by means of statistical methods. The identified lower and upper parameter limits help achieve uniformity in large-scale production where worse-case scenarios are tested to ascertain homogeneity. The following are some of these parameters and their selection process:

- Upstream process.
- Seed flask and fermenter culture is tested for pH, conductivity, and temperature, and the tested parameter is cell density.
- Bioreactor is monitored additionally by oxygen supply, nitrogen supply, nutrient supply, dissolved oxygen, aeration rate, agitation rate, pCO_2, methanol concentration, ethanol concentration, and holding time. The tested parameters are cell density, viability, respiration quotient, biomass, cell number, and target protein concentration.
- Centrifugation is monitored by pH conductivity, temperature, rotations per minute, g-force, time, and holding time. The tested parameters are recovery and volume of supernatant.
- Filtration is monitored by pH, conductivity, temperature, inlet flow velocity, cross-flow velocity, filtrate flux, retentate flux, re-circulation rate, back pressure, inlet pressure, outlet pressure, holding time, and load. The tested parameters are transmembrane pressure, volume of filtrate, volume of retentate, protein concentration, protein stability, amount of process-related impurities, bioburden, and yield.
- Precipitation is monitored by pH, conductivity, temperature, protein concentration, and holding time. The tested parameter is recovery.
- Chromatography conditions are monitored by pH, conductivity, load, linear flow, temperature, bed height, column diameter, and holding time. The tested parameters are back pressure, recovery, protein concentration, protein stability, amount of process related impurities, ultraviolet profile, selectivity, and resolution.

571

16.10.2 Robustness

Robustness studies are conducted using a fractional factorial design, wherein variables are tested at two levels, usually a low and a high value, to allow statistical variance analysis. The process takes several well-defined steps:

Identifying the goals of the unit operation or process: The purpose and expected outcome (e.g., recovery, protein stability, impurity profile) of the unit operation are defined in terms of minimally acceptable performance.

Choosing operational parameters: The number of variables to investigate is often large; however, this can be reduced by excluding extremely well-controlled parameters (e.g., narrow-range parameters) or parameters not expected to interact or influence the process outcome. On the other hand, parameters with strong process impact need investigation. Also, some parameter interactions can be predicted, for example, interaction of pH and conductivity in ion-exchange chromatography.

Defining ranges: Parameter ranges are difficult to define in early stages; however, narrow ranges can jeopardize large-scale operations, for example, adjusting pH in large volume tanks to a narrow range is more difficult than in liter flasks, which requires a broader range. Broader validated ranges add to robustness and allow for optimization. An acceptable range developed earlier is narrowed down to control or operating range. The limits are used to create worst- and best-case scenarios and are within 2–3 standard deviations.

Defining responses: Responses are unit operation/process outputs that measure performance against the predetermined goals, for example, specific biological activity, recovery, target protein stability, and content of specific impurities (e.g., DNA, endotoxins, viruses). Operational parameters are associated to specific responses in the process control (in process analytical control).

Designing the experiment: In many cases, it is sufficient to consider the factors affecting the production process at two levels. For example, the temperature for a fermentation process may be set either a little higher or a little lower; the amount of solvent in a chromatographic eluant can be either slightly increased or decreased. The experimenter would like to determine whether any of these changes affect the results of the production process. The most intuitive approach to study those factors would be to vary the factors of interest in a full factorial design, that is, to try all possible combinations of settings. This would work fine, except that the number of necessary runs in the experiment (observations) will increase geometrically. For example, if you want to study 7 factors, the necessary number of runs in the experiment would be $2^7 = 128$. To study 10 factors, you would need $2^{10} = 1,024$ runs in the experiment. Because each run may require time-consuming and costly setting and resetting of machinery, it is often not feasible to require that many different production runs for the experiment. In these conditions, *fractional factorials* are used that "sacrifice" interaction effects so that main effects may still be computed correctly. In general, it will successively "use" the highest-order interactions to generate new factors. For example, consider the following design that includes 11 factors but requires only 16 runs (observations) (see Tables 16.5 through 16.7).

Table 16.5 Example of Fractional Factorials for Determination of Ideal Process Parameters

Run	A	B	C	D	E	F	G	H	I	J	K
				Design: $2^{(11-7)}$, Resolution III							
1	1	1	1	1	1	1	1	1	1	1	1
2	1	1	1	−1	1	−1	−1	−1	−1	1	1
3	1	1	−1	1	−1	−1	−1	1	−1	1	−1
4	1	1	−1	−1	1	1	1	−1	1	1	−1
5	1	−1	1	1	−1	−1	1	−1	−1	−1	1
6	1	−1	1	−1	−1	1	−1	1	1	−1	1
7	1	−1	−1	1	1	1	−1	−1	1	−1	−1
8	1	−1	−1	−1	1	−1	1	1	−1	−1	−1
9	−1	1	1	1	−1	1	−1	−1	−1	−1	−1
10	−1	1	1	−1	−1	−1	1	1	1	−1	−1
11	−1	1	−1	1	1	−1	1	−1	1	−1	1
12	−1	1	−1	−1	1	1	−1	1	−1	−1	1
13	−1	−1	1	1	1	−1	−1	1	1	1	−1
14	−1	−1	1	−1	1	1	1	−1	−1	1	−1
15	−1	−1	−1	1	−1	1	1	1	−1	1	1
16	−1	−1	−1	−1	−1	−1	−1	−1	1	1	1

Note: The example is a $2^{(11-7)}$ design of resolution III. Overall, there are 11 factors and 7 of those factors are from a full factorial design, which indicates that 7 of the factors are confounded (i.e., they cannot be determined independently of other factors).

Table 16.6 Additional Example of a Resolution III Design

Run	A	B	C	D	E	F	G
			Design: $2^{(7-4)}$ Design				
1	1	1	1	1	1	1	1
2	1	1	−1	1	−1	−1	−1
3	1	−1	1	−1	1	−1	−1
4	1	−1	−1	−1	−1	1	1
5	−1	1	1	−1	−1	1	−1
6	−1	1	−1	−1	1	−1	1
7	−1	−1	1	1	−1	−1	1
8	−1	−1	−1	1	1	1	−1

Note: This time the example is $2^{(7-4)}$ and will be converted to the more robust resolution IV design in Table 16.7.

The foregoing design should be interpreted as follows. Each column contains +1's or −1's to indicate the setting of the respective factor (high or low, respectively). So, for example, in the first run of the experiment, set all factors A through K to the positive setting (e.g., a little higher than before); in the second run, set factors A, B, and C to the positive setting, factor D to the negative setting, and so on. Note that there are numerous

Table 16.7   Using Foldover to Convert the Resolution III Design in Table 16.6 to a Resolution IV Design

	Design: $2^{(7-4)}$ Design (+Foldover)							
Run	A	B	C	D	E	F	G	New: H
1	1	1	1	1	1	1	1	1
2	1	1	−1	1	−1	−1	−1	1
3	1	−1	1	−1	1	−1	−1	1
4	1	−1	−1	−1	−1	1	1	1
5	−1	1	1	−1	−1	1	−1	1
6	−1	1	−1	−1	1	−1	1	1
7	−1	−1	1	1	−1	−1	1	1
8	−1	−1	−1	1	1	1	−1	1
9	−1	−1	−1	−1	−1	−1	−1	−1
10	−1	−1	1	−1	1	1	1	−1
11	−1	1	−1	1	−1	1	1	−1
12	−1	1	1	1	1	−1	−1	−1
13	1	−1	−1	1	1	−1	1	−1
14	1	−1	1	1	−1	1	−1	−1
15	1	1	−1	−1	1	1	−1	−1
16	1	1	1	−1	−1	−1	1	−1

options provided to display (and save) the design using notation other than ± 1 to denote factor settings. For example, you may use actual values of factors (e.g., 90°C and 100°C) or text labels (*low* temperature and *high* temperature). Because many other things may change from production run to production run, it is always a good practice to randomize the order in which the systematic runs of the designs are performed. This design is described as a $2^{(11-7)}$ design of *resolution* III (three). This means that you study overall $k = 11$ factors (the first number in parentheses); however, $p = 7$ of those factors (the second number in parentheses) were generated from the interactions of a full $2^{[(11-7)=4]}$ factorial design. As a result, the design does not give full *resolution*; that is, there are certain interaction effects that are confounded with (identical to) other effects. In general, a design of resolution R is one where no l-way interactions are confounded with any other interaction of order less than $R-l$. In the current example, R is equal to 3. Here, no $l = 1$-way interactions (i.e., main effects) are confounded with any other interaction of order less than $R-l = 3 - 1 = 2$. Thus, main effects in this design are confounded with two-way interactions, and consequently, all higher-order interactions are equally confounded. If you had included 64 runs and generated a $2^{(11-5)}$ design, the resultant resolution would have been $R = IV$ (four). You would have concluded that no $l = 1$-way interaction (main effect) is confounded with any other interaction of order less than $R-l = 4 - 1 = 3$. In this design, main effects are not confounded with two-way interactions but only with three-way interactions. What about two-way interactions? No $l = 2$-way interaction is confounded with any other interaction of order less than $R\text{-}l = 4 - 2 = 2$. Thus, two-way interactions in that design are confounded with each other. One way in which a resolution III design can be enhanced and turned into a resolution IV design is via *foldover*. Suppose you have a 7-factor design in 8 runs, see Table 16.6.

This is a resolution III design, that is, two-way interactions will be confounded with the main effects. A typical design would test pH (7.5–8.5), conductivity (15–20 mS/cm), temperature (18°C–25°C), flow (100–130 cm/h), and load (10–15 mg/mL); the responses measured could be recovery, DNA content, and target protein stability. When critical parameters have been identified, further factorial studies link different unit operations, providing information of the entire process. This type of experimental design can be used to show process robustness during process validation at phase III manufacture.

You can turn this design into a resolution IV design via the foldover (enhance resolution) option. The foldover method copies the entire design and appends it to the end, reversing all signs (see Table 16.7).

Thus, the standard run number 1 was −1, −1, −1, 1, 1, 1, −1; the new run number 9 (the first run of the "folded-over" portion) has all signs reversed: 1, 1, 1, −1, −1, −1, 1. In addition to enhancing the resolution of the design, we have gained an 8th factor (factor *H*), which contains all +1's for the first eight runs and −1's for the folded-over portion of the new design. Note that the resultant design is actually a $2^{(8-4)}$ design of resolution IV. To summarize, whenever you want to include fewer observations (runs) in your experiment than would be required by the full factorial 2^k design, you "sacrifice" interaction effects and assign them to the levels of factors. The resulting design is no longer a full factorial but a *fractional* factorial. The $2^{(k-p)}$ designs are the "workhorse" of industrial experiments. The impact of a large number of factors on the production process can simultaneously be assessed with relative efficiency (i.e., with few experimental runs). The logic of these types of experiments is straightforward (each factor has only two settings). The simplicity of these designs is also their major flaw. As mentioned before, underlying the use of two-level factors is the belief that the resultant changes in the dependent variable (e.g., fabric strength) are basically *linear* in nature. This is often not the case, and many variables are related to quality characteristics in a nonlinear fashion. In the aforementioned example, if you were to continuously increase the temperature factor (which was significantly related to fabric strength), you would of course eventually hit a "peak," and from there on the fabric strength would decrease as the temperature increases. While this type of *curvature* in the relationship between the factors in the design and the dependent variable can be detected if the design included centerpoint runs, one cannot fit explicit nonlinear (e.g., quadratic) models with $2^{(k-p)}$ designs (however, central composite designs will do exactly that). Another problem of fractional designs is the implicit assumption that higher-order interactions do not matter; sometimes they do, for example, when some other factors are set to a particular level, temperature may be *negatively* related to fabric strength. Again, in fractional factorial designs, higher-order interactions (greater than two way) particularly will escape detection.

Statistical analysis: Frequency diagrams indicate the distribution of all outputs. Pareto plots estimate the relative strength of each variable and interaction. Analysis of variance (ANOVA) determines the statistical significance of the effects.

16.11 VIRUS VALIDATION

Virus safety evaluation requires selecting virus-free cell lines, testing unprocessed bulk, assessing the capacity of the downstream process to remove or clear viruses, and finally testing the product to assure absence of contaminating viruses.

16.11.1 Cell Substrates and Animals

Viruses are introduced into the cell bank by several routes such as derivation of cell lines from infected animals, use of viruses to establish the cell line, use of contaminated reagents (e.g., animal serum), and use of contaminants during handling of cells. Extensive screening for both endogenous and non-endogenous viral contamination is performed on the master cell bank (MCB). The working cell bank (WCB) test program very much depends on the extent of MCB characterization, and a complementary approach should be used. Cells at the limit of in vitro cell age should be evaluated once for those endogenous viruses that may have been undetected in the MCB and WCB. Another serious source for viral contamination is the feeding during fermentation. The test program, as detailed in the WHO requirements for the use of in vitro substrates for the production of biologicals and the ICH guidelines Q5A, B, and D, should always be complied. Serum and trypsin should be free of infectious viruses. Viral agents are tested using cell cultures to test monolayer cultures; the use of polymerase chain reaction (PCR) technology is getting good acceptance by regulatory authorities; the testing of viruses is also performed in animals and eggs to test for pathogen viruses that are not able to grow in cell cultures (e.g., suckling mice, adult mice, guinea pigs, fertilized eggs). Tests for retroviruses, endogenous viruses, or viral nucleic acid include infective assays, transmission electron microscopy (TEM), and reverse transcriptase (Rtase) of cells cultured up to or beyond in vitro cell age. Induction studies are generally not very useful. Testing for specific viruses is done for murine cell lines using mouse, rat, and hamster antibody production tests (MAP, RAP, HAP). In vivo testing for lymphocytic choriomeningitis virus is required. Human cell lines are screened for human viral pathogens (Epstein–Barr virus, cytomegalovirus, human retroviruses, hepatitis B and C viruses with appropriate in vitro techniques). PCR technology may be useful in specific virus testing. Transgenic animals used for the production of biotechnological products should be kept according to good agricultural practice (GAP). Adequate testing for viruses such as the test methods listed earlier should be performed.

16.11.2 Unprocessed Bulk

Adventitious agent contamination is tested at the end of the cell culture in the unprocessed bulk (if multiple harvest pools are prepared at different times, the culture shall be tested at the time of the collection of each pool). Test for adventitious viruses in continuous cell line cultures used for expression of recombinant proteins should include inoculation onto monolayer cultures of the same species and tissue type as that used for production, cultures of human diploid cell line, and cultures of another cell line from a different species. If appropriate, a PCR test or another suitable method may be used. The primary harvest material (milk) from animals is to be considered an equivalent stage of manufacture to unprocessed bulk harvest from a bioreactor.

16.11.3 Virus Inactivation and Removal

The validation of the virus removal during downstream processing is arrived from the evaluation of cell substrates, raw materials used, virus inactivation/removal, and testing of the final product. A retrovirus or adventitious virus contamination leads to concerns on product safety. Even if no virus infectivity or Rtase activity can be detected for MCB or WCB, the presence of virus-like particles (VLPs) can often be demonstrated by electron microscopy. The microscopic evaluation gives no answer on the biological relevance of suspicious particles, especially regarding their infectivity such as the presence of high numbers of A-type particles in hybridoma cells, where infectivity is extremely low or not detectable at all. Despite this discrepancy between the number of VLPs and infectivity, it is the general recommendation to calculate the overall reduction factor based on the particle number.

The presence of a virus of unknown origin cannot be excluded: An unidentified virus might have unknown and potentially harmful physiological effects, and it is the unknown nature of the virus contaminant, which complicates the development of a specific assay. Without a specific and sensitive assay, it is impossible to monitor the presence as well as the removal or inactivation of the virus along the downstream process of the protein drug. Preventive measures include extensive testing of the producer cells for specific viruses and testing for adventitious virus at a number of stages during fermentation.

The assessment of viral clearance or inactivation requires process evaluation using viruses, which are identical to or from the same genus or family as the virus(es), which are closely related to the known or suspected virus or nonspecific viruses. The process quantitatively estimates the overall level of relevant virus reduction obtained in the process (of viruses known to be present). It is not necessary to evaluate every unit operation of the downstream process if adequate clearance has been demonstrated in selected steps by deliberate addition of virus to the unit operation application sample. Due to the complexity of carrying out viral clearance studies and that log reduction factors of one do not contribute to the overall clearance factor, focus is on a few but efficient unit operations for virus removal (typically 2–3 in a downstream process). It may be difficult to assess the excess clearance (clearance measured minus risk measured), but this should be a central part of the effort to reduce the risk from viral contamination.

It is not recommended to perform the virus-spiking experiments in the cGMP facility. This is one exception in scaling large-scale manufacturing. It is acceptable to perform the virus validation studies in small-scale studies (with scalable equipment) preferably around the capture and intermediary steps to avoid any potential virus burden at the polishing step. Steps, which are likely to clear virus, should be individually assessed with sufficient virus present for adequate assessment. Chromatographic columns and filter devices used repeatedly should be validated with respect to cleaning in place and performance. Downscale factors of 100–1,000 can be achieved. Studies are best conducted under fractional factorial designs.

Virus inactivation is usually a complex two-phase event (fast phase 1 and slow phase 2). Samples are taken at different time intervals, and an inactivation curve is constructed including at least one time point less than the minimum exposure time. Quantitative infectivity assays should have adequate sensitivity and reproducibility and should be performed with sufficient replicates to ensure adequate statistical validity of the results. Assays for the detection of viral contamination produce highly variable results due to the biological nature of the test methods and comprehensive validation with respect to assay accuracy, reproducibility, repeatability, linearity, limit of quantitation, and limit of detection if needed. The need for objective statistical evaluation has been emphasized by FDA in "Points to Consider," EMEA in "Notes for Guidance," and ICH guidelines and otherwise widely in the literature. The two main in vitro assay methods used quantitative virus clearance studies are the plaque formation assay and the cytopathic assay. Both assays have been validated, and they are routinely used to determine virus titers. The ICH harmonized tripartite guideline Q5A, step 4, further describes details of assays.

The selection of model viruses for the purpose of validation is critical and must take into account the nature and origin of the producer cell line; the model virus should be close to identical to a virus suspected in the cell line or closely related to viruses that might infect the cell, for example, retroviruses for recombinant or hybridoma cells. To achieve a maximum reduction factor for virus, the model virus should be grown to high titers and should be detectable in a simple but sensitive assay. Care has to be taken when concentrating a virus solution to increase the volumetric titer: The aggregation of viral particles might lead to an increased but not relevant mechanical removal by means of filtration or a decrease in inactivation due to protection of viral particles in the core of the aggregate. Examples of useful model viruses used as unknown source of infection are SV40, human polio virus 1, animal parvovirus, a parainfluenza virus or influenza virus, Sindbis virus, RNA viruses, and murine retroviruses.

The downstream processing provides clearance of virus when using mammalian cell culture or when using components of biologic origin; the efficacy of these processes is verified just like the sterility testing is done for bacterial contamination, and thus, a statistical sample of the lot can be tested in accordance with sterility testing protocols. The effect of virus clearance is determined by spiking experiments for the respective unit operations. Virus distribution is monitored and balanced for the individual intermediates of such an operation: The virus titer of the load is measured and compared to the (residual) virus titer of the product containing fraction after processing, for example, the flow-through or eluate of a chromatographic process or the permeate of a filtration process.

Prior to the titration of process samples, the potential effect of the applied buffer solutions has to be investigated regarding interference with the detector cells or reduction of infectivity of the model virus. Typical detector cells for the titration of viruses are SC-1 cells (retrovirus), CV-1 cells (SV 40), L 929 cells (reovirus), and Vero cells (PI3). For an extended detection for retroviruses, the XC plaque assay can be applied, where SC-1 cells are inoculated with the respective sample; after a defined period of cultivation, the cell layer is UV irradiated and overlaid with XC cells. After plaque formation, the cell layer is fixed and stained and plaques are counted. With reference to the morphological shape of a retrovirus-infected cell monolayer, the titer is expressed in plaque or focus-forming units (pfu/FFU). Viruses not leading to the formation of plaques or foci are measured by their CPE (cytopathic effect) on the detector cells, and the titer is expressed as $TCID_{50}$ (tissue culture infectious dose for 50% of the entire cell number). The balance of virus distribution throughout the complete process step, that is, including corresponding fractions such as washing and regeneration steps of chromatography or the retentate of filtration, is unlikely for most processes due to the denaturation of virus by caustic solutions typically used for regeneration or due to capture of virus particles within the membrane matrix of a filter. The demonstration of virus clearance for a single validation experiment is limited mainly by two factors: the maximum available titer for the accepted viruses is in the range of 10^7 to 10^9/mL; it is further reduced by 1 log by the required spike of 1:10–20. Another limitation is the technical difficulty to titrate the entire process fluids: The volume of a sample is depending on the detector cell. Typically, the titration is performed using a sample volume of 0.1–1.0 mL.

The reduction factor of a unit operation is calculated upon the volumes of the process fluids and the virus titers measured for the load and the product containing fraction after processing. The reduction factor is typically expressed in log 10 units, the "individual reduction factor" R_i for each unit operation. The overall reduction factor for a virus within the entire purification process is the cumulation of the individual reduction factors. However, the cumulation of virus clearance can only be claimed for process steps, which represent different physicochemical measures. Based on a cell assay variability, which is measured in a logarithmic scale, a logarithmic reduction factor in the order of 1, that is, a 90% reduction in titer, is considered to be not significant for virus clearance. To set a numerical figure for the virus burden of a cell culture fluid at the time of harvest, electron microscopy is applied for counting viral particles in a distinctive volume. However, this approach raises additional questions: How representative can a few milliliters of sample be for a few hundred liter to several thousand liter scale of cell culture fermentation? Furthermore, the cells in culture are grown to densities between 10^6 and 10^7/mL; the number of cells investigated by electron microscopy (EM) is reduced by several logs and is about 10^3/mL. The identification of virus particles and their differentiation from particulate matter due to the preparation procedure requires extensive experience, and a confirmation of the viral nature is impossible. Examples are artifacts, which are originated from sample preparation, for example, high-speed centrifugation of cell culture supernatant; the pellets derived from centrifugation typically harbor complex aggregates that often conceal those details necessary to identify virus structures.

16.12 TESTING OF PRODUCT

It is usually not necessary to assay for the presence of noninfectious virus particles in the purified bulk if cell lines (e.g., CHO cells), which have been extensively characterized, have been used to express the protein, and if adequate clearance has been demonstrated.

16.12.1 Analytical Method Validation

QA systems assure that the analytical procedures are reliable and suitable for the intended use. GMP considerations require that not only should the quality of raw materials, personnel, equipment, and suppliers be assessed, but the analytical methods be fully validated. The extent of validation depends on the stage of development; in early phases, the methods are evolving and the main interest is in testing for efficacy and toxicity. However, prior to manufacturing clinical test batches, the methods must be fully validated. The elements of validation include specificity, linearity, range, accuracy, precision, detection limit, quantification limit, robustness, and system suitability testing. These requirements are identical to those used for any other testing method used as part of CMC preparation; details can be found elsewhere. For example, the validation of analytical procedures is described in the ICH harmonized tripartite guideline Q2B (http://www.ich.org/fileadmin/Public_Web_Site/ICH_Products/Guidelines/Quality/Q2_R1/Step4/Q2_R1__Guideline.pdf). Revalidation may be necessary if the manufacturing process is changed, if the drug product composition is changed, or if the analytical method is changed. The degree of revalidation required depends on the nature of changes. An analytical validation plan is a description of how the validation will be carried out. It is a part of the master validation plan. A formal report on analytical method description including sample preparation instructions, raw material and equipment list, method description, data collection procedure, results, and data interpretation should be provided. A formal validation protocol including specific sample and control replicate analysis sequences, validation characteristics, method of data analysis and reporting, working values for system suitability, assay performance requirements, assay limitations, and reference standard identification should be provided.

16.12.2 QC Systems

The testing of therapeutic proteins follows similar methods and protocols as used for chemically derived products including the in-process testing, as discussed under QA issues. The testing as a part of a comprehensive QC program monitors various parameters and responses, definition of critical parameters, in-process control of intermediary compounds, and tests of drug substance and drug product. In its usual description, QC comprises in-process control, control of drug substance/product, and a description of analytical methods used to characterize intermediary and final products. The most common in-process tests include measure for pH, conductivity, total protein, and redox potential. The drug substance/product testing follows the ICH guidelines in which the product is characterized with respect to identity, biological activity, immunoreactivity, purity, and quantity comparing data with specified acceptance criteria. Where a compendium monograph exists such as in the case of interferon, erythropoietin, growth hormone, or insulin, the testing on the final product and the concentrate is performed accordingly. The methods used are validated (and verified where there exists a compendium method), and an appropriate documentation is created to support this.

16.13 IN-PROCESS CONTROL

For biological products, safety is considered a larger issue than in the case of chemical products; impurities in the system are of lesser concern in chemical system than in biological systems as they can alter the three-dimensional structure of protein affecting its immunogenicity; so, while the levels of impurities may be well below what is considered unsafe or even undetectable, they can adversely affect the product. As a result, the product quality is inevitably linked to the process design, process robustness, process compliance with cGMP, and extensive QC programs including product specifications, process specifications, in-process control, drug substance and drug product testing, regulatory policies, and scientific understanding. In-process controls apply to control of raw materials, control of process variables, analytical testing of intermediary compounds, end-of-production test after termination of cell culture, and so on. In addition, in-process controls are included to control quality by monitoring process parameters and responses. This requires complete characterization of the process where the parameters and their action limits are well defined. This is accomplished in early stages of process development and scale up in the manufacturing of phases I and II clinical supplies and finalized with completion of process validation during manufacture of phase III material including regulatory and operating ranges. Retrospective validation, though routinely used in pharmaceutical manufacturing, may not be sufficient to assure that all essential parameters have been optimized to monitor in-, on-, and/or at-line processes during manufacture.

The goal of PAT (process analytical techniques of the FDA) is to understand and control the manufacturing process, which is consistent with our current drug quality system: *quality cannot be tested into products; it should be built-in or should be by design*. PAT is a system for designing, analyzing, and controlling manufacturing through timely measurements (i.e., during processing) of critical quality and performance attributes of raw and in-process materials and processes with the goal of ensuring final product quality. It is important to note that the term *analytical* in PAT is viewed broadly to include chemical, physical, microbiological, mathematical, and risk analysis conducted in an integrated manner. There are many current and new tools available that enable scientific, risk-managed pharmaceutical development, manufacture, and QA. These tools, when used within a system, can provide effective and efficient means for acquiring information to facilitate process understanding, develop risk-mitigation strategies, achieve continuous improvement, and share information and knowledge. In the PAT framework, these tools can be categorized as

- Multivariate data acquisition and analysis tools
- Modern process analyzers or process analytical chemistry tools
- Process and endpoint monitoring and control tools
- Continuous improvement and knowledge management tools

An appropriate combination of some, or all, of these tools may be applicable to a single-unit operation or to an entire manufacturing process and its QA. A desired goal of the PAT framework is to design and develop processes that can consistently ensure a predefined quality at the end of the manufacturing process. Such procedures would be consistent with the basic tenet of quality by design and could reduce risks to quality and regulatory concerns while improving efficiency. Gains in quality, safety, and/or efficiency will vary depending on the product and are likely to come from

- Reducing production cycle times by using on-, in-, and/or at-line measurements and controls.
- Preventing rejects, scrap, and re processing.
- Considering the possibility of real-time release.
- Increasing automation to improve operator safety and reduce human error.
- Facilitating continuous processing to improve efficiency and manage variability:
  - Using small-scale equipment (to eliminate certain scale-up issues) and dedicated manufacturing facilities.

- Improving energy and material use and increasing capacity.
- Using a combination of increased automation and real-time analysis reduces human error, facilitates continuous processing, and shortens process time.

16.13.1 Parameters

The biological manufacturing processes are clearly divided into distinct unit operations, normally comprising a single technical procedure (e.g., filtration) in which a sample is treated according to a protocol resulting in an output pool, precipitate, supernatant, and filtrate (e.g., sample ⇒ procedure ⇒ output). The sample and procedure parameters can be controlled, but the output is difficult to control because of a large number of parameters that control the upstream and downstream operations. In typical upstream processes, parameters such as pH, redox potential, and dissolved oxygen affect cell growth and stability; temperature, agitation rate, and flow rates affect cell growth, redox potential, and metabolic activity, which is further controlled by the supply of glucose and glutamine. Similarly, the parameters of importance in the downstream process and how they affect the outcome include

- Back pressure affects protein aggregates or other high-molecular increase pressure (should be kept constant).
- Conductivity affects stability, binding to chromatographic media, viscosity, turbidity, and holding time.
- Filtration inlet pressure affects flux, fouling, and cross-flow velocity.
- Filtration outlet pressure affects flux, fouling, and cross-flow velocity.
- Holding time affects stability and solubility.
- Linear flow affects protein binding ability in chromatographic media.
- Load affects capacity of chromatographic media (adjust accordingly).
- pH affects stability, precipitation reactions, formulation of des-amido forms, β-elimination, racemization, disulfide bond and cleavage, binding to chromatographic media, solubility, and holding time.
- Protein concentration affects stability, solubility, viscosity, turbidity, and holding time.
- Redox potential affects stability of inter- and intramolecular disulfide bonds, formation of oxidized forms, and holding time.
- Temperature affects stability, solubility, formation of protein derivatives, enzymatic activity of proteolytic enzymes, reaction kinetics, and holding time.
- Transmembrane pressure affects filtrate flow, flux, and fouling.
- Turbidity affects ability to pass filters and chromatographic media.
- Viscosity affects ability to pass filters and chromatographic media.

Because of complex composition of the sample, it is frequently difficult to fully characterize the sample, a prerequisite to operation control because the procedure applied can have unpredictable responses such as cell density, cell viability, specific production rate, ammonia concentration, expression level, specific amino acid concentration, NADH/NADPH ratio, and lactate dehydrogenase activity in the upstream process and yield, retention time, UV profile, protein stability, and biological activity in the downstream process.

The parameters are stated in terms of intervals and not set points to allow for adjustments particularly in large-scale operations, defining lower and upper limits, to allow for statistical multivariate data analysis, and to allow for process optimization without process redesign. The specified range intervals as specified in regulatory documents are further refined with internal action limits that are a PAR based on small-scale experiments and with compliance in the case of worst-case scenarios as dictated by the U.S. FDA. The statistical methods applied to validating the interval ranges are arrived at using factorial designs.

The intermediate products are tested analytically extensively in the process development stages to obviate such testing during manufacturing operations. Typical in-process control analyses are test for microbial agents, test for fungi, test for mycoplasmas, test for viruses, test for endotoxins, one-dimensional sodium dodecyl sulfate polyacrylamide gel electrophoresis (1D-SDS PAGE), high-performance ion exchange chromatography (HP-IEC), high-performance reversed phase chromatography (HP-RPC), high-performance size exclusion chromatography (HP-SEC), and ELISA. The following are details on some of these tests and their limitations.

Parameters are often monitored using a continuous probe system such as those found in the many automated controls offered in a modern fermenter. An unusual situation arises in the monitoring of biological manufacturing because the properties of the medium monitored changes with time; for example, the pH change may be accompanied by change in temperature, ionic strength, other solute strengths, and redox potential; the pH probes therefore should be validated to take into account all these factors. This type of work will likely be conducted as part of PAT exercise; however, it will be impossible to select all pertinent factors ahead of the completion of the process development, requiring revalidation of the probes. Another problem arises in the stability and robustness of the probes itself. In many instances, the solutions can alter the probes because of chemical or biological reactions, and thus, a shelf life of each probe must be predetermined. Other aspects that must be examined include the common factors in the measurement of parameters. For example, pH measurements are affected by the ionic strength of the solution and temperature (which should be the same as used during calibration). When measuring redox potential, it is often impossible to obtain stable measurements. Instead, the potential will shift toward more negative values (e.g., biological systems). The reason for the slow exchange of electrons with the platinum electrode as the redox center is because the electrode is often being shielded by protein. A rapid measurement can be achieved by adding a redox mediator capable of making rapid exchanges of electrons with the electrode. In practice, a mediator is chosen having E_{m7} (the midpoint redox potential at pH 7.0) close to the estimated redox potential of the solution at a given pH (these E_m values can be used at a different pH considering $\Delta pH[2 - 10]$) ~ −400 mV or approximately −50 mV per increase in pH unit). The volume of the mediator must be small compared to the volume of the solution. Good results are often obtained with a mediator volume of a few drops of a 0.05% solution to 100 mL of test solution. It is common practice to perform redox titration in both oxidative and reductive sequences, vary the concentration of mediators in 10^{-6} to 10^{-3} range, and use mediators in the range of E_m (± 60 mV) to the redox couple being measured.

As is well known for the pKs of the pH buffers, the E region of greatest resistance is close to the redox E_m value of the mediator. Because of temperature fluctuations in the process, one must ensure that all redox potential measurements include a temperature reference. Special precautions must be taken regarding the influence of oxygen, for example, by use of an oxygen-free protective gas such as nitrogen.

16.13.2 Total Protein

In testing protein content, sensitivity is not an issue, and method chosen is a matter of convenience, sample, amount, purity, interfering compounds, sensitivity, accuracy, and assay time. The chromogenic assays are used for a fast evaluation of protein content in crude samples, but they may later on be exchanged with quantitative methods, such as Kjeldahl. The UV spectrometry assay is preferably used in purified samples with a high content of target protein, and amino acid analysis is typically used for the quantification of drug substance reference standards. It may be a useful strategy to use two different methods for the determination of total protein and compare the results.

The methods of choice are the following:

- The bicinchoninic acid (BCA) assay, a copper-based spectrophotometric assay, is often preferred to the biuret or Lowry assay because of its simplicity and ruggedness toward many buffer components. The accuracy is good, but protein-to-protein differences in reactivity can occur. Major interfering agents are strong acids, ammonium sulfate, and lipids.
- The copper-based biuret assay is among the oldest of the total protein assays offering low sensitivity (1–10 mg/mL) and is still used frequently in more concentrated solutions. The major interfering agents are ammonium salts.
- The Bradford assay uses the ability of the Coomassie brilliant blue G-250 dye to bind to peptides and proteins. Upon binding, the dye undergoes a color shift from 465 to 595 nm. This assay can be used in dilute solutions.
- The Lowry assay and its modifications (Hartree–Lowry) are enhancements of the biuret reaction making use of the Folin–Ciocalteu reagent. The color reaction is time dependent, and protein-to-protein variations may occur. The accuracy is good. Numerous buffer components can interfere with the assay (e.g., strong acids, ammonium sulfate).
- The Kjeldahl assay is a quantitative method for nitrogen determination, also in crude samples. The method is based on the fact that nearly all proteins contain approximately 16.5% nitrogen by weight, which gives a conversion factor between nitrogen and protein content of approximately 6. The sample must be free of interfering nitrogen-containing compounds.
- UV spectrometry measures the absorbance at 277–280 nm (tyrosine and tryptophan), which is an indirect measure of the protein concentration. In protein mixtures, an average extinction coefficient must be used, and the method is consequently semi-quantitative if not used relative to a quantitative method such as Kjeldahl. Major interfering agents are detergents, nucleic acids, particulates, and lipid droplets.

The accuracy of the assay depends on the validity of the standard curve and thereby the quality of the standard solution used (stability, purity, protein). In addition, the buffers used for the standard curve must reflect the buffer of the sample to be analyzed. Interfering compounds should preferably be identified and the signal from blank samples monitored. Time of reaction is of importance for some assays (e.g., Lowry), and test samples must be treated accordingly. Common practice is to prepare a minimum of five standard points in duplicate or triplicate across a 5- to 10-fold range of concentration. It is important to realize that good performance in calibration with single, fairly pure proteins does not necessarily translate into reliable performance with real samples. Samples are generally dialyzed, desalted, or precipitated with trichloroacetic acid (TCA) prior to analysis to remove interfering compounds where suspected; for example, nucleic acids are precipitated with polyethyleneimines (PEI).

16.13.3 Specifications

Specifications comprise a list of tests, references to analytical procedures, and appropriate criteria that are numerical limits, ranges, or other criteria for the test described to establish the set of criteria to which a drug substance or drug product or an intermediary compound should conform to; this conformity of batch data to specified test acceptance criteria is an important part of the batch QC release (COA).

The specifications are developed in the early part of process and product development (process design, scale up, non-GMP manufacture, and cGMP manufacture for clinical phases I and II), wherein the active drug is fully characterized for its physiochemical properties, biological activity, immunochemical properties, purity, and quantity. The acceptance criteria are related to the analysis method chosen and established as early as possible; however, throughout the development process, these specifications change, partly as a result of scale up and partly as a result of a better understanding of the relevance of the parameters to activity including the identification of product and process impurities. Examples of the ICH recommendations of characterization parameters include appearance (color, clarity), identity (amino acid composition, amino acid sequence, circular dichroism, differential scanning calorimetry, electron paramagnetic resonance, mass spectrometry [MS], isoelectric focusing, isoform pattern, native electrophoresis, near-infrared spectroscopy, nuclear magnetic resonance spectroscopy (NMR), peptide map, 2D electrophoresis, X-ray diffraction), biological activity (animal assays, cell assays, receptor assays, as applicable), immunochemical properties (antigen-binding assays), purity (capillary electrophoresis [CE], ELISA-HCP, HP-IEC, HP-RPC, HP-SEC, Limulus amebocyte lysate [LAL] test, PCR), quantitative amino acid analysis (Kjeldahl analysis, UV absorbance), sterility, pH, and osmolality.

Identity of the active product is established using tests for primary, secondary, and tertiary structure, posttranslational modifications, and physiochemical properties of the drug substance/product. These tests include determination molecular weight (MW), isoform pattern, extinction coefficient, electrophoretic patterns, liquid chromatography patterns, and spectroscopic profiles. The structural characterization program often includes amino acid sequence, amino acid composition, terminal amino acid sequence, peptide map, sulfhydryl group(s) and disulfide bridges, X ray diffraction, NMR analysis, and carbohydrate structure. Animal, cell, receptor, ligand, and biochemical assays may be used to determine the biological activity of the product. Potency (expressed in units) is the quantitative measure of biological activity. When possible, the biological activity should be compared to that of the natural product.

Additional tests required for therapeutic proteins include tests for potential to induce immunogenicity, which is difficult to assess, and the only real test of the immunogenicity potential is ascertain once the drug goes into actual use where millions of doses administered over a longer period of time provide the only correct evaluation of immunogenicity. Early studies can only identify significant hypersensitivity and allergic reactions. However, assays such as binding to antibodies are becoming increasingly accepted, and the FDA has been emphasizing development of highly sensitive assays to detect antibodies at below nanogram levels. The immunogenicity potential becomes more relevant when the molecules are modified from their natural state, such as PEGylation, wherein unexpected immunogenic responses can be expected.

Impurities in biological products can be adventitious agents, process impurities, and product impurities. Virus infection risk is a lesser concern if a bacterial expression system has been used, but the presence of scrambled forms of the target protein arising from the in vitro folding could be an issue. Therefore, protein purity should not be related to a few analytical methods but rather be analyzed on the basis of the expression system used, the process design, and the derivatives of the target protein arising as a consequence of upstream and downstream processing.

Impurity identification and quantitation is more important for biological products because even small concentrations of impurities can significantly alter the protein structure, though they themselves may not be harmful. The host cell–related impurities arrive from the construction of the recombinant organism, from eventual infections of the cell, from compounds co-expressed with the target protein, or from cells undergoing apoptosis and lysis. Examples of host cell–related impurities are endotoxins, viruses, prions nucleic acids, host cell lipids and proteins, and proteolytic enzymes. The process-related impurities encompass those that are derived from the manufacturing process (upstream, downstream, and formulation). Examples of process-related impurities are bacteria, yeast, fungi, mycoplasmas, viruses, prions endotoxins, raw materials, and cell culture substrates. This category also includes adventitious agents not intentionally used in the process such as mycoplasma infections of the cell culture. The product-related impurities are target product derivatives such as des-amido forms, oxidized forms, scrambled forms, glycoslylated forms, cleaved forms, carbamylated forms, acylated forms, and polymeric forms. These forms may be physically and chemically closely related to the target protein and may also exhibit full or partly biological activity. Especially, the polymeric forms may be immunogenic. In a regulatory sense, some of these derivatives are not regarded as impurities if they have similar properties (activity, efficacy, safety) as the desired product.

Quantity is usually measured as amount of total protein present in the sample of highly purified recombinant products. Quantitative methods such as amino acid analysis, Kjeldahl, or UV absorbance are used for quantity determination. In less-pure products, immunogenic assays (e.g., ELISA) may be used to determine the quantity of the active drug.

16.13.4 Identity

An important part of the overall characterization program for a recombinant-derived protein is the identity tests confirming MW, isoelectric point (pI), primary structure, secondary structure, tertiary structure, quaternary structure, possible posttranslational modifications, liquid chromatography patterns, and biomolecular interactions. Identity is generally a qualitative measure of the physical and chemical target protein properties favoring specificity over sensitivity.

Protein structure and function is closely related. Even minor deviations in the three-dimensional conformation or in the posttranslational modifications (e.g., glycosylation, phosphorylation, or acylation pattern) may result in altered biological activity or in an adverse immunogenic/allergic response.

During the drug development phase, extensive characterizations programs are exerted on reference materials (often of the drug substance level) to confirm the chemical and physical properties of the protein and to compare the recombinant product with its natural counterpart, if possible. Only a minority of the identity tests will be used for batch release.

The standard methods for the determination of MW are electrospray MS, matrix-assisted laser desorption ionization time-of-flight, HP-SEC, and ultrafiltration. The MW can be determined if the sedimentation coefficient is known. Various ultrafiltration sedimentation velocity measurements (sedimentation velocity, difference sedimentation, and sedimentation equilibrium) are used to gain information on shape and conformation. This is a useful check of homogeneity. Scanning TEM is used for the determination of MW of large particles.

The pI is the pH, where the protein has no net charge. The standard methods for the determination of pI are isoelectric focusing (IEF) in polyacrylamide gels and CE-IEF. The separation principle is based on charge heterogeneity caused by differences in amino acid residue charges. It is common practice to include a sample of the natural protein, if possible. The pI may also be determined by means of 2D electrophoresis, where molecules are separated according to pI and MW.

The primary structure provides information of the amino acid sequence of the protein. For most proteins, a primary structure analysis comprises N-terminal sequencing by Edman degradation, C-terminal analysis, and peptide mapping followed by HP-RPC purification and subsequent determination of the MW of the fragment by mass spectroscopy. Peptides and smaller proteins may be sequenced by means of only Edman degradation. The amino acid sequence is often supported by total amino acid analysis in comparison with the cloned gene sequence and the MW determination. Comparative fingerprints between the natural and the recombinant protein are also used to confirm primary structure identity.

The secondary structure provides information on disulfide bond arrangement, α-helix, and β-sheet content. The standard methods for the determination of disulfide arrangements are peptide mapping by HP-RPC or sodium dodecyl sulfate polyacrylamide electrophoresis (SDS-PAGE). Structural information is obtained by means of fluorescence, far UV circular dichroism, Raman scattering, and infrared absorption using Fourier transform infrared spectroscopy (FTIR). The spectroscopic methods are very powerful when used for comparison analysis with the natural counterpart. The confirmation of correct disulfide linkage is usually carried out on appropriate enzymatic or chemical digests of the target protein followed by HP-RPC purification of the fragments and subsequent mass analysis using electrospray ionization mass spectrometry (ESI-MS) or matrix-assisted laser desorption ionization time-of-flight. The analysis may be challenged by close neighboring cysteinyl residues, making it difficult to cleave the protein at least once between successive Cys residues. Cleavage techniques must take the possibility of disulfide bond interchange into consideration at pH above 7, where some proteolytic enzymes have their optimum. Scrambling is catalyzed by the presence of free cysteinyl residues or free cysteine, but these can be blocked before digestion.

The tertiary structure is the three dimensional structure of the molecule. The standard methods for tertiary structure determination are NMR (in solution), X-ray diffraction using crystals at high atomic resolution (<3 Å), and near-UV circular dichroism. The latter method is very powerful for comparison analysis with the natural counterpart

The quaternary structure of a protein is the structure that results from interaction between individual polypeptide chains to yield larger aggregates. The individual chains are often referred to as subunits. The standard methods for the determination of quaternary structure are HP-SEC, Raman scattering, light scattering useful for the determination of large macromolecular assemblies, and scanning TEM for the determination of MW of large particles.

Posttranslational modifications are chemical modifications of side groups (e.g., oxidation of Met, de-amidation of Asn of Gln), phosphorylation, glycosylation, fatty acid acylation, farnesylation, sialic acid capping, N-methylation, and acetylation. Typical standard methods for the detection of posttranslational modifications are HP-RPC, HP-IEC, or mass spectroscopy. In mass spectroscopy, the MW of the molecule can be determined with high accuracy and precision (better than 0.01%). This performance is normally sufficient to identify modifications such as missing residues or additional groups. Peptide mapping using specific enzymes and subsequent HP-RPC purification of the fragments prior to MW detection is also used for the determination of glycosylation patterns. Heterologous glycosylated products are often identified by their IEF slab gel pattern or more rarely by 2D electrophoresis. A thorough carbohydrate structural analysis may include glycosylation site(s), the carbohydrate chain structure, the oligosaccharide pattern, and the content of neutral sugars, amino sugars, and sialic acids.

The extinction coefficient can be determined from a known protein quantity (protein concentration) and the absorbance at 277–280 nm.

In chromatography evaluation, the target protein retention time using HP-IEC or HP-RPC can be used as an identity marker. For biomolecular interaction analysis, the method uses surface plasmon resonance to detect biomolecular interactions.

16.13.5 Biological Activity

The biological activity describes the ability or capacity of the drug substance to achieve a defined biological effect. Examples of procedures used to measure the biological activity include animal-based biological assays, cell culture–based biological assays, biochemical assays, ligand assays, and receptor-binding assays. A biologic assay may be replaced by physicochemical tests, provided sufficient information and correlation between the bioassay and the said tests can be given and there exists a well-established manufacturing history (ICH harmonized tripartite guideline Q6B). In some cases, the specific biological activity may provide additional useful information.

16.13.6 Purity

Protein purity has been historically linked to the specific biological activity in terms of units of biological activity per mass unit of the product. The purest product was that of the highest specific biological activity. In contrast to drugs based on small molecules, which could be controlled on the drug product level, protein-based pharmaceuticals were closely linked to the process itself because of the complexity of the active pharmaceutical ingredient and the lack of proper characterization of the final product. With the introduction of recombinant technology and modern analytical methods, a much better drug substance/product characterization became possible, resulting in the well-characterized protein concept and the widespread use of comparability studies. The importance of stronger focus on the presence of adventitious agents and specific impurities was also recognized, as the presence of even minor amounts of toxic, immunogenic, or adventitious compounds proved to have severe side effects. Unless otherwise specified, the level of impurities acceptable depends on the nature of the drug product and the dose.

16.13.7 Endotoxins

Endotoxins come from gram-negative bacteria (e.g., *E. coli*), if it is used as the expressions system. The presence of endotoxins indicates bacterial contamination in raw materials, columns, water, and buffers. Endotoxins bind strongly to anion exchange media even at high ionic strength, and thus, hydrophobic interaction chromatography (HIC) and cation exchange chromatography (CEC) are used for their removal, provided the target protein binds to the matrix. Binding of the target protein to cation exchange also allows effective endotoxin clearance. SEC can remove endotoxins, provided the differences in MW between the endotoxins and the protein are sufficient. However, SEC may be an unpredictable method, because endotoxins range in size from subunits of 10–20 KDa in the presence of detergents to vesicles of 0.1 Pm in diameter in the presence of divalent cations. In the absence of significant levels of divalent cations and surface-active agents, they dissociate into micelles of 300–1,000 KDa.

Traditional inactivation methods (CIP) against endotoxins include acid hydrolysis, base hydrolysis, oxidation, alkylation, heat, and ionizing radiation. To ensure complete removal from chromatographic columns, the use of NaOH is recommended (the concentration depends on the matrix used). Endotoxins are destroyed by exposure to NaOH or peracetic acid but are not affected by ethanol.

16.13.8 Nucleic Acids

Nucleic acids contamination comes from host cell DNA/RNA or retroviral RNA. Molecules with more than 150–200 base pairs will behave as flexible coils in SEC, whereas molecules up to 18 base pairs will behave as globular proteins. In between, the rigid rod structure should be expected. Their presence results in increased viscosity of the solution. Circular DNA is often supercoiled and will elute as a molecule of smaller size. Nucleic acid free biopharmaceutical products are obtained by using nucleases (e.g., Benzonase) and/or by minimizing release of nucleic acids from the host cell organism. Anion exchange chromatography (AEC) has been shown to be effective in binding the highly charged nucleic acids at ionic strength at which most proteins elute. Because of the negative net charge and hydrophilic character binding of the target protein to a cation exchanger, hydrophobic interaction or affinity matrix may reduce the nucleic acid content. DNA binds to hydroxyapatite at low to moderate phosphate concentrations. Precipitation of nucleic acids with PEI or magnesium chloride has been reported. Use of 1 M NaOH is recommended (make sure that equipment, filters, and chromatographic media are not affected by NaOH) for CIP. Nucleic acids are detected by monitoring the absorption of light at 260 nm. The residual content in drug substance and/or drug product is usually measured by PCR or amplification techniques. The maximum allowable content of nucleic acid per dose has been under continuous evaluation because the initially proposed content of 10 pg per dose was suggested by the CBER. The World Health Organization (WHO) has stated that 100 pg per dose is acceptable. CBER now states that "Lot-to-lot testing for DNA content in biological products produced in cell lines should be performed and lot release limits established that reflect a level of purity that can be achieved reasonably and consistent."

16.13.9 Host Cell Proteins

HCPs come from the host organism and constitute a major purification problem due to variability structure and surface properties. The amount released into the culture medium depends on the expression system used, the culture conditions, and whether the cells are disrupted or not to extract intracellular expressed target protein. Notice that "foreign" cellular proteins can be introduced by means of recombinant derived raw materials (e.g., enzymes) used in the downstream process. The range of preventive actions include the use of expression systems with direct expression of the target protein to the culture medium, gentle handling of intact cells, purification procedures such as chromatography, filtration, precipitation, and crystallization. If milk from transgenic animals is used as the product source, the presence of the animal equivalent to the target protein should be of concern (as it might co-purify with the target protein). Protein impurities should be considered on a case-by-case basis and be relegated to process validation rather than final product testing. Because of molecular diversity, no specific purification method can be recommended, as the separation depends on difference in affinity (selectivity) between HCP and the target protein for chosen chromatographic media and operating conditions. Use of a combination of different chromatographic principles is recommended. Most proteins will be removed (CIP) by means of 0.1–1 M NaOH (make sure that equipment, filters, and chromatographic media are not affected by NaOH). Several analytical methods have been used to monitor HCP including SDS-PAGE, 2D electrophoresis, Western blot (WB), and immunoassays. SDS-PAGE separates molecules according to the MW of the protein. The method, which is semi-quantitative, has a sensitivity of 100 pg/band (silver staining). 2D-electrophoresis (IEF in combination with SDS-PAGE) provides the most powerful separation of protein mixtures. The method, which is semi-quantitative, provides the widest window of the methods used with a sensitivity of 100 pg/spot. The WB method provides information of immunological identity. The sensitivity is 0.1–1 ng/band, and the method is qualitative. Immunoassays are widely used for HCP analysis in drug substances and drug products. The method depends on the nature and quality of antibodies used, and not all proteins (regardless of quantity) are detected. The method, which is semi-quantitative, provides the highest sensitivity (<0.1 ng/mL). Two types of assays have been used to detect HCPs: generic and specific assays. In generic assays, HCPs typical for a given expression system are detected. If the assays are based on competently produced antibodies raised against cell lysates, the quality may be adequate or better than those produced by individual companies. Generic assays are typically used during process development, as process-specific assays by definition are not available before the process has been locked. However, it is recommended also to use generic HCP assays for lot release for several reasons. First, the protein patterns are highly conserved between strains, and second, a generic HCP assay will be a very strong tool for the detection of variations in the process, which could lead to a different impurity profile. Process-specific assays are directed against HCPs co-purifying with the target protein. The assays are typically developed by purifying the cell lysate without target protein using the exact like process to be used for the licensed product. By definition, the process-specific assay cannot be developed before the process is locked. The assay, which typically takes from 1 to 2 years to develop, may thus be a time-delaying factor. The process-specific assays provide a much narrower window than do generic assays, and their value at lot-release test has recently been challenged, because these assays will most probably fail to detect atypical HCP contaminants. There are some significant differences between WB technology and immunoassays. In WB, the denaturation and solubilization steps can destroy some native epitopes, whereas the immunoassay technology relies on reaction with the native protein. The immunoassay technology provides an objective result, whereas the WB depends on a subjective interpretation. Finally, the sensitivity of immunoassays is generally higher than for WB assays. None of the methods mentioned are quantitative. They are at best semi-quantitative. Even the commonly used HCP immunoassay lack the linear accuracy applied to single analyte immunoassays due to variance in relative affinities between antibodies and HCP antigens and HCP concentrations. Instead assay results are correlated with clinical conditions and to process control. The amount of HCP to be accepted depends on the antigenicity of the co-purifying proteins. Recognizing the complexity of the task and the inability of quantitative measurements, it is not possible to state a general acceptable level.

16.13.10 Viruses

Virus contamination comes from the host cell, the culture medium, and infections during manufacture. The host cell may contain a genomic virus or virus vectors used to transform the cell line. The type of viral genome and/or vector depends on the cell line history. Continuous cell lines are extensively characterized, but chronic or latent viruses may be present. The retroviruses associated with continuous cell lines are noninfectious but oncogenic. Epstein–Barr virus or Sendai virus are often used for cell transformations. Contaminants such as BVDV, IBR, reovirus, PI-3, bovine leukemia virus, and bovine polyomavirus should be expected from serum supplemented media. Virus control is executed on several levels. The cell line history reveals all information on the origin and identity of the cell line and the host genome vectors used to establish the cell line. The MCB is extensively characterized using viral identity tests, in vitro tests, and in vivo tests to assure freedom of adventitious viruses. The end-of-production test of the cell culture is carried out to assure that the cells are free of viruses. Viruses are brought into the process from the environment because of contaminated equipment, infected raw materials, water, or non-sterile handling procedures. Working in closed systems and avoidance of raw materials of animal origin will help reduce the risk of infection. Strict control of equipment cleaning and sanitization procedures during processing will also help reducing contamination risk. Viruses may be inactivated by heat, radiation, chemical compound, or low pH or removed by chromatography or filtration techniques. Because of molecular diversity, no specific chromatographic purification method can be recommended and virus reduction factors must be determined for selected unit operations. Nanofiltration is a very efficient virus removal step often resulting in logarithmic reduction factors of 5–8. A commonly used reagent for cleaning of chromatographic media is 0.1–1 M NaOH. Viruses can be destroyed successfully with peracetic acid (make sure that equipment, filters, and chromatographic media are not affected by NaOH or peracetic acid). A variety of purity analyses are available: monolayer cultures; test for pathogen viruses not able to grow in cell cultures in both animals and eggs; test for retroviruses, endogenous viruses, or viral nucleic acid; test for selected viruses using mouse, rat, and hamster antibody production tests. It is necessary to document the utilization of adequate virus removal and inactivation strategies to ensure the exclusion of contaminating viruses. Different modes of action should ensure overlapping and complementary levels of protection. The purification process is validated with respect to virus removal and inactivation. The final product is rarely tested if continuous mammalian cell lines have been used as an expression system.

16.13.11 Prions

Prions come from transmissible spongiform encephalopathies (TSE) including scrapie in sheep and goats, chronic wasting disease in mule deer and elk, bovine spongiform encephalopathy (BSE) in cattle, and kuru and Creutzfeldt-Jakob disease (CJD) in humans. The disease-causing agents (prions) replicate in infected individuals generally without evidence of infection detectable by available diagnostic tests applicable in vivo. The major source of contamination of a recombinant product is the use of animal-derived raw materials, which could harbor bovine prions (BSE agent). Currently, there are no assays that are sensitive or specific enough to test raw materials or sources, and the only reliable prevention is to include barriers, such as avoidance of animal or human raw materials (e.g., trypsin, serum, transferrin, bovine/human serum albumin, protein supplements, peptones). However, this is not always possible (e.g., in the propagation of cells for the establishment of cell banks), and inactivation and removal procedures during downstream processing become of interest. Milk is unlikely to present any risk of prion contamination. Filtration has proven efficient in the removal of prion particles. Thus, size exclusion partitioning of abnormal prion particles using normal flow filtration or tangential flow filtration resulted in significant reduction of the infectious agent. The most effective inactivation methods include chloride dioxide, glutaraldehyde, 4 M guanidium thiocyanate, sodium dichloroisocyanurate, sodium metaperiodate, 6 M urea, and autoclaving at 121 qC for 15 min, of which several will not be suited if the target protein is present. Biological assays such as in vivo infection of susceptible animals are time consuming (months to years). They will not be of practical use in the test of biopharmaceutical products. The best semiquantitative biochemical assays include WB, capillary immunoelectrophoresis, conformation-dependent immunoassay, and dissociation-enhanced, time-resolved fluoroimmunoassay. The infectious dose is not known. Acceptance criteria must be decided upon on a case-by-case basis.

16.13.12 Proteolytic Enzymes

Proteolytic enzymes are released to the medium because of cell death, mechanical stress, or induced cell lysis. Their presence should be expected during fermentation and initial downstream unit operations. Measures taken are to work fast at low temperatures and to avoid working near the pH optimum of the enzyme. The most rewarding strategy is to prevent proteolysis already during fermentation either by using mutant strains or by optimizing the conditions toward minimum enzymatic activity. Most enzymes of the vacuoles and lysosomes will be minimally active at slightly alkaline pH (7–9), a pH interval strongly recommended for the extraction of proteins expressed in bacteria. Proteins are probably more resistant toward proteolytic attacks in their native state, and stabilizing factors (e.g., co-factor, correct parameter interval, co-solvent) should always be considered optimized. Use of protein inhibitors is not recommended for safety reasons. Proteolytic enzymes are typically removed during the capture and intermediary purification steps, and they rarely co-purify with the target protein throughout the downstream process. Despite the variety of enzymes present in the cell cytosol, proteolytic enzymes rarely constitute a problem in final products. Selective removal (e.g., affinity chromatography) of specific enzymes should be considered. Most proteins will be removed by means of 0.1–1 M NaOH (make sure that equipment, filters, and chromatographic media are not affected by NaOH). Suited analytical methods for early control are SDS-PAGE and WB. Purified preparations may be analyzed by means of HP-IEC, HP-RPC, MS, and peptide mapping. Ascertain that the degradation observed is not a function of the analytical assay. Enzyme inhibitors can be used for the prevention of enzymatic activity in analytical assays.

16.13.13 Lipids

Lipids (lipoproteins, triglycerides, phospholipids, cholesterol) are brought to the medium by cell lysis. If transgenic animals are used, the protein is expressed into the milk containing up to 4% fat. Lipids can be removed from the feedstock by centrifugation, by specific adsorption of hydrophobic compounds such as Hyflow by precipitation with dextran sulfate, by binding to anion exchangers, or by affinity chromatography allowing for specific binding of the target protein. Lipids will bind to hydrophobic media and surfaces. Lipids are retarded (2–3 column volumes) by adsorption of Sephadex. Milk fat is usually removed by centrifugation. Lipids are removed by means of NaOH or organic solvents (make sure that equipment, filters, and chromatographic media are not affected by NaOH or organic solvents).

16.13.14 Microbial Agents

Microbial agents and fungi come from infection of the bioreactor during cell culture. Other sources are contaminated water, buffers, raw materials, chromatographic columns, and equipment. Fermentation and cell culture bioreactors are prone to microbial infections. As the use of antibiotics in large-scale operations should be avoided, strict demands to the design of bioreactors and handling procedures are the key measures to avoid microbial infections. Test for microorganisms at end of production assures that no infections have taken place during culture. The nature of samples and buffers used during downstream processing makes these excellent growth substrates for microorganisms. For that reason, water QC, sterile filtration of buffers prior to use, sterile filtration of intermediary products, and effective cleaning and sanitization procedures are key elements of the downstream operations. Sterile filtration can be accomplished by filtering water, the desired buffer or intermediary product through 0.22μm filters. Bacterial spores are typically removed by means of 0.1 pm filters. Cleaning with 60%–70% v/v ethanol is a commonly used disinfectant against microbial agents; often 20% v/v ethanol is used as a storage solution for chromatographic resins, but the solution has no sporicidal effect while 0.1–1.0 M NaOH is widely used to kill microorganisms. Peracetic acid has both bacterial and sporicidal effect. Viable cells can be identified by spread out of the cell suspension or sample solution on agar plates.

Mycoplasmas have for long been recognized as a contaminant of continuous cell cultures caused by an infection of the cell line or bioreactor. Working in closed systems under GMP will reduce the risk of infection. The end-of-production test includes screening for mycoplasmas. Mycoplasmas are extremely sensitive to osmotic shock and pH extremes and should not constitute a problem in downstream processing, provided sanitization and cleaning in place procedures are carried out according to good manufacturing practices. Mycoplasmas are resistant to most antibiotics. Frequent testing (at every passage) is recommended. The cell culture is discarded upon infection. Cleaning with 0.1–1 M NaOH will inactivate mycoplasmas. Mycoplasmas are difficult to detect; the only reliable way of demonstrating infection is by agar plating, fluorescent dying of DNA, or PCR. Recently, a selective biochemical test that exploits the activity of certain mycoplasma enzymes has been made commercially available.

16.13.15 Raw Materials

Raw materials are themselves considered impurities, which should be removed from the final product. They include cell culture substrates, enzymes, reagents, amino acids, peptides, proteins, chromatographic media, inhibitors, and antibiotics. Raw materials should not be of animal origin because of the potential virus and prion infection risk. They are intentionally introduced in the process. The basic quality concepts include assurance of the identity, purity, suitability, and traceability of all the raw materials used in the manufacturing process. The quality of the raw materials used should meet standards appropriate for their intended use. Quality requirements for raw materials are met somewhat differently in the production of clinical batches (process evolution) and manufacturing of licensed product. Special attention should be paid to raw materials of animal or human origin. They should, as a general rule, be avoided. Chromatographic media must be supplied with a regulatory support file. Specific analytical assays may be required to detect residual amounts of critical raw materials in the final product. Critical reagents such as toxic compounds, enzymes, detergents, and stabilizers must be accounted for and their removal validated. Large amounts of hydrophobic reagents may affect HIC. Drug substance and/or drug product should be tested for residual content by specific assays. Detection-specific assays are required. Be aware of ligand leakage from chromatographic media and be prepared for setting up specific assay for their detection (ELISA or TOC).

16.13.16 Des-Amido Forms

Des-amido forms are target protein derivatives in which one or several of the glutamyl or asparagyl amino acid residues are converted to the corresponding acids (glutamyl and asparagyl). The deamidation reaction is slow at pH 3–5, at low temperatures, and at low conductivity. Deamidated forms are removed by HP-IEC and HP-RPC. Des-amido forms are detected by analytical HP-IEC, HP-RPC, native PAGE, IEF, MS, or CE. The content accepted depends on the nature of the drug product and the dose.

16.13.17 Oxidized Forms

Oxidized forms are target protein derivatives in which one or several of the Met, Cys, His, Trp, and Tyr residues have been oxidized. The oxidation of cysteinyl residues results in the formation of a disulfide bond (cystinyl residue). The oxidation reaction is slow at low pH and low temperature. Formation of disulfide bonds will take place above 0 mV. Oxidized forms are removed by HP-IEC and HP-RPC. Disulfide aggregates can be removed by SEC. Oxidized forms are detected by analytical HP-IEC, HP-RPC, native PAGE, IEF, MS, or CE. The content accepted depends on the nature of the drug product and the dose.

16.13.18 Carbamylated Forms

Carbamylated forms are target protein derivatives in which one or several of the primary amino, sulfhydryl, carboxyl, phenolic hydroxyl, imidazole, and phosphate groups react with cyanate to form a derivative. The blocking may change the pI of the protein. Cyanate is formed spontaneously in urea solutions, which is the primary source. The formation is slow at low temperatures, but it is nevertheless strongly recommended to purify the urea solution by means of mixed ion exchangers before use. Carbamylated forms are removed by HP-IEC and HP-RPC and detected by analytical HP-IEC, HP-RPC, native PAGE, IEF, MS, or CE. The content accepted depends on the nature of the drug product and the dose.

16.13.19 Aggregates

Aggregates are target protein derivatives in which two or more molecules are linked together either by covalent inter-disulfide bonds or by hydrophobic interaction. Target protein aggregates are formed as a result of hydrophobic intermolecular reactions or intermolecular disulfide bond formation under oxidizing conditions. Aggregates are very often antigenic, resulting in the formation of target protein antibodies. Proteins exposed to even mildly denaturing conditions may partially unfold, resulting in exposure of hydrophobic residues to the aqueous solvent favoring aggregation. The aggregation process is assumed to be controlled by the initial dimerization step in a second-order reaction. Consequently, high protein concentrations will increase the aggregation rate. Intermolecular disulfide bond formation between cysteinyl residues takes place at alkaline pH under oxidizing conditions. Proteins with reactive-free thiol groups should be purified under reducing conditions (typically 1–10 mM reducing agent) in the presence of ethylenediaminetetraacetic acid (EDTA). Even proteins with disulfide bonds may participate in intermolecular disulfide bond reactions due to disulfide bond shuffling at neutral and alkaline pH. The aggregation reaction based on intermolecular disulfide bond formation is prevented at pH < 6 and under reducing conditions. The hydrophobic aggregation reaction strongly depends on the hydrophobicity of the molecule. Preventive actions are to keep the protein in its native conformation during processing to avoid unfolding and exposure of hydrophobic sites. Hydrophobic proteins (e.g., certain membrane proteins) may be kept soluble by addition of specific co-solvents (e.g., detergents). Aggregates may be removed by filtration or SEC. Disulfide-based aggregates can be detected by nonreducing (no boiling of sample) 1D-SDS, HP-SEC, MS, or CE. Hydrophobic aggregates may be detected by HP-SEC. The content accepted depends on the nature of the drug product and the dose.

16.13.20 Scrambled Forms

Scrambled forms are target protein molecules with a disulfide bond pattern different from that of the native molecule. They are typically formed during in vitro folding of proteins, but disulfide bond shuffling at neutral pH or above also occurs. This requires studies on control of protein stability during downstream processing. The formation of scrambled forms is closely linked to the folding procedure. The best preventive action is to optimize said procedure. As the folding reaction is protein specific, no general rules can be given. Scrambled forms are removed by HP-IEC and HP-RPC. Scrambled forms are detected by analytical HP-IEC, HP-RPC, CE, or peptide mapping. The content accepted depends on the nature of the drug product and the dose.

16.13.21 Cleaved Forms

Cleaved forms are typically used for target protein derivatives with almost identical MW (± a few hundred daltons), where a peptide bond is cleaved resulting in loss of a N- or C-terminal site or where an internal peptide bond is cleaved while at the same time the resulting fragments are kept together by means of disulfide bonds. Gentle handling of cells, low temperatures, and working in pH intervals where enzymatic activity is low reduce proteolysis. The use of enzyme inhibitors is not recommended for safety reasons. Removal of proteolytic enzymes during capture prevents the formation of cleaved forms as well. Cleaved forms are removed by HP-IEC and HP-RPC. Cleaved forms are detected by analytical HP-IEC, HP-RPC, native PAGE, IEF, MS, peptide mapping, or CE.

16.13.22 Glycosylated Forms

Glycosylated forms appear in the yeast, insect cell, mammalian cell, transgenic animal, and plant expression systems. The glycosylation pattern is a consequence of the molecular biology and the fermentation conditions. Unwanted glycoforms are removed by HP-IEC or HP-RPC methods. Glycosylated forms are detected by analytical HP-IEC, HP-RPC, native PAGE, IEF, MS, peptide mapping, or CE.

16.13.23 Quantity

The quantity of target protein is determined as the total peptide/protein content in a given sample excluding any inactive derivatives such as des-amido forms, oxidized forms, and polymeric forms. High-performance chromatographic methods are used to quantitate both the target protein and its derivatives using UV detection and determination of peak areas. If the extinction coefficient is not known (e.g., analogues), amino acid or Kjeldahl analysis is used as a primary reference method. Bioassays are often replaced with quantity determination partly because the usual high costs associated with biological assays and partly because of the much higher accuracy of quantitative assays. The subject is of great interest to regulatory authorities as the principle goal of biogeneric manufacturers is to reduce cost of product, and much work has been done to create surrogate tests for target proteins. The commonly used quantity methods are amino acid analysis, Kjeldahl analysis, UV spectrometry, and high-performance chromatographic procedures.

16.13.23.1 Amino Acid Analysis

Amino acid analysis involves hydrolysis of peptides and proteins into free amino acids followed by derivatization and separation (or vice versa) of the amino acid derivatives. The method is in principle independent of protein shape, charge, hydrophobicity, or MW because the peptide/protein is fully degraded. Protein hydrolysis is commonly accomplished by acid hydrolysis of the peptide bonds under vacuum and heat, typically at 110°C–165°C for 1–24 h. Only 16 of the common 20 amino acids are usually measured by this technique because Cys, Trp, Ser, and Tyr are degraded during acid hydrolysis. Seven amino acid residues (Asp, Glu, Asn, Gln, Leu, Lys, and Gly) are well recovered, and they are commonly used for protein quantitation. The sample must be highly purified; ideal sample would contain from 1 to 10 nmol protein in a volume of 10–100 pL water or very low concentration of defined buffer. If interfering compounds are present, dialysis of the sample prior to analysis is recommended. In the pre-column method, the hydrolysis is followed by derivatization of the free amino acids with reagents such as phenylisothiocyanate (PITC), o-phtalaldehyde (OPA), or Fmoc chloride before the chromatographic separation (e.g., HP-RPC-C18). In the post-column method, the hydrolysis is followed by chromatographic separation (HP-IEC) of the free amino acids, which are then mixed with ninhydrin at approximately 135°C. The reaction forms a blue derivative detectable at 570 nm. The preferred post-column method is the more precise of the two but is less sensitive (picomolar quantities). It is strongly recommended to establish an internal standard such as norvaline or norleucine to minimize the variability of the assay and to provide an additional parameter in the event of method problems. Hydrolysis and analysis of a protein standard (e.g., bovine serum albumin available from the National Institute of Standards and Technology: http://www.nist.gov) should be compared to predefined suitability requirements and acceptance criteria. Theoretically, the yield of just one well-recovered amino acid in a protein sample can be used for quantitation. However, using an average of several stable residues is preferred to assure accurate and precise measurements. The amount of protein can be correlated to the absorbance at maximum wavelength (typically 280 nm) with the purpose of determination of the extension coefficient and protein concentrations in solution. A comparative study between amino acid analysis, Kjeldahl analysis, and UV spectroscopy for the determination of protein content yielded a strong correlation between methods for proteins in the range of 6–22 kDa. For larger proteins such as immunoglobulins (150 kDa), amino acid analysis may underestimate the total protein concentration (evaluation of amino acid analysis as reference method to quantitative highly purified proteins). The AAA technology also provides support to primary structure studies (amino acid composition), identification of odd or modified residues, and identification of proteins by way of computer database searches. This method should be the primary method for measuring the protein content. The range of sensitivity is about 1 pmol of each amino acid.

16.13.23.2 Amino Acid Sequencing

Amino acid sequencing is divided into N-terminal and C-terminal sequencing. Amino terminal (N-terminal) sequence analysis is based on the modification of the unmodified N-terminal amino group of the peptide/protein with PITC followed by acid cleavage of the peptide bond releasing the phenylthiohydantoin (PTH) derivative of the amino acid. A new amino group of the next amino acid is now available to react with PITC, and the protein sequencing will thus take place in a cyclic manner (Edman degradation). The resulting PTH-amino acid derivative is thereafter analyzed on a PTH amino acid analyzer based on HP-RPC separation technology. The cyclic reaction is not 100% effective, and in practice from 20 to 40 amino acid residues can be sequenced by the method described in the low picomol range. Entire sequences may be obtained by cleavage of the protein with specific proteases such as trypsin, V8 protease, or chymotrypsin followed by HP-RPC separation, MALDI-MS, and Edman sequencing of the peptides separated. Carboxy-terminal (C-terminal) sequence analysis is used for confirmation of the C-terminal part of the peptide or protein. Typically, the peptide/protein is digested with enzymes such as carboxypeptidase A, P, or Y, which are exopeptidases removing one amino acid residue, one at a time, from the C-terminus of the peptide/protein. The enzymes have different specificity, and mixtures may be used. After digestion, the released amino acids are removed from the residual peptide/protein and analyzed by amino acid analysis. The reaction is followed over time allowing for the determination of relative amounts released. Recently, an automated procedure has been introduced consisting of two principal reaction events. First, the D-carboxylic acid group of the C-terminal amino acid residue is activated with trifluoroacetic acid (TFA) and coupled with diphenyl phosphoroisothiocyanatidate (DPP-ITC) in the presence of pyridine. The resulting peptide/protein thiohydantoin is then cleaved with potassium trimethylsilanolate to release the thiohydantoin amino acid from the now-shortened peptide/protein. The thiohydantoin derivative is identified by RP-HPC analysis at 269 nm. The method is currently able to provide three to five cycles of sequence information. The range of sensitivity is from 10 to 20 pmol of protein.

16.13.23.3 Bicinchoninic Assay

The assay is a modification of the biuret assay. BCA sodium salt is a stable water-soluble compound capable of forming an intense purple complex with cuprous (Cu) ions under alkaline conditions. The maximum absorbance is at 562 nm. The end product is stable for hours, and the assay is not affected by detergents and denaturing agents such as urea. This, combined with the simplicity of the assay (only one reagent), makes the BCA assay very attractive compared with the Lowry and biuret assays. Compounds interfering with the assay are EDTA, sucrose (>10 mM), glucose (>10 mM), glycine (1 M), ammonium sulfate (>5%), sodium acetate (2 M), sodium phosphate (>1 M), and reducing mercapto reagents. Samples containing lipids show high absorbencies. The sensitivity range is from 0.2 to 1 mg/mL. The sample may be treated with TCA or deoxycholate-TCA to precipitate the protein before analysis as most proteins are almost quantitatively precipitated even from dilute solutions. The TCA precipitate should be dissolved in base or appropriate buffer prior to analysis. Samples may also be dialyzed against a suited buffer to remove substances interfering with the assay. Desalting is also recommended, but a loss of protein in the range from 10% to 15% should be expected. The BCA assay is typically used during the development of in-process control.

16.13.23.4 Biuret Assay

The assay is based on polypeptide chelation of cupric ion in strong alkaline solution. The reaction of the peptide bond with copper sulfate reduces copper, resulting in a color shift (deep purple) to 540 nm. Although the assay is less susceptible to chemical interference than other copper-based assays, tris, glycerol, glucose, ammonium sulfate, sulfhydryl compounds, and sodium phosphate containing buffers may interfere with the assay. Samples should contain from 1 to 10 mg/mL of protein. The sample is diluted about 5-fold upon addition of reagent to give a concentration of 0.2–2 mg/mL final assay volume.

The biuret assay is relatively independent on the protein standard of choice as the reaction chemistry is based on polypeptide structure and not on the composition of amino acid residue side chains. The sensitivity range is from 0.5 to 10 mg/mL, making the assay the least sensitive among the colorimetric assays. The sample may be treated with TCA or deoxycholate-TCA to precipitate the protein before analysis as most proteins are almost quantitatively precipitated even from dilute solutions. The TCA precipitate should be dissolved in base or appropriate buffer prior to analysis. Samples may also be dialyzed against a suited buffer to remove substances interfering with the assay. Desalting is also recommended, but a loss of protein in the range from 10% to 15% should be expected.

16.13.23.5 Bradford Assay

The semi-quantitative assay is based on the dye, Coomassie brilliant blue G-250, which undergoes a shift from 465 to 595 nm when binding to peptide bonds under acidic conditions. The binding of the dye to protein is a very rapid process (approximately 2 min) and the protein-dye complex remains dispersed in solution for up to an hour. Some variability in response between different proteins should be expected. The protein is irreversibly denatured by the reaction. The assay is relatively insensitive to most commonly used buffer components. However, detergents such as SDS and Triton X-100 interfere with the assay although small amounts of detergent may be eliminated by the use of proper control. By comparison of four different methods (Kjeldahl, biuret, Lowry, and Bradford), an underestimated protein content by a factor of 2 was observed relative to other assays. The reliability of the Coomassie dye binding assay should therefore be verified case by case. The sensitivity is about 25 pg/mL. The sample may be treated with TCA or deoxycholate-TCA to precipitate the protein before analysis as most proteins are almost quantitatively precipitated even from dilute solutions. The TCA precipitate should be dissolved in base or appropriate buffer prior to analysis. Samples may also be dialyzed against a suited buffer to remove substances interfering with the assay. Desalting is also recommended, but a loss of protein in the range from 10% to 15% should be expected.

16.13.23.6 Capillary Electrophoresis

The basic principle to CE is to apply high voltage to a fused silica capillary filled with an appropriate electrolyte and with both ends dipped in the same solution. The separation occurs due to the combination of electrophoretic migration and electro-osmotic flow. The fused silica capillary column may be derivatized or filled with different types of material (polyacrylamide, agarose) or filled with ampholyte solutions allowing for separation according topI. CE can be viewed as a combination of traditional electrophoresis and HP-RPC offering rapid, precise, and highly efficient analysis of complex mixtures (amino acids, peptides, DNA). Protein analysis is difficult to carry out. Proteins bind to uncoated columns, and each protein tend to have its own set of optimal separation parameters (pI, stability, solubility, hydrophobicity), not easily transferred to other proteins. However, the afore mentioned separation techniques based on charge alone (IEF-CE), on MW (CE in the presence of SDS), or by means of derivatized columns have made CE a reliable technique for characterization of recombinant proteins as demonstrated in the separation of human growth hormone and insulin molecular forms. CE offers several separation modes. Capillary zone electrophoresis (CZE) is based on the differences in the electrophoretic mobility of sample ions, which migrate with a linear velocity proportional to their charge–mass ratio. SDS is often used to form a protein–SDS complex, allowing for separation according to molecular radius. Micellar electrokinetic capillary electrophoresis (MECC) is based on a separation of molecules (according to hydrophobicity) between an aqueous phase and a micellar pseudo-stationary phase comprising a surfactant in an amount above its critical micellar concentration. Capillary isoelectric focusing (CIEF) is based on separation according to IEF using a background electrolyte to establish the pH gradient. Charged molecules will migrate to their pI's. Capillary isotachophoresis (CITP) is based on sample separation at constant velocity.

The sample is applied between two solutions of different ionic mobilities with an electrolyte that is more mobile than any sample ion and a terminating electrolyte that is least mobile. The peak capacity is in the range of 18 peaks per minute (compared to HP-RPC of 3 peaks per minute). Unlike conventional electrophoresis, the method is highly efficient with small sample requirements. The CE methods are quantitative. Small sample sizes are required (from 1 to 10 pL).

16.13.23.7 High-Performance Ion Exchange Chromatography

Analytical HPLC offers high level of resolution and precision, making the technology available for identity, purity, and quantity determinations. HP-IEC is based on highly specific analytical columns comprising mono-disperse particles with a diameter of 5–10 pm separating proteins according to their electrical charge. The resolution may be comparable to that of HP-RPC, and the technology will apply to almost all types of globular proteins. The HP-IEC is used for the detection of target protein-related compounds (e.g., desamido forms, oxidized forms, scrambled forms, cleaved forms), which may be present in amounts from 1 ppt (part per thousand) and upward. The resulting UV diagram provides an impurity profile within the relatively narrow window offered by the technology, but it should be kept in mind that not all impurities are detected by this or similar methods. Impurities present in 0.1% or higher should be fully characterized no later than phase III manufacture. HP-IEC offers two separation modes: CEC and AEC. In CEC, positively charged biomolecules are typically retained due to interaction with negatively charged groups (e.g., sulfonic acid) on the surface of the chromatographic resin. The buffer pH must favor a net charge of the biomolecule lower than pI to maintain separation. CEC primarily retains biomolecules by the interaction with histidine, lysine, and arginine (pKa about 6.5, 10, and 12, respectively). In AEC, negatively charged biomolecules are typically retained due to interaction with positively charged groups (e.g., quaternary amine) on the surface of the chromatographic resin. The buffer pH must favor a net charge of the biomolecule higher than pI to maintain separation. AEC primarily retains biomolecules by the interaction with aspartic or glutamic acid side chains (pKa about 4.4). The separation is affected by temperature (due to structural changes of the protein molecule), presence of displacer ions such as Na and Cl, presence of denaturing agents, presence of organic solvents, and hydrophobic interactions with the resin. HP-IEC is used for in-process control analysis of target protein identity (retention time), quantity (peak area), and purity (215 nm or 280 nm profile). The method is also used for drug substance/product impurity profiles and determination of quantity.

16.13.23.8 High-Performance Reversed Phase Chromatography

Analytical HPLC offers high level of resolution and precision, making the technology available for identity, purity, and quantity determinations. HP-RPC is based on highly specific analytical columns comprising mono-disperse particles with a diameter of 5–10 pm separating proteins according to their hydrophobicity. The high-resolution methodology is restricted to analysis of hydrophilic or semi-hydrophobic proteins of a MW of 3,000–100,000. Retention of molecules of interest can be controlled by manipulating the properties of the mobile phase, and the separation of molecules with only small differences in hydrophobicity can be performed. The HP-RPC is used for the detection of target protein-related compounds (e.g., des-amido forms, oxidized forms, scrambled forms, cleaved forms), which may be present in amounts from 1 ppt and upward. The resulting UV diagram is said to provide an impurity profile within the relatively narrow window offered by the technology, but it should be kept in mind that not all impurities are detected by this or similar methods. Impurities present in 0.1% or higher should be fully characterized no later than phase III manufacture. HP-RPC is used for in-process control analysis of target protein identity (retention time), quantity (peak area), and purity (215 nm or 280 nm profile). The method is also used for drug substance/product impurity profiles and determination of quantity.

16.13.23.9 High Performance Size Exclusion Chromatography

HP-SEC is based on highly specific analytical columns comprising uniform particles of a given diameter depending on the MW of the target protein. The principal feature of SEC is its gentle noninteraction with the sample, enabling high retention of biological activity, while separating multimers that are not easily distinguished by other chromatographic methods.

The resolution is less than for HP-IEC and HP-RPC techniques. The technology applies for almost all types of globular proteins. HP-SEC can be coupled directly to ESI and MS by means of ammonium formate buffer (typically 50 mM), making direct determination of MWs possible.

HP-SEC is used for the detection of di- and polymeric target protein content in the drug substance/product. It is a purity analysis.

16.13.23.10 Isoelectric Focusing

IEF is one of the electrophoretic methods comprising SDS-PAGE, native electrophoresis, IEF, 2D-electrophoresis, and CE. One-dimensional SDS-PAGE offers separation of proteins according to their MW. Samples run under denaturing but nonreducing conditions will provide information of presence of other molecular species and of disulfide intermolecular di- and polymers. Samples run under denaturing and reducing conditions will provide information on monomeric compounds. Notice that in the latter procedure, it is common practice to boil the sample in the denaturing and reducing buffer before application. The boiling procedure must not be used if information of aggregates is required (denaturing but nonreducing conditions). Native electrophoresis separates proteins according to charge, MW, shape, and other factors (samples are typically applied under conditions maintaining the tertiary structure). IEF separates proteins according to the pI (samples may be applied under native or denaturing conditions). The method offers very high resolution and is often used to provide information of the presence of closely related derivatives (e.g., des-amido forms) or presence of glycosylated derivatives of the target protein. 2D-electrophoresis separates proteins according to the protein's pI (first dimension) and its MW (second dimension). The method is a combination of IEF and SDS-PAGE. The resulting coordinate (pI, MW) provides a unique identification of the protein. Differences in posttranslational modifications (e.g., phosphorylation) will often result in separate spots (slightly different pI and MW). CE offers similar separation technologies. The CE methods can be used as a purity analysis. In IEF, the movement of the protein through the gel matrix is modulated by a pH gradient created by soluble ampholytes, which are small organic molecules with various pI's and buffering capacities. The pH gradient is produced when the soluble ampholytes migrate in the gel matrix until they reach their pI's. Stable pH gradients are difficult to establish outside the range of 3.0–8.0, and nonequilibrium conditions are required. Commercial carrier ampholyte mixtures comprise hundreds of individual polymeric species with pI's spanning a specific pH range. When a voltage is applied across a carrier ampholyte mixture, the carrier ampholytes with the lowest pI (and the most negative charge) move toward the anode, and the carrier ampholytes with the highest pI (and the most positive charge) move toward the cathode. The other carrier ampholytes align themselves between the extremes, according to their pI's, and buffer their environment to the corresponding pH. The result is a continuous pH gradient. An attractive alternative to soluble ampholytes is the use of immobilized pH gradient gels (IPG), where buffering side chains are covalently incorporated into the acrylamide matrix. The pH gradient is stabilized by an electric field allowing the proteins to migrate until they reach their pI's, where the protein has no net charge. Because reproducible linear gradients with a slope as low as 0.01 pH units/cm can separate proteins with pI differences of 0.001 pH units, the resolution possible with immobilized pH gradient gels is 10–100 times greater than that obtained with carrier ampholyte–based IEF. IEF can be run in either a native or a denaturing mode. Native IEF is the more convenient option, as precast native IEF gels are available in a variety of pH gradient ranges. This method is also preferred when native protein is required, as when activity staining is to be employed. The use of native IEF, however, is often limited by the fact that many proteins are not soluble at low ionic strength or have low solubility close to their pI's. In these cases, denaturing IEF is employed. Urea is the denaturant of choice, as this uncharged compound can dissolve many proteins, not otherwise soluble under IEF conditions. Detergents and reducing agents are often used in conjunction with urea for more-complete unfolding and solubilization. Urea is not stable in aqueous solution, so precast IEF gels are not manufactured with urea. Dried precast gels are a convenient alternative; they have been cast, rinsed, and dried and can be rehydrated with urea, carrier ampholytes, and other additives before use. Samples are typically dialyzed against buffer comprising a nonionic detergent (e.g., TX-100), urea, a reducing agent (DTT or 2-ME), and ampholytes before electrophoresis. Multi-subunit proteins dissociate, and each polypeptide migrates as a single species, according to its mass and charge. Specific isoelectric focusing standards are included in the electrophoretic run. The standards have a range of pI's and will carry a net positive, negative, or zero charge depending on the pH of the system. The IEF slab gel method is very powerful, and even closely related derivatives such as phosphorylated or glycosylated forms are detected. The method is primarily used for identification of glycosylation patterns (protein micro-heterogeneity) and for determination of product-related impurities (des-amido forms, oxidized forms, scrambled forms, blocked amino groups). However, the method is semi-quantitative only, at its best, and one must be very careful about method validation, if the method is used for purity purposes. The IEF tube gel method is typically used for the first-dimension 2D-electrophoresis run. Coomassie blue and silver staining are the two most common staining methods used for band detection on slab gels. Coomassie staining has a sensitivity of 0.05–0.5 pg of protein per band. Silver staining is about 10–100 times more sensitive enabling detection of 1–5 ng of protein per band. IEF is used as a target protein identity method according to the pI of the molecule. The powerful resolution of closely related derivatives makes the method suited for pattern recognition of, for example, glycosylated forms. One should in general be careful to use electrophoretic methods as purity analyses because of difficulties in quantifying the method.

16.13.23.11 Kjeldahl Analysis

The Kjeldahl analysis is used for quantitative determination of the nitrogen content in protein samples. In the Kjeldahl analysis, nitrogen is converted to ammonium sulfate by digestion of the protein in a mixture of concentrated sulfuric acid, copper sulfate (to raise the boiling point), and a catalyst (typically copper II, mercury II, or selenium salts) under high temperatures. Sample nitrogen is converted to ammonium sulfate by this procedure. Ammonia is released by change in pH to alkaline conditions (addition of NaOH), and steam distillation is followed by a titration to determine the quantity of ammonia released. To account for potential environmental contaminants, a reagent blank without protein is run. An ammonium sulfate reference can be used as a standard to ensure assay accuracy. An alternate method is the Nessler assay in which hydrogen peroxide is used to accelerate the oxidation of nitrogen to ammonium sulfate. After digestion, the Nessler reagent (mercury and potassium chloride in sodium hydroxide) is added to produce a colored complex. Both methods exploit the observation that nearly all proteins contain approximately 16.5% nitrogen by weight. Multiplication of the weight of nitrogen determined by a factor of 6 should provide a valid benchmark measure of the weight of protein. The methods are not as sensitive as the other methods described. However, the accuracy is high, and the indirect determination of the nitrogen content may be one of the most reliable methods for the determination of total protein in crude samples. This type of assay does not demonstrate the protein-to-protein variation of colorimetric methods. Note that mg amounts are required for analysis. Also, make sure that the sample does not contain non-protein nitrogen-based compounds such as tris and amino acids; precision can be decreased because of loss of ammonia by leakage or adsorption. The Kjeldahl analysis quantitatively determines the total amount of protein present in a sample. The method is typically used for total protein determination in crude samples.

16.13.23.12 Limulus Amebocyte Lysate Assay
The LAL test is used for the determination of endotoxin. Pyrogens are a group of chemically diverse substances that cause fever and shock in severe cases. The most important pyrogenic substances in pharmaceutical industry are bacterial endotoxins. There are two methods of detection: the Pyrogen test, which is based on the measurement of body temperature of rabbits before and after injection of the specimen, and the LAL test, which is based on the clotting reaction of an enzyme complex of cells of the horseshoe crab together with bacterial endotoxins (in vitro test). Although the LAL test is widely used, a total replacement of the Pyrogen test is still not possible because on one hand the LAL test will only detect bacterial endotoxins and on the other hand not all specimen can be tested with the LAL test because of interference with the test. LAL is the aqueous extract obtained after the lysis of the blood cells from the horseshoe crab. Limulus polyphemus contains blood proteins causing clotting of the crab blood when exposed to lipopolysaccharides (LPS) from gram-negative bacteria (e.g., *E. coli*). The presence of LPS located within the cell wall, also named *endotoxins*, is an indicator of bacterial contamination in water, buffers, chromatographic columns, and raw materials. There are currently three LAL methods in use: the gel clot test, the turbidimetric test, and the chromogenic test method. All methods allow for reading after a fixed time interval (end point tests). The turbidimetric and chromogenic test methods can also be read continuously (kinetic tests). The gel clot test is the simplest and most widely used form. A mixture of test sample and LAL reagent is mixed in a test tube and incubated for a given time interval (typically 1 h at 37°C) and then read for the presence or absence of a firm gel clot. The turbidimetric test is a spectrophotometric method based on the optical density (at 340 or 405 nm). End point tests do not require very many data points, whereas kinetic assays will require a computer for data handling. Optical density values must be collected without disturbing the integrity of the coagulation matrix formed. It is therefore advisable to use optical readers where the samples are fixed. The chromogenic test is a spectrophotometric method based on measurement of the optical density of the leaving group (e.g., *para*-nitroaniline). End point tests do not require very many data points, whereas kinetic assays will require a computer for data handling. For most chromogenic assays, turbidity develops along with the increase in color intensity. It is advisable to fix the samples in the optical reader in order not to disturb the coagulin

matrix formed. The kinetic assays make use of the time period after mixing sample and LAL reagent in which the optical density increases. The differences in the rate of increase in optical density are a function of the endotoxin concentration: The rates of increase in optical density increase with increasing concentration of endotoxin. The endotoxin concentration is calculated from a standard curve constructed by linear regression of the log of the onset time, on the log of the endotoxin concentration. The absolute coefficient of correlation recommended by FDA is 0.980. One of the most important aspects of LAL test is that the test is in accordance with the latest demand of the European Pharmacopoeia Commission for the replacement of the animal-based tests in favor of alternative methods where possible. The USP Reference Standard for endotoxin has a defined potency of 10,000 EU per vial. It must be demonstrated that the sample does not inhibit or enhance the LAL reaction. The LAL assay determines the endotoxin content. It is used as and in process control procedure, typically during development, and as a purity test of the drug substance/product.

16.13.23.13 Lowry Assay

The Lowry assay is a colorimetric method based on cupric ions and the Folin-Ciocalteu reagent for phenolic groups. The phosphomolybdate-phosphotungstate salts are reduced to produce a maximum absorbance at 750 nm. Little variation between different proteins is observed by this method making it very useful for protein mixtures. The color reaction is light sensitive and can vary from protein to protein. The protein is irreversibly denatured. Numerous buffer components can interfere with the Lowry assay including potassium, ions, magnesium ions, EDTA, GuCl, Triton X-100, SDS, Brij 35, tris (>0.1 M), ammonium sulfate, sodium acetate (>1 M), sodium phosphate (>1 M), thiol reagents, and carbohydrates2,3. The two-step nature of the Lowry assay, the instability of the reagent in alkaline solutions and the different compounds interfering makes it a complex and cumbersome assay to use. The Hartree version of the Lowry assay makes use of three reagents instead of five. The method is less laborious than the original method, and it maintains the sensitivity of the original. The sensitivity range is from 0.01 to 1 mg/mL.

Sample treatment The sample may be treated with TCA or deoxycholate TCA in order to precipitate the protein before analysis as most proteins are almost quantitatively precipitated even from dilute solutions. The TCA precipitate should be dissolved in base or appropriate buffer prior to analysis. Samples may also be dialyzed against a suited buffer in order to remove substances interfering with the assay. Desalting is also recommended, but at loss of protein in the range from 10% to 15% should be expected. Note that most of the interfering substances can be removed by precipitating the protein with deoxycholate-TCA prior to running the assay; color development reaches a maximum in 20–30 min; lipids can be removed by chloroform extraction; the reaction is pH dependent, and it is important to keep pH in the range from 10 to 10.5. The Lowry assay is typically used during development for in process control of total protein, preferentially in crude samples.

16.13.23.14 Native Electrophoresis

Native electrophoresis is one of the electrophoretic methods comprising SDS-PAGE, native electrophoresis, IEF, 2D-electrophoresis, and CE. One-dimensional SDS-PAGE offers separation of proteins according to their MW. Samples run under denaturing, but non-reducing conditions, will provide information of presence of other molecular species and of disulfide intermolecular di- and polymers. Samples run under denaturing and reducing conditions will provide information on monomeric compounds. Notice that in the latter procedure, it is common practice to boil the sample in the denaturing and reducing buffer before application. The boiling procedure must not be used if information of aggregates is required (denaturing but non-reducing conditions). Native electrophoresis separates proteins according to charge, MW, shape and other factors (samples are typically applied under conditions maintaining the tertiary structure). IEF separate proteins according to the pI (samples may be applied under native or denaturing conditions). The method offers very high resolution and is often used to provide information of presence of closely related derivatives (e.g., des-amido forms) or presence glycosylated derivatives of the target protein. 2D-electrophoresis separates proteins according to the proteins pI (first dimension) and its MW (second dimension). The method is a combination of IEF and SDS-PAGE. The resulting coordinate (pI, Mw) provides a unique identification of the protein. Differences in posttranslational modifications (e.g., phosphorylation) will often result in separate spots (slightly different pI and Mw). CE offers similar separation technologies. The CE methods can be used as a purity analysis. In native electrophoresis proteins are separated according to charge, shape and MW in the absence of denaturants, ampholytes or other reagents, which can influence the molecular properties or electric field. The sample is typically transferred to or solubilized in 5% (w/v) sucrose or dilute gel buffer (1–5 mM). The gel pH and the pI of the protein(s) to be analyzed must match, as the net charge of the protein(s) may change from positive to negative or vice versa affecting the protein's ability to enter the gel (i.e., if gel pH < protein pH, the protein will have a net positive charge; if gel pH > protein pH, the protein will have a net negative charge). Note that severe solubility problems can be experienced for certain proteins in the absence of denaturing and solubilizing agents such as urea or SDS. IEF standards can be used for native electrophoresis as well. Coomassie blue and silver staining are the two most common staining methods used for band detection on slab gels. Coomassie staining has a sensitivity of 0.05 to 0.5 Pg protein per band. Silver staining is about 10–100 times more sensitive enabling detection of 1–5 ng of protein per band. Native electrophoresis is used as a target protein identity method and to evaluate product related impurities (e.g., des-amido forms, oxidized forms) during process development. One should in general be careful to use electrophoretic methods as purity analyses due to difficulties in quantifying the method.

16.13.23.15 SDS-PAGE

SDS-PAGE is one of the electrophoretic methods comprising SDS-PAGE, native electrophoresis, IEF, 2D-electrophoresis, and CE. One-dimensional SDS-PAGE offers separation of proteins according to their MW. Samples run under denaturing, but non-reducing conditions, will provide information of presence of other molecular species and of disulfide intermolecular di- and polymers. Samples run under denaturing and reducing conditions will provide information on monomeric compounds. Notice that in the latter procedure, it is common practice to boil the sample in the denaturing and reducing buffer before application. The boiling procedure must not be used if information of aggregates is required (denaturing but non-reducing conditions).

Native electrophoresis separates proteins according to charge, MW, shape, and other factors (samples are typically applied under conditions maintaining the tertiary structure). IEF separate proteins according to the pI (samples may be applied under native or denaturing conditions). The method offers very high resolution and is often used to provide information of presence of closely related derivatives (e.g., des-amido forms) or presence glycosylated derivatives of the target protein. 2D-electrophoresis separates proteins according to the proteins pI (first dimension) and its MW (second dimension). The method is a combination of IEF and SDS-PAGE. The resulting coordinate (pI, Mw) provides a unique identification of the protein. Differences in posttranslational modifications (e.g., phosphorylation) will often result in separate spots (slightly different pI and Mw). CE offers similar separation technologies. The CE methods can be used as a purity analysis. SDS-PAGE under denaturing (and reducing) conditions separates proteins according to the molecular size as they move through the gel toward the anode (positively charged electrode). The system comprises a large pore stacking gel (in which the sample is loaded) and a running gel (in which the proteins are separated). Because of the high resolution obtainable with discontinuous buffer systems, the SDS discontinuous system is usually used. In the discontinuous system, protein mobility, a quantitative measure of the migration rate of a charged species in an electric field is intermediate between the mobility of the buffer ion of the same charge (usually negative) in the stacking gel (leading ion) and the mobility of the buffer ion in the upper tank (trailing ion). When electrophoresis is started, the ions and the proteins begin migrating into the stacking gel. The proteins concentrate in a very thin zone, called the stack, between the leading ion and the trailing ion. The proteins continue to migrate in the stack until they reach the separating gel. At that point, due to a pH or an ion change, the proteins become the trailing ion and "unstack" as they separate on the gel. Although a continuous system is slightly easier to set up than a discontinuous system and tends to have fewer sample precipitation and aggregation problems, much greater resolution can be obtained with a discontinuous system. Only minimal concentration of the sample takes place with continuous gels, and proteins form zones nearly as broad as the height of the original samples in the sample wells, resulting in much lower resolution. Other buffer systems can be used, for example the Tris™-tricine system for resolution of polypeptides in the size range below Mr 10,000. The sample may be treated in different ways according to the type of information the electrophoresis should reveal in presence of SDS and no boiling (separation according to size—disulfide bonds are intact and aggregates with intermolecular disulfide bonds will separate from the monomer) or in presence of SDS and a reducing agent (50–100 mM DTT) and boiling (only monomers will appear). SDS is an anionic detergent that denatures proteins by wrapping the hydrophobic tail around the polypeptide backbone. For almost all proteins, SDS binds at a ratio of approximately 1.4 g SDS per gram of protein, thus conferring a net negative charge to the polypeptide in proportion to its length. The SDS also disrupts hydrogen bonds, blocks hydrophobic interactions, and substantially unfolds the protein molecules, minimizing differences in molecular form by eliminating the tertiary and secondary structures. DTT is a reducing agent. DTT of 50–100 mM will cleave protein disulfide bonds and in presence of SDS the protein will unfold. Standard proteins of known MW are included in the electrophoretic run. Coomassie blue and silver staining are the two most common staining methods used for band detection on slab gels. Coomassie staining has a sensitivity

607

of 0.05 to 0.5 μg protein per band. Silver staining is about 10 100 times more sensitive enabling detection of 1–5 ng of protein per band. SDS-PAGE is used as a target protein identity method (separation according to MW). The method may also be used under non-reducing conditions to evaluate the pattern of di and polymeric target protein impurities One should in general be careful to use electrophoretic methods as purity analyses due to difficulties in quantifying the method.

16.13.23.16 2D-Electrophoresis

2D-electrophoresis is one of the electrophoretic methods comprising SDS-PAGE, native electrophoresis, IEF, 2D-electrophoresis and CE. One-dimensional SDS-PAGE offers separation of proteins according to their MW. Samples run under denaturing, but non-reducing conditions, will provide information of presence of other molecular species and of disulfide intermolecular di- and polymers. Samples run under denaturing and reducing conditions will provide information on monomeric compounds. Notice that in the latter procedure, it is common practice to boil the sample in the denaturing and reducing buffer before application. The boiling procedure must not be used if information of aggregates is required (denaturing but non-reducing conditions).

Native electrophoresis separates proteins according to charge, MW, shape, and other factors (samples are typically applied under conditions maintaining the tertiary structure). IEF separate proteins according to the pI (samples may be applied under native or denaturing conditions). The method offers very high resolution and is often used to provide information of presence of closely related derivatives (e.g., des-amido forms) or presence glycosylated derivatives of the target protein. 2D-electrophoresis separates proteins according to the proteins pI (first dimension) and its MW (second dimension). The method is a combination of IEF and SDS-PAGE. The resulting coordinate (pI, Mw) provides a unique identification of the protein. Differences in posttranslational modifications (e.g., phosphorylation) will often result in separate spots (slightly different pI and Mw). CE offers similar separation technologies. The CE methods can be used as a purity analysis. Two-dimensional electrophoresis is a combination of IEF (first dimension) and SDS-electrophoresis (second dimension) revealing information about a proteins charge and molecular coordinates (pI, Mw). It is very unlikely that two different proteins will have identical pI and Mw making 2D-electrophoresis a very powerful protein identification technique. Further, 2D-electrophoresis offers unique separation and identification even of complex protein mixtures making comparability analyses possible. From 1,000 to 2,000 well-resolved spots can be expected, when sensitive detection methods are used. There are, however, some restrictions to the methods usability, as proteins normally are reduced and denatured prior to IEF electrophoresis in the first dimension. One should therefore be careful to interpret the results obtained correctly, as pI and Mw may not be that of the native protein. Further, even when extreme care is taken in producing first and second dimension gels, some gel-related variability among gel casts occurs. The comments related to IEF and SDS electrophoresis will apply for 2D-electrophoresis as well. The method will apply for determination of target molecule pI and Mw, purity analysis with respect to target molecule derivatives, identity of post translational forms and as a method for determination of HCP patterns supporting immunoassay methods. However, the method is semi-quantitative only, at its best, and one must be very careful about method validation.

A specific feature of the method is diagonal gel electrophoresis for investigation of subunit composition of multi-subunit proteins containing inter chain disulfide bonds. Very basic proteins must be analyzed by non-equilibrium pH gradient electrophoresis (NEPHGE) developed by O'Farrell. The major difference between this and typical 2D systems is in the first dimension. Instead of applying the sample to the basic end of the gel, it is applied to the acidic end. In order to avoid the proteins to run to the end of the gel, short run times are used before an equilibrium state is reached. Coomassie blue and silver staining are the two most common staining methods used for band detection on slab gels. Coomassie staining has a sensitivity of 0.05 to 0.5 Pg protein per band. Silver staining is about 10–100 times more sensitive enabling detection of 1–5 ng of protein per band. 2D-electrophoresis is used as a target protein identity method (separation according to MW and pI). One should in general be careful to use electrophoretic methods as purity analyses due to difficulties in quantifying the method.

16.13.23.17 UV Absorbance

The method is based on the absorbance of tyrosine, tryptophan, and phenylalanine residues at 275–280 nm (ultraviolet region). Phenylalanine is only weakly absorbing and is usually neglected for most purposes. The protein structure is not affected by the method making on-line measurement a possibility. Pigments, organic cofactors and phenolic compounds interfere with the assay. The protein concentration measurement is based on Beer's law: $280 = E \times C \times L = H \times C \times L/Mw$, where OD is the optical density at 280 nm E is the absorptivity (nm × mL)/(mg × cm); C is the protein concentration in mg/mL; L is the light pathway (cm); H is the molar extinction coefficient; Mw is the MW (g/mol). The curve is normally linear between an O.D. of 0.05 and 0.8. It is common practice to use an extinction coefficient of 1 for protein mixtures accepting the great variability in the extinction 1% coefficient between different proteins. Weight absorbance coefficients, E (gram dry protein per 100 mL), range between 3 and 30 OD280 units for most proteins. The sensitivity range is from 0.05 to 1.0 mg/mL. Note that the presence of nucleic acids in the sample will interfere with the absorbance, the extinction coefficient of a protein is pH dependent. The UV absorbance method is used for determination of total protein in semi- and purified samples. The assay may be used as an on-line in process control method, for determination of total protein in intermediary samples and in the drug substance/product.

16.14 REGULATORY AFFAIRS

The regulatory filing of biological products is made in accordance with the rules established by the regulatory agencies. The main regulatory authorities and their current status regarding biogeneric products is given below.

16.14.1 United States Food and Drug Administration (http://www.fda.gov)

On October 1, 2003, FDA transferred certain product oversight responsibilities from the CBER to the CDER). This consolidation provides greater opportunities to further develop and coordinate scientific and regulatory activities between CBER and CDER, leading to a more efficient, effective, and consistent review program for human drugs and biologics.

FDA believes that as more drug and biological products are developed for a broader range of illnesses, such interaction is necessary for both efficient and consistent agency action. Under the new structure, the biologic products transferred to CDER will continue to be regulated as licensed biologics. The therapeutic biological products now under CDER's review include the following:

- Monoclonal antibodies for in vivo use
- Cytokines, growth factors, enzymes, immunomodulators; and thrombolytics
- Proteins intended for therapeutic use that are extracted from animals or micro-organisms, including recombinant versions of these products (except clotting factors)
- Other non-vaccine therapeutic immunotherapies

The IND filings and filings of BLA for therapeutic proteins are now received at CDER and not at CBER (http://www.fda.gov/cder/biologics/default.htm). Even though the therapeutic proteins mentioned above have been moved to CDER, the requirement for filing BLA continues. In the past, the approved biological products were not listed on the Orange Book as there was no generic equivalent so the information was not readily available on these products. Now a new listing method at FDA (http://www.accessdata.fda.gov/scripts/cder/drugsatfda/index.cfm) shows a listing of all approved products. The U.S. FDA has not yet developed a mechanism to accept generic applications for biological products. By the time this book goes to press, it is expected that the FDA will release a limited guideline on the filing of some specific proteins, most likely insulin and growth hormone. Sandoz has filed generic biological applications for growth hormone at both EMEA and FDA but at both of these agencies the review process has been held back and the matter is in the courts. To begin the process of developing guidelines for biogeneric products, the U.S. FDA had held a Public Workshop: Scientific Considerations Related to Developing Follow-On Protein Products, on September 14–15, 2004. It was open for comments till 12 November, 2004. The presentation made at this public hearing reveals the many hurdles that the bio-generic manufacturer is likely to face and these can be read at: http://www.fda.gov/cder/meeting/followOn/followOnPresentations.htm. In 1984, Congress created a mechanism for the approval of generic chemistry-based drugs in the Hatch–Waxman Amendments to the federal Food, Drug, and Cosmetics Act. Under Hatch–Waxman, once a drug reaches the end of its patent life, a competitor can get approval to market the same product using much of the first manufacturers' formulas and testing data. Without making the investment in drug discovery and clinical testing, generic manufacturers can offer their products at a much lower price than the company that did the original research. When a generic competitor enters the pharmaceutical market, prices for an already existing drug typically fall 70%. Biotech analysts say the price differential will be less for biologics because of the complexities of manufacturing protein-based drugs. Up until now most biotech companies believed their drugs, spawned by recombinant technology that evolved in the 1970s and 1980s, would remain free of generic competition because no similar pathway existed for abbreviated approvals. In the United States, most biotech drugs have been approved for market under the Public Health Service Act (PHSA), which was used to regulate vaccines and serums in the early 1900s. When bioengineered products began to come through the approval process, they fell under a different center in the FDA than did chemical-based drugs, which had been governed by the Food, Drug, and Cosmetics Act and later, Hatch–Waxman. In June, those centers merged to streamline administration, but the move provided FDA with an opportunity to examine its policy on generics. The agency's current review began with insulin and human growth hormone, because those products are easier to characterize than the more complex biotech drugs; also, they had always been regulated under the drug laws and not the PHSA.

Some relevant documents at FDA include the following:

- Guidance for Industry: Monoclonal Antibodies Used as Reagents in Drug Manufacturing (March 29, 2001);
- Guidance for Industry: Content and Format of Chemistry, Manufacturing and Controls Information and Establishment Description Information for a Biological In Vitro Diagnostic Product (March 8, 1999)
- Points to Consider in the Manufacture and Testing of Monoclonal Antibody Products for Human Use (February 28, 1997);
- Guidance for Industry for the Submission of Chemistry, Manufacturing, and Controls Information for a Therapeutic Recombinant DNA-Derived Product or a Monoclonal Antibody Product for In Vivo Use (August 1996). 21 CFR 120: *Hazard Analysis and Critical Control Point Systems*
- 21 CFR 210: Current Good Manufacturing Practice (GMP) in Manufacturing, Processing, Packing, or Holding of Drugs, General
- 21 CFR 211: Current GMP for Finished Pharmaceuticals
- 21 CFR 610: General Biological Products Standards
- 21 CFR 809: In Vitro Diagnostic Products for Human Use
- Draft Guidance for Industry: Drug Substance—Chemistry, Manufacturing, and Controls Information (January 6, 2004)
- Draft Guidance for Industry: Comparability Protocols—Protein Drug Products and Biological Products: Chemistry, Manufacturing, and Controls Information (September 3, 2003)
- Draft Guidance for Industry: Sterile Drug Products Produced by Aseptic Processing—Current Good Manufacturing Practice (September 3, 2003)
- Draft Guidance for Industry: Comparability Protocols—Chemistry, Manufacturing, and Controls Information (February 20, 2003)
- Draft Guidance for Industry: Drug Product—Chemistry, Manufacturing, and Controls Information (January 28, 2003)
- Draft Guidance for Industry: Preventive Measures to Reduce the Possible Risk of Transmission of Creutzfeldt-Jakob Disease (CJD) and Variant Creutzfeldt-Jakob Disease (vCJD) by Human Cells, Tissues, and Cellular and Tissue-Based Products (HCT/Ps) (June 14, 2002)
- Draft Guidance for Industry: Biological Product Deviation Reporting for Licensed Manufacturers of Biological Products Other than Blood and Blood Components (August 10, 2001)
- Guidance for Industry: Content and Format of Chemistry, Manufacturing and Controls Information and Establishment Description Information for a Biological In Vitro Diagnostic Product (March 8, 1999)

- Guidance for Industry: Content and Format of Chemistry, Manufacturing and Controls Information and Establishment Description Information for a Vaccine or Related Product (January 5, 1999)
- FDA Guidance Concerning Demonstration of Comparability of Human Biological Products, Including Therapeutic Biotechnology-Derived Products (April 1996)
- FDA Guidance Document Concerning Use of Pilot Manufacturing Facilities for the Development and Manufacturing of Biological Products
- Draft Points to Consider in the Characterization of Cell Lines Used to Produce Biologicals (July 12, 1993)
- Supplement to the Points to Consider in the Production and Testing of New Drugs and Biologics Produced by Recombinant DNA Technology: Nucleic Acid Characterization and Genetic Stability (April 6, 1992)
- Guideline on General Principles of Process Validation (May 1987)
- Points to Consider in the Production and Testing of New Drugs and Biologicals Produced by Recombinant DNA Technology (April 10, 1985)

16.14.2 European Medicines Evaluation Agency (http://www.emea.eu.int/)

On October 25, 2004, the EU accepted BioPartner's interferon as first "biosimilar" filing. If approved, the "biosimilar" could be on the market as early as next year. BioPartner's filing represents the first occasion that the EMEA has accepted an application for a bio-similar drug for review. This development comes shortly after the U.S. government turned down an application to market Omnitrop/Omnitrope (somatropin), a generic version of recombinant human growth hormone developed by Sandoz, citing problems in establishing an appropriate regulatory route for "biogeneric" products. Last year, the European Parliament approved new pharmaceutical legislation that, among other things, set out a legal framework for the registration of so-called biosimilars, biological therapies that are therapeutically the same as existing, approved biological products. Sandoz had also filed for approval with the European Medicines Evaluation Agency for Omnitrop, but was unable to progress the application. Documents of interest at EMEA include the following:

- 3AB4A: Production and Quality Control of Monoclonal Antibodies
- 3AB8A: Virus Validation Studies—The Design, Contribution and Interpretation of Studies validating the Inactivation and Removal of Viruses
- 3AB9A: *Validation of Virus Removal/Inactivation Procedures—Choice of Viruses* Regulation No. 1946/2003 of the European Parliament and of the Council of 15 July 2003 on Transboundary Movements of Genetically Modified Organisms
- 21/04/02 EudraLex Volume 4: Medicinal Products for Human and Veterinary Use—Good Manufacturing Practices
- 2000/608/EC: Commission Decision of 27 September 2000 Concerning the Guidance Notes for Risk Assessment Outlined in Annex III of Directive 90/219/EEC on the Contained Use of Genetically Modified Microorganisms (notified under document number C[2000] 2736)

- Commission Directive 91/356/EEC, of June 13, 1991, Laying Down the Principles and Guidelines of Good Manufacturing Practice for Medicinal Products for Human Use
- Council Directive 90/219/EEC of April 23, 1990 on the Contained Use of Genetically Modified Microorganisms
- 3AB1A: Production and Quality Control of Medicinal Products Derived by Recombinant DNA Technology
- 3AB2A: Quality of Biotechnological Products—Analysis of the Expression Construct in Cells Used for Production of r-DNA Derived Protein Products
- 3AB3A: Production and Quality Control of Cytokine Products Derived by Biotechnological Process
- 3AB6A: Gene Therapy Product Quality Aspects in the Production of Vectors and Genetically Modified Somatic Cells
- 3AB10A: Minimizing the Risk of Transmitting Agents Causing Spongiform Encephalopathy via Medicinal Products
- 3AB14A: Harmonization of Requirements for Influenza Vaccines

Japanese Ministry of Health and Welfare (MHW): http://www.nihs.go.jp Japanese health authorities mainly follow the ICH guidelines (see below).

World Health Organization (WHO): http://www.who.int/biologicals/. WHO provides International Biological Reference Preparations which serve as reference sources of defined biological activity expressed in an internationally agreed unit. These preparations are the basis of a uniform reporting system, helping physicians and scientists involved in patient care, regulatory authorities and manufacturing settings to communicate in a common language for designating the activity or potency of biological preparations used in prophylaxis or therapy and ensuring the reliability of in vitro biological diagnostic procedures used for diagnosis of diseases and treatment monitoring. This concept of using well-characterized preparations as references against which batches of biological products are assessed remains fundamental to ensuring the quality of biological products as well as the consistency of production and are essential for establishment of appropriate clinical dosing. These preparations are generally intended for use in the characterization of the activity of secondary reference preparations (regional, national or in-house working standards). The National Institute of Biological Standards and Control (http://www.nibsc .ac.uk/) is an international laboratory of WHO that supplies standards. WHO (www.who .int) has published a general guide to Good Manufacturing Practices for Pharmaceutical Products (Technical Report Series No. 823, Geneva, 1992), which is a good place to start when looking for regulatory guidance.

International Conference on Harmonization (ICH): http://www.ich.org. There are currently no official guidelines for the development of recombinant products. However, the rationale and views expressed by The International Conference on Harmonisation of Technical Requirements for Registration of Pharmaceuticals for Human Use (ICH) on licensed products are relevant. ICH is a project that brings together the regulatory authorities of Europe, Japan, and the United States and experts from the pharmaceutical industry in the three regions to discuss scientific and technical aspects of product registration. The purpose is to make recommendations on ways to achieve greater harmonization in the interpretation and application of technical guidelines and requirements for product registration in order to reduce or obviate the need to duplicate the testing carried out during the research and development of new medicines. The ICH quality web page is available at http://www.ich .org/TxtServer.jscr?@_ID=476&@_TYPE=HTML&@_TEMPLATE=616 and should be consulted for all aspects of biogeneric product filing. Some of the most relevant documents include the following:

- ICH harmonized tripartite guideline Q5B, Analysis of the expression construct in cells used for production of r-DNA derived protein products, Step 4 (http://www .ich.org/ich5q.html)
- ICH harmonized tripartite guideline Q5D, Derivation and characterization of cell substrates used for production of biotechnological/biological products, Step 4 (http://www.ich.org/ich5q.html)
- ICH Guidance on Viral Safety Evaluation of Biotechnology Products Derived From Cell Lines of Human or Animal Origin (September 24, 1998), ICH Draft Guidance: Q5E Comparability of Biotechnological/Biological Products Subject to Changes in Their Manufacturing Process (March 29, 2004)
- ICH Guidance: Q7A Good Manufacturing Practice Guide for Active Pharmaceutical Ingredients (September 25, 2001)
- ICH Guidance on Quality of Biotechnological/Biological Products: Derivation and Characterization of Cell Substrates Used for Production of Biotechnological/ Biological Products (September 21, 1998)
- ICH Final Guideline on Quality of Biotechnical Products: Analysis of the Expression Construct in Cells Used for the Production of r-DNA Derived Protein Products (February 1996)

16.15 REGULATORY ISSUES

Regulatory issue are mostly related to product safety, which is assured not only by product control but also in use of established and extensively tested cell banks, process robustness, well-characterized raw materials and in process control procedures generally decided on a case-by-case basis. The newest guidelines of the FDA related to PAT go into great detail on how to assure process robustness. The risks related directly to the use of recombinant technique relate either to contamination or immunogenicity, over and above the risks of manufacturing that are common and well-defined in the cGMP guidelines. The contamination results from viruses and other transmissible agents, cellular DNA and HCPs (e.g., growth factors). The potential introduction of adventitious agents such as fungi, bacteria, viruses and prions in cell culture media is of major concern and has prompted constant improvements in media and raw materials used. Thus raw materials possessing high contamination risk (e.g., hydrolysates and peptones produced from animals or by means of animal derived enzymes) should be avoided. The use of antibiotics is discouraged and when used, the selection markers are selected with care (e.g., kanamycin). Content of endotoxins (gram negative bacteria), nucleic acids, HCPs, and correct N-terminal in the drug substance/product are of major regulatory concern.

One of the most important components of regulatory scrutiny is the MCB and a thorough cell line characterization is required. The testing of the cell substrate is the first part of bio-safety program carried out for each biopharmaceutical drug substance/product used in clinical trials. For example, mammalian cell line characterization would typically include the following:

- Rodent retrovirus assays including RT, mus Dunni, XC, S + L−, and ERV
- Human pathogens including HIV-I and II, HBV, HCV, HAV, HSV-I, HSV-2, HSV-6, HTLV-I, HTLV-II, and CMV
- Primate pathogens including SIV, STLV, foamy agent, and SMRV
- Mycoplasma testing
- In vivo and in vitro adventitious agents testing
- Karyology and isoenzymes
- Electron microscopy

16.15.1 Sterility

Further issues are end of production tests, test of raw materials, and QC analyses of drug substance and drug product (the latter are rarely tested for viruses if produced in continuous cell lines). The potential risks associated with the use of microbial or metazoan expression systems are partly related to contaminants from the cells and partly from raw materials used to propagate the cells. Cell related impurities are nucleic acids and HCPs. Metazoan cells may be infected with viruses or other transmissible agents and they may produce growth-promoting proteins. Insect cells has been introduced as the baculoviral vector does not infect mammals, but the transfected insect cell line cannot be considered completely free of contaminating viruses (e.g., Flaviviridae), and it strongly advised to set up test programs similar to those of metazoan cells. It should be mentioned that mycoplasma infections might constitute a greater problem than previously anticipated. The extensive characterization of the MCB does to some point overcome the concerns of using serum and perhaps other raw materials of animal origin. It is strongly advised not to use raw materials of animal origin at any point after MCB characterization as safety could be compromised by such an act.

The downstream process is required to be fully validated for regulatory submissions. Some of the documents that may be required to establish the validation include the following:

- Batch records (downstream part)
- Development report (downstream part)
- In process control analytical method descriptions including typical data
- Laboratory notebooks
- List of raw materials used
- Protocol for validation
- Strategy and rationale report for the downstream part
- Summary reports
- Unit operation description

16.15.2 Purity Control Program

Purity of target protein is the most important consideration in supporting a regulatory filing. The analytical program is product specific and the rationale of the suggested program is to analyze the drug substance extensively in the early phases to ensure safety and to prevent unintended process redesign later on. It is highly recommended that biogeneric product manufacturer discuss the regulatory analytical procedures with the official authorities as early as possible; however, in those instances where compendial monographs exist, the choice of analytical methodology is well established. The manufacturers, however, must still demonstrate its plan for purity control. The purity control program depends on the expression system and the intended use of the material produced. In a typical microbial expression system, identity and biological activity are required for all four phases of development, preclinical, phase I–III; immunogenicity is not required at the preclinical level but must be evaluated at all other stages. Similarly, all tests related to purity are required at all levels, except viruses and prions. Virus clearance is performed prior to phase I and is not repeated until prior to phase III unless process is changed in a way that invalidates the preclinical study. The prion test program is yet unclear. Virus and prions testing is required in phase I and phase three when using insect cell, mammalian cell, and transgenic animal expression The tests for impurity that are required include HCPs, DNA, endotoxins, bioburden, co-solvents, leachable (if affinity chromatography has been used or if a new polymeric matrix has been introduced) components, and the impurity profile (impurities exceeding 0.1%) should normally be fully characterized prior to phase III clinical studies. If the impurity comprises less than 0.5% it is suggested to suspend the characterization program until phase III. Transgenic animals may co-express the equivalent animal protein. Its removal must be documented by means of specific test procedures. The target protein requires quantification at all stages but the toxicity is evaluated only at the preclinical stages. When preparing a regulatory filing for the biogeneric product, many of these analyses may be redundant and it is recommended that the regulatory authorities be consulted with in the early phase of development.

16.15.3 Immunochemical Properties

Immunogenicity is the ability of therapeutic protein products to elicit immune responses; antibodies are the most frequent measure of immune response to soluble protein products.

Cell-mediated immune responses to proteins may be critically important to generation of antibodies. The T-cell dependent antibody responses are generally required for antibodies to proteins or generally required for class switching to IgG and affinity maturation. T cells and B cells are activated by different segments of the same protein. The clinical concerns for antibodies to therapeutic proteins fall into several categories (Table 16.8):

Several recent case examples need to be reviewed to understand the potential and extent of the immunogenicity potential.

PEG-MGDF: The biologically unique function of MGDF/TPO is its megakaryocyte/ platelet growth and development potential. Literature reports that its neutralizing antibody caused thrombocytopenia in healthy platelet donors (4%) and oncology patients (0.5%). This illustrates effect of immune status of host. Furthermore, in

Table 16.8 Effect of Antibodies on Clinical Outcome

Clinical Concern	Clinical Outcome
Safety	Neutralize endogenous counterpart with unique function causing deficiency syndrome; hypersensitivity reactions
Efficacy	Inhibition or enhancement of product efficacy
Pharmacokinetics	Changes in dosing level due to PK changes.
None	Despite generation of antibodies, no discernable impact.

healthy donors, tolerance was easily broken (2–3 doses) in some cases and TCP developed in all animal models tested, including non-human primate using species specific product; however, antibody was present in some patients prior to treatment.

Erythropoietin: The neutralizing antibody to erythropoietin induces PRCA and approximately 300 cases have occurred from 1997 to 2003. Incidentally, nearly all cases are related to use of Eprex brand of erythropoietin and nearly all cases developed following packaging changes (prefilled syringes), formulation changes (delete HSA), and shift in route of administration (to SC from IV). These cases turned out not to be an isolated group, but clearly part of a more pervasive problem. By December 2003, a total of 262 cases reported.

The reason why it is possible to break immunologic tolerance to endogenous proteins is because mammals are not fully tolerant to endogenous proteins and forms the basis for autoimmune diseases such as autoimmune thyroiditis, MS, and RA as well as the basis for regulation of inflammatory cytokines and fail-safe mechanism for potent growth factors (Epo, TPO, G-CSF). As a result, the immune response can abort efficacy of life saving or life enhancing protein therapeutics to glucocerebrosidase in Gaucher's disease where most patients tolerize with continued treatment and in a small percentage high titer antibodies persist and neutralize activity, to Factor VIII in Hemophilia A where approximately 30% develop "inhibitors" or neutralizing antibody, to alpha-glucosidase in Pompe's disease, and to mAbs in treatment of autoimmune disease.

As a result, regulatory agencies like the FDA assess the risk of immune responses to therapeutic proteins by estimating the likelihood of development of an immune response as learned from known product and patient risk factors, potential clinical sequelae resulting from generation of immune response from understanding of biological function and redundancy of protein; alternative products for indication if available; ability to terminate immune response. Predicting immunogenicity is a difficult task and factors such as evaluation if it is derivation, self or foreign, product-specific attributes, patient/immune system specific attributes and the results of animal immunogenicity testing. Immunogenicity is expected from proteins of foreign origin as it would neutralize the product and produce hypersensitivity; in the case of immunogen created by the body itself, there is a potential for immunogenicity and would neutralize endogenous protein and produce severe deficiency syndrome. The product-specific factors of importance are: molecular structure, aggregation, novel epitopes > epitope spreading, degradation, oxidation/deamidation, glycosylation.

The important factors to assess the potential of a product to raise an immune response include product specific factors and patient specific factor that impact on decisions regarding testing. Aggregation remains one of the most important factors. It is important to remember that there can be covalently bonded aggregates, which may be measured by standard means in current use, and there can be non-covalently bonded aggregates resulting from hydrophobic or weaker ionic interactions, which are difficult to quantitate using standard techniques. Covalent aggregates are mostly affected by the molecular structure while non-covalent aggregates are a result of formulation effects. Recently, greater understanding has been developed about the role of aggregation in inducing immunogenicity. The presence of aggregates precludes tolerance in naïve immune system and that the product changes associated with enhanced immunogenicity (oxidation, degradation) are associated with protein aggregation. For example, tolerance to interferon alpha breaks when aggregates are formed at room temperature storage; IL-2 exists as microaggregates (average size 27 mols) and is highly immunogenic resulting in antibody development in 47%–74% instances; in a study on mAb, the elimination of aggregates eliminated immunogenicity. The methods to detect aggregation include methods that disrupt non-covalent or weak aggregates and include SDS-polyacrylamide gel electrophoresis, CE, size exclusion HPLC. Methods that better detect weak aggregates include analytical ultracentrifugation, field flow fractionation, and atomic force microscopy. The problem of aggregate formation requires studies using sensitive methods to quantitate product aggregation for covalently bonded and weak aggregates. The effects of product aggregates in in vitro and in vivo systems should be assessed to understand what level of aggregates can break tolerance? And obviously, the processing steps should be designed such as to minimize product aggregation.

The product specific factors also include the inherent immunomodulatory activity. The example of immune suppression include anti-CD4 mAb CTLA4-Ig and of immunostimulatory, GM-CSF; Flt-3L;CpG oligos. The formulation factors are also product specific factors that may arise from novel epitope formation with protein adducts, patient/immune System factors, immune competency is more likely to generate response than immune compromised. The route of administration takes its importance in the following hierarchy: SC/ID > IM > IV. The dose and frequency of administration also play an important role; for example, it was demonstrated that frequent intravenous dosing of Factor VIII resulted in generating therapeutic counterpart of endogenous leading to tolerance.

The usefulness of animal immunogenicity testing depends on homology of human to animal protein. For example, studies with TPO and PEG-MGDF precisely predicted immunogenicity results in humans; however, it is not generally useful if homology is low as a result of xenogeneic responses. Other uses of animal models include deliberate provocation of immunity to assess effects of neutralization of endogenous product; the use of knock out animals may predict effect of loss of endogenous product due to antibody neutralization.

The risk of immunogenicity is determined by analysis of factors critical for generation of immune responses, how they apply to the product in question and the clinical consequences of such responses. For products that are critical components of therapy for life threatening or debilitating diseases, sensitive immunogenicity assays should be in place at earliest stages of product development. This should include evaluation of the change of manufacturing changes (formulation, specification, virus or adventitious agent removal/inactivation, establishment of MCB) on immunogenicity. Examples of formulation changes that have demonstrated impact on aggregation-related effects include the observation that addition of sucrose to buffer eliminated aggregation in mAb products, in the case of Eprex removal of human serum albumin increased immunogenicity while removal of human serum albumin from interferon alpha reduced immunogenicity; heat denaturation when virus/adventitious agent increased product aggregation in the case of urokinase, shear force from product filtration increases product aggregation and so does low pH as shown in the case of interferon alpha; renaturation or refolding induces protein aggregation and in some instances protein overexpression in some systems can theoretically lead to aggregation; even such changes as storage commodity have shown impact on aggregation. The syringe material may affect hydrophobic interaction and thus aggregation of product. Additionally, in one instance leaching from syringe gasket activated metalloprotease-product truncation or leaching from syringe barrel caused product oxidation regaling in aggregation. There are reported incidences where prefilled syringes stored at home storage condition alter immunogenicity of photo and heat labile molecules like erythropoietin; even mechanical agitation would induce or disrupt structure for most proteins.

Testing for immunogenicity for high risk manufacturing changes can take many routes; the most important being up front testing but it is generally insufficiently powered to detect relatively rare events, that is, <1/1,000; this leaves post-marketing adverse event assessment, passive AE surveillance programs, epidemiologic studies and post-marketing commitments for active data collection as only viable choices. Requirement for further in vivo testing depends on the product, the manufacturing change, results of extended comparability assessment including comprehensive aggregate analysis.

As elaborated earlier, one of the most important concerns of the regulatory authorities is the immunogenic potential of generic proteins. During recent considerations by the U.S. FDA, this has been the prime concern, over and above all other considerations. The first generation of protein drugs was based on tissue extracts from animals (e.g., bovine insulin, porcine insulin) or from human extracts (pituitary glands). The foreign origin and the lack of purity of these earlier preparations often resulted in immune responses in patients. With the introduction of the recombinant technology, it was hoped that the near identity with the human "natural" protein and better purification procedures would reduce the problem due to immunological tolerance of "self" proteins. Although replacement of the animal protein with the human species reduced the problem, it still persisted, and it was learned that the incidence of immunogenicity does not necessarily correlate with the sequence homology to the human protein. Interestingly, it has been observed that the target protein may induce an immune response even in individuals not being deficient in the protein, but merely produces an insufficient amount. Furthermore, individuals with no predisposition to auto-immunity often produce antibodies against the target protein. Even minor amounts of protein impurities may raise an antigenic response (the limit for presence of bovine proinsulin in bovine insulin preparations can be 1 ppm) making it mandatory to use well-designed, robust, and controlled downstream processes to produce the product and to use validated HCP assays to detect for content of HCP in the drug substance/product. Apparently modern process technologies and designs cope well with the challenge resulting in a reduction of immunogenic responses due to HCPs. Product derived impurities such as target protein aggregates may also be antigenic making protein stability during processing and storage a central safety issue.

The target protein may be immunogenic for several reasons:

- It has a different amino acid sequence from the human protein equivalent.
- It has an incorrect 3D structure.
- It has incorrect posttranslational modifications.
- It is aggregated.
- It is chemically modified.
- It is administered together with an adjuvant.
- The protein is administered in large amounts.
- The protein is delivered by a method raising an immune response.

An immune response should be expected if there is a sequence difference between the target protein and the human equivalent. However, an indication of the complexity of immunogenicity is illustrated by lack of antibody response in patients having received animal proteins even after years of use. Further, administration of de-aggregated non-self proteins without adjuvants has induced immunological tolerance. Foreign proteins may also be of bacterial or plant origin, for example, introduced as impurities. In some diseases the patient lack the human protein (e.g., hemophilia patients carrying a homozygous deletion) and the recombinant human protein must be considered foreign. Human protein analogues comprise a specific class of proteins having high homology with the native protein. These products predominantly induce immune responses in patients, who lack immune tolerance because of an innate insufficiency of the native gene.

Incorrect native structure is often associated with scrambled forms resulting from in vitro folding of proteins expressed in *E. coli*. Posttranslational modifications (e.g., glycoproteins) not resembling those of the natural product may also be immunogenic. It is a common observation that several different forms are expressed and co-purified resulting in a mixed product. A consistent pattern at IEF or peptide mapping should be provided to demonstrate identity between batches.

Protein aggregates have been shown repeatedly to cause immunogenicity in patients. The immune response is usually weak and is generally observed after long-term treatment. The clinical consequence is usually minor and loss of efficacy can be compensated for by increased doses. In rare cases the antibody neutralizes the native protein with severe biological consequences. Formation of protein aggregates is a function of upstream processing, downstream processing, formulation, and storage conditions making protein stability a key issue not only in process design but also in broader aspect. It should be noted that animals rendered fully tolerant to monomeric proteins will not mount an immune response when challenged with and aggregated version of the protein. Chemically modified forms such as des-amido and oxidized forms may also be antigenic. Interestingly chemically modified analogues (e.g., PEGylated products) have been introduced with the purpose of altering the protein half-life and the immune reactive response. The effect on the immune system is still unclear. Administration of self-proteins to patients can break immunological tolerance due to the presence of adjuvants such as LPS. Administration of the protein in large amounts may induce an immunogenic response. The route of administration also influences the local inflammatory response or induction of antibodies in patients.

The formation of antibodies may have several, sometimes severe consequences for the patient. Those cases with the most serious adverse events have been those instances where antibodies raised against product cross react with endogenous proteins as seen with inhibition of endogenous thrombopoietin and subsequent development of autoimmune thrombocytopenia. Examples of therapeutic proteins resulting in antibody formation in patients are streptokinase, staphylokinase, bovine adenosine deaminase, calcitonin, trichosanthin, gonadotropin, erythropoietin, interleukin 2, TNF receptor 2-Ig, and Denileukin diftitox. Other clinical consequences are hypersensitivity reactions including fever, nausea, chills, and allergic reactions. Immediate hypersensitivity responses that cause anaphylactic or anaphylactoid responses are of major concern.

Better process design, control of protein stability, generation of soluble non-aggregated native proteins, high purification factors of immunogenic substances, avoidance of contaminating adjuvants, and better formulations are examples of process related preventive actions. The impact of the process, also on long-term product stability, should be taken into consideration throughout the drug development program.

Covalent binding with polymers such as polyethylene glycol (e.g., in PEG-Intron) and dextran may reduce the antigenicity and immunogenicity of proteins. The effect of proteins, which are homologous with human proteins, is unclear as exemplified in the serious clinical consequences observed with PEGylated TNF-β treatment. Sequence modifications, especially where T-cell epitopes have been removed or changed, are of interesting modifications meant to reduce the immune response.

The ability to predict immunogenicity is the key issue at most regulatory authorities. The approaches include bioinformatics, screening for T-cell epitopes, detection of antibiotics, the use of animal models and ultimately, the response in patients. Bioinformatics approaches are based on identification of super motifs present across different MHC alleles or to identify "promiscuous" epitopes capable of binding different MHC alleles regardless of "super type" family. Algorithms allow for the construction of a matrix of all possible amino acid side chain effects for a single MHC binding motif. The screening of T-cell epitopes rely on the induction of T-cell activity from cells derived from previously exposed subjects or the identification of priming T-cell epitopes using a dendritic cell based assay—the i-mune assay. The detection of antibodies is a common methodology to confirm an immune response in patients. Typical immunoassays are ELISA (direct binding and competitive ELISA), ELISA in combination with bioassays and surface plasmon resonance (BIAcore technology), electrochemiluminescense (ECL), SDS-PAGE, and WB technology. However, it should be noticed that the antibody level might be too low for detection in some of the assays mentioned (lack of sensitivity). The goal of antibody testing include detection of all antibodies capable of binding to the target protein, to identify all antibodies of clinical relevance, to determine whether the antibodies can neutralize the drug's biological effect, to characterize the antibodies of relevance and to assess the impact of antibodies on the therapeutic protein program. The animal models have in general not been able to predict the immunogenicity of recombinant biopharmaceuticals in humans, the main issue being that the administration of a human protein into an animal species is likely to be immunogenic. In addition, the said biopharmaceutical cannot be expected to be biologically active, which can affect the immunogenicity. The use of transgenic animals is a promising technology as shown for interferon-α studies in human interferon-α transgenic mice.

Since therapeutic proteins can provoke life threatening autoimmuno response, regulatory agencies will expect, prior to licensure, detailed clinical evaluation of the potential for immunogenicity. CBER (and now CDER) considers immune responses to biological therapeutic agents in a hierarchy, structured by clinical effects. The greatest concern regards immediate hypersensitivity responses that cause anaphylactic or anaphylactoid responses. Also the presence of neutralizing antibodies is of major concern as seen in patients exhibiting pure red blood cell aplasia and immune-mediated thrombocytopenia after treatment with recombinant erythropoietin and thrombopoietin. Of importance, but posing less threat, is generation of binding antibodies, which can diminish product efficacy. The Concerted EU Action started in 1993 with the purpose to coordinate research on the immunogenicity of biopharmaceuticals is an important learning exercise.

Immunochemical properties are described in the ICH Harmonized Tripartite Guideline. Specifications: Test Procedures and Acceptance Criteria for Biotechnological Products (Q6B) on 10 March 1999, for example, see http://www.ich.org/TxtServer.jser?@_ID=476&&@_TYPE=HTML&&@_TEMPLATE=616 and in Preclinical safety evaluation of biotechnology derived pharmaceuticals, ICH topic S6, see: http://www.ich.org/TxtServer.jser?@_ID=501&&@_TYPE=HTML&&@_TEMPLATE=616.

16.15.4 Documentation

Regulatory filings often comprise truck-loads of documentation. This documentation is supposed to support technology transfer from research over to manufacturing of material for clinical trials. Although the major part of the development information and data gathered is not a part of the material submitted to regulatory authorities, it was a natural choice to use the structure of the Common Technical Document, ICH, Section 3.2. A comprehensive regulatory filing will include documents related to authentication (sponsor's identification), the identification of the project (including the identification of the staff and facility participating), general characteristics of the protein, the description of manufacturing and testing facilities (see The Common Technical Document, ICH Section 3.2.S., NTA 2B, CTD module 3, July 2001).

The control of materials (reagents, enzymes, substrates, solvents, catalysts, etc.) used in the process must be described in detail. It is common practice to establish a list of raw materials prior to the up-scaling program. The required information about the raw materials includes the following:

- Raw material name
- Manufacturer
- Lot number
- Batch number
- Raw material description
- Raw material acceptance criteria
- Analytical test methods
- Stability of the raw material
- Release procedure(s)
- Regulatory support files for chromatographic media

- Reference to EP and USP
- Where in the process is the raw material used?
- Clearance control of adventitious agents
- Control of source and starting materials of biologic origin
- Source, history, and generation of cell substrate
- Cell banking system, characterization, and testing

The process is presented in the form a flow sheet which is a rather detailed overview of the downstream process preferably using diagrams and boxes that identifies Unit operations in sequential order; Unit operation number; Protocol reference; Where in the process is the raw material introduced; Where is the raw material removed?; Parameter intervals of each unit operation; Critical parameters; Buffer composition and description; Chromatographic media used; Filters and membranes used. The details about this arrangement are available in the ICH CTD (www.nihs.go.jp/dig/ich/m4index-e.html; Section 3.2.S., NTA 2B, CTD module 3, July 2001).

The rationale and strategy report is a final document describing the rationale and strategy behind the drug development program and process design. The report should be written at the initiation of the experimental process development work. The rationale and strategy report is part of a suggested process development documentation system comprising the rationale and strategy report, the laboratory notebooks, the summary reports, the unit operation reports, the unit operation protocols, and the development report.

The laboratory notebook is a written record of the laboratory work performed. It is a final document. The laboratory notebooks are part of a suggested process development documentation system comprising the rationale and strategy report, the laboratory notebooks, the summary reports, the unit operation reports, the unit operation protocols and the development report. Specific rules regarding keeping records in laboratory books should be observed.

A summary report describes a study related to the process development, the development of an analytical method, or other specific development issues that need to be addressed during drug substance development. Usually, the summary report is a short and concise final document that summarizes the results from a development study shortly after the study has been performed. Typical examples are: reports describing a factorial design experiment, a unit operation optimization, chemical modifications of the protein, semi-synthesis, and technical investigations. The summary reports are part of a suggested process development documentation system comprising the rationale and strategy report, the laboratory notebooks, the summary reports, the unit operation reports, the unit operation protocols and the development report.

The unit operation document describes the development work related to a given unit operation. The aim is to collect all information of relevance in one document giving easy access to overview the rationale of the unit operation protocol. The report is a final document providing a status at the time of tech transfer from development to pilot. The unit operation reports are part of a suggested process development documentation system comprising the rationale and strategy report, the laboratory notebooks, the summary reports, the unit operation reports, the unit operation protocols, and the development report.

The unit operation protocol is a live document describing the state of the art of the unit operation. The combined collections of unit operation protocols comprise the manufacturing procedure of the drug substance batches produced. The summary reports are part of a suggested process development documentation system comprising the rationale and strategy report, the laboratory notebooks, the summary reports, the unit operation reports, the unit operation protocols, and the development report.

The development report is the overall development document summarizing the drug development program. The development report is part of a suggested process development documentation system comprising the rationale and strategy report, the laboratory notebooks, the summary reports, the unit operation purports, the unit operation protocols, and the development report.

A structural characterization report describes the analytical method used to characterize the structure of the drug substance. The structural characterization reports are part of the suggested drug substance QC program comprising QC and characterization methods.

The report on control of drug substance suggests the content of an analytical method report. The report will develop from a method description over qualification to a fully validated report.

The reference material is an internal standard used as a working standard during development and early phase production for clinical trials. The reference material precedes the reference standard normally established during production for phase III clinical material.

16.16 PROTEIN DEGRADATION

Proteolysis is a selective, highly regulated process that plays an important role in cellular physiology. *Escherichia coli* contains a large number of proteases that are localized in the cytoplasm, the periplasm, and the inner and outer membranes. These proteolytic enzymes participate in a host of metabolic activities, including the selective removal of abnormal proteins. Protein damage or alteration may result from a variety of conditions, such as incomplete polypeptides, mutations caused by amino acid substitutions, excessive synthesis of subunits from multimeric complexes, posttranslational damage through oxidation or free-radical attack, and genetic engineering. Such abnormal proteins are efficiently removed by the bacterial proteolytic machine. To date, the mechanisms of protein degradation are incompletely understood, and it is unlikely that all proteolytic pathways or enzymes operating in *E. coli* have been identified yet. For example, a new protease associated with the outer membrane was recently discovered and a fascinating new mechanism for the degradation of abnormal proteins in *E. coli* has just been uncovered. Nevertheless, the intense scientific interest in this area has generated new tools and strategies for minimizing the degradation of heterologous proteins in *E. coli*.

Although the precise structural features that impart lability to proteins are not known, some determinants of protein instability have been elucidated. In a series of systematic studies, Varshavsky and colleagues formulated the "N-end rule" that relates the metabolic stability of a protein to its amino-terminal residue. Thus, in *E. coli*, N-terminal Arg, Lys, Leu, Phe, Tyr, and Trp conferred 2 min half-lives on a test protein, whereas all the other amino acids except proline conferred more than 10 h half-lives on the same protein. As discussed above, amino acids with small side chains in the second position of the polypeptide facilitate the methionine aminopeptidase catalyzed removal of the N-terminal methionine. Therefore, these studies suggest that Leu in the second position would probably be exposed by the removal of the methionine residue and would destabilize the protein.

The second determinant of protein instability is a specific internal lysine residue located near the amino terminus. This residue is the acceptor of a multiubiquitin chain that facilitates protein degradation by a ubiquitin-dependent protease in eukaryotes. Interestingly, in a multisubunit protein, the two determinants can be located on different subunits and still target the protein for processing.

Another correlation between amino acid content and protein instability is presented in the PEST hypothesis. On the basis of statistical analysis of eukaryotic proteins that have short half-lives, it was proposed that proteins are destabilized by regions enriched in Pro, Glu, Ser, and Thr, flanked by certain amino acid residues. Phosphorylation of these PEST domains leads to increased calcium binding, which in turn facilitates the destruction of the protein by calcium-dependent proteases. It was suggested that PEST-rich proteins may be produced efficiently in *E. coli*, which apparently lacks the PEST proteolytic system.

Strategies for minimizing proteolysis of recombinant proteins include protein targeting to the periplasm or the culture medium, the use of protease-deficient host strains, growth of the host cells at low temperature, construction of N-and/or C-terminal fusion proteins, tandem fusion of multiple copies of the target gene, coexpression of molecular chaperones, coexpression of the T4 *pin* gene, replacement of specific amino acid residues to eliminate protease cleavage sites, modification of the hydrophobicity of the target protein, and optimization of fermentation conditions.

Although the variety of approaches for protein stabilization attests to the ingenuity of the investigators, the usefulness of some of the above methods may be limited, depending on the intended use of the recombinant protein. Thus, for example, the presence of fusion moieties on the target protein may interfere with functional or structural properties or therapeutic applications of the product. The engineering of enzymatic or chemical cleavage sites for the subsequent removal of the fusion partners is a complex process that involves numerous considerations: the accessibility of the cleavage sites to enzyme digestion; the purity, specificity, and cost of the commercially available enzymes; the authenticity of the N or C termini upon enzymatic digestion; the possible modification of the target protein upon chemical treatment, and so forth. For the large-scale production of fusion proteins, some of these difficulties are amplified. Similarly, the fusion of multiple copies of the target gene to create multidomain polypeptides requires the subsequent conversion to monomeric protein units by cyanogen bromide cleavage. In this case, the target protein must not contain internal methionine residues and must be able to withstand harsh reaction conditions. Moreover, a limited extend of amino acid side chain modification may occur, and the toxicity of cyanogen bromide presents a significant issue for large-scale cleavage reactions. Similarly, the rational modification of a protein sequence requires extensive structural information which may not be available. Molecular chaperones have been used successfully to stabilize specific proteins, but this approach remains a hit-or-miss affair.

The cytoplasm of *E. coli* contains a greater number of proteases than does the periplasm. Therefore, proteins located in the periplasm are less likely to be degraded. For example, proinsulin localized to the periplasm was 10 fold more stable that when produced in the cytoplasm. However, proteolytic activity in the periplasm is substantial. Secretion into the culture medium would provide a better alternative in terms of protein stability. Unfortunately, the technology for secretion of proteins from *E. coli* into the culture medium is still in its infancy. A major catalyst of protein degradation in bacteria is the induction of heat shock proteins in response to a variety of stress conditions, such as the thermal induction of gene expression or the accumulation of abnormal or heterologous proteins in the cytoplasm. Under these conditions, the production of the *lon* gene product, protease La, and other proteases is enhanced. This problem is minimized by the use of host strains deficient in the *rpoH* (*htpR*) locus. The *rpoH* gene encodes the RNA polymerase 32 subunit, which regulates several proteolytic activities in *E. coli*. Hosts that carry the *rpoH* mutation have been patented and have been demonstrated to dramatically increase the production of foreign proteins in *E. coli*. Strain SG21173, which is deficient in proteases La and Clp and the *rpoH* locus, is particularly effective in protein production. A large number of protease-deficient hosts exists, including some that are deficient in all known protease loci that affect the stability of secreted proteins.

Before leaving this section, it is worth repeating a caveat on the use of protease-deficient strains: proteolysis may be an effect rather than a cause of folding problems, serving as a disposal system to remove misfolded and aggregated material. Therefore, it is possible that the absence of proteases will result in increased toxicity to the host as a result of the accumulation of abnormal proteins.

Like other small molecules, protein drugs are subject to demonstration of stability (providing a predetermined minimum potency) to the time of use and in addition, a safety profile since the degradation products of protein drugs can be immunogenic, compared to small molecules where the concern is mainly creation of toxic molecules. The stability studies for therapeutic proteins are conducted at three levels: preformulation, formulation development, and formal GMP studies. The preformulation studies determine basic stability properties of bulk protein or peptide and the accelerated studies at this stage are primarily intended to establish stability indicating assays and other analytic methods. The formulation development studies are intended for the candidate formulation and encompass large studies that evaluate the effects of excipients, container/closure systems, and where lyophilized, a study of myriad factors that can alter the characteristics of products. The data generated in the formulation development studies is used to select final formulation and to design the studies that follow: formal GMP studies. The formal stability studies are used to support clinical use, IND and then all the way through a Biological License Application (submitted to CDER; effective June 2003, therapeutic proteins are now handled by CDER). When preparing supplies for the clinical use, it is important to know that there is no need to demonstrate shelf-life for the commercial dosage form and only stability demonstration is required during the testing phase, such as six months; many manufacturers used frozen product to assure adequate stability; this may create a logistics problem of assuring that the clinical sites can store the produce frozen. Obviously, for products which may be adversely affected by freezing will not be subject to this method of reducing the clinical startup time. Also, at this stage of initial clinical testing under an IND, the test methods need not be fully validated or having demonstrated robustness; as long as reproducibility and repeatability is demonstrated, this should be acceptable to FDA. The formal GMP studies monitor commercial lots and clear ICH guidelines are available to follow the protocols of these studies in ICH Stability Guidelines for Biologics, Federal Register July 10, 1996, Volume 61, No. 133, pp. 36466–36469.

16.17 STABILITY CONSIDERATIONS

Commercial viability of recombinant production processes depends on the final product yield; this is a particularly more significant issue as biogeneric manufacturer will bring their line of products which will be sold at a lower price than the innovator's products; the issue of yield becomes more important now. A primary cause of poor yield is neither the quality of the gene construct nor the nature of molecule but the degradation of the product during the manufacturing process. Protein degradation therefore becomes a key factor that must be thoroughly understood and steps taken to minimize this degradation step wherever possible. This chapter deals with this significant issue and makes suggestions on how to avoid the degradation of proteins in the downstream processing.

16.17.1 Proteolysis

In contrast to the cellular environment, where enzymatic degradation of proteins is highly controlled, extra cellular proteases is the cause of uncontrolled protein degradation. The result of the proteolytic attack may vary from complete hydrolysis, single breaks within the peptide chain, or loss of a few N- or C-terminal amino acid residues. Besides loosing the product, presence of truncated forms may seriously challenge the purification design.

Proteolytic enzymes are released to the medium because of cell death, mechanical stress, or induced cell lysis. Their presence should be expected during fermentation and initial downstream unit operations. Most enzymes of the vacuoles and lysosomes will be minimally active at slightly alkaline pH (7–9), a pH interval strongly recommended for extraction of proteins expressed in bacteria.

Proteins are probably more resistant toward proteolytic attacks in their native state and stabilizing factors (e.g., co-factor, correct parameter interval, co-solvent) should always be considered optimized. Use of protein inhibitors is not recommended for safety reasons. The primary mechanism of proteolysis is the enzymatic hydrolysis of the peptide bond. The indicators of this reaction taking place in the system include loss of product or poor yield, lack of expected activity, changes in specific activity, change in MW, high background staining in 1D SDS electrophoresis, smeared bands and many lower Mw bands of poor resolution, bands may disappear, discrepancies in Mw. The preventive actions that can be taken to prevent proteolysis are listed in Table 16.9.

The use of enzyme inhibitors is not recommended as they are harmful to human beings. Ascertain that the degradation observed is not a function of the analytical assay. Enzyme inhibitors can be used for prevention of enzymatic activity in analytical assays. Mild denaturation may accelerate enzymatic digestion. Selective removal (e.g., affinity chromatography) of specific enzymes should be considered, too.

Table 16.9   Preventive Actions against Proteolysis

Factor	Comment
pH	There is no specific pH range in which all enzymes are considered inactive; At slightly alkaline pH the non-specific enzymes of the vacuoles and lysosomes will be minimally active. Use strong buffers for extraction to prevent unintended shift in pH as a result of cell disruption. Some yeast enzymes are least active in the pH range of 4–5, but active in the pH range of 7–9. Phosphate may exhibit a stabilizing effect on proteins
Temperature	Low temperature decreases the proteolytic activity. It is recommended to store harvest at 4°C–8°C or frozen.
Time	Enzymatic protein degradation is a function of time. Lengthy procedures and long storage times should be avoided during harvest, capture, and initial purification steps.
Conductivity	Non-critical
Redox potential	Reducing and oxidizing conditions may alter the disulfide bridge arrangement and state of free cysteine residues thus influencing the protein secondary and tertiary structure.
Co-solvents	Presence of other proteins in excess (e.g., albumin) will reduce the proteolytic damage. Co-solvents such as glycerol or dimethylsulfoxide may have a stabilizing effect, but will probably be too expensive for large-scale operations.
Low Mw compounds	Substrates, substrate analogues, and co-factors can help stabilizing the protein. Potential proteinase activators (e.g., divalent metal ions) should be excluded from the extraction buffer.
Techniques	Careful cell disruption and specific extraction procedures may lower the enzymatic cleavage.
Denaturation	The proteolytic enzymes lose their biological activity upon denaturation. However, some enzymes are stable under mild denaturing conditions leading to increased activity if the target protein is partly denatured under the same conditions.

16.17.2 Deamidation

Two amino acid residues are involved in the deamidation reaction: Asparagine and glutamine. The conversion to the corresponding carboxylic acid residues results in a shift in net charge of the protein at pH above the pKa. As the deamidation may influence the biological activity and the stability of the molecule the maximal content of des-amido forms in bulk materials and in biopharmaceutical preparations is constantly being debated. The list of proteins undergoing deamidation is comprehensive and includes well-known proteins such as insulin, human growth hormone, and cytochrome C.

Asparagine residues tend to be more susceptible to deamidation that glutamine residues. Further, the deamidation reaction is strongly sequence specific in model peptides with the half-life of the -Asn-Pro- sequence being 100-fold greater than that of -Asn-Gly.

Table 16.10 Preventive Actions against Deamidation

Factor	Comment
pH	Deamidation should be expected above pH 5. The optimal working range in which to avoid deamidation is probably between 3.0 and 5.0.
Temperature	The deamidation rate increases with increasing temperature.
Time	The deamidation rate is a function of time. Presence of des-amido forms is a marker for drug product stability and shelf life.
Conductivity	The ionic strength of the solution should be kept low. At high ionic strength the deamidation reaction can be fast even at neutral pH.
Redox potential	Non-essential parameter.
Co-solvents	In general the buffer species and the buffer strength will influence the rate of deamidation. High solvent dielectrics favor deamidation. In model peptides the protein stability was higher in Tris buffer than in phosphate buffer.

To some extent these observations can also be used on proteins taking the structural steric factors and nearby amino acid residues into consideration.

At pH above 5, deamidation of asparagyl or glutamyl occurs via a relatively slow intermediate succinimide formation. The succinimidyl derivative is rapidly hydrolyzed at either the α- or β-carbonyl group to generate a mixture of normal- and iso-residues. Under strongly acidic conditions, asparagine or glutamine residues are hydrolyzed to the corresponding carboxyl residue. The indicators of deamidation include extra bands in electrophoresis and extra peaks in chromatographic recordings. Table 16.10 lists preventive actions against deamidation.

16.17.3 Oxidation

The amino acid residues histidine, methionyl, cysteine, tryptophan, and tyrosin are potential oxidation sites at neutral at slightly alkaline conditions. Oxidation of the said residues often results in loss of immunological and/or biological activity. The list of proteins that have been oxidized is comprehensive and includes biopharmaceutical products such as albumin, growth hormone, glucagons, interleukin-1β and interleukin 2. In many cases, the immunological and/or biological activity was only partially lost. In general, oxidation of methionyl to methionyl sulfoxide does not affect protein antigenicity, probably because the conformational structure of the oxidized protein is close to the native structure. On the other hand oxidation of a single amino acid residue often causes changes in the biological activity and all efforts should be taken to minimize oxidation reactions.

The mechanism of oxidation involves methionyl residues which are converted to methionyl sulfoxide residues under mild oxidizing conditions. The most reactive residues are those exposed to the solvent, while those residues buried within the hydrophobic regions

Table 16.11   Preventive Actions against Oxidation

Factor	Comment
pH	The oxidation rate is assumed low at slightly acidic pH.
Temperature	Working at low temperatures decreases the rate of oxidation.
Time	The oxidation reaction is a function of time.
Conductivity	No data available.
Redox potential	Disulfide bond formation will take place at a redox potential above 0 mV. A high redox potential indicates presence of oxidizing agents.
Co-solvents	Avoid oxidizing agents and protect against light. Addition of chelating agents (EDTA, citric acid, thioglycolic acid), antioxidants (BHT, BHA, propyl gallate, Vitamin E) and/or reducing agents (Cys, DTT, methionine, ascorbic acid, sodium sulfite, thioglycolic acid, thioglycerol) may reduce oxidation.

are fairly inert to oxidation (e.g., methionine residues in myoglobin and trypsin). Methionine residues are susceptible to auto oxidation, chemical oxidation, and photooxidation.

The cysteinyl residues are easily oxidized and the reaction is usually accelerated at alkaline pH, where the thiol group is deprotonated. Under mild oxidizing conditions the reactions are oxidation of cysteinyl residues to sulfenic/sulfonic acid (alkaline conditions), cysteinyl residues to dehydroalanyl residues (alkaline conditions), cysteinyl to cystine residues (neutral to alkaline conditions). In the absence of a thiol reagent or a nearby thiol, the cysteine may instead oxidize to sulfenic acid.

The oxidation reaction is strongly catalyzed by divalent metal ions (e.g., copper). The indicators of oxidation include extra bands in gel electrophoresis and extra peaks in chromatographic recordings. Preventive actions against oxidation are listed in Table 16.11.

The degradation rate is often governed by trace amounts of peroxides, divalent metal ions, light, base, and free radicals. There are three classes of antioxidants:

- Phenolic compounds: BHT, BHA, propyl gallate, Vitamin E
- Reducing agents: Cysteine, DTT, methionine, ascorbic acid, sodium sulfite, thioglycolic acid, thioglycerol
- Chelating agents: EDTA, citric acid, and thioglycolic acid

16.17.4 Carbamylation

Cyanate is able to react with amino, sulfhydryl, carboxyl, phenolic hydroxyl, imidazole and phosphate groups in proteins according to the general scheme, $RXH + HNCO = RXCONH_2$. Cyanate is easily soluble in water. Most reactions have a pH optimum around 7. Acidic pH should be avoided as acidic conditions are ideal for modifications of carboxyl groups. For the same reason reactions with cyanate should not be terminated with acid. At high concentrations, cyanate may react with itself to form cyanuric acid and cyamelide and it is recommended to work at concentrations about 0.2 M. Cyanate reacts rapidly with amino groups. At neutral pH and below the α-amino group can be expected to react about

100 times faster than the ε-amino group. The resulting carbamoylamino groups are stable even in dilute NaOH. Typical reaction conditions are 3 mg/mL protein, 0.1 M cyanate at pH 8, 25°C for 1 h. Cyanate also reacts even more rapidly with sulfhydryl groups than amino groups resulting in the formation of S-carbamylcysteine residues. Since cyanate reacts rapidly with sulfhydryl groups, labile disulfide bonds may be ruptured. The resulting carbamylmercaptans decompose readily to free mercaptan and cyanate at alkaline pH. Consequently, cyanate can be used as reversible blocking agent for –SH groups. At acidic pH cyanate reacts with carboxylic groups under formation of a mixed anhydride, which can react with many nucleophiles (e.g., formation of amides). The reaction can be avoided entirely at pH 7 to 8. Aliphatic hydroxyl are resistant to carbamylation even at high cyanate concentrations at low pH. However, the reactive hydroxyl groups of chymotrypsin and other proteases react with cyanate to give urethans. Phenolic hydroxyl groups react more readily than aliphatic groups in a reversible reaction that is quite analogous to the one that occurs with –SH groups.

Cyanate present in aqueous urea solutions reacts with the free amino and sulfhydryl groups of proteins. Urea is often tacitly assumed to be a reagent, which alters the structure of the protein and may be used to keep target proteins on their monomeric form during purification. However, at pH 6 and above urea hydrolyses under formation of cyanate leading to carbamylation reactive groups in proteins.

The equilibrium $(NH_2)_2CO = NH_4CNO$ between an undissociated urea and dissociated cyanate in aqueous urea solutions is the main course of unintended carbamylation of primary amino groups in proteins. As the protein concentration normally is from 0.1 to 30 mg/mL corresponding to the μM range, a considerable part of the protein mass is expected to undergo carbamylation under these conditions. Thus, the exposure of ribonuclease to cyanate in aqueous solution leads to a considerable loss of enzymatic activity. Formation of cyanate is prevented by storage of neutral urea solutions at 4°C or by buffering the solution at pH 4.7. Thus, acifidication of urea solutions just before use will decompose any cyanate present. Cyanate can be removed from urea solutions by mixed IEC. The method of Salinas describes a sensitive and specific method for quantitative estimation of carbamylation in proteins.

16.17.5 β-Elimination

The β-elimination reaction is caused by the abstraction of a β-hydrogen from cysteinyl, seryl and threonyl residues under alkaline conditions. The cystinyl residue decomposes as a result of β-elimination under formation of HS⁻ and free sulfur thus affecting the redox potential of the solution. Several studies indicate that the rate of reaction is proportional to the hydroxide ion concentration and pH should consequently be kept low (use dilute NaOH solutions to adjust pH preferably below 0.1 M NaOH). In alkaline solutions the abstraction of β-hydrogen from cystine, serine, and threonine residues result in formation of a carbanion. Depending on the nature of the side chain, the carbanion can rearrange to form an unsaturated derivative (dehydroalanine or β-methyl-dehydroalanine) or add a proton to give the L- and D-amino acid residues (racemization). The derivatives formed are reactive with a number of nucleophilic protein groups. The reaction is independent of the primary structure of the protein. The indicators of β-elimination include degradation

Table 16.12   Preventive Actions against β-Elimination

Factor	Comment
pH	PH should be kept below 10. Do not use NaOH solutions above 0.1 M to adjust pH.
Temperature	High temperature even at pH 4–8 results in β-elimination.
Time	The β-elimination reaction is a function of time.
Conductivity	Increased ionic strength increases the rate of β-elimination.
Redox potential	Cystinyl rich proteins may decompose under formation of HS^-, which will lower the redox potential of the solution. Reduction of disulfide bonds may result.
Co-solvents	Removal of divalent metal ions with EDTA.

of the protein, cleavage of disulfide bridges, and smell of sulfur. Preventive actions against β-elimination are listed in Table 16.12.

16.17.6 Racemization

All amino acid residues except glycine are subject to racemization at alkaline pH resulting in formation of the D-enantiomers of the residue. Racemization is inevitably associated with conformational changes and thereby loss of function. The racemization of proteins has been described in several reports. The initial step of the reaction is abstraction of the β-hydrogen by hydroxide ions. By uptake of a proton this will result in either the L- or D- amino acid residue. The carbanion formed may also undergo β-elimination. At pH 5–12 Asn, Asp, Gln, and Glu may modify via a succinimidyl intermediate resulting in both the D- and L- derivatives. The indicators of racemization include change of protein structure and loss of biological activity. The change in optical rotation correlates with the rate of racemization. The amino acid residues undergo racemization at different rates. Preventive actions against racemization are listed in Table 16.13.

Table 16.13   Preventive Actions against Racemization

Factor	Comment
pH	High pH will favor abstraction of the β-hydrogen under formation of a carbanion. pH should be kept below 10 and use of NaOH in concentration above 0.1 M should be avoided when adjusting pH.
Temperature	The temperature should be kept low.
Time	The reaction is a function of time.
Conductivity	No data are available.
Redox potential	No data are available.
Co-solvents	No data are available.

16.17.7 Cysteinyl Residues

The reactive site of the cysteinyl residue is the thiol group, which is deprotonated at alkaline pH (pKa around 8.5). The residue is under oxidizing conditions (and neutral to alkaline pH) able to react with a similar residue under formation of a disulfide bond. Many proteins are stabilized by intramolecular disulfide bonds (e.g., insulin, growth hormone, IGF-1), but intermolecular bonds may also result from the reaction under formation of aggregates. In order to avoid unintended disulfide bond formation/cleavage, the redox potential of the solution must be monitored and controlled. In practice, aqueous buffers contains micro-molar amounts of dissolved oxygen assuring a redox potential of 200–600 mV, which is sufficient to maintain the intramolecular disulfide bonds. Proteins with free cysteines may prefer slightly reducing conditions, which can be obtained by addition of micromo-lar amounts of reducing agent (e.g., cysteine or DTT). The number of proteins containing both –SH groups and disulfide bonds are relatively small (e.g., albumin, β-lactoglobulin). In many cases the disulfide bond stabilization is essential for maintaining the biological activity. Ribonuclease, for example, loses almost all activity when the four disulfide bonds are reduced. The mechanism of reaction involves cysteinyl and cystinyl residues in the disulfide bond formation by oxidation or reduction, conversion of a cystinyl residue to a cysteinyl residue and a sulfenic/sulfonic acid residue at alkaline pH and decomposition to a dehydroalanine residue at alkaline pH (β-elimination reaction). Disulfide bond formation is often catalyzed by the presence of a mercapto reagent (e.g., DTT, cysteine) in mM concentra-tions (typically 1–10 mM). Controlled disulfide bond formation has gained much attention in the biopharmaceutical industry in connection with in vitro folding of proteins expressed in *E. coli*. Presence of divalent metal ions (typically Cu^{++}) may result in oxidation of cysteinyl residues by an ill-defined reaction mechanism. Cleavage of the disulfide bond is initiated by an attack on a sulfur atom by a nucleophile reagent (HS^-, RS^-, CN^-, SO_3^-, OH^-). The reac-tion, which takes place at neutral to alkaline pH, consists of two steps with a formation of a mixed disulfide as the intermediary step. The indicators of cysteinyl residues include inter-molecular disulfide bond formation resulting in aggregation, under reducing conditions the disulfide bonds destabilizing resulting in conversion of cystinyl to cysteinyl residues (in vitro refolding may be the only solution to re-establish the correct disulfide bonds), presence of scrambled and structural altered forms, smell of sulfur. Be careful when adjusting pH with high concentrations of NaOH. Locally high pH may facilitate β-elimination. Table 16.14 summarizes the preventative actions against cysteinyl residue loss.

16.17.8 Hydrolysis

The peptide bond is not undergoing significant hydrolysis in the pH interval (3–9.5) usu-ally used in industrial downstream processing. However, in dilute acid, where the carboxyl group of aspartyl residues is not dissociated, the peptide bond is cleaved 100 times faster than other peptide bonds and especially the –Asp-Pro- sequence is prone for degradation. The guanidinium group of arginine is hydrolyzed by OH^- to give ornithine and possi-bly some citrulline, depending on the nature of the protein. The mechanism of hydrolysis includes hydrolysis of the peptide bond, hydrolysis of the amide group of Asn and Gln, hydrolysis of the guanidine group from Arg residues resulting in the formation of ornithine

Table 16.14 Preventive Actions against Cysteinyl Residue Loss

Factor	Comment
pH	Minimum reactivity should be expected in the pH range of 3–7. The reactivity of the –SH group is at maximum above the pKa (8.5), where the group is deprotonated. In strongly acidic media the reaction is expected to take place via a sulfenium cation by an electrophilic displacement.
Protein concentration	The intramolecular disulfide bond formation is a first order reaction and thus independent of protein concentration. Intermolecular reactions via the cysteinyl residue may be affected by the protein concentration (aggregation). The aggregation rate is favored by high protein concentration.
Temperature	The temperature should be kept low (4°C–20°C) especially at pH above 9.5.
Time	The reaction is a function of time.
Conductivity	No data available.
Redox potential	Reducing conditions favor free cysteinyl residues. Oxidizing conditions favor disulfide bonds. The redox potential is a function of pH (60 mV/pH unit).
Co-solvents	Cysteine (non-animal origin) is recommended as a reducing agent for large-scale operations. Divalent metal ions should be removed by EDTA.

Table 16.15 Preventive Actions against Hydrolysis

Factor	Comment
pH	The Asp-peptide bonds are prone to degradation at acidic pH. Deamidation of Asn and Gln at pH above 5. Arg is converted to ornithine by OH$^-$ in a concentration-dependent manner.
Temperature	The deamidation rate increases with increasing temperature.
Time	The degradation reactions are a function of time.
Conductivity	The ionic strength of the solution should be kept low in order to prevent deamidation. At high ionic strength the deamidation reaction can be fast even at neutral pH.
Redox potential	No data available.
Co-solvents	No data available.

residues (hydroxide ion catalyzed). The indicators of hydrolysis include formation of split products and formation of a split product of identical MW (the peptide fragments are linked via disulfide bonds). Table 16.15 summarizes the preventative actions against hydrolysis.

16.17.9 Denaturation

The native protein molecule is losing its tertiary structure upon denaturation resulting in a population of partially unfolded molecules. In practice the denaturation process will lead to a mixture of more or less unfolded molecules comprising residual secondary structure elements (helix, β-sheet, β-turn, *cis-trans* isomery around the prolinyl residue). A population of random coil molecules should not be expected even under strong denaturing and reducing conditions. Upon denaturation the inner hydrophobic core of the protein molecule is exposed to the hydrophilic environment (solvent water) often resulting in (irreversible) aggregation of the target protein. The cooperativity of the denaturation process results in an abrupt transition from the native to the unfolded state within a narrow range of pH, temperature, ionic strength, and denaturant concentration meaning that protein denaturation may come fast and unexpected. As globular proteins are only marginally stable in aqueous solutions, parameter interactions should be well understood and described using, for example, factorial design experiments. Proteins with disulfide bonds may undergo unfolding under reducing conditions, where the covalent bond is cleaved.

A denatured protein may be brought back to its native form by in vitro folding. The folding process is often slow and yields can be poor. As each protein is unique, the in vitro folding conditions must be determined case by case often using specific co-solvents as additives. An example is the group of proteins where disulfide bonds must be reestablished as part of the renaturation process.

Hydrogen bonds and intramolecular interactions (electrostatic, van der Waals) are stabilizing the native structure of the protein in a co-operative manner. Upon denaturation, the co-operative effect is lost resulting in unfolding of the molecule and exposure of the inner hydrophobic core to the hydrophilic aqueous environment. For small globular proteins, denaturation is an almost all-or-none process approximated rather well by the two state transition. Thermodynamically, the denaturation process can be observed by an increase of molar heat capacity and a rapid enthalpy increase with increasing temperature. The primary structure (amino acid sequence) is not affected by denaturation. The indicators of denaturation include loss of structure and loss of biological activity and aggregation. Table 16.16 summarizes the preventative actions against denaturation.

16.17.10 Aggregation

Protein aggregation is a major problem in the purification and formulation of protein biopharmaceuticals. Two types of intermolecular reactions dominate: aggregation resulting from hydrophobic interactions, and aggregation stemming from inter-molecular disulfide bond formation between cysteinyl residues.

Proteins exposed to even mildly denaturing conditions may partially unfold resulting in exposure of hydrophobic residues to the aqueous solvent favoring aggregation. The aggregation process is assumed to be controlled by the initial dimerization step in a second-order reaction. Consequently, high protein concentrations will increase the aggregation rate.

Intermolecular disulfide bond formation between cysteinyl residues takes place at alkaline pH under oxidizing conditions. Proteins with reactive free thiol groups should be purified under reducing conditions (typically 1–10 mM reducing agent) in the presence of EDTA. Even proteins with disulfide bonds may participate in intermolecular disulfide bond reactions due to disulfide bond shuffling at neutral and alkaline pH.

Expression of proteins in *E. coli* often results in the formation of insoluble aggregates called inclusion bodies, probably comprising fully or partially unfolded protein. Inclusion bodies are brought to their monomeric form by extraction with a denaturant (e.g., 8 M urea) under reducing conditions (e.g., 0.1 M cysteine).

Table 16.16   Preventive Actions against Denaturation

Factor	Comment
pH	Loss of tertiary structure should be expected at pH above 9.5. Proteins tend to be most stable near the pI.
Temperature	The unfolding process is a function of temperature. Many proteins have optimal stability in the temperature range of 10°C–30°C. Loss of structure should be expected both at low temperatures (cold denaturation) and at elevated temperatures. The reason that many protein biopharmaceuticals are stored at low temperatures is to minimize chemical degradation (e.g., deamidation).
Time	The denaturation reaction can be very fast.
Conductivity	No data available.
Redox potential	Cleavage of disulfide bonds should be expected under reducing conditions. A redox potential below 100 mV is considered unstable for some proteins (e.g., insulin). Not all proteins will undergo conformational changes upon reduction of the disulfide bond(s).
Co-solvents	Sucrose, mannose, glucose, glycine, alanine, glutamine, and ammonium sulfate are examples of compounds acting as protein stabilizers (weak or no binding to the protein surface).
	Magnesium sulfate, guanidinium sulfate, sodium chloride and other weakly interacting salts will exhibit an effect depending on protein charge and concentration.
	Polyethylene glycol (PEG) and 2-methyl-2,4-pentanediol (MPD) act as stabilizers due to steric exclusion and repulsion from charged groups. Both PEG and MPD may destabilize the protein under certain circumstances, where binding is favored over exclusion.
	Co-solvents such as urea or guanidinium chloride, which binds strongly to the protein surface, are strong denaturants.

The mechanism of reaction is primarily hydrophobic interaction or interaction via disulfide formation. Exposure of hydrophobic residues to the surface of the molecule leads to disorganization of the surrounding water molecules, thus increasing the entropy of the system. In order to avoid the change of the hydration shell structure, the protein molecules are forced to aggregate. The aggregation reaction can be very fast and will, in severe cases, lead to formation of insoluble polymers. The dominant mechanism is presumably specific interaction of certain conformations of intermediates rather than non-specific co-aggregation. Proteins comprising free thiol groups may form intermolecular disulfide bonds leading to aggregation of the protein. The reaction takes place at alkaline pH (presence of $-S^-$) under oxidizing conditions. Indicators of aggregation include loss of structure and loss of biological activity, turbid solution, presence of fibrils in the solution, precipitation, formation of gels. Formation of inclusion bodies in *E. coli* is an example of in vivo protein aggregates. Hydrophobic protein aggregates will often dissolve at high pH (>11). Intermolecular disulfide aggregates may dissolve under reducing conditions (presence of DTT, cysteine, or the like). Table 16.17 summarizes the preventative actions against aggregation.

Table 16.17   Preventive Actions against Aggregation

Factor	Comment
pH	High pH should be avoided in order to prevent protein unfolding. Some proteins do change conformation as a function of pH and certain pH intervals should be avoided. pH < 7 will protect the protein from intermolecular disulfide bond formation.
Temperature	The unfolding process is a function of temperature. Many proteins have optimal stability in the temperature range of 10°C–30°C. Loss of structure should be expected both at low temperatures (cold denaturation) and at elevated temperatures.
Protein concentration	Low protein concentrations should be favored.
Time	The aggregation reaction can be very fast.
Conductivity	No data available.
Redox potential	Oxidizing conditions results in formation of disulfide bonds and intermolecular interactions should be expected. Reducing conditions will prevent intermolecular disulfide bond formation.
Co-solvents	Denaturing or destabilizing agents (e.g., urea, certain alcohols, organic solvents) should be used with care. Detergents may prevent aggregation, but they often bind strongly to the protein.

16.17.11 Precipitation

Protein precipitates are aggregates large enough to be visible. However, in practice aggregates not visible by the naked eye may result in severe problems as filters and chromatographic columns can be blocked.

Protein precipitation is typically observed at high ionic strength, in the presence of organic solvents or close to the pI, where solubility is low due to the zero net charge of the protein. Presence of precipitates is not always easily observed. Typical markers are presence of large often white particles or flocculates, a turboid appearance, fibrils, or increased viscosity.

Unintended precipitation can be difficult to predict as the effect depends on a combination of the distribution of hydrophilic and hydrophobic residues on the proteins surface, the pH, ionic strength, protein concentration, temperature, and composition of the aqueous phase. A perfectly clear solution may gradually become turbid during application to a chromatographic column resulting in column blocking.

The mechanism of precipitation involves salting out, iso-precipitation or the presence of polar solvents. In most cases high salt concentrations will lead to precipitation of the protein. The process is largely dependent on the hydrophobicity of the protein, and the optimal salts are those favoring dehydration of the non-polar regions without binding to the protein. At zero net charge of the protein, the electrostatic repulsion between the molecules is minimal. Therefore, proteins tend to precipitate near the pI of the molecule. Additions of non-polar organic solvents reduce the water activity. The organic solvent reducing the hydrophobic attraction will displace the water molecules around hydrophobic areas. The principal forces leading to precipitation are, therefore, likely to be electrostatic forces and di-polar van der Waals' forces. The indicators of precipitation include cloudy solution and precipitation of solid material (the precipitates often appear white). The Hoffmeister series provides the impact of various cations and anions:

Cations:

$$NH_4^+ > K^+ > Na^+ > Li^+ > Mg^{++} > Ca^{++} > Gdn^+$$

Anions:

$$SO_4^{--} > HPO_4^{--} > CH_3COO^- > Cl^- > NO_3^- > SCN^-$$

The ions to the left in the series exert a stabilizing effect on proteins. The ions to the right may bind to the protein surface and thereby destabilize the protein. The effect of the ions is additive. Ammonium sulfate is a stabilizing salt often used for precipitation of proteins (2–3 M solution). Gdn-sulfate is a stabilizing salt, while Gdn-chloride is a strong denaturant.

Precipitation is commonly used as a purification tool in downstream processing as the biological activity is rarely affected by this procedure (organic solvents may result in denaturation). Iso-precipitation becomes more effective by adding alcohols or polyalcohols to the solvent. pH adjustment may result in unintended iso-precipitation of the protein. Passing the isoelectric point does not affect the biological activity or stability of the protein (in most cases) and the protein will normally enter into solution again 2–3 pH units from the pI. Precipitates may form hours after the protein solution has been prepared or adjusted. The precipitates are not always visible. As the particles may result in blocking of filters and chromatographic columns, unintended precipitation in application samples constitutes a great problem in downstream processing. Table 16.18 summarizes the preventative actions against precipitation.

Table 16.18 Preventive Actions against Precipitation

Factor	Comment
pH	The protein solubility is minimal near the isoelectric point. A change in pH may affect the redox potential of the solution, the protein solubility, and the protein stability.
Temperature	High temperature increases the conformational flexibility, for example organic, solvents may more easily penetrate the internal structure of the protein.
Protein concentration	Low protein concentration will protect the protein from precipitation; concentrations below 0.1 mg/mL may be necessary to avoid precipitation.
Time	Precipitation is a function of time. Always determine the holding time for a given sample to assure precipitates are not formed during storage.
Conductivity	High ionic strength normally results in protein precipitation. Keep the salt concentration low to moderate, but at the same time, be aware of the "salting in" effect. Ions such as NH_4^+ do stabilize the protein upon precipitation.
Co-solvents	Typical protein precipitation agents are salts (e.g., ammonium sulfate), polyethylene glycols (e.g., PEG 20000), polyelectrolytes (e.g., carboxymethyl cellulose), and organic solvents (e.g., acetone).

Questions

1. What is the difference between QC and QA?

    Answer: QC is primarily concerned with testing the product, while QA has a broader responsibility of oversight of the process which includes the paperwork required.

2. While a QC department or individual should be established within a company, list some of the other units that need to play active roles in ensuring the production of a quality product.

3. Describe the controls that should be in place for inputs to a process.

4. When a batch of product is found to not be in conformance to the quality standards, before a decision is made about how to deal with the batch, what should be done to prevent inadvertent shipping of the product to consumers?

    Answer: Mark and separate the batch so that it is held until a decision on the appropriate action can be made.

5. Name some sources of information that should be used to develop a corrective action plan.

6. Describe steps in developing a robust process. While it may be desirable to test all combinations of parameters, what is the common practice to establish statistical bounds on a parameter?

    Answer: Identify the process steps that are going to affect the quality of the product to establish ranges for such parameters, … Bounds are often established using a low and high value.

7. When concern that a process is contaminated, a scaled down system test called virus spiking, with same or similar virus as is suspected of being contaminated, is performed. Is it required to perform this process in the cGMP environment?

    Answer: No, in fact it is usually better to do it outside to prevent inadvertent further contamination.

8. What are the nine elements of validation?

9. In determination of the indenting of a recombination protein, the primary and secondary structure are followed by what methods to determine the tertiary or quaternary structure?

    Answer: NMR, X-ray diffraction, near-UV circular dichroism, and for quaternary structure HP SEC, Raman scattering, light scattering useful for determination of large macromolecular assemblies and scanning TEM.

10. Why might one choose CE instead of conventional electrophoresis?

17

Intellectual Property

LEARNING OBJECTIVES

1. Recognize the benefit and protection provided by provisional patents.
2. Understand that U.S. patents do not provide global protection.
3. Realize how the time to bring a pharmaceutical to market necessitates the subsequent high cost because of current patent laws.

17.1 INTRODUCTION

"The Congress shall have Power ... To promote the Progress of Science and useful Arts, by securing for limited Times to Authors and Inventors the exclusive Right to their respective Writings and Discoveries."—U.S. Constitution.

"Everything that can be invented has been invented."—Charles H. Duell, U.S. Patent Office Director, telling President McKinley to abolish the office in 1899. (Note: Till 1836, U.S. Patent and Trademark Office had issued 9,957 patents; from 1837 to November 2004, it issued over 6.8 million patents.)

The development of new pharmaceutical or biotechnology-derived products undergoes a lengthy and expensive cycle, which is adequately described elsewhere in the book. Given the cost of development now hovering around the billion-dollar mark for each new drug, amortized over all other molecules racing, the only way to protect this investment is to create intellectual property claims to not only the active molecule but wherever possible, each and every step of its production, processing, and testing. Almost 4% of the development cost is spent on filing and prosecuting patents.

Typically, the research-based pharmaceutical companies spend about 15%–20% of their total sales revenue on developing new drugs, as compared with less than 4% for industry overall; the cost of patent protection ranges between 1% and 3% of the R&D expenditure. Successful patenting, patent protection, and exploitation of expired patents involve a complex interaction among scientists and lawyers. Generally, the development teams should have a basic understanding of the patenting process to be able to make the best use of legal expertise in the field; the complex the field is, the more input from scientists becomes valuable. In this chapter, I have described the fundamentals of patenting that I consider important enough for scientists, administrators, and marketing personnel to understand well.

17.2 PATENTING SYSTEMS AND STRATEGIES

A patent is a grant by the state of exclusive rights for a limited time in respect of a new and useful invention, and a right to prevent others from making or selling the invention (see later on making vis-à-vis the Food and Drug Administration) in a limited territory as defined by the patent issuing authority. It is not necessarily a right to practice an invention by the inventor. The word *patent* means "open," from the word *letters patent*, meaning an announcement to all that the inventor has been awarded rights to the invention. *Open* here means without having to break any seal as was the custom in the decrees issued by the sovereign governments and royalties. Note that *letters patent* are not restricted to inventions, as even today these are issued to appoint judges in the United Kingdom. Historically, patents were issued on elaborate stationary, as they still are to some extent. The point about the rights to exercise an invention vis-à-vis prevent others from practicing needs further elaboration. The new chemical entity patent for sildenafil citrate expired in March 2003; the use and composition patents listed for sildenafil citrate in the Orange Book (Food and Drug Administration) extend to 2012 and 2019; 17 U.S. patents were issued to Pfizer on various aspects of sildenafil citrate; a total of 44 patents make claims for sildenafil citrate including its use in Tourette's syndrome to its chewing gum formulations that require chewing the gum for not less than two minutes; and so on.

The example of erythropoietin demonstrates how the patent laws can create great difficulties for biogeneric offering. For example, the following issued claims exemplify the numerous ways in which patent protection relating to a protein may be obtained.

U.S. Patent No. 5,621,080: An isolated erythropoietin glycoprotein having the *in vivo* biological activity of causing bone marrow cells to increase production of reticulocytes and red blood cells, wherein said erythropoietin glycoprotein comprises the mature erythropoietin amino acid sequence of Figure 6 and has glycosylation which differs from that of human urinary erythropoietin.

U.S. Patent No. 6,048,971: A secretable mutant human erythropoietin protein having an amino acid residue which differs from the amino acid residue present in the corresponding position in wildtype human erythropoietin, the amino acid residue of said wildtype erythropoietin selected from the group consisting of: amino acid residue 103, amino acid residue 104, and amino acid residue 108.

U.S. Patent No. 5,955,422: A pharmaceutical composition comprising a therapeutically effective amount of human erythropoietin and a pharmaceutically acceptable diluent, adjuvant or carrier, wherein said erythropoietin is purified from mammalian cells grown in culture.

U.S. Patent No. 4,703,008: 1. A purified and isolated DNA sequence encoding erythropoietin, said DNA sequence selected from the group consisting of: a. the DNA sequences set out in Figures 5 and 6 or their complementary strands; and b. DNA sequences which hybridize under stringent conditions to the DNA sequences defined in (a). ... 4. A prokaryotic or eukaryotic host cell transformed or transfected with a DNA sequence according to claim [1] in a manner allowing the host cell to express erythropoietin.

U.S. Patent No. 5,618, 698: A process for the preparation of an in vivo biologically active erythropoietin product comprising the steps of growing, under suitable nutrient conditions, host cells transformed or transfected with an isolated DNA sequence selected from the group consisting of (1) the DNA sequences set out in Figures 5 and 6, (2) the protein coding sequences set out in Figures 5 and 6, and (3) DNA sequences which hybridize under stringent conditions to the DNA sequences defined in (1) and (2) or their complementary strands; and isolating said erythropoietin product therefrom.

U.S. Patent No. 5,641,670: A homologously recombinant cell having incorporated therein a new transcription unit, wherein the new transcription unit comprises an exogenous regulatory sequence, an exogenous exon and a splice-donor site, operatively linked to the second exon of an endogenous gene, wherein the homologously recombinant cell comprises said exogenous exon in addition to exons present in said endogenous gene.

The homologously recombinant cell of claim [1] wherein the endogenous gene encodes a protein selected from the group consisting of erythropoietin, calcitonin, growth hormone, insulin, insulinotropin, insulin-like growth factors, parathyroid hormone, beta-interferon, gamma-interferon, nerve growth factors, FSH-beta, TGF-beta, tumor necrosis factor, glucagon, bone growth factor-2, bone growth factor-7, TSH-beta, interleukin 1, interleukin 2, interleukin 3, interleukin 6, interleukin 11, interleukin 12, CSF-granulocyte, CSF-macrophage, CSF-granulocyte/macrophage, immunoglobulins, catalytic antibodies, protein kinase C, glucocerebrosidase, superoxide dismutase, tissue plasminogen activator, urokinase, antithrombin III, DNAse, alpha-galactosidase, tyrosine hydroxylase, blood clotting factor V, blood clotting factor VII, blood clotting factor VIII, blood clotting factor IX, blood clotting factor X, blood clotting factor XIII, apolipoprotein E, apolipoprotein A-I, globins, low density lipoprotein receptor, IL-2 receptor, IL-2 antagonists, alpha-1 antitrypsin, immune response modifiers, and soluble CD4.

U.S. Patent No. 6,048,524: A method of expressing erythropoietin in a mammal, comprising the steps of:

Obtaining a source of primary cells from a mammal;

Transfecting primary cells obtained in (a) with a DNA construct comprising exogenous DNA encoding erythropoietin and additional DNA sequences sufficient for expression of the exogenous DNA in the primary cells, thereby producing transfected primary cells which express the exogenous DNA encoding erythropoietin;

Culturing a transfected primary cell produced in (b), which expresses the exogenous DNA encoding erythropoietin, under conditions appropriate for propagating the transfected primary cell which expresses the exogenous DNA encoding erythropoietin, thereby producing a clonal cell strain of transfected secondary cells from the transfected primary cell;

Culturing the clonal cell strain of transfected secondary cells produced in (c) under conditions appropriate for and sufficient time for the clonal cell strain of transfected secondary cells to undergo a sufficient number of doublings to provide a sufficient number of transfected secondary cells to produce erythropoietin; and

Introducing transfected secondary cells produced in (d) into a mammal of the same species as the mammal from which the primary cells were obtained in sufficient number to express erythropoietin in the mammal.

U.S. Patent No. 4,397,840: A method for the preparation of an erythropoietin product having no inhibitory effect against erythropoiesis which comprises the steps of:

Adsorbing a crude erythropoietin product obtained from the urine of healthy human on to a weakly basic anion exchanger from a neutral or weakly acidic aqueous solution in the presence of an inorganic neutral salt in a concentration in the range from 0.1 to 0.2 mole per liter, and

Eluting the thus adsorbed erythropoietin product with an aqueous eluant solution containing an inorganic neutral salt in a concentration in the range from 0.5 to 0.7 moles per liter.

U.S. Patent No. 4,667,016: A process for the efficient recovery of erythropoietin from a fluid, said process comprising the following steps in sequence: subjecting the fluid to ion exchange chromatographic separation at about pH 7.0, thereby to selectively bind erythropoietin in said sample to a cationic resin; stabilizing materials bound to said resin against degradation by acid activated proteases; selectively eluting bound contaminant materials having a pKa greater than that of erythropoietin by treatment with aqueous acid at a pH of from about 4.0 to 6.0; and selectively eluting erythropoietin by treatment with an aqueous salt at a pH of about 7.0; and isolating erythropoietin-containing eluent fractions.

U.S. Patent No. 6,001,800: A method for preparing spray dried recombinant human erythropoietin (rhEPO), comprising:

Providing an aqueous solution of rhEPO having a concentration within the range of about 20 mg/ml to about 100 mg/ml;

Atomizing said solution into a spray;

Drying said spray with hot drying air in order to evaporate the water from the spray to form a dried rhEPO; and

Separating dried rhEPO from the drying air to provide biologically active spray dried rhEPO.

U.S. Patent No. 5,629,175: A method for producing a mammalian peptide which comprises: growing tobacco plant cells containing an integrated sequence comprising, a first expression cassette having the direction of transcription (1) a transcriptional and translational initiation region functional in said plant cells, (2) a structural gene coding for said mammalian peptide, and (3) a termination region, whereby said structural gene is expressed to produce said mammalian peptide.

U.S. Patent No. 5,780,709: A method to increase water stress resistance or tolerance in a monocot plant, comprising: (a) introducing into cells of a monocot plant an expression cassette comprising a preselected DNA segment comprising an mtlD gene, operably linked to a promoter function in the monocot plant cells to yield transformed monocot plant cells; and (tb) regenerating a differentiated fertile plant from said transformed cells, where in the mtlD gene is expressed in the cells of the plant so as to render the transformed monocot plant substantially tolerant or resistant to reduction in water availability that inhibits the growth of an untransformed monocot plant.

17.3 PATENT LAWS

It is noteworthy that patents are awarded for things or *res*, which must have some use; there need not be any rationale provided why an invention works, obviously it must meet all statutory requirements to be eligible for patenting. The patent laws are extremely complex, often inexplicably irrational and in almost all instances questionable in their enforcement.

The following definitions and terms are commonly used in describing patent laws:

- Invention: An invention is the conception of a new and useful article, machine, composition, or process.
- Patent application: A document describing an invention in detail, which is to be submitted to a patent office with the aim of obtaining a patent on the invention.
- Patent: Right of ownership granted by the government to a person that gives the owner the right to exclude others from making, selling, or using the claimed invention.
- Reduction to practice: An in-depth description of how the invention works, described in concrete terms.
- Prior art: The existing or publicly available knowledge available before the date of an invention or more than one year prior to the first patent application date.
- Utility: This is the most common type of patent. It includes inventions that operate in a new and useful manner.
- Design: The emphasis of this type of patent is on the design of the invention, not on its functionality. What is important with this type of patent is the invention's unique ornamental and aesthetic properties.
- Plant: This type of patent includes new varieties of asexually reproduced plants.
- Actual reduction to practice: Constructing the machine or article, synthesizing the composition or performing the method and testing sufficiently to demonstrate that the invention works for its intended purpose. Testing is *not* required if one of ordinary skill in the art would recognize that it will work.
- Constructive reduction to practice: Filing U.S. patent application—in compliance of first paragraph of §112.
- Diligence: Working on reducing the invention to practice, or else it is considered abandoned.

The patenting of inventions is a complex process that has historically been confused, particularly by inventors who may not be practitioners of patent law. For example:

- Patents are valuable only if they can be used to protect a profit stream by excluding others from making, using, or selling whatever is covered by the patent's claims.

- A patent does not mean that the invention works as verified by the government, it is left for the licensors to evaluate; it is suspected that as many as 10% of all issued patents are invalid for being nonfunctional as claimed.
- You cannot get a provisional patent as there is nothing like this. You can file a provisional patent application for a small fee that allows you 12 months to file a regular application while protecting your priority. A provisional application is not "just describing the idea," it is a complete application except the required claim(s). You may not change anything in the body of application when you file the regular application if you want to take priority advantage.
- You cannot get a patent for an idea or mere suggestion. Patents are granted to people who (claim to) "invent or discover any new and useful process, machine, manufacture, or composition of matter, or any new and useful improvement thereof," to quote the essence of U.S. statute governing patents. Complete and enabling disclosure is also required.
- A patent can be enforceable from the time it issues till it expires, not necessarily 20 years. New rules provide some guarantee that the enforceable term of a utility patent will be at least 17 years and that some royalties may be collectable when a patent is published before it issues. Design patents are only good for 14 years and only cover the ornamental appearance of the item and not its structure or functionality.
- A patent does not give the owner the exclusive right to make, use, and sell his or her invention; it gives its owner the right to *exclude* others from making, using, and selling exactly what is covered by his or her patent claims. A holder of a prior patent with broader claims may prevent the inventor whose patent has narrower claims from using the inventor's own patent. A patent right is exclusory only.
- A U.S. patent is only enforceable in the United States. It can be used to stop others from importing into the United States what the patent covers, but other people in other countries are free to make, use, and sell the invention anywhere else in the world even if the inventor does not have a patent. This is the reason why one must consider filing Patent Cooperative Treaty and follow it up with either individual state filings or consortium filing such as European Patent Office.
- A patent does not protect an invention because only a patent in conjunction with a legal opinion of infringement will give the owner(s) of the patent the right to sue in a civil case against the alleged infringer. The U.S. government does not enforce patents (however, the Customs Service can help block infringing imports), and infringement of a patent is not a crime. The responsibility, and all expenses, for enforcing the rights granted by a patent (and securing Customs Service help) lie with the patent owner(s).
- Filing for a patent is not the only way to protect an invention. When properly used, the U.S. Patent and Trademark Office Disclosure Document Program ($10), Non-Disclosure Agreements (free), and Provisional Applications for Patent ($80) along with maintaining good records and diligent pursuit can keep your patenting rights intact until you do.
- A patent attorney or agent is not needed to file your patent; an inventor may choose to go *pro se* (on one's own). However, given the complexity of the law, advice from professionals always proves invaluable.

17.4 TYPES OF PATENT LAWS

There are two types of patent laws: the world laws and U.S. laws. The U.S. Congress had many options in enacting laws in accordance with the constitution; it chose to include many unique features not found in the laws of other countries. For example, the laws in the United States give the inventor the recognition and that the United States is the only country where the patent applications must be filed by the inventor and not by an assignee such as the inventor's employer. It is for this reason, correct designation of inventorship plays such an important role in U.S. patenting, whereas in most other countries it has little or no effect on patent validity, although it may be important for other reasons such as compensation for employee inventors. This issue is of particular importance in the pharmaceutical industry where a team of researchers often work on the same invention, often members of this team move to other companies and at times they are not available or cooperative in the filing of a patent for an invention. U.S. patent laws go into fine detail on how to handle all these situations. U.S. law further distinguishes from the world law by establishing the precedence between two patent applications claiming the same invention on the simple basis that the first to invent has priority contrary to the rest of the world where the party who files first has the precedence. This creates significant legal issues often leading to lengthy and cumbersome "interference practice," in the prosecution of patent applications establishing when was the invention made vis-à-vis when was it filed. Not only is the date of filing important, the date when a "workable" model was conceived, the period when the inventor did not "diligently" follow the development, the dates when the inventor began working again and whether this renewed interest was in response to knowledge that someone else may be working on the same invention, and host of other related factors exemplify the complexity of legal proceedings in the practice of patent law, particularly in the United States.

There is no requirement of a working model to declare that an invention has been made; it can be a mental process wherein all essential elements of invention are present, U.S. laws assert. One of the most interesting recent court decision on this issue pertained to the legal battle between Amgen and Chugai. Chugai filed prior to Amgen, but Amgen could show completion of invention prior to Chugai's date of invention; Amgen won and made billions. Legal cases such as this establish interpretation of the laws—the so-called patent case law history.

The development of U.S. patent law has been strongly influenced by decisions of the courts, particularly of the U.S. Supreme Court. For example, the question "how much invention is needed to support a patent" was resolved by the U.S. Supreme Court. It was said that it is clearly wrong that patents should be granted for improvements so minor that any competent mechanic or chemist could make them as a matter of course, for this would restrict all the normal day-to-day work of the workshop or laboratory. On the other hand, it was also ascertained to be wrong that patents should be granted only for outstanding inventions that revolutionize the society. Many inventions are ingenious and at least potentially useful without being world shattering, and one great merit of the patent system is that the value of the patent grant is left to be determined by market forces. It is not as if the state, in granting a patent, guarantees to the patentee that he or she will profit by it; by and large a patent for a poor invention will not be very valuable. The extreme position that only outstanding inventions should be patentable was nevertheless adopted by the Supreme Court in 1941, when Justice Douglas condemned the grant of patents for "gadgets" as being superfluous. The Cornell University Library provides an excellent resource on patent law.

Of great importance to the pharmaceutical industry is the Drug Price Competition and Patent Restoration Act of 1984, commonly known as the Hatch–Waxman Act, which provided for extensions of patent term for human drugs, food additives, and medical devices the commercialization of which had been delayed by regulatory procedures (in the Food and Drug Administration) and at the same time made registration easier for competitors when patent protection expired and provided that testing for regulatory approval involving a patented drug did not amount to patent infringement. Amendment of this act is in the process right now to support the generic drug industry; more on this amendment later in this chapter. Several legislative changes to U.S. patent law have been made, but the most important was certainly the Uruguay Round Amendments Act (URAA) of 1995, which made changes necessary to bring U.S. law into line with the TRIPS (Trade-Related Intellectual Property) agreement.

17.5 ANATOMY OF A PATENT

A published patent (is published every Tuesday in the United States) is a legal document, not unlike the deed for a real property that describes its boundaries. Each of the printed information on the patent has a special meaning, and although it is most useful for the attorneys, the scientists have much to gain by understanding the anatomy of a patent. This will teach them how to design their searches and how to interpret the findings of invention (see Figure 17.1).

- (10) Patent Number: The number assigned to the issued patent is the best place to branch out your search, particularly the patent numbers quoted in the front page of the patent which served as related reference
- (12) Publication type and inventor's family or Sir name
- (45) Date of Patent: The date the patent was issued (always on a Tuesday) is when it becomes effective; however, know that the date when the application was published under the new rules determines if the inventors of an issued patent are eligible to claim royalties to a marketed invention if it reads of the patent claims. This date also tells you the period of exclusivity remaining in the patent
- (54) Title: Patent title describes the broadest area of invention description; it is often misleading but very useful in determining the broadest classification of the invention. Most often the title is chosen for (the) express purpose of making a random search difficult to reveal the content of a patent
- (76) Inventor: Inventor's name and address can be a very useful lead if you know your competitor; the same inventor files often a series of patents on an invention; this information also helps track down reissues and reexamined patents. Given under the inventor information is a notice with an asterisk indicating patent term extension or reduction granted during prosecution delays by either the United Sates Patent and Trademark Office or the applicant. Almost invariably this entry would include any additional patent term extensions granted based on regulatory delays in the approval of a healthcare product, which can be found in the Official Gazette or through other searches as shown below

US006447820B1

(12) **United States Patent**
Niazi

(10) **Patent No.:** **US 6,447,820 B1**
(45) **Date of Patent:** **Sep. 10, 2002**

(54) **PHARMACEUTICAL COMPOSITION FOR THE PREVENTION AND TREATMENT OF SCAR TISSUE**

(76) Inventor: **Sarfaraz K Niazi**, 20 Riverside Dr., Deerfield, IL (US) 60015

(*) Notice: Subject to any disclaimer, the term of this patent is extended or adjusted under 35 U.S.C. 154(b) by 0 days.

(21) Appl. No.: **09/681,137**

(22) Filed: **Jan. 22, 2001**

(51) Int. Cl.[7] **A61K 35/78**; A61K 9/00; A61K 9/50; A01N 25/00

(52) U.S. Cl. **424/767**; 424/400; 424/502; 424/725; 514/946; 514/947

(58) Field of Search 424/400, 502, 424/725, 767; 514/946, 947

(56) **References Cited**

U.S. PATENT DOCUMENTS

5,405,608 A * 4/1995 Xu 424/195.1

6,126,950 A * 10/2000 Bindra et al. 424/401

OTHER PUBLICATIONS

Johnson, T. CRC Ethnobotany Desk Reference, 1999, CRC Press LLC, p. 568.*

* cited by examiner

Primary Examiner—Leon B. Lankford, Jr.
Assistant Examiner—Kailash C. Srivastava
(74) *Attorney, Agent, or Firm*—Welsh & Katz, Ltd.

(57) **ABSTRACT**

The disclosed is a treatment of existing and prevention of new skin scars in humans and animals using a topical application containing alcoholic extracts of *Cortex Phellodendri* and *Opuntia ficus indica* in a specific combination.

5 Claims, No Drawings

Figure 17.1 Example documentation from a filed patent.

(21) Application No: The Application Number assigned to a patent application can be useful in tracking down its publication prior to issuance of patent to compare if there were any changes made in the application during prosecution (something you may get through file wrapper as well)

(22) Patent Filing Date: The date the application was filed with the Patent and Trademark Office is a critical date for §102e prior art reference; this date also tells you about how long your competitors have been working on this project; since the patent wrapper (all correspondence between the United Sates Patent and Trademark Office and the inventor or whoever is prosecuting the patent is public information, you may want to request the wrapper, particularly if there was a long delay between the filing and issuance of patent—meaning there was some admission by the filer, which may be of use to you in establishing the patentability of your invention)

(51) International Classification. This is an important field as it allows you to do comparable international searches (more on it later); notice that there is a conversion of classification available between the United States and the International System

(52) United States Classification: Class and subclass information, the categories that the United Sates Patent and Trademark Office uses to classify or sort the various types of inventions. These numbers means a lot for any patentability search

(58) Field of Search: This indicates the class or subclasses that were searched for the purpose of determining patentability

(56) Reference Cited: During the prosecution, the examiner may bring several references (patents and publications) that formed the basis of defining the scope of invention, given here are the patent number and class/subclass of patents that were brought up during prosecution; most likely, you would also want to see the full text of these patents. Other publications are also cited here. It is further indicated whether these references were brought up by the examiner (marked with an asterisk). Combined with the information in the file wrapper, these references provide the most significant data on evaluating the proposed invention. The names of examiner and primary examiner are also given here; chances are if your invention is similar you will see correspondence from the same examiner or primary examiner

(74) Attorney, Agent of Firm: Identification of who did the prosecuting can be important if you want to track down what other patents were prosecuted by the same attorney, agent or firm. If no name is listed here or the category is not listed, this patent was filed as a pro se patent

(57) Abstract: This is usually one concise paragraph summarizing the invention in plain English (no legalese or technical jargon is preferred here). Since this appears on the front page of the issued patent, it is the most frequently referenced section of a patent. This is one of the most craftily written pieces of language in the patent; as you prepare patent searches, you will learn how to read between lines in an abstract

Drawings: Drawings of the invention from different perspectives; also disclosed here is the number of drawings and claims in the patent. If there are no drawings reported, you may not want to switch to patent image (unless there are chemical structures or other graphic information). The text format of a patent is more suitable for cutting and pasting in your search document; the patent image is in a non-editable *. tiff format

Background of the Invention: This section discusses any previous inventions related to the patented invention—prior art, in legal terms. Since you are allowed to incorporate other patents by reference, you may also include this material in your own application if it suits the purpose as well. A recent patent with an extensive background section provides a wealth of information and saves great effort on the part of the filer. Read it carefully as it may disclose information that may later be used by the patent examiner as §103e information

Summary of the Invention: This is a discussion of the invention that captures its essential functions and features; this must be read first before reading the background section

Brief description of Drawings: A one-sentence description of each drawing figure is useful in ascertaining whether you want to switch to image of patent. It is noteworthy that the United Sates Patent and Trademark Office website allows searching of patents from 1790 through 1975 only by Patent Number and Current United States Classification; later patents are searchable by text entries. Online patent images were made available recently

Detailed Description: This section is generally an in-depth discussion of the various aspects of the claimed invention. Detailed references to drawings are made in this section; here you see exactly what is invented

Claims: Analogous to the boundaries of a real estate described in a deed, the claims layout the legal scope of the patent, going down from the broadest claim to the narrowest claim. This section determines if your invention infringes on a patent (reads onto claims). This section also provides you with the vocabulary you may want to use for your own invention. Often searches are made of the claims section only to determine patentability

17.6 PATENTABILITY

The following are the three principal requirements for an invention to be patented as set out in the European Patent Convention:

- That the invention must be new
- That it must involve an inventive step
- That it must be capable of industrial application

The same three requirements are met in one form or another in the United States, in Japan, and, indeed, in practically every country that has a patent system. Some countries and conventions exclude certain inventions, but these exclusions may be forbidden under TRIPS.

17.6.1 First Requirement: Novelty

Patent issued for what is already known would deprive the public of its use; it is thus not permitted. In fact, the very reason a patent is awarded is to encourage new technology to come forth. Though the concept of novelty is rather basic in the human mind, its interpretations are not. Absolute novelty as applied by European Patent Commission is that an invention is new if it is not part of the "state of the art"; the state of the art is defined as everything that was available to the public by written or oral publication, use, or any other way, in any country in the world, before the priority date of the invention. The law, particularly U.S. law, goes into great detail in describing what is considered "prior art." This is exemplified by a situation where U.S patent application is rendered invalid by written publication anywhere in the world, however; prior use in a foreign country would not invalidate if there was no written description. Under the absolute novelty system, which is now the law in the United Kingdom, and under the European Patent Commission, prior use of an invention anywhere in the world would invalidate a British or European patent application, if that use made the invention available to the public. The situation is clear if the invention is a machine, a gadget, or a chemical compound or composition that can be analyzed and reproduced by skilled people "without undue burden." In this case, sale makes the invention available to the public, and it is immaterial whether in fact anyone did investigate the workings of the machine or analyze the compound or even whether or not anyone would have any motivation for doing so. However, the use, or even the widespread sale to the public, of a complex mixture, which cannot be precisely analyzed, may not be held to make the invention that it represents available to the public. A special situation is that of so-called selection inventions in which an earlier publication discloses a broad class, and the invention is or is characterized by a narrower subclass. This situation may occur in mechanical inventions in which the class is a group of structural elements, one of which is selected as being particularly useful. More usually, however, selection inventions are found in the field of chemistry, where a narrow group of compounds is selected from a known broad group. So long as no members of the narrow subgroup are specifically disclosed in the publication, it is generally considered, at least in the United Kingdom, the United States, and the European Patent Office, that the compounds are novel, even though they may have been described in general terms. The narrow subgroup of compounds will, however, be patentable only if it has some nonobvious advantage over the other members of the broad class, that is, if there is an inventive step in choosing that particular subgroup from all those generally disclosed.

An important question in considering novelty and inventive step is the position of earlier patent applications that were not published at the priority date of a later application. Unpublished patent applications are not available to the public, and on this basis, one would expect that he or she should not be considered as part of the state of the art. On the other hand, it has been a principle of patent law from the earliest times that not more than one patent should be granted for the same invention, because if this were not the rule, licensees could be forced to pay twice over to obtain the same rights, and the term of patent protection for one invention could be extended beyond the statutory period.

In the European Patent Office, an earlier unpublished European application is prior art against a later one, so long as it is not withdrawn before publication, and to the extent that it validly designates the same countries. This means that the earlier application may be effective in respect of some states designated in the later application, but not against others. Unpublished European patent applications designating the United Kingdom can be prior art against a later British national application, and an earlier unpublished British application is prior art against a granted European patent (United Kingdom) under British law. In the European Patent Office, however, earlier unpublished national applications are not considered as prior art against European applications.

Although under the whole-contents approach the earlier unpublished application is considered to be part of the state of the art, this applies only to considerations of pure novelty, and not to the question whether or not there is an inventive step. The existence of an earlier unpublished application can destroy the novelty of an invention, but it cannot be used to argue that the invention is obvious. This possibility means that under the Patents Act 1977 lack of novelty and obviousness must be clearly distinguished from each other. In early reported cases in England this was often not the case, and many patents were found invalid for lack of novelty or "anticipation," whereas the real reason was lack of an inventive step. Nowadays the term *anticipation* is normally used to mean lack of novelty and is considered to occur when a piece of prior art (i.e., a publication or use that was part of the state of the art before the priority date of the patent application in question) either is or describes something that would be an infringement of one or more of the claims in the application. That is, the test for anticipation is essentially the same as the test for infringement and is met in the case of a written publication if the publication clearly describes something having every feature of the claim or gives instructions to do something that, if carried out, would give something falling within the scope of the claim.

Thus, a claim to a chemical compound may be anticipated by a description of a process if carrying out the process will inevitably give that compound, even if the compound itself was not described. However, anticipation requires "more than a signpost upon the road to the patentee's invention … the prior inventor must be clearly shown to have planted his flag at the precise destination."

Japan also has a system in which earlier unpublished Japanese applications are part of the state of the art, but with the difference that earlier unpublished applications of the same applicant are excluded. In the United States, a pending patent application of earlier date is a priori prior art against a later application, unless the later applicant can show that he or she had an invention date earlier than the date of filing of the earlier application. If it is prior art, it can be applied to attack both novelty and inventive step.

A disclosure formed by combining two documents together is not novelty destroying, although it may be relevant to the question of inventive step. Indeed, it is not even permissible in the European Patent Office to attack novelty by combining two different embodiments described in the same document, unless the document itself indicates that they should be combined. Nevertheless, the prior art document must be interpreted in light of the common general knowledge of the skilled worker in the relevant field as at the date of publication of the document. Needless to say, there is a gray area between what is clearly common general knowledge (e.g., something in a standard reference book used by everyone in the field) and what is simply another publication, and there have been many decisions on this point both in the United Kingdom courts and in the European Patent Office.

Conception is the formation in the mind of the inventor of a definite and permanent idea of the complete and operative invention as it is thereafter to be applied in practice. An invention date is the date when diligence began and leads to reduction to practice. §104 prohibited evidence outside of the United States prior to December 8, 1993, except for filing of a Patent Cooperative Treaty or foreign application or acts domiciled in the United States but serving outside of United States on government business. After December 8, 1993, but prior to January 1, 1996, North American Free Trade Agreement countries included, and on or after January 1, 1996, all countries of WTO included. If there were events prior to these dates, they are taken to the dates the privileges became available. This is important for overcoming 102(a) rejections.

U.S. patent law goes into great detail in describing various events that can be novelty defeating, as described in 35 USC §102:

§102 Events include

- Novelty defeating events occurring prior to invention: 102(a), (e), and (g): AGE
- Time barring events occurring more than fixed time (e.g., 1 yr) prior to United States filing date: 102(b) and (d): ABSOLUTE TIME BAR
- Miscellaneous: 102(c) and (f): OTHERS

§102(a) events include
Events by OTHERS; public knowledge and use only in United States or patented or printed publication anywhere in the world—all prior to date of invention. By definition, the inventor himself cannot trigger a 102(a) event. Applicant's own publication is not but if someone else describes applicant's invention without learning anything from the applicant then it is a 102(a) event if it happened prior to date of invention.

653

"Knowledge" means the claimed invention must have been publicly known to a sufficiently large segment of the public, the size depending on the number of persons skilled in the art that have such knowledge—the more likely it is then for the invention to be in public knowledge.

"Use by others" means in use before date of invention and by more than one person and the use must have been accessible to the public without deliberate attempt to keep the use secret, although it need not be "visible" to the public—a hidden device, such as.

"Printed publication" is a reference only for what it discloses and enables (it can not be a passing remark); the effective date of publication is when the document is indexed or cataloged in a library or disseminated by mail—the test being if one of ordinary skill would have had access to the document with reasonable diligence to locate it. The number of copies distributed, whether recipients constitute a significant portion of those interested in the subject matter and whether the disclosure was an oral paper only at a conference, determines "Publication" status. It need not be in a classic printed form—the key is public accessibility, even if stored in a remote location in a remote library, even if no one read the document in the library. Electronic publication such as online databases or internet resources are "printed publication" if accessible.

"Patent" is a reference the date it becomes enforceable but if it is kept secret (as in some countries) then it is the date it becomes sufficiently accessible to the public; if patent is published before its rights are exercisable, the date is when it becomes exercisable, not the date of publication. The published patent is treated as "printed publication" not a patent until such time. The patented subject matter includes, in addition to claimed subject matter, subject matter disclosed in the specification that is covered by the claims: unclaimed species are covered by a genus claim. Specification that relates to the subject matter is also "patented" matter. The disclosure need not be enabling, quite unlike the requirements for a "printed publication."

Priority can be claimed to avoid 102(a) rejection based on earlier foreign, continuation, provisional or nonprovisional filing for any claim (establishing its effective filing date) in the later United States application if the earlier application provides §112 ¶1 support, it is filed within one year (or 6 month for design) of the earlier application and it makes a claim to priority.

§102(b): Events by ANYONE (including inventor); public use and on sale only in United States or patented or printed publication anywhere in the world, more than 1 year before filing date—the earliest United States filing date of application; also called "the critical date." If anniversary date of the critical date falls on a weekend or a federal holiday in the DC, the application may be filed on the next business day to avoid statutory bar. §102(b) is a statutory time bar—it cannot be removed or antedated regardless of date of invention or who was responsible.

A §102(b) event anticipates a claim if and only if all elements and limitations recited in the claim (under application) are present in the subject matter of the event, i.e., if the claim reads on the subject matter of the event.

A single public use of the claimed invention by a single person is sufficient for this bar. Hidden from sight but public uses are sufficient. Intentionally concealing (making it available on a restricted basis and confidentiality obligation) is not public use. Misappropriated use is still a public use. Experimental use is not public use (where necessary to demonstrate the workability and where the profit was incidental to the experimental use). Experimentation must be the primary purpose (control by the inventor, confidentiality agreements, record of performance and progress report kept, necessity of public testing, length of test period, whether payments were made, changes made as a result of use). Product acceptance by the market is NOT experimental use.

On sale bar applies when offered for sale in the United States and the invention was "ready for patenting," reduced to actual practice or the inventor had prepared drawings or other descriptions of the invention sufficient to enable a person skilled in the art to practice the invention. The product sold need not be on hand or in physical existence. The sale offer can be made by anyone (inventor, assignee or a third party). Published abstracts may qualify for on sale rejection if they identify product's vendor, contain information useful for potential buyers (contact, price, warranties, etc.), along with date of product release or installation before the critical date. Note it can also be a §102/§103 bar as well (obviousness based on sale activity). A sale can be: conditional, secret (phone or discrete), without profits, an offer from the United States to an offeree abroad or vice versa, offer originating but not received prior to critical date, an offer that never reaches, rejected offer, not consummated, single sale, sale between two related entities not controlled by each other, or even sale made without inventor's consent or in violation of any confidentiality agreement. NOT a sale event: incidental sale to experimental use is NOT a sale even if yields profit provided the primary purpose was experimental study (see above for conditions); assignment of rights is not an "on sale" event, the "res" of invention must be sold.

Patents on the date of their availability become §102(b) bar. A foreign fling within 12 month of §102 event and then filing United States patent within one year of the foreign filing does not remove §102(b) bar—It must be filed in the United States within 12 months either as provisional or nonprovisional. Foreign priority does not remove this bar, the United States priority does. A continuation application is governed by its ancestral filing date and thus it can avoid §102(b) bar.

§102(c): Events by INVENTOR—abandonment of invention, expressed, implied, by action or by inaction. Unreasonable delays in filing the United States patent, developing invention, coupled with other evidence such as spurring into activity if someone else has commercialized or about to commercialize the product of invention. Delay alone is not sufficient to demonstrate abandonment. Disclosing but not claiming a distinct embodiment; can be overcome by filing another application claiming the disclosed embodiment within one year of the issue date of the patent or filing a broadening reissue application within two years of the patent. Abandoned invention may be recaptured by proceeding diligently to obtain a United States patent prior to another's invention of the same subject.

§102(d): Events by INVENTOR or AFFILIATE (as allowed in foreign filings)—filing abroad more than 1 year (six months for design) before United States filing date and patent must issue before United States filing date (unlike §102(a) and (b)), the date of patent is the date rights attach even if the patent is kept secret. The same invention must be involved but not necessarily claimed in the United States application; a different aspect of the invention might be claimed.

§102(e): The default date of invention of a pending application is its filing date (constructive reduction to practice) unless otherwise proven. Events by OTHERS; published application in United States or in English if Patent Cooperative Treaty and designating United States or an issued United States patent filed before the date of invention of application in question. Note: the only date of the United States Patent and Trademark Office has for a pending application is the filing date of application (constructive reduction to practice), which must then be challenged through affidavits if contested If rejection is based on §102(e). "Another" means an inventive entity different from the application's inventive entity. An inventive entity is different if not ALL inventors are the same. Rule 132 declaration can be used to establish this. §102(e)(2)[A]. A United States patent to "another" stemming from a domestic application (not a Patent Cooperative Treaty filing designating United States) has the effective date as a reference as of its United States filing date (with claim extending to its provisional or continuation application if applicable) as a prior art

reference but NOT its foreign priority date, where applicable, against a pending United States application. On the contrary, the pending United States application against which the reference is used CAN use its foreign priority date as a SHIELD provided the reference's United States filing date is later than the foreign filing date of the application. This is applicable even if the reference has a foreign filing date prior to the foreign filing date of the application since the foreign filing date of the reference is immaterial. However, if the reference has domestic priority date prior to the applicant's foreign priority date then the foreign priority date of applicant cannot be used to overcome §102(e)(2)[A] rejection. §102(e)(2)[B]. A United States patent to "another" stemming from a national stage-Patent Cooperative Treaty application has the priority date depending on the filing dates of the pending applications against which it is used. If the application under examination was filed: for a pending United States Patent and Trademark Office application filed prior to November 29, 2000 and NOT voluntarily published, the priority date of the United States patent as a reference is the date when the Patent Cooperative Treaty application for this reference patent entered the national stage in the United States. For a pending United States Patent and Trademark Office application filed before November 29, 2000 and published voluntarily, the United States patent stemming from a national stage-Patent Cooperative Treaty filing has no effect on this application. (Meaning that the United States patent reference has no effective filing date. It does not exist.) For a pending United States Patent and Trademark Office application filed on or after November 29, 2000, the United States patent stemming from a national stage-Patent Cooperative Treaty filing has no effect on this application. (Meaning that the United States patent reference has no effective filing date. It does not exist.) §102(e)(1)[A]. Published domestic United States Patent Application is an anticipatory reference as of its filing date, even if it were subsequently abandoned. The §102(e) reference must contain an enabling disclosure relative to the application claim against which it is applied; an issued United States patent has a statutory presumption of validity, a published application does not. If the reference is not enabling, it cannot be a §102 event but can still be a §103 event. §102(e)(1)[B]. Published Patent Cooperative Treaty patent application (by WIPO or by United States Patent and Trademark Office—entering national stage) is a reference as of the Patent Cooperative Treaty filing date if it did designate United States and was published by WIPO in English. The United States Patent and Trademark Office-published national stage is a reference as of its Patent Cooperative Treaty filing date but only if the Patent Cooperative Treaty application was published by WIPO in English. If a Patent Cooperative Treaty application does meet these requirements, it can be a §102(a) or (b) event but not §102(e).

§102(f): The inventor is the one who conceives the invention, not derives it from someone else—disclosed by someone else or getting the idea from someone else.

§102(g): §102(g)(2). A patent bar arises if the invention was made in this country by another inventor who did not abandon, suppress or conceal it. An interference proceeding or an *ex parte* examination decides and thus §102(g) becomes applicable ONLY after these evaluations. Five conditions apply: the invention must have been made, i.e., reduced to practice, in this country (§104—invention in foreign countries does not apply), by another, before the applicant's date of invention and that the other did not abandon, suppress or conceal it. Reasonable diligence is a major key to these decisions. §102(g)(1). Applies only in an interference proceeding to establish than the invention was made within the limits of §104—North American Free Trade Agreement country after Dec 7, 1993 or WTO country after December 31, 1996. Other conditions of abandoning, suppressing and concealing apply as above. Countries outside North American Free Trade Agreement or WTO are not considered regardless of date of activity in those countries. Even in North American Free Trade Agreement and WTO countries the latest date of activity is the date given above

when they entered the jurisdiction; all prior dates are shifted to these dates. *§102 Special Forms*: Abandoned Applications: If an issued patent refers to an abandoned application, the content of that application become evidence of public-knowledge (§102[a]). If an issued application expressly incorporates the disclosure of an abandoned application by reference, then the contents become part of the disclosure effective as of the patent's filing date under §102(e)(2). Material cancelled from an application is not part of the patent for the purposes of §102(e)(2), however the prosecution history becomes available to the public as of the issue date of the patent and becomes §102(a) event. Incipient §102(e) references: Unpublished applications cannot be cited as prior art under §102(e), however, claims in a later-filed application may be provisionally rejected over an earlier application under §102(e) if the two applications have a common inventor or assignee. Oral testimony alone, without at least some documentary corroboration, is generally insufficient to prove invalidity. SIRs (Statutory invention registration) examined in compliance with §112, ¶1 are treated the same as a patent for §102(e)(2) purpose—defensive purpose. The Doctrine of Forfeiture states that a commercial, purposely hidden use of a process or a machine by an applicant (but not by a third party) more than one year before the filing date of the application, coupled with a sale of the res precludes the application from obtaining a patent.

17.6.2 Second Requirement: Inventive Step

The question whether or not something for which a patent is applied for involves an inventive step is one that is intrinsically much more difficult, because to some extent judgment of what is or is not obvious must be a subjective matter. Because the question is such a contentious one, there have been a great many patent cases in which obviousness has been at issue, and a great many judges have tried at various times to define what is meant by "obviousness," or to pose questions such as "is the solution one which would have occurred to everyone of ordinary intelligence and acquaintance with the subject matter who gave his mind to the problem?" or, more bluntly, was it "so easy that any fool could do it?" Thus, the person to whom the invention must be nonobvious if it is to be patentable is "the person skilled in the art": a competent worker but without imagination or inventive capability. In the days when the great majority of patents were for relatively simple mechanical devices, it was common to describe the person skilled in the art as an "ordinary workman." This is no longer appropriate in view of the increasing technical sophistication of industry. For chemical patents, the person skilled in the art may normally be considered as the average qualified industrial chemist, and for complex inventions such as in the field of biotechnology, the "person skilled in the art" may be considered to be a team of highly qualified scientists. When attacking a patent, it behooves to bring in a witness, who is an ordinary worker rather than a Nobel Laureate, whose testimony will be challenged and likely thrown out as he or she is expected to know more than what is "a person of ordinary skills."

The inventive step need not be a giant stride nor a result of any planned research; there is also no need to demonstrate a flash of genius in the process. An oft-asked question is that if this was obvious, why did not anyone else come up with this invention before. The answer to that is that this is that person. The patent examiners are also warned to look not only at the invention in the hindsight as this may appear too obvious but also in light of the art available at the time of invention; this is particularly true of fields of invention that are fast growing.

The European Patent Office applies a "problem and solution approach" to an inventive step. The invention must attempt to solve a technical problem, a slightly better objective method than what U.S. Patent and Trademark Office practices. Anything in the state of the art, other than unpublished earlier patent applications, may be taken into account. It was not allowed to use different publications, reconstructing the invention by taking a piece from one and another piece from another, unless, for example, one document directly referred to the other. The documents can be combined together in considering obviousness if a person skilled in the art would naturally consider them in association; thus, it may be enough if they simply relate to the same technical field. The jurisprudence of the European Patent Office is similar; it is permissible to combine documents in assessing inventive step only if it would have been obvious for the skilled person to do so at the time of filing. In the United States, it is allowed to combine any number of prior art documents including earlier filed applications.

The issue of obviousness is dealt under 35 USC §103 of U.S. patent law. If the difference between the claimed invention and the prior art is such that the invention as a whole would have been obvious *at the time of invention* to a person having ordinary skill in the art to which said subject matter pertains, a patent will not be granted. The manner in which the invention is made does not negate patentability (e.g., an invention made someone not familiar with the field of invention or making an accidental invention). The famous "*Graham v. John Deere*: Fundamental Inquiry" invokes the scope and content of the prior art, the difference between the prior art and the claims at issue, the level of ordinary skill in the pertinent art, and secondary considerations, that is, objective indicia of nonobviousness. These measures may include commercial success, long-felt but unresolved needs, failure of others, recognition of problem, failure to resolve problem, competitors' prompt copying, licensing of patent to industry, teaching away, unexpected results, and disbelief and incredulity.

Prima facie obviousness is the level of showing that the Patent and Trademark Office must achieve in order to shift to the applicant the burden of going forward with the production of evidence or arguments tending to prove nonobviousness. The examiner, on the basis of prior art, proposes a combination that would be possible for one of ordinary skills to make. To protect applicant:

- Hindsight is impermissible.
- Examiner must step back before invention.
- Knowledge of applicant's disclosure is put aside.
- Only the facts gleaned from the prior art may be used.

Examiner bears the initial burden of supporting prima facie conclusion; otherwise, the applicant has no obligation to submit evidence of nonobviousness. Once so produced, the burden shifts to applicant to submit additional evidence, for example, commercial success and unexpected results. The prima facie requirements state that there must be some suggestion or motivation, either in the references themselves or in the knowledge generally available to one of ordinary skill in the art, to modify the references or to combine reference teachings. Prima facie does not hold if it is shown that (Niazi, 2003)

- Teachings can be modified or combined.
- Prior art does not suggest the desirability of combination.
- One of ordinary skill is merely capable of combining the teachings.
- Modifications or combinations destroy the intended function.
- There is a change in the principle of operation of the prior art.

- Modification or combination of prior art teaches away from such modification or combination.
- Applicant's invention is the discovery of problem or the source of problem. There must be a reasonable, not absolute, expectation or predictability of success of the proposed modification or combination of the prior art at the time of invention was made, not when the examiner does evaluate it. The prior art reference(s) must teach or suggest *all* the claim limitations. This includes indefinite limitations (not meeting §112, ¶2) and limitations unsupported by the specification in the application. (Thus there may be rejection on §112 basis but not §103 in these situations.) Unclaimed features are not germane to the obviousness determination. The prior art must be "analogous" to invention—either in the field of invention or reasonably pertinent to it. Only the teachings of prior art, which must be combinable. It is not necessary that the specific structure be physically combinable; prima facie obviousness is not negated for business reasons not to combine; the issue is technologic combination. Prior art need not suggest same advantage or results as the invention; motivation to modify or combine the prior art may be stimulated by a purpose different from that of the claimed invention, or the solution of a problem different from that solved by the claimed invention. Routine manipulative steps cannot be prima facie obvious when the claimed material it uses or produces is patentable, i.e., where either the starting or the ending material is patentable.

§102(e), (f), and (g) Events as §103 Prior Art: Prior art under §102(e), (f), and (g) may be modified or combined to establish obviousness, except when the subject matter of prior art and the invention claimed in the application under examination were, at the time the claimed invention was made (not when it was filed), owned by the same person or subject to an obligation of assignment to the same person. With respect to §102(e), §103(c) is effective as of November 29, 1999 (AIPA). Rejections on §102(e)/§103 can be obviated using an affidavit if the ownership is same by an affidavit for an application filed after November 29, 1999. For applications filed prior to this date, a continuation application may be filed to take advantage of this ruling change. Whereas references in §103 are as of the date of invention, an exception arises when using a §102(e) event are applied, wherein the prior art is applied as of the date of the filing of the application vis-à-vis the filing date of the reference.

Admission as Prior Art Under §103: If an applicant admits a reference as prior art it cannot be reversed in a traversal; admissions include labeling drawings are prior art and any written admission during prosecution in addition to whatever has been submitted in the specification. A Jepsen claim however is rebuttable.

17.6.3 Third Requirement: Be Patentable

The third basic requirement of patentability is that the invention should be capable of industrial application, broadly defined, and includes making or using the invention in any kind of industry, including agriculture. Methods of medical treatment or diagnosis performed on the human or animal body are defined as being incapable of industrial application, although substances invented for use in such methods are patentable.

There are certain specific exceptions to patentability, which apply whether or not the invention is capable of industrial application. Artistic works and esthetic creations are not patentable and are generally not industrially applicable either, but scientific theories and mathematical methods, the presentation of information, business methods, and computer programs are also unpatentable, although they may very well be applied in industry.

Animal and plant varieties are not patentable in countries adhering to the European Patent Commission, although in the U.S. plants may be protected either by normal utility patents or by special plant patents for plant varieties. In the United Kingdom and certain other European countries, new plant varieties, although not patentable, can be protected by plant breeders' rights granted under the UPOV (International Union for the Protection of New Varieties of Plants) convention. Transgenic plants and animals are in principle patentable only if they do not constitute a variety raising a difficult and uncertain situation. A further exception applies to offensive, immoral, or antisocial inventions, which need not just be an article prohibited by the law; if it is abhorrent to society, it is unpatentable, though it may be legal. A portable nuclear device would be such an example. Also excluded are inventions contrary to well-established natural laws, for example, a perpetual motion machine, though European Patent Commission does not spell it out like this.

According to U.S. laws, the patentable inventions are defined as any new and useful process, machine, manufacture, or composition of matter or any new and useful improvement thereof. The requirement that the invention be useful is rather stronger than the European Patent Commission requirement that it be capable of industrial application and is more like the old British utility requirement.

17.7 PATENTABILITY AND TECHNICAL INFORMATION SEARCH

Before a patent application is filed, a thorough search of the subject matter is conducted to unearth prior art; this is, however, an excellent means for scientists to learn about the state of science as well. Though many scientist remain skeptical about the correctness of information vis-à-vis refereed publications, there is no doubt that much time can be saved in conducting research if a thorough analysis of the invention and related inventions is made by the scientists. With the availability of Internet, it has now become routine for the scientists to present the most comprehensive analysis of the state of the art prior to beginning the process of patenting. This search does not replace the search conducted by the patent attorneys.

17.7.1 Patent Office Resource

The patent offices worldwide have opened their databases to the public; there is no better place to start the search for patentability with these free databases; know that the same databases are packaged by other vendors who provide additional services and literature search. The U.S. Patent and Trademark Office (http://www.uspto.gov) has created one of the world's largest electronic databases that include every patent issued; recently published applications are also available in the database. Scientists are strongly urged to develop strong skills on interacting with the database study of the U.S. Patent and Trademark Office. The search at the U.S. Patent and Trademark Office can be most beneficial if the scientist learns how to use the patent classification system. (Tutorials are available at the U.S. Patent and Trademark Office website; alternately, consult *Filing Patents Online: A Professional Guide* by Sarfaraz K. Niazi, CRC Press, 2002.)

The U.S. Patent Office Classification 435 includes the following subcategories related to therapeutic proteins:

CLASS 435: CHEMISTRY: MOLECULAR BIOLOGY AND MICROBIOLOGY, provides for methods of purifying, propagating or attenuating a micro-organism; e.g., a virus, bacteria, etc., except for propagating a micro-organism in an animal for the purpose of producing an antibody containing sera. Class 435, provides for methods of propagating animal organs, tissues or cells; e.g., blood, sperm, etc., and culture media therefor. Class 435 is the generic home for processes of (1) analyzing or testing which involve a fermentation step or (2) qualitative or quantitative testing for fermentability, or fermentative power.

435. Chemistry: Molecular Biology and Microbiology, see appropriate subclasses: for processes in which a material containing an enzyme or micro-organism is used to perform a qualitative or quantitative measurement or test; for compositions or test strips for either of the stated processes; for the processes of making such compositions or test strips; for processes of using micro-organisms or enzymes to synthesize a chemical product; for processes of treating a material with micro-organisms or enzymes to separate, liberate, or purify a preexisting substance or to destroy hazardous or toxic waste; for processes of propagating micro-organisms; for processes of genetically altering a micro-organism; for processes of tissue, organ, blood, sperm, or microbial maintenance; for processes of malting or mashing; for micro-organisms, per se, and subcellular parts thereof; for recombinant vectors and their preparation; for enzymes, per se, compositions containing enzymes not otherwise provided for and processes of preparing and purifying enzymes; for compositions for microbial propagation; for apparatus for any of the processes of the class; for composting apparatus; and subclasses 4+ for in vitro processes in which there is a direct or indirect, qualitative or quantitative, measurement or test, by or of a material which contains an enzyme or micro-organism (for the purposes of Class 435, micro-organism includes bacteria, actinomycetales, cyanobacteria [unicellular algae], fungi, protozoa, animal cells, plant cells, and virus). Class 424 definition contains controlling statements on the class lines.

93.2 Genetically modified micro-organism, cell, or virus (e.g., transformed, fused, hybrid, etc.): This subclass is indented under subclass 93.1. Subject matter involving a micro-organism, cell or virus which (a) is a product of recombination, transformation, or transfection with a vector or a foreign or exogenous gene or (b) is a product of homologous recombination if it is directed rather than spontaneous or (c) is a product of fused or hybrid cell formation. (1) Note. Examples of subject matter included in this and the indented subclass are compositions containing micro-organisms, cells, or viruses resulting from (a) a process in which the cellular matter of two or more fusing partners is combined producing a cell which initially contains the genes of both fusing partners or (b) a process in which a cell is treated with an immortalizing agent which results in a cell which proliferates in long term culture or (c) a process involving recombinant DNA methodology. (2) Note. Excluded from this subclass are products of unidentified or non-induced mutations; products of microbial conjugation wherein specific genetic material is not identified and controlled; and products of natural, spontaneous, or arbitrary

conjugation or recombination events. These products are not considered genetically modified for this subclass and therefore will be classified as unmodified
micro-organisms, cells, or viruses.

93.21: Eukaryotic cell: This subclass is indented under subclass 93.2. Subject matter
involving an eukaryotic cell, such as an animal cell, plant cell, fungus, protozoa,
or higher algae which has been genetically modified. (1) Note. An eukaryotic cell
has a nucleus defined by a nuclear membrane wherein the nucleus contains chromosomes that comprise the genome of the cell.

93.3: Intentional mixture of two or more micro- organisms, cells, or viruses of different genera: This subclass is indented under subclass 93.1. Subject matter involving
a mixture consisting of two or more different microbial, cellular, or viral genera. (1) Note. A mixture of E. coli and Pseudomonas or a mixture of Aspergillus
and Bacillus would be considered proper for this subclass while a mixture of
Bacillus cereus and Bacillus brevis would be classified under Bacillus rather than
in this subclass since they are both in the genus, Bacillus. (2) Note. Rumen, intestinal, vaginal, etc., microflora mixtures are mixtures appropriate for this subclass
unless mixture constituents are disclosed and are found to be contrary to the
subclass definition.

133.1: Structurally-modified antibody, immunoglobulin, or fragment thereof (e.g.,
chimeric, humanized, CDR-grafted, mutated, etc.): This subclass is indented
under subclass 130.1. Subject matter involving an antibody, immunoglobulin,
or fragment thereof that is purposely altered with respect to its amino acid
sequence or glycosylation, or with respect to its composition of heavy and light
chains or immunoglobulin regions or domains, as compared with that found
in nature; or wherein the antibody, immunoglobulin, or fragment thereof is
part of a larger, synthetic protein. (1) Note. Structurally-modified antibodies
may be made by chemical alteration or recombination of existing antibodies,
or by various cloning techniques involving recombinant DNA or hybridoma
technology. (2) Note. Structurally-modified antibodies may be chimeric (i.e.,
comprising amino acid sequences derived from two or more nonidentical
immunoglobulin molecules, such as interspecies combinations, etc.). (3) Note.
Structurally-modified antibodies may have domain deletions or substitutions (e.g., deletions of particular constant-region domains or substitutions of
constant-region domains from other classes of immunoglobulins). (4) Note.
Structurally-modified antibodies may have deletions of particular glycosylated amino acids, or may have their glycosylation otherwise altered, which
may alter their function. (5) Note. While expression of cloned antibody genes
in cells of species other than from which they originated may result in altered
glycosylation of the product, compared with that found in nature, this subclass
and indented subclasses are not meant to encompass such antibodies or fragments thereof unless such cloning is a deliberate attempt to alter their glycosylation. However, such antibodies or fragments thereof may still be classified
here or in indented subclasses if they are structurally-modified in other ways
(e.g., if they are single chain, etc.). (6) Note. It is suggested that the patents
of this subclass and indented subclasses be cross-referenced to the appropriate subclass(es) that provide for the binding specificities of these antibodies, if
disclosed.

141.1: Monoclonal antibody or fragment thereof (i.e., produced by any cloning
technology): This subclass is indented under subclass 130.1. Subject matter
involving an antibody or fragment thereof produced by a clone of cells or cell

line, which clone of cells or cell line is derived from a single antibody-producing cell or antibody-fragment-producing cell, wherein said antibody or fragment thereof is identical to all other antibodies or fragments thereof produced by that clone of cells or cell line. (1) Note. This and the indented subclasses provide for bioaffecting and body-treating compositions of antibodies or fragments thereof as well as bioaffecting and body-treating methods of using said compositions, said antibodies, or said fragments, which antibodies or antibody fragments are produced by any cloning technology that yields identical molecules (e.g., hybridoma technology, recombinant DNA technology, etc.). (2) Note. Monoclonal antibodies, per se, are considered compounds and are provided for elsewhere. See the search notes below. (3) Note. Monoclonal antibodies are sometimes termed monoclonal receptors or immunological binding partners.

1.49 and 1.53, for methods of using radiolabeled monoclonal antibodies or compositions thereof for bioaffecting or body-treating purposes and said compositions, per se.

9.1+ for methods of using monoclonal antibodies or compositions thereof for in vivo testing or diagnosis and said compositions, per se.

178.1+ for bioaffecting or body-treating methods of using monoclonal antibodies or fragments thereof that are conjugated to or complexed with nonimmunoglobulin material; bioaffecting or body-treating methods of using compositions of monoclonal antibodies or fragments thereof, which monoclonal antibodies or fragments thereof are conjugated to or complexed with nonimmunoglobulin material; and said compositions, per se.

199.1: Recombinant virus encoding one or more heterologous proteins or fragments thereof: This subclass is indented under subclass 184.1. Subject matter involving a virus into whose genome is integrated one or more nucleic acid sequences encoding one or more heterologous proteins or fragments thereof. (1) Note. A heterologous protein is one derived from another species (e.g., another viral species). (2) Note. Such genetically-modified viruses may be used as multivalent vaccines.

200.1: Recombinant or stably-transformed bacterium encoding one or more heterologous proteins or fragments thereof: This subclass is indented under subclass 184.1. Subject matter involving a bacterium into whose genome is integrated one or more nucleic acid sequences encoding one or more heterologous proteins or fragments thereof; or involving a bacterium that carries stable, replicative plasmids that include one or more nucleic acid sequences encoding one or more heterologous proteins or fragments thereof. (1) Note. A heterologous protein is one derived from another species (e.g., another bacterial species). (2) Note. Such genetically-modified bacteria may be used as multivalent vaccines.

201.1: Combination of viral and bacterial antigens (e.g., multivalent viral and bacterial vaccine, etc.) This subclass is indented under subclass 184.1. Subject matter involving a combination of viral and bacterial antigens, such as that found in a multivalent viral and bacterial vaccine.

202.1: Combination of antigens from multiple viral species (e.g., multivalent viral vaccine, etc.): This subclass is indented under subclass 184.1. Subject matter involving a combination of antigens from multiple viral species, such as that found in a multivalent viral vaccine. (1) Note. A combination of antigens from multiple variants of the same viral species should be classified with that viral species.

203.1: Combination of antigens from multiple bacterial species (e.g., multivalent bacterial vaccine, etc.): This subclass is indented under subclass 184.1. Subject matter involving a combination of antigens from multiple bacterial species, such as that found in a multivalent bacterial vaccine. (1) Note. A combination of antigens from multiple variants of the same bacterial species should be classified with that bacterial species.

801: INVOLVING ANTIBODY OR FRAGMENT THEREOF PRODUCED BY RECOMBINANT DNA TECHNOLOGY: This subclass is indented under the class definition. Subject matter involving an antibody or fragment thereof produced by recombinant DNA technology.

A search under CCL/"435/69.1" yields 8898 patents including the earliest patents wherein insulin was produced by genetically modified fungi from the University of Minnesota and the two classic patents from Stanford and Columbia.

Second to the U.S. Patent Office, the largest database is accessed through the European Patent Office, where one should conduct a similar classification search as suggested above for the U.S. Patent and Trademark Office (http://ep.espacenet.com). The World Intellectual Property Organization at http://ipdl.wipo.int/ offers many useful features including complete details of the Patent Cooperative Treaty and its gazette. The Canadian Patent Office can be reached at http://patents1.ic.gc.ca/srch_bool-e.html.

17.7.2 Information Portals

- The Library of Congress is the best place to start as it is the world's largest library: http://lcweb.loc.gov
- Gateway to all government information: http://www.firstgov.gov/
- The Scout Report is one of the Internet's longest-running weekly publications, offering a selection of new and newly discovered online resources: http://scout.cs.wisc.edu/
- Internet Public Library—an annotated collection of high-quality Internet resources for their usefulness in providing accurate, factual information on a particular topic or topics: http://www.ipl.org/ref/RR/
- A highly artistic website on the patenting process with much support for independent inventors: http://www.invent.org/
- The Canadian Innovation Center: http://www.innovationcentre.ca
- The 150-million volume British Library is a good source; search here the key word *patent*: http://www.bl.uk/
- Knowledge Express provides business development and competitive intelligence resources—including intellectual property, technology transfer, and corporate partnering opportunities—to organizations involved with science/technology research and new inventions: http://www.knowledgeexpress.com/
- New product information on thousands of products weekly: http://productnews.com
- Aimed at manufacturers and inventors: http://www.techexpo.com
- Health and medical information: http://www.pubcrawler.ie/
- National Library of Medicine consumer site on health: http://medlineplus.gov/
- Info on all U.S. clinical trials underway and you can branch out to learn about how to do clinical trials: http://clinicaltrials.gov/

- A major archive of free online life science journals: http://www.pubmedcentral.nih.gov/
- Free online journals in science, technology, and medicine: http://highwire.stanford.edu/lists/freeart.dtl
- Reliable health information from government agencies: http://www.healthfinder.gov/
- The Centers for Disease Control and Prevention: http://www.cdc.gov/
- Food and Drug Administration regulations: http://www.fda.gov
- USDA Food and Nutrient Information Center: http://www.nal.usda.gov/fnic/
- Medical design technology for devices: http://www.mdtmag.com
- Medical information from WebMD: http://www.medscape.com/
- Consumer healthcare information from Harvard: http://www.intelihealth.com
- British Medical Journal; prestige medical issues: http://www.bmj.com
- Medical devices: http://www.devicelink.com/
- The human genome project: http://www.ornl.gov/hgmis/

17.7.3 Technical Databases

- National Institutes of Health offers over 12 million research papers mainly in the biomedical sciences, which are available through the National Library of Medicine. This free database allows download of abstract in an ASCII format for direct placement into programs such as Microsoft Word to develop a comprehensive bibliography: http://www.ncbi.nlm.nih.gov/PubMed
- Derwent is one of the most widely used databases, from which the U.S. Patent and Trademark Office examiners benefit as well: http://www.derwent.com
- Dialog is another large database that allows you to search without having to register an account; you pay as you go alone using your credit card. You cannot do this if you are searching for trademarks: http://www.dialog.com
- Nerac: http://www.nerac.com

17.7.4 Patent Search and IP Services

- Investor's Digest is a resource for inventors: http://www.inventorsdigest.com/
- The MIT has provided an elaborate and detailed website for invention development: http://web.mit.edu/invent/

17.7.5 Patent Copies, Search Facilities

- Questel: http://www.questel.orbit.com/
- Faxpat: http://www.faxpat.com
- Lexis-Nexus: http://www.lexis-nexis.com

17.8 COMPONENTS OF A PATENT APPLICATION

A patent specification (not specifications) is a legal document that ends up getting published as the patent, if allowed. Great care and detail goes into writing this document in defining the scope of invention, deciding what is claimed, and wording the claims (which are part of specification) such that they can withstand challenges.

Deciding on what is "invented" is the job of the research scientist, but the decision is made in light of prior art; for example, if there is a discovery of a new group of chemicals, the breadth of group should be ascertained in light of the prior art available and obviously what can be reasonably predicted regarding the structure of chemicals and the ability to synthesize representative chemicals, if not all. Where a completely new molecular structure has been invented, a broad scope, including all kinds of derivatives of the basic structure that the inventor thinks may be useful, is possible. It is surprising how many times scientists who are sure of the novelty of a structure, composition, or application find out when a thorough search is made of the possible prior art. It is worth realizing that with the availability of databases in electronic format, the Internet, and generally a faster access to remove publications (even brochures for promotion in remote countries), what a thorough search would reveal; know that the patent examiners have access to these same channels of information and then some. The author has been humbled more than once on what the patent examiner can dig out. So, scientists are advised not to jump the gun in making very broad claims until so advised by the patent attorneys after conducting a thorough patent search. Obviously, the scope is narrowed down gradually as more and more prior art emerges. The goal is not to narrow it down to a point where it loses its commercial importance. The scope of protection that it is commercially important to achieve varies from one field to another. In extreme situations, it is sufficient to have a scope that includes a singular compound, if that is what the company wishes to market. The strength in this approach comes from the regulatory control of pharmaceutical products. Once a company received marketing authorization from the Food and Drug Administration, at a great expense, imitators would like only to reproduce the invention, which they cannot do through the course of patent term and any other extensions granted by the Food and Drug Administration. So, while there may be other molecules, perhaps better ones, available, imitators are unlikely to invest in their development because they are unprotected, and there is no guarantee that the Food and Drug Administration will approve them. So, in the field of new drug development, a single chemical entity does have substantial value. Such is not the case in other industries where regulatory costs are not involved, such as in the chemical industry.

Once a decision is made about what is invented, how much to claim, and what specifically to claim, the process of drafting specification begins. One method is to draft the main claim, defining the scope of the invention in the form of the statement of invention, which is the heart of the patent specification, then the rest of the specification and claims will be drafted.

Specification begins with a title. Newcomers to the field of patenting would be amazed or perhaps amused at the choice of patent titles and even the language used to describe an invention. Historically, inventors kept the titles vague to keep the searchers (who then did manual searches) out of finding about their inventions. Today, as most patent offices have gone electronic, this is no long an issue, nevertheless the practice continues.

Patent applications have fixed formats that often vary between patent offices but nevertheless require a similar information submission: a background, a summary, a detail of invention, and so on. The patent application must be comprehensive to demonstrate novelty and the inventive step in light of prior art; it should be understood that the purpose is not to fool the patent examiner into allowance but to protect the invention from competitors who will challenge it, should it be worth anything. A full disclosure is required to keep the infringers out as the chance of their success in knocking out a patent goes down. Additional statements are included defining the features of the invention for use as basis for specific claims. Examples of stating that are "In one aspect the invention provides ...," "In another aspect the invention provides ...," and "The above defined widgets are new and form part of the invention." Attorneys have their preferences and standard statements that fill the specification write up quickly.

After the statements of invention, there is a description of indication of what are the preferred parts of the scope, and one or more formulae may be given defining narrower subgeneric scopes. This section fulfils the requirement of adequacy of description. The specification must also describe how the invention is to be carried out, an essential part of a patent application. This is a critical stage in deciding how and what to disclose. As discussed earlier, often at this stage a decision may be made not to file for a patent application for the disclosure will inevitably cause the invention to escape from the hands of inventors, and if there were no certain ways to determine infringement, this would make patenting useless. It is also not a smart move to be deceptive when it comes to describing how the invention works; many a patent applications have been declared invalid, after the companies have made significant investment in marketing the invention, because a competitor was able to demonstrate that the inventors hid certain critical facts. It must be understood that the disclosure need not be for a commercial model of invention and thus need not include many fine details generally required for a large-scale production of the invention, such as in-process specifications, certain handling conditions, and the grade of excipients used, which may be material to produce a product fit for a particular purpose, such as human consumption. As long as the competitor can manufacture the article, not necessary for the commercial production, using the details provided, the requirement of sufficiency of disclosure is met. This becomes more important in the discovery of new chemical entities where chemical synthesis can be described adequately, but not necessarily for the grade of material required; for example, the impurity profile of an NCE (New Chemical Entity: Food and Drug Administration) is critical for the purpose of an NDA (New Drug Application: Food and Drug Administration); manufacturers often are able to produce a product that would meet the Food and Drug Administration's requirement for quality, yet not report this method in the patent, which would allow the competitor to manufacture the product with impurities only. The reason why the companies are able to get away with this trick is for the reason that the patent claims a chemical compound, not necessarily what would be suitable for ingestion by humans. Obviously, if the molecule turns out to be a blockbuster, many will imitate the process and may challenge the patent; case law on this aspect is silent. It is well known, as a result, that once an NCE comes to the end of its patent cycle, new sources of active pharmaceutical ingredient are developed with greater difficulty than what would be anticipated from the disclosures in the patent.

Next comes an indication of what the invention is useful for, a part of the specification usually called the utility statement. Whereas in the case of mechanical inventions it is often obvious, it requires explanation for chemical inventions along with any peculiar or particular advantages. It is important to know that there is no requirement to explain how and why the invention works; thus, it is best not to offer any hypothesis about the invention. However, if a theory must be given, one should leave room for a change of mind later, for example, by wording such as "whilst we do not intend to be bound to any particular theory, it is believed that …." In a chemical case, a number of examples are given with detailed instructions for the preparation of at least one of the compounds within the scope and for the use of the compounds.

After these comes the heart of patent, the claims. There is no limitation on how many claims are made; however, redundant and superfluous claims are frowned upon by the examiners and should be avoided. It is important to know that all dependent claims are narrower in scope and written exclusively for the purpose of protecting the invention, or any part of it, should the broader claim or claims be knocked out in court proceedings.

Other parts of a patent application such as priority dates, affidavit requirements, assignment, and appointment of attorney or agents are best left to patent practitioners and the company legal department to worry about; however, there may be some interaction with the inventor in filling out certification documents. The filing of an application is followed by numerous communications, office actions, from the patent office, the responses to which are drafted in full consultation with the scientists and their approval for accuracy of information and its interpretation. A word of caution is needed here. In the United States, there is a clause of "estoppel," under which admissions made in the specification or in responses to office action about what is actually taught by the prior art may be binding upon the applicant. A wrong statement about accepting an article as prior art may be reversed later. Court proceedings will have the entire text of correspondence available for examination, and the "file wrapper" becomes part of the patent. The safest rule is to admit nothing and say as little about the prior art as possible. Of course, all relevant prior art known to the applicant or his or her attorney must be brought to the attention of the U.S. Patent and Trademark Office, but this does not mean that it has to be mentioned in the specification.

There must be at least one claim in each patent application. Claims define the scope of subject matter for which protection is sought. A competitor does not infringe and cannot be stopped unless he or she makes, sells, offers for sale, imports, or does something falling within the scope of at least one claim of the granted patent; in other words, if the infringing object "reads onto claim," then it is an infringement. How claims are interpreted keeps the courts filled with opportunities to create case laws. Claims are always read in light of the published specification, and thus, the issue of prior art comes up again; had there been a mistake in allowing a claim in light of prior art, the claim will be thrown out and, in some cases, the entire patent rendered invalid.

All claims fall into one of two broad categories: they claim either a product (a mechanical device, a machine, a composition of matter, etc.) or a process (a method of making, using, or testing something). For chemical patents, this may include the chemical per se as a useful intermediate, as a composition in a pharmaceutical product, as a specific form (optical isomer, crystal form, etc.), or for direct use. The process claims would include process of synthesis, isolation, or purification as the case may be; the methods of use may be the first or a subsequent use such as a method of medical treatment or diagnosis or testing and analysis methods.

4.1 Drawing(s) (§113)

When necessary, most likely in mechanical or electrical and some chemical applications. Filing date not assigned if drawings not provided at the OIPE level of evaluation; examiner may require drawings but filing date not affected; drawings MUST show all of the claimed elements; drawings may be added later by amendment if already described in the specification or claim as originally filed; no need for manufacturing drawings (such as tolerances or in-process controls).

4.3 Specification (§112 ¶1)

The written description, the manner and process of making and using, in such full, clear, concise, and exact terms as to enable any personal skilled (with ordinary skills) in the art to which it pertains, or with which it is most nearly connected, to make and use the invention and setting forth the best mode contemplated by the inventor for carrying out his invention. There are three requirements of disclosure.

4.4 Description

- Must described what is claimed clearly
- Focus is on the claimed invention only
- Scope commensurate with scope of claim(s): disclosure of a single species may or may not support a generic claim
- Critical or essential element MUST be recited in claims
- The vantage point is one of ordinary skill in the art
- The inventor may be his/her own lexicographer; spell out but not befuddle, not use in a contrary manner to what is commonly acceptable
- Theory need not be set forth; if theory is wrong, the error is not fatal (unless theory is claimed invention)
- Manner of invention is not important (how the invention was made)

4.5 Enablement

- To one of ordinary skills to make and use
- Without undue experimentation
- Not necessarily for commercial production
- This requirement different from §101 requirement of being useful
- Claim not reciting essential matter may be rejected for lack of enablement or failing to claim the subject matter applicant regards as the invention
- Publications after filing date may not be used to support enablement but may be used to defeat enablement (such as by examiner)
- Scope of enablement must be commensurate with scope of claims(s)
- Amount of disclosure required depends on the state of the art and predictability—the more is known and the greater is the predictability, the less the disclosure is required

4.6 Best Mode

- What inventor considers best mode not what anyone or everyone else considers and not what is objectively best
- At the time of application is filed; need not and cannot be updated by amendment (as it will be considered new matter) even in a division or continuation but can be updated in CIP if it pertains to a new claim made

- Must be disclosed though not necessarily identified as such; embodiment disclosed is automatically considered as the best mode; several embodiments may be disclosed without identifying which one is the best

4.7 Paragraph 1 35 USC §112 Requirement

Description, enablement and best mode for each claim as filed or else it renders claims invalid if contested. Mythical person is one of ordinary skills in the art not a layperson. Need to disclose what is considered as required knowledge of one of ordinary skill. Any one or more of can satisfy each of these three requirements: specification, drawing(s) and claims as originally filed. Unclaimed inventions need not satisfy this requirement.

4.8 Paragraph 2 35 USC §112 Requirement: Parts of a Claim

- Preamble sets for the invention's technical environment and class (composition, process or apparatus, etc: A method of …, Apparatus for …, A composition …). It is not limiting if it only it merely states the purpose of the invention; however if it breathes life and meaning into the claim (such as if it is essential to tell what is claimed of if the body of claim refers to it as antecedent support) it can become limiting.
- Transitional phrase connects the body of the claim to preamble: comprising, consisting of, consisting essentially of, etc. Three types: open-ended: comprising, including, containing, characterized by, etc; closed: consisting of, also composed of, having, being etc, some of these can be interpreted differently; partially closed: consisting essentially of … wherein it allows only those additional elements that do not affect the basic and novel characteristics of invention. No synergism. The applicant has burden of proof to show that additional elements in prior art would materially change the characteristics of the invention. If ABCD is known and ABC is claimed; absence of D must be demonstrated to affect materially the invention.
- Body is a list of elements such as ingredients of a composition, components of the apparatus; all elements must be interconnected. (There must a reason why a component is recited; not just to list it.)

4.9 Reading a Claim

Claim reading onto prior art is to prove validity of claim., a device or process to indicate infringement or own specification satisfies §112 ¶1 requirements. Claim does not read on prior art with elements ABCD if the claim is ABC and closed (consisting of) but it reads if the transitional phrase is open such as "comprising" and may or may not read if it is "consisting essentially of."

4.10 Punctuation of Claim

One sentence, comma after preamble; colon after transitional; each element gets own paragraph; semicolon at the end of each paragraph; "and" between last two elements. More than one period means more than one sentence and thus an indefinite claim (¶2 §112).

4.11 Definiteness of Claim

- Without proper antecedent basis a claim is rendered indefinite. "A" or "an" introduces an element for the first time except in a means-plus-function format. "Said" or "the" refers back to previously introduced elements or limitations or refer to inherent properties (not required to be recited for antecedent purpose; example, "the surface of said element" when "surface" is not defined earlier).
- Inferential claiming where interconnectivity of elements is not certain—does not tell if the element is part of combination or not.

4.12 Narrowing of Claim

Narrowed by adding an element or limitation to a previously recited element; narrow claim can be dependent or independent. Adding a step narrows method claims. Adding an element to a closed (such as Markush Group) claim broadens not narrows claim.

4.13 Dependent Claims (§112 ¶3 ¶4)

- Claim can be dependent or independent; a dependent claim incorporates by reference all the limitations of the claims to which it refers and is always narrower; must depend from a preceding claim not a following claim (numbering of claims is readjusted during prosecution).
- "Further comprising" or "further including" used to narrow a claim by adding another element or step.
- Claimed narrowed by further defining an element or the relationship between elements. Transitional element "wherein" used to add limitation. Narrowing can be both adding an element and further defining their relationship.
- Defining a step further narrows method claim.

4.14 Multiple Dependent Claims (§112 ¶5)

- A claim referring to more than one previously set forth claim but only in the alternative ("or") and narrows the claim from which it depends.
- Cannot serve as a basis for another multiple dependent claim; may refer to other dependent claim and a dependent claim may depend from a multiple dependent claim.
- Incorporates by reference all the limitations of the particular claim in relationship to which it is being considered (individually and not collectively).
- It takes place of writing several dependent claims—in its spirit.
- A flat special fee is charged at the time of filing application if multiple dependent claim or claims are included.

4.15 Dominant-Subservient Claims

Dominant (Subcombination or genus)-Combination (Subservient-species). Need two members (species) to have genus, which is illustrated by the selection of species; genus is an inherent commonality among embodiments (species).

4.16 Means-Plus-Function Clauses §112 ¶6

Claim defining an element by its function not what it is. Means for performing a function. Interpreted by the literal function recited and corresponding structure or materials described in specification and equivalents thereof. Does not cover all structures for performing the recited function. A claim reciting only a single means plus function clause without any other element is impressible. Must have the phrase, "means for," which then must be modified by functional language but not modified by the recitation of structure sufficient to accomplish the specific function. If specification does not adequately disclose the structure corresponding to the "means" claimed the claims fails to comply with paragraph 2 requirement for "particularly pointing out and distinctly claiming" the invention. If disclosure is implicit (for those skilled in the art), an amendment may be required or stated on record what structure performs the function. Equivalents: examiner must explain rationale; prior art must perform, not excluded by explicit definition in the specification for an equivalent, prior art supported by:

- Identical function, substantially same way, substantially same results
- Art-recognized interchangeability
- Insubstantial differences
- Structural equivalency

4.17 Process Claims

A method for making a product, comprising the steps of ...; a method of using a specified or known material, comprising the steps of ...; recitation of at least one step required and a single step method claim is proper.

4.18 Step-Plus-Function Clauses

- Functional method claims reciting a particular result but not the specified act—i.e., techniques used to achieve results—adjusting pH, raising temperature, reducing friction, etc.
- No recital of acts in support required.
- Typically introduced by words like "whereby," "so that" or "for."
- Addition of a functional description alone is not sufficient to differentiate claim—rejected under §102.
- Functional language without recitation of structure, which performs the function, may render the claim broader (rather than narrower) and rejected under §112 ¶1.

4.19 Ranges

Commonly used for temperature, pressure, time and dimensional limitations. "Up to" means from zero to the top limit; "at least" means not less than (does not set upper limit, which must be fully disclosed in specification); specification must support eventual ranges. A dependent claim cannot broaden the range. Range within range is indefinite in a claim but acceptable in specification.

4.20 Negative Limitations

Permissible if boundaries set forth definitely, such as free of an impurity or a particular element or incapable of performing a certain function. Absence of structures cannot be claimed: holes, channels, etc as structural elements.

4.21 Relative and Exemplary Terminology

Imprecise language may satisfy definiteness requirement (for one of ordinary skill). "So dimensioned" or "so spaced" can be definite if it is as accurate as the subject would permit; "about" is clear and flexible but rendered indefinite if specification or prior art does not provide indication about the dimensions anticipated. "Essentially," "substantially," "effective amount" are definite if one of ordinary skills would understand. Exemplary terminology is always indefinite: such as, or like material, similar—all rejected.

4.22 Markush Group

Closed form. Two forms: wherein P is a material selected from a group consisting of A, B, C, and D; or wherein P is A, B, C or D. Members must belong to a recognized class, possess properties in common as disclosed in specification and these properties mainly responsible for their function or the grouping is clear from their nature or the prior art that all members possess the property.

Adding members broadens claim. Prior art with one of the members anticipates the claim.

4.23 Markush Alternates

"Or" terminology if choices are related: one or several pieces; made entirely or part of; red, blue or white. If unrelated choices, the use of "or" will lead to indefinite interpretation. "Optionally" if definite if there are no ambiguities in the scope of claim as a result of choices offered.

4.24 Jepson-Type Claims—Improvement Claims

Preamble defines what is conventional; transitional phrase, "wherein the improvement comprises"; body builds on preamble; can add element or modify element in preamble. Preamble is limiting.

4.25 Mixed-Class Claims

Mixed elements are improper: methods claims should have no structural elements; apparatus claims should have no step elements. Limitations can be mixed, such as method step may include a structural limitation and an apparatus may include a process limitation.

4.26 Product-by-Process Claims

A product claim that defines the claimed product in terms of the process by which it is made: A product made by the process comprising of steps …. Patentability based on product itself and NOT on method of production. If the product is same (as prior art) using another process does not make it patentable. If examiner shows that product appears to be the same or similar the burden shifts to applicant; United States Patent and Trademark Office bears lesser burden of proof in making out a case of prima facie obviousness. One step method claims acceptable but claims where body consists of single "means" elements are not acceptable.

4.30 Patent Term Adjustment

The United States Congress passed legislation known as the Hatch–Waxman Act in 1984 that weakened patent law for pharmaceuticals, making it easier for generic copies to enter the market based on the innovator's safety and effectiveness data. Under the Act, pharmaceutical research companies lost nearly all of their rights to defend their unexpired patents before generic copies enter the market. Patent holders can sue to defend their unexpired patents *only* when a generic drug manufacturer submits a filing to the Food and Drug Administration seeking to bring the generic copy to market. The Act also created a 30-month stay procedure to allow patent holders the opportunity to obtain a court ruling on whether the generic copy infringes their patent. Thirty-month stays do not extend patents—they are triggered *before* the patent expires and provide a period of time during which patent infringement cases can be resolved.

Patent lawsuits based on the Act are rare because generally challenges to patents on prescription medicines are rare. Food and Drug Administration reports that of 8,259 generic applications filed between 1984 and 2001, only 6 percent raised a patent issue, the necessary condition for patent litigation. According to the Federal Trade Commission, more than one-quarter of patent challenges studied did not result in a lawsuit by the innovator company. Since enactment of the law, generic company share of prescription medicine use has increased from 19% of prescription units in 1984 to 50% today.

The average effective patent life for prescription medicines under the Hatch–Waxman Act is 11–12 years, compared to an average of 18.5 years for other products.

Effective August 18, 2003, The Food and Drug Administration has revising its regulations to:

Permit only one 30 month stay in the approval process for a generic drug pending resolution of patent litigation. Past regulations acquiesced to the delayed launch of generic versions beyond 30 months when there were multiple, consecutive patent challenges that were made against the launch of the generic versions, even if the challenges were frivolous.

Clarify the types of patents that may be listed in the "Orange Book", which is the Food and Drug Administration 's official register of approved pharmaceutical products that provides notice to generic drug makers of name brand patent rights. Patents may no longer be listed that cover drug packaging or other minor matters not related to effectiveness. Patents are to be listed that pertain to active ingredients, drug formulations/compositions and approved uses of a drug. A more detailed, signed attestation will be required to accompany a patent submission. False statements in the attestation can lead to criminal charges.

For patents that are granted after the drug application is filed, the brand name drug maker has 30 days to list the patent(s) from the grant date.

To seek approval for a generic, the generic drug maker must certify to the Food and Drug Administration that either (1) there are no Orange Book listed patents for the name brand drug or (2) the patent(s) has (have) expired or (3) will expire by the time approval is sought or (4) the listed patent(s) is(are) invalid or will not be infringed. If the latter, notice of the certification is given to the patent owner and to the brand name drug maker with an explanation as to why the patent(s) is(are) invalid or not infringed. If the patent owner does not bring a patent infringement suit against the generic drug maker within 45 days, the Food and Drug Administration may approve the generic version. Otherwise, the approval process is stayed for the shorter of 30 months or the date when a court concludes the patent(s) is(are) either invalid or not infringed.

Require generic manufacturers to demonstrate to the Food and Drug Administration that their generic drug is therapeutically equivalent to an approved brand name drug. That is, equivalence in terms of safety, strength, quality, purity, performance, intended use and other characteristics. Review drug applications for generics more quickly. The Food and Drug Administration is hiring 40 generic drugs experts to expedite the approval process and to institute targeted research to expand the range of generic drugs available to consumers.

Improve the review process for generic drugs by instituting internal reforms. The reforms include making early communications with generic drug manufacturers who submit applications and guiding generic manufacturers in preparing and submitting quality, complete applications.

The recent decision in the United States patent infringement case Madey v. Duke is very important to academic researchers as well as the industry. The Duke University had challenged the general assumption that academic research using a patented device or method cannot constitute infringement. The subject matter was a laser device which had originally been developed and patented by Duke University. When the inventor left the University to pursue commercial applications for the laser, Duke University continued to use their model for research purposes. Duke claimed that it was entitled to continue using the laser for non-commercial purposes under the experimental use exception in United States patent law. However, the court held that Duke University's use of the laser "unmistakably" furthered its commercial goals, including facilitating the education of students. The court further held that research using the laser had helped the University to obtain research grants. The equivalent provision in English law is section 60(5)(b) of the Patents Act 1977 which states that an act relating to the subject matter of a patent which is done for "experimental purposes" will not constitute infringement. The provision does not set out whether the exemption is available to those whose experimental purposes have a commercial element. There is no United Kingdom equivalent, however, of the United States exemption which permits the unauthorised use of a patented device or method by a person seeking Food and Drug Administration approval to market a new product. The exemption applies only while the application is pending but extends to the use of patented devices or drugs in clinical trials, their sale for use in trials, demonstrations at trade shows and the reporting of clinical data to potential investors.

The United States Patent Office prescribes specific regulations regarding patent term adjustment:

–   Application filed prior to June 8, 1995: 17 years from the date of issuance regardless of the length of prosecution.
–   Application filed June 8, 1995-May 28, 2000 The Uruguay Round Agreements Act (URAA): 20 years from filing date but with up to 5 years extension for delays resulting from secrecy orders, interferences and/or successful appears.
–   Application pending or patent in force on June 8, 1995: 17 years from issue date or the period between the issue date and the 20th anniversary of the filing date, whichever is greater.
–   Application filed on or after May 29, 2000 American Inventors Protection Act (AIPA) may be entitled to patent term adjustment (PTA) in a continuing application including Continued Prosecuting Application (CPA), Request for Continued Examination (RCE) filed after May 29, 2000 in an application filed before May 29, 2000 does NOT provide PTA eligibility; Patent Cooperative Treaty's eligibility depends on its filing date, not its national stage entry date (Patent Cooperative Treaty must be filed on or after May 29, 2000 to be eligible for PTA).
–   PTA: termination date (20th anniversary from filing date) is extended by number of days Patent and Trademark Office delays minus the number of days applicant delays.

4.31 Patent and Trademark Office Delays: Guaranteed Adjustment Basis (GAB)

GAB1: Patent and Trademark Office failure to take certain actions within 14 months from filing date and 4 month from other events: Patent and Trademark Office must mail an examination notification (first Office action including Quayle action or notice of allowability, restriction requirement and request for information, but NOT OIPE notice of incompleteness of application or other such notices) to applicant within 14 months of filing date; Patent and Trademark Office must also respond within 4 month to applicant's reply to an office action or applicant's opening appeal brief, Patent and Trademark Office must act within 4 months of a BPAI or court decision where allowable claims remain in the application; Patent and Trademark Office must issue the patent within 4 months of date the issue fee is paid and all outstanding requirements are satisfied.

GAB2: Patent and Trademark Office delays due to interference, secrecy order or successful appellate review (where BPAI or court reverses determination of patentability of at least one claim [allowance by examiner after a remand from BPAI is not a final decision]). GAB2 were also the bases of PTA under URAA but for a maximum of 5 years, AIPA removes 5-year limit.

GAB3: Patent and Trademark Office fails to issue a patent within 3 years excluding time consumed in RCE, secrecy order, interference, or appellate review (whether successful or not), time consumed by applicant requested delays (e.g., suspension of action up to six months for "food and sufficient cause," up to three month delay request at time of filing RCE or CPA, up to three year deferral of examination requested by applicant). Filing an RCE for an application filed on or after May 29, 2000 cuts off any additional PTA due to failure to issue patent within 3 years but it does NOT eliminate PTA in GAB 1 and 2.

4.32 Required Reduction Basis (RRB)

Applicant's delay for failure to engage in reasonable effort to conclude prosecution of the application is subtracted from GAB1—3: failure to reply within 3 months to any notice from the office making any rejected, objection, argument or other request (even though applicant pays for and received extension), days in excess of 3 months are deducted; reinstatement of deduction of up to 3 months can be made by applicant showing that "in spite of all due care, the applicant was unable to reply," due perhaps to testing to demonstrate unexpected results, death of applicant's sole practitioner or a natural disaster. (Do not confuse the 3 months concession with 3 months required to respond.) Additional RRBs are generated because of: suspension of action under Rule 1. 103, deferral of issuance under Rule 1. 3114, abandonment or late payment of issue fee, petition to revise more than 2 months after notice of abandonment, conversion of provisional to nonprovisional, preliminary amendment within one month of office action that requires supplemental office action (i.e., a response is sent when an office action was to come within one month)*, inadvertent omission in reply to office action*, supplemental reply not requested by examiner*, submission filed after BPAI or court decision within one month of office action that requires supplemental office action*, submission filed after notice of allowance* and filing a continuing application to continue prosecution. Note that in instances marked with an asterisk (*) IDS submission will not create reduction if information is received from foreign patent office within the last 30 days (i.e., the applicant responds within 30 days of receiving such information).

4.33 Notification

Notification of PTA is first given in the notice of allowance assuming that the applicant WILL pay the fee within 3 months and that the patent will issue within 6.5 months of Notice of Allowance; applicant may request revision or correction of PTA before payment of issue fee by showing that failure to reply within 3 months occurred "in spite of all due care," for reinstatement (a three months maximum is available for this reinstatement), the applicant may also point to Patent and Trademark Office miscalculations; in either case (even if it were Patent and Trademark Office error) a fee is required. Final PTA is listed in the Issue Notification that comes about two weeks prior to issue of patent—this includes any corrections made; applicant may request Patent and Trademark Office reconsideration (with payment of fee) for until 30 days after patent issues; no third party challenge to PTA is permitted in the Patent and Trademark Office. If correction accepted, it is printed in Certificate of Corrected; if applicant dissatisfied, applicant may appeal to United States District Court for the DC within 180 days of patent grant.

Summary: Patent term begins the day of patent issuance; terminal disclaimer date ends patent term; failure to pay a post issuance maintenance fee ends patent term (notice: no such fee required for design and plant patents); term extension beyond statutory period only through private congressional legislation or by showing government agency delays (e.g., Food and Drug Administration); 20-yr term begins from the earliest ancestral application from which priority is claimed (does not include provisional application or a foreign application for term running purpose); design applications excluded from URAA and AIPA as they have fixed 14 year term from issue.

4.34 Food and Drug Administration

A listing of drugs for which the patent term had been extended by the United States Food and Drug Administration is available at http://www.uspto.gov/web/offices/pac/dapp/opla/term/156.html. The longest patent term extension given by the United States Food and Drug Administration to any drug belongs to United States Patent 3,737,433 (Trental) for 2,494 days.

The point in the development program at which a patent application is filed will vary somewhat from company to company, but will normally be at an early stage in the process, when the substance has been made and been shown to be active in early screening. For a patent with a nominal term of 20 years from filing the effective term during which the patentee has exclusive rights to a marketed product is only eight to 12 years. This explains the importance attached by the pharmaceutical industry to provisions to extend the patent term, whether directly, as in USA and Japan, or indirectly by way of the SPC in Europe, in order to compensate for this loss of effective patent term. It also explains the importance to the industry of the minimum 20-year term guaranteed by the TRIPS Agreement. The SPC for medicinal and plant protection products by the United Kingdom Patent office does not extend the entire scope of the patent on which it is based, but is limited to the product covered by the marketing authorization, and for any medicinal use of the product that has been authorized before the expiry of the certificate. Thus sales of the product for non-medicinal uses do not infringe, but the SPC would be infringed by sales of a medicinal product by a third party even if that party had a marketing authorization for a different indication. Apart from this, the SPC confers the same rights as the basic patent, and is subject to the same limitations and obligations to allow existing licenses under the basic patent to continue under the SPC. The scope of protection given by a United States patent during the Hatch–Waxman extension period is essentially the same.

17.9 INVENTIONS OF INTEREST TO PHARMACEUTICAL SCIENTISTS

Chemical compounds per se, a main requirement of TRIPS, is a relatively recent development in many countries even in Germany, Japan, the Netherlands, Switzerland, Scandinavian countries, Austria, Spain, and Greece, with several countries still not awarding patents for chemicals per se, though they may recognize the process being patentable. (Much of this would change on January 1, 2005, WTO deadline when the countries must adopt the TRIPS requirements.) The process patents are notoriously difficult to write and defend. The strength emanates from whether it is a "product-by-process" or a pure process or whether in a given country the onus lies on the infringer to prove innocence (a requirement of TRIPS). A process method can have value if the options available for synthesis are limited such as in the case of diazo coupling to produce azo dyes, but if a compound can be synthesize alternately, the patent becomes very weak indeed; in some instances, the process of patenting opens up the opportunity for others to "design around" a given patent, something that is widely practiced today as the chemical processes have become more sophisticated; the same applies to the production of chemical through biotechnology.

Pharmaceutical compositions remain at the top of the list of inventions patented by pharmaceutical companies. It is important to design these patents such that the claims provide a range of components, beyond which the product will not be effective; however, such tight ranges are not necessary and often not allowed by the patent office or for reasons such as prior art. However, the fact that a product may have to be approved by the Food and Drug Administration makes such patents very valuable, meaning that a generic equivalent cannot be filed until the expiry of patents. Of great importance to pharmaceutical research is the Hatch–Waxman Act of 1984, which allows patent term extension; this is described in detail later.

This use of a new strain of microorganism, whether this is found in nature, selected from organisms produced by artificially induced random mutation, or transformed by recombinant DNA technology, often presents special problem of sufficient disclosure (a requirement), requiring depositing of the strain in a bank, which can result in loss of control, and as a result, many companies decide not to pursue a patent filing. The products of rDNA are getting easier to disclose sufficiently.

Patents have historically been denied for an invention of a method of treatment of the human or animal body by surgery or therapy or of diagnosis practiced on the human or animal body as it is not considered to be capable of industrial application. However, this does not prevent a compound for specific use to have a useful application. Novel compounds that have a pharmaceutical utility are patentable per se in all countries that have implemented TRIPS.

Prodrugs are compounds that break down into active drugs in the body, anywhere along the delivery path. If the discovery of prodrug is made after the active drug, this may be infringing on the patent of the active drug if there are no additional benefits in using the prodrug; for example, hetacillin, an acetone adduct of ampicillin, which quickly hydrolyzes into penicillin, would infringe a patent for ampicillin. As long as it was not known that hetacillin converts to ampicillin, use of hetacillin would not have infringed ampicillin patent.

A patent claiming "a novel cephalosporin, its salts and a pharmaceutically acceptable bioprecursors thereof" is apparently a very broad claim and may lack sufficiency of disclosure because it will require an undue amount of experimental work to determine whether or not a given compound could fall under the vague definition of "bioprecursor." It is nevertheless possible to draft allowable claims to drugs that literally cover prodrugs, for example, one can claim "physiologically hydrolysable and acceptable esters" of alcohols or acids. The situation is different when a compound is patented as a drug and subsequently found to be only a precursor of the real active substance, the active metabolite. This should not affect the patentability of the substance; if a pharmacological result is obtained by administering the substance, it is immaterial by what process the result is obtained; the mechanism need not be determined to be a patentable invention. However, if claims to the first substance do not include the second, they cannot be construed to cover it indirectly. The active metabolite, if novel and inventive, can be patented separately, and then the question arises whether sales of the original drug substance infringe the patent claiming the active metabolite. A classic example is that of terfenadine and fexofenadine, the active metabolite of terfenadine. The U.S. Patent 6,558,931 concerns a method for preparing fexofenadine from terfenadine by a bioconversion process using *Absidia corymbifera* LCP

63-1800 or *Stepromyces platensis* NRRL 2364 strain. However, before this patent, Merrell Dow had patented fexofenadine, as an attempt to obviously extend the life of terfenadine patent. When a generic competitor began to sell terfenadine, Merrel Dow contended infringement (effectively, contributory infringement) under the metabolite patent, meaning that as terfenadine converts to fexofenadine, administering terfenadine is like administering fexofenadine—an audacious attempt. To prevent this misuse of patent system in this case (*Merrell Dow v. Norton* [1996] RPC 76 [HL]), the United Kingdom House of Lords, the U.S. district court, and courts in Germany declared that the patent holds but there is no infringement—perhaps the most bizarre judgment ever rendered. The arguments that lead to this conclusion are interesting and worth examining here. Obviously, there is never an "inherent lack of novelty" in any invention, so that patent could not be rendered invalid. It was suggested that fexofenadine was manufactured prior to Merrell Dow's knowledge about what is happening in the liver of patients taking terfenadine; however, they did not know this so this could not be a novelty-destroying event. However, the disclosure of the terfenadine patent specification though did not mention the active metabolite, it made available to the public the invention of the acid metabolite because it "enabled the public to work the invention by making the active metabolite in their livers," that is, by taking terfenadine. Accordingly, the patent was held invalid to the extent that it covered this way of making the claimed metabolite. For the patent to be valid, it should include a disclaimer to the substance when prepared by ingestion and metabolism of terfenadine. Obviously, Merrell Dow did not have any further interest in the patent after these decisions.

Generally, whatever is available in nature is not patentable; however, if the claimed product is different from what is found in the nature, it can be patented. For example, a purified or extracted form of a natural product can be patented, wherein the "specification" section of patent application would include limits of purity and so on. For example, adrenal gland could not be patented, but pure adrenaline from the gland was patented. A large number of patents have been granted covering newly isolated hormones, cytokines, and other substances occurring in the human body. Whereas all antibiotics are natural products, identification and purification of these molecules allows their patenting. Even when purity limitations are not known, the natural products can be patented, provided they are described in the claim in such a way that it would not include or cover the product as it is found in nature. To test this, one needs to determine if the claim infringes on the natural product; if it does not, then in the patent jargon, "the claim is not anticipated" and thus allowed. Remember that only a claim is read onto a product and not vice versa. Where the chemical structure of a natural product is discovered, this can be patented as a new chemical, but this would exclude the product from nature and thus it does not provide any significant protection.

In the grand scheme of delivering new chemical entities, the pharmaceutical research relies heavily on novel techniques besides the classical method of synthesizing related structures based on known structure–activity relationship and test them pharmacologically. Some of these techniques include the following:

> Rational drug design is based on the dependence of a great many biochemical processes on specific interaction of a receptor molecule with a corresponding ligand. This interaction requires exact three-dimensional configuration of the receptor

and ligand molecules, which must fit closely together. By X-ray diffraction and other physical methods, it is often possible to determine exact three-dimensional structures of even large protein molecules. Sophisticated computer modeling enables scientists to predict which molecules, existing or hypothetical, would mimic the effect of the natural ligand or to block the receptor-ligand interaction, whichever is desired. Whereas the industry has invested large sums of money in this science, the results have not been very promising compared to other most traditional methodologies of drug discovery.

Random screening of large number of chemicals used in other trades or industries or found in nature often turn up with excellent lead compounds. Plant extracts, soil samples, or fermentation broths from microorganisms are good examples. If activity is found, the active compound can be isolated and identified subsequently. This is indeed a long-shot strategy.

Combinatorial chemistry involves simultaneous synthesis of hundreds or even thousands of different compounds by a combination of different starting materials, reaction steps, and reagents to produce a "library" of compounds that are screened using such methods as reactions on a solid surface, for example, a plastic bead, or "tagging" the bead in some way so as to identify the sequence of reactions and reagents to which the original compound on the bead was subjected, and hence the structure of the final compound on the bead. Patenting a library or groups within the library presents some interesting options and problems. Generic claims to a group of compounds may include compounds known in prior art and chances are many of members of group may be inactive. The library may be claimed the way it was synthesized or tagged in testing, and the only way to overcome the utility question is to show that there is a use (or value) for these libraries; recently, an assertion was made that because this database can be sold, there is an inherent value in it and thus "useful" in generating income; case law has yet to validate this concept.

Patentable pharmaceutical compositions and modalities can be as follows:

Combination preparations comprising two or more known pharmaceutically active ingredients: Whereas it is easier to make such claims in chemical compositions (see earlier), pharmaceutical compositions are more difficult to patent in the United States as these may easily be rendered prima facie obvious unless the patentee can demonstrate some synergism or a definite additive effect, not just the sum effect that is anticipated. Unlike the combinations in the chemical industry, the pharmaceutical compositions must further pass the regulatory test; however, this does not obviate the patenting objections of usefulness, and the patent office need not agree with the argument that if the Food and Drug Administration has approved a product, this proves its utility. Synergism between two drugs is difficult to prove in the absence of knowledge about what to predict if they were given separately. This would require long dose–response studies of individual components and in combination to prove synergism, if at all measurable. The costs of these studies in the experimental stage can be prohibitive. However, the inventor may exploit any advantageous and unpredictable results to support the inventive steps. For example, a patent issued to the author is for the reduction of side effects in the use of orlistat (a patent product of Roche); the use of natural fibers results in a dramatic decrease in the rectal leakage of oil—a patent was granted. However, based on the arguments presented earlier, this invention cannot be exercised until the use patent on orlistat (Xenical; Roche) expires. This also demonstrates the basic concept of patenting—to prevent others from practicing—as Roche cannot use this invention but neither can the inventor because of the protection in place.

New drug delivery systems or forms such as a new kind of tablet giving a controlled rate of release of drug when swallowed can be patented. Here the inventive step lies not in the active drug but in other constituents that enable it to be administered in a particular way to achieve such effects as a sustained blood level. Other examples would include using adhesive patches to deliver drugs, bypassing the first-pass phenomenon using buccal delivery, and using nasal sprays for hormones like insulin.

Compositions comprising a compound not previously used as a drug, together with any conventional pharmaceutical carrier or excipient: A routine claim for this type of invention would be, "a pharmaceutical composition comprising a compound of formula X in association with a pharmaceutically acceptable diluent or carrier," which would include all forms in which the compound could be administered, from a complex drug delivery system to a simple tablet or solution. Care must be exercised not to include claims that are not novel, for example, if the compound were reportedly used in a solution form, then its claim in the same form will be inadmissible, regardless of the newly found application of composition.

Compositions involving first-time use of a substance can be easily patented; however, if the compound is disclosed for another use, finding another (new) use does not allow patenting of the substance. The only solution then is to patent the substance in a pharmaceutical composition containing the active ingredient. These claims would not be limited to any specific pharmaceutical indication and would cover all delivery systems. An alternative approach would be to claim the use of the compound as a pharmaceutical or therapeutic agent, provided the claims do not render it a medical treatment, which is not patentable. As an example, one way to claim it is to state "an invention consisting of a substance or composition for use in a method of treatment of the human or animal body by surgery or therapy." Claims in the form "compounds of formula X for use as an active therapeutic substance" are allowable and cover all therapeutic uses of the substances and are not restricted to a specific indication that is disclosed. Know that the patent applies to the substance when packaged as a pharmaceutical preparation and does not apply to the bulk substance.

Second or later uses of a new compound is exemplified by the patenting of sildenafil citrate for the treatment of male erectile dysfunction while it was already patented for use in the treatment of hypertension and also covered under new chemical entity claim. There is no limitation to how many new uses can be invented for an existing moiety, provided it is not "taught" or disclosed in prior art. In some instances, a contrary claim to what is "taught" in the literature forms enough basis for the inventive step. A patent on the use of apomorphine in alleviating male erectile dysfunction (which was in prior art) was allowed when the patentee claimed a sublingual dosage form, which was otherwise listed as a "poor delivery system." Additional patents were secured listing the range of plasma concentration to be obtained from the sublingual tablet composition.

Method treatment claims take the form: "[a] method of treating disease X by administering compound Y"; however, if this were written as "the use of compound Y in treating disease X," this will be a claim for medical treatment, which is not allowed under the assertion that a doctor must be free to treat his or her patient as he or she sees fit, without having to worry about being sued for patent infringement. The British Patents Act provides that a claim to a pharmaceutical substance or composition is not infringed by a pharmacist making up an individual prescription written by a doctor or dentist. In the United States, claims to medical treatment of humans have been allowed for a long time. A typical claim of this type relating to a new use of a pharmaceutical would read "[a] method of treatment of disease Y comprising the administration, to a human in need of such treatment, of an effective dose of compound X." Claims to surgical procedures are also patentable, and this caused controversy when a U.S. surgeon patented a new type of incision for eye operations, demanded royalty payment from hospitals carrying out this technique, and in 1993 sued a clinic in Vermont for patent infringement. Besides the fact that it made AMA furious over the physician's behavior, this led to the introduction of a bill in the House of Representatives, which, after undergoing a lot of political activity, resulted in a new subsection of U.S. patent law, 35 USC 287(c), to exempt from infringement performance of a medical activity by a medical practitioner and a "related health care entity," for example, the hospital where the doctor works. "Medical activity" does not include the use of patented drugs or equipment, patented uses of drugs, nor biotechnological processes, so that in practice only surgical procedures are protected from infringement suits. Other patenting agencies have yet to reciprocate with such specific declaration.

17.10 BIOTECHNOLOGY INVENTIONS

Biotechnology inventions generally fall into one of two classes:

New compositions of matter related to newly discovered isolated genes or proteins or to pharmaceutical inventions based on those genes or proteins: One cannot patent a naturally occurring gene or protein as it exists in the body, but one can patent a gene or protein that has been isolated from the body and is useful in that form as a pharmaceutical drug, as a screening assay, or in other application.

Methods of treating patients with a given disease through the use of a particular gene or protein: Even if someone has a patent on a gene or protein, a second inventor can obtain a patent on a new use of that gene or protein, if the second inventor discovers a new use for the substance.

The world patent authorities give extreme importance to biotechnology-related inventions. The *Manual of Patent Examination Procedures* used by U.S. patent examiners contains an entire chapter on biotechnology-related inventions; a critical review of this document is highly recommended (http://www.uspto.gov/web/offices/pac/mpep/documents/2400 .htm).

Biotechnology means the production of useful products by living microorganisms and includes such examples as the production of ethanol from yeast cells or production of various industrial chemicals such as acetic acid and acetone by fermentation processes. The dairy industry represents the best example of biotechnology implementation. The first "biotechnology" patent was awarded to Louis Pasteur in 1873 claiming "yeast, free from organic germs of disease, as an article of manufacture." The antibiotics and the therapeutic proteins industry is based on the isolation of products from selected strains of microorganisms or mammalian cells, natural or mutated, such as fermentation of cyclosporine and CHO-cell-derived recombinant erythropoietin. The modern biotechnology, as distinct from the classical fermentation technology, began in the 1970s with the two basic techniques: recombinant DNA (rDNA) and hybridoma technology. The rDNA is also referred to as gene splicing or genetic engineering where genetic material from an external source is inserted into a cell in such a way that it causes the production of a desired protein by the cell; in the hybridomea technology, different types of immune cell are fused together to form a hybrid cell line producing monoclonal antibodies. More recently, the techniques of genetic engineering have been applied to higher organisms to produce transgenic animals and plants, and even to humans (gene therapy), for example, to replace missing or defective genes coding for a protein required by the body or to introduce genes into cancer cells that will render them easier to kill. The early completion of the human genome project has allowed the identification of genes that could make useful protein products, the implementation of gene therapy, the elucidation of disease mechanisms, designing of novel diagnosis tests, and better selection of drugs based on sensitivity to different molecules. A large number of new biotechnology-related study tools have been developed, which are also patentable.

The patent law and practice have had serious difficulties in keeping up with the rapid scientific progress in this field, and issues such as inventive step, sufficiency of disclosure, and permissible breadth of claims have proved challenging. As a result, the patent law has undergone significant changes to accommodate the inventions made in biotechnology. One question that arose was to define the "person of ordinary skills," as the science was new; the other was to define what is considered prior art and to resolve the argument that biotechnology products are natural products and not patentable.

Patentability of microorganisms generally involves the use of a new strain of microorganism to produce a new compound or to produce a known compound more efficiently (e.g., in higher yield or purity). The new organism may be found in nature (e.g., by screening of soil samples) or may have been produced in the laboratory by artificially induced random mutation or by more specific techniques such as genetic engineering or gene splicing. If the microorganism produces a novel product, such as a new antibiotic, of which the structure has been determined or which can be characterized by a "fingerprint claim," then the novel product may be claimed as a new chemical compound. If the end product is already known, the patentee may rely on the process protection, but this protection is weak and it would be preferable to patent the new microorganism itself as did the Lilly company for the production of human insulin and General Electric for the cleanup of oil spills.

Whereas the plant and animal varieties are excluded from protection, as are the biological processes for their production, the microbiological process or the product of such a process including the microorganism are not excluded. The TRIPS agreement makes it obligatory for all WTO members to grant patents for microorganisms. If the microorganism intended for patenting exists in nature, it will be necessary to claim it in the form of an isolated strain to avoid possible novelty objections. It must be remembered that the term *microorganism* is interpreted broadly to include not only bacteria and fungi but also viruses and animal and plant cells. The interpretation on patenting of microorganisms went through a total turnaround at the U.S. Patent and Trademark Office after the famous Chakrabarty case was decided by the Supreme Court (though by a narrow 5 to 4 majority), wherein General Electric claimed a bacteria useful in removing oil spills, which in itself was not a useful product, though it did have a useful property.

Patent disclosure requires complete description of invention to enable others to reproduce it. This is a relatively simple subject when it comes to chemicals or pharmaceutical compositions, but it is almost impossible to define a strain of microorganism. This difficulty in adequately describing the invention has resulted in a worldwide requirement that the strain be deposited in a recognized culture collection. The designated centers will maintain the strain in a viable condition and make samples of it available to the public, when required. The deposit can be made at any time while the application is pending. The majority of developed countries have now adopted the solution of requiring deposit of strains, and the Budapest Treaty on International Recognition of the Deposit of Microorganisms for the Purpose of Patent Protection (1977), which came into force in 1980 and as of 2002 has been ratified by 56 countries; the European Patent Office provides a list of international depository authorities where a single deposit made will suffice for all signatory states. A redeposit of strain is required if it becomes nonviable on storage; the minimum storage period is 30 years from the original deposit is required. Whereas the depositories provide a means of fulfilling the most important requirement of patenting, the practice creates a serious problem associated with this type of disclosure. For example, if the patentee does not get the patent and the competitors get hold of the strain 18 months after the application is filed and published, when the strain becomes public, this will be like giving away highly proprietary information. It is important to differentiate this from the disclosure made for chemical or pharmaceutical inventions where adequate disclosure can be made. In the case of the deposited strain, the pubic has access to the "real" product that may have taken millions of dollars to create. This is of greater concern if the strain is mutated (genetically engineered) to produce specific molecules. Whereas the patent offices have modified rules requiring that deposits will be made available only to experts and not the competing parties, it is almost impossible to guarantee that the strain will not disseminate as it is very easy to do. After the fall of the Russian Empire, it was not difficult to locate vendors offering clandestine test tubes containing modified bacteria.

17.10.1 Recombinant DNA Technology—Therapeutic Proteins

The patents describing secretion of therapeutic compounds from biological cells number over 66,000 dating from 1976 in the U.S. Patent Office; one of the earliest molecule for which such a patent exists is urokinase (Nicol, U.S. Patent 3,930,944, January 6, 1976), wherein the addition of specified amounts of pronase to the production medium for urokinase using live cells increases the production of urokinase by 50%–100%. The first patent (dating back to April 27, 1976) that uses recombinant technology is that of Peetermanc (U.S. Patent 3,953,592): live influenza virus vaccines and preparation thereof.

There are two basic types of patentable invention in the field of recombinant DNA technology. The first relates to techniques and methods that are generally applicable to the production of a wide range of gene products; the second relates to specific products, both the proteins and the DNA sequences coding for them. The complexity involved in patenting product of recombinant technology requires some understanding of the history of technology development. The basic invention of gene-splicing techniques was made by Cohen at Stanford University and Boyer at the University of California, and Stanford University filed patent applications to cover their invention, but because publication in a scientific journal had already taken place before filing, patents could be granted only in the United States (see 35 USC §102 bar events, which allow 12 months to file patents after disclosure). The patent (U.S. Patent 4,237,2240) was issued in December 1980 and claimed a method of producing a protein by the expression of a gene inserted into any unicellular host. This covered the great majority of all genetic engineering processes and, before expiring in December 1997, earned hundreds of millions of dollars in royalty payments for the two universities. Though not so broad, other key patents cover the purification process, novel vector systems (e.g., plasmids), or promoter systems to regulate inserted genes into high expression rates of product. Most of the early patents are now nearing expiry, including patents on drugs such as human insulin, erythropoietin, and growth colony-stimulating factor kicking off a race for biogeneric drugs with stakes into billions of dollars. Table 17.1 lists some key drug patent expiry in the recombinant field.

Another field of recombinant DNA technology relates to the production of a specific protein product by a transformed microorganism. The structure (amino acid sequence) may be known, or may have been isolated in pure state but whose structure is not yet elucidated, or a product known only by its activity in some impure mixture. In the last of these cases, the product can be claimed per se as a new compound characterized by its structure (which will generally be known once the gene has been obtained and sequenced). The gene itself, or at least the c-DNA coding for the protein, can also be claimed.

Where the product has previously been obtained in the pure state, a per se claim is no longer possible, but the invention can still be claimed in a variety of ways having the effect of covering the product whenever made by recombinant DNA techniques. In the European Patent Office, for example, the patentee could claim the isolated gene for the product, a vector containing the gene, the host cell transformed with the vector, the process for obtaining any of these, and finally the process for obtaining the end product, which would be infringed by sale of the product obtained by that process. It may be possible to claim the unglycosylated protein per se even when the natural glycosylated form is known.

Table 17.1   Patent Expiration Dates for Several Key Drugs Currently on the Market

Brand Name (Generic Name)	Marketing Company	Indication	2002 Sales ($, Millions)	U.S. Patent Expiry
Robetron combination therapy (Ribavirin and Interferon alfa-2b)	Schering-Plough	Chronic hepatitis C	1,361	2001
Ceredase (aglucerase)	Cenzyme	Gaucher disease	537	2001
Cerezyme (imiglucerase)	Cenzyme	Gaucher disease	537	2001
Humulin (human insulin)	Novo Nordisk	Diabetes	500	2002
Intron A (interferon alfa-2b)	Schering Plough	Leukemia, hepatitis B and C, melanoma, lymphoma	2,700	2002
Avonex (interferon beta-1a)	Biogen	Multiple sclerosis	1,034	2003
Humatrope (somatropin)	Eli Lilly & Co	Growth hormone deficiency	329	2003
Nutropin/Nutropin AQ (somatropin)	Genentech	Growth hormone deficiency	226	2003
Epogen (epoetin alpha)	Amgen	Anemia	2,300	2004
Procrit (epoetin alpha)	Johnson & Johnson	Anemia	4,283	2004
Geref (sermorelin)	Serana Laboratories	Growth hormone deficiency	0.07	2004
Synagis (palivizumab)	Abbott	Respiratory syncytial viral	480	2005
Activase (alteplase)	Genentech	Myocardial infarction, stroke, pulmonary embolism	180	2005
Protropin (somatrem)	Genentech	Growth hormone deficiency	2,100	2005
Neupogen (filgrastim)	Amgen	Neutropenia	1,400	2005
Albutein (human albumin)	Enzon	Shock and hemo-dialysis	4,509	2006

Source: IMS Health, ABN AMRO estimates, and Food and Drug Administration Orange Book (patent expiry as quoted by Carl Peck, Center for Drug Development Science, Georgetown University, at the presentation on Principles of Clinical Pharmacology, NIH, 2003; updated sales figures from http://www.i-s-b.org/business/rec_sales.htm).

In the United Kingdom, it is possible to go further and claim, for example, "human tissue plasminogen activator as produced by recombinant DNA technology."

What constitutes an inventive step has changed rapidly in the field of biotechnology since the days of Cohen and Boyer. Genentech's European patent claiming a recombinant DNA process for the preparation of known tPA was upheld by the Board of Appeal, albeit in restricted scope in the European Patent Office, but turned down in England stating that it was obviously desirable to create a recombinant form of a known protein. The U.S. Patent Office used to take the position that the gene coding for a protein of known amino acid sequence was prima facie obvious and unpatentable, but in 1993 the CAFC (Court of Appeals for Federal Circuit) held otherwise, considering that the redundancy of the genetic code meant that there were over 1,036 distinct DNA sequences coding for the protein in question (insulin-like growth factor) and that the prior art may not suggest any particular one of these sequences. It is therefore now possible to patent a recombinant form of a known protein.

A claim to a recombinant product defined by one specific amino acid sequence is likely to give a scope of protection that is too narrow because for any natural protein, there are some regions in which it is possible to change one or two amino acids without affecting the function of the protein and other regions where any change in the exact amino acid sequence will alter or destroy the activity. Thus, although porcine and bovine insulin differ slightly from human insulin, they have essentially the same activity in humans. To solve this problem, claims are drafted for proteins that have a certain degree of homology with the defined amino acid sequence or that may have a certain number of possible amino acid deletions, additions, or substitutions (some of which have been so broad as to claim practically all possible proteins). However, such a claim must necessarily cover a large number of useless products in view of the fact that a change of one amino acid may cause complete loss of activity and is likely to be invalid for this reason. A better claim combines such possibility of structural variation with a requirement that the product must have a certain defined activity. Wishfully, the courts need to interpret a claim to a specific protein structure as covering also minor variations such as might be expected to occur in nature and which do not alter the properties of the claimed product.

The claims to DNA sequences may be placed in four categories of increasing breadth:

- A "Picture" claim to one specific DNA sequence
- Including other DNA sequences coding for the same protein (genetic code redundancy)
- Including DNA sequences coding for modified proteins having the same function
- Including DNA sequences coding for significantly modified proteins, some of which may not be functional, or including noncoding DNA sequences

The first two comprise the majority of patents issued in the United States. In the United States, it is not only the literal wording of the claim granted by the U.S. Patent and Trademark Office that is important but also the extent to which the courts will broaden the wording by application of the Doctrine of Equivalents. In the litigation between Genentech, Wellcome, and Genetics Institute (GI) over the clot-dissolving drug tissue plasminogen activator (tPA), Genetics Institute had developed a modification of tPA called FEIX, which had 15% fewer amino acids than did natural tPA, as well as several minor changes, and as a result stayed active in the blood 10 times longer than the natural product. Genentech's claims literally covered only the natural sequence and naturally occurring variants, but before the District Court a jury found infringement by equivalence. However, the CAFC reversed on appeal, "on the basis that there was no evidence that FEIX functioned in the same way as natural tPA."

U.S. courts frequently find broad claims to proteins and DNA sequences to be invalid for lack of enabling disclosure. Thus, for example, in the litigation between Amgen and Chugai over erythropoietin (European Patent Office), a claim of category 3, claiming any purified and isolated DNA sequence "encoding a polypeptide having an amino acid sequence sufficiently duplicative of that of erythropoietin to allow possession of (biological properties of European Patent Office)" was held invalid for lack of an adequate disclosure of how to make other DNA species in this broad genus. However, the court made it clear that broad generic claims could be valid if they corresponded to a proper disclosure of the invention. A situation frequently arises where a patent application is written at an early stage of the work, when sufficient data are not available yet based on the prior art and extrapolations, it is possible to guess how the results may turn out. In such cases, risk is taken and broad speculative claims are drafted, which may be allowed by the patent office. In the United States, such claims, once granted, have at least until recently been very difficult to attack, but in the infringement litigation between the University of California and Eli Lilly, the CAFC dealt a serious blow to broad claiming. The university inventors had isolated and sequenced only the gene for rat insulin, and the patent claimed genes for all mammalian insulin, including human. The description was sufficient in that the reader would be able to isolate human insulin gene using the method described in the patent. But it did not meet the "written description" requirement of 35 USC §112 because the inventors did not make the human insulin gene and did not describe its structure. In the European Patent Office, it has been difficult to attack overbroad claims because the violation of Article 84 is not a ground of opposition, and for some time it was difficult to allege insufficiency of disclosure because of the Genentech case, which was interpreted to mean that a single working example establishes sufficiency for the entire scope, no matter how broad. Later cases now agree that the description has to be sufficient over the whole claimed scope. This situation exemplifies the dilemma a researcher and his company may face at the time of filing a patent; if you go too broad, you may be knocked out later; if you claim too narrow, you will soon have a competitor nevertheless.

For inventions in a rapidly moving field, it is often critical to file a patent application as early as possible so that the art appearing in the literature could not be used to invalidate the claims. This was shown in the United Kingdom in the case of *Biogen v. Medeva*, which illustrated the difficulty of upholding the validity of broad biotech claims. The patent claimed a recombinant DNA molecule characterized by a DNA sequence for a polypeptide displaying HBV (hepatitis B virus) antigen specificity and covered the genes for both core and surface antigen, although only one of these had been developed. In the European Patent Office, the patent was opposed, but the Board of Appeal ruled that it was sufficient disclosure as it enabled the user to make both core and surface antigens. The patent was upheld despite publication of methods during the prosecution of the patent that would have made the patent invalid, had it not been filed earlier. Priority date (date when the claim is made) was also an issue in a case relating to a whooping cough vaccine, in which the inventor had discovered that a certain known protein was a protective antigen; however, by the time the European application was filed, it had been realized that the antigen that had been discovered was in fact a different protein, and even though the patentee argued that both proteins could be manufactured by the described method, the application was turned down for lack of adequate disclosure compared to the breadth of claims.

17.10.2 Monoclonal Antibody Technology

Biotechnology products are also derived from the workings of the immune system responsible for producing white blood cells, or lymphocytes. These cells originate as stem cells in the bone marrow and then differentiate and mature either in the bone marrow to B lymphocytes (B cells) or in the thymus gland to T lymphocytes (T cells). The main task of the B cells is to produce antibodies in response to exposure to foreign substance through interaction on the surface receptors of B cells. Upon activation, the activated B cell undergoes rapid division and develops into a clone of identical plasma cells, all of which secrete antibody molecules that have the same specificity to the antigen as did the original B cell. The antibodies thus produced (immunoglobulin [Ig] molecules) are complex proteins having the approximate shape of the letter Y with binding sites in its branches for a particular antigen. The antibodies react with antigen molecules and form a cross-linked insoluble structure, removing the antigen from circulation. Where the antigen is located on the surface of a foreign cell like a bacterium, the antibodies bind to the surface (opsonization) rendering the cell ready for destruction by macrophages or other components of the immune system.

Antibodies isolated from human blood, particularly in the form of immunoglobulin-G (IgG or gamma-globulin), have been used therapeutically for a long time such as to provide immunity against viral infections; the potency will depend on how recent had the donor experience the infection. Antibodies are also a powerful tool in the diagnosis of disease and in the identification of biological organisms. Recently, a test method has been developed to test for contamination with anthrax using an antigen-antibody reaction (http://www.osborn-scientific.com/); the pregnancy test kits routinely exploit this technique. Historically, antibodies were produced commercially from mice immunized with human T cells; however, the antisera would contain a mixture even if pure antigen were used to immunize mice. Individual B cell specific for a particular antigen isolated and cultured would provide a single antibody, but the normal B cells cannot be kept alive in culture. It was discovered that myeloma, malignant tumors of the immune system, all derived from B cells, sometimes produced large quantities of a single monoclonal antibody. Cloning of tumor cells thus represented an opportunity to produce monoclonal antibodies except the fact that in a natural myeloma, the antibody actually produced was a matter of chance. To overcome this problem, in 1975, Milstein and Kohler fused a malignant mouse myeloma cell with a normal B cell from the spleen of a mouse to obtain a hybrid cell line, a hybridoma, which had the properties of both parent cells, producing antibody and growing in culture amounting to immortalization of B cells. Choosing a myeloma that did not produce antibodies of its own, this technique will allow production of the antibody from the normal B cell only. The technique was further refined by Kohler and Milstein using spleen cells from a mouse immunized with sheep erythrocytes (red blood cells), and monoclonal antibodies (MAbs) against sheep erythrocytes were obtained. The importance of this work was only realized years later when MAbs against a desired antigen in a mouse or rat immunized with the antigen were obtained by recovering lymphocytes from the spleen of the animal and fusing them with cells from a suitable myeloma line to create individual hybridoma cells. Clones that produce the desired MAb may then be selected and the hybridoma line cultured to manufacture the MAb in commercial quantities.

Initial inventions could not characterize the sequence of the amino acid in the antibody molecules, and the hybridoma lines were deposited as part of patent application disclosure; later, as more refined methods became available, the sequencing of the antibodies was submitted in lieu of or in addition to cell line deposits. Characterization of amino acid sequencing of antibodies also allowed use of recombinant DNA technologies to produce antibodies. The use of recombinant DNA addressed another problem with the therapeutic use of monoclonal antibodies where mouse proteins upon repeated administration reacted with the patient's immune system, reducing their effectiveness or even causing harmful allergic reaction. Antibodies produced by recombinant (rDNA) methods using chimeric MAbs, in which the variable regions (the arms of the Y) remain murine but the constant regions (the base of the Y) are replaced with the constant regions of a human antibody. Another advancement in the technology came when there was replacement of all but the actual hypervariable regions, which give the specificity, to give a humanized antibody.

More advances in technology allowed use of fragments of antibody genes to be expressed on the surface of a carrier such as a bacteriophage-enabling fragments coding for hypervariable regions of desired specificity for selection and incorporation into genes that can be expressed to give fully human monoclonal antibodies. This made the technology for the production of chimeric and humanized antibodies obsolete by the time the first of these products came on the market. The phage display technique can also be used to find large or small molecules that bind to a particular structure, for example, one corresponding to a receptor or its ligand. Antibodies having certain specificities are also used as catalysts by holding two reagent molecules together in the correct configuration for reaction to proceed.

Whereas the work of Cohen and Boyer (for recombinant DNA technology) was patented only in the United States (as described earlier), the work of Kohler and Milstein could not be patented for mere lack of foresight. Many patents have been granted claiming MAbs directed to particular antigens, or classes of antigens in light of the case of Wistar Institute. Patent was at first denied in the United Kingdom to Wistar, which claimed broadly monoclonal antibodies to any viral antigens. It was allowed in the United States and Japan. Though several patents claim any MAbs to specific antigens (e.g., to alpha-interferon) or to certain groups of cells (e.g., certain groups of human T cells), their validity is questionable. Once the general applicability of the hybridoma technique was recognized, it was argued that there was no longer any invention in producing MAbs to any previously known antigen, in the absence of special difficulties that had to be overcome. If the antigen was unknown at the time, inventive step may not be an issue, but there are serious problems of sufficiency of disclosure given that fusion to produce hybridomas is a random process that is inherently nonreproducible and that finding one MAb with a specific affinity does not necessarily make it any easier to find a second one.

In the case of Ortho before the European Patent Office Board of Appeal, the patent contained broad claims to antibodies reacting with certain human blood cells but not others, but there was only a single example, and it was shown not to fall within these claims. Not only were the broad claims invalid, a claim limited to the deposited hybridoma was also rejected because the written description did not correspond to what was deposited.

Where the new and useful individual MAbs have defined structure and the hybridoma deposited, patents can be obtained but only if they have some advantageous properties.

The dilemma of depositing hybridoma (vis-à-vis a recombinant bacteria) is a moot point with the availability of sequencing of amino acids in antibodies.

17.10.3 Antisense Technology

If a particular gene has a role in disease, and the genetic code of that gene is known, one could use this knowledge to stop that gene specifically. Genes are made of double-helical DNA. When a gene is turned on, the genetic code in that segment of DNA is copied out as a single strand of RNA, called messenger RNA. The messenger RNA is called a *sense* sequence, because it can be translated into a string of amino acids to form a protein. The opposite strand in a DNA double helix (A opposite T, T opposite A, C opposite G, G opposite C) is called the *antisense* strand. The antisense coding sequence of a disease gene can be used to make short antisense DNAs to work as a drug that works by binding to messenger RNAs from disease genes, so that the genetic code in the RNA cannot be read, stopping the production of the disease-causing protein.

Generally, a fragment of 20 baselength will be specific for one particular gene and therefore will not interfere with the expression of other genes. Several difficulties arise in developing antisense drugs that range from the instability of single-stranded DNA in vivo to finding suitable delivery systems. The stability problem may be overcome by chemical modification of the backbone of the DNA chain, for example, replacing the phosphate groups by groups that are hydrolyzed less easily, and these modifications can be patented. The first antisense drugs was approved in 1998: the first antisense therapeutic for treating CMV retinitis, Vitravene. In 2003, there were over 1,500 patents making claim for products related to antisense technology. The impact of biotechnology on antisense technology is expected to increase dramatically as the links between genetics, protein production, and disease are better understood. The application of antisense technology is not limited to human and veterinary medicine. It is also used to make biotechnology food products. For example, in agriculture, this technology was used to develop the Flavr Savr tomato.

17.10.4 Cell Therapy

A nontherapeutic use of monoclonal antibodies is in characterizing cells, particularly cells that are present in the blood, lymphatic system, and bone marrow for the cell-specific molecules carried on their surfaces. This is done by tagging monoclonal antibodies tagged with fluorescent molecules and differentiating and separating cells by the FACS (fluorescence activated cell sorting) technique. In this way, the development of the various types of blood cell (the hematopoietic system) can be traced back to a single type, the hematopoietic stem cell (HSC), which can give rise to all other types. Also, mesenchymal stem cells (MSCs) differentiating into all types of connective tissue such as cartilage, bone, and tendon can be isolated from bone marrow. These cells are patentable where claims are not made to cover the cells in their natural state in the human body. Such stem cells can have direct therapeutic uses, for example, HSCs may be administered to cancer patients whose hematopoietic system has been damaged by chemotherapy or radiotherapy, and MSCs may be useful, for example, to regenerate cartilage damaged by injury or arthritis. Most likely these treatments would require harvesting cells from the patient, isolating them, expanding the culture, and infusing back into patients. These cells may also be used in gene therapy (see next).

17.10.5 Gene Therapy

Genes, which are carried on chromosomes, are the basic physical and functional units of heredity. Genes are specific sequences of bases that encode instructions on how to make proteins. Although genes get a lot of attention, it is the proteins that perform most life functions and even make up the majority of cellular structures. When genes are altered so that the encoded proteins are unable to carry out their normal functions, genetic disorders can result, such as hemophilia and cystic fibrosis.

Gene therapy is a technique for correcting defective genes responsible for disease development. Researchers may use one of several approaches for correcting faulty genes:

- A normal gene may be inserted into a nonspecific location within the genome to replace a nonfunctional gene. This approach is most common.
- An abnormal gene could be swapped for a normal gene through homologous recombination.
- An abnormal gene could be repaired through selective reverse mutation, which returns the gene to its normal function.
- The regulation (the degree to which a gene is turned on or off) of a particular gene could be altered.

In most gene therapy studies, a "normal" gene is inserted into the genome to replace an "abnormal," disease-causing gene. A carrier molecule called a vector must be used to deliver the therapeutic gene to the patient's target cells. Currently, the most common vector is a virus that has been genetically altered to carry normal human DNA. Viruses have evolved a way of encapsulating and delivering their genes to human cells in a pathogenic manner. Scientists have tried to take advantage of this capability and manipulate the virus genome to remove disease-causing genes and insert therapeutic genes. Target cells such as the patient's liver or lung cells are infected with the viral vector. The vector then unloads its genetic material containing the therapeutic human gene into the target cell. The generation of a functional protein product from the therapeutic gene restores the target cell to a normal state.

Besides virus-mediated gene-delivery systems, there are several nonviral options for gene delivery. The simplest method is the direct introduction of therapeutic DNA into target cells. This approach is limited in its application because it can be used only with certain tissues and requires large amounts of DNA.

Another nonviral approach involves the creation of an artificial lipid sphere with an aqueous core. This liposome, which carries the therapeutic DNA, is capable of passing the DNA through the target cell's membrane.

Therapeutic DNA also can get inside target cells by chemically linking the DNA to a molecule that will bind to special cell receptors. Once bound to these receptors, the therapeutic DNA constructs are engulfed by the cell membrane and passed into the interior of the target cell. This delivery system tends to be less effective than other options.

Researchers also are experimenting with introducing a 47th (artificial human) chromosome into target cells. This chromosome would exist autonomously alongside the standard

46—not affecting their workings or causing any mutations. It would be a large vector capable of carrying substantial amounts of genetic code, and scientists anticipate that, because of its construction and autonomy, the body's immune systems would not attack it. A problem with this potential method is the difficulty in delivering such a large molecule to the nucleus of a target cell.

The Food and Drug Administration has not yet approved any human gene therapy product for sale. Current gene therapy is experimental and has not proven very successful in clinical trials. In January 2003, the Food and Drug Administration placed a temporary halt on all gene therapy trials using retroviral vectors in blood stem cells. Whereas the progress has been slow, it is anticipated that with greater advances in the technology there will eventually be a treatment found for diseases such as cystic fibrosis, just to name one. There will definitely be many opportunities of patenting not just the products but also the methods to study gene therapy.

17.10.6 Life Patenting

Techniques such as microinjection can be used to introduce extraneous genetic material into a fertilized mammalian ovum, or insert the ovum into a pseudopregnant female, and obtain offspring in which the genetic material has become incorporated into the genome. By combining this process with classical breeding steps such as back-crossing, it is possible to obtain a strain of animal that stably transmits the new gene to subsequent generations, which will display the corresponding phenotype according to the laws of Mendelian genetics. Two possible uses can be made for such transgenic animals: as models for research and as a source for useful materials such as large quantities of therapeutic proteins where gene expression takes place randomly throughout the body, and the proteins may be secreted in milk, for example. This technique can be useful in producing human serum albumin and alpha-trypsin in larger animal species. Another use of transgenic animals is in supplying organs for transplantation. For example, if a pig is transformed with a human gene so that the cells in its organs express a human surface protein, it is expected that the hyperacute rejection upon transplant of pig organs into humans would be blocked or reduced.

The Oncomouse was developed in the 1980s at Harvard Medical School, through DuPont funding. It was patented by Harvard and licensed exclusively to DuPont. *Onco* is derived from oncogene, a name geneticists give to a damaged or mutated gene, which can cause cancer if these genes are responsible for the regulation of cell growth. When oncogene meets mouse, the result is Oncomouse, and when two such mice breed, the cancer-causing genes are passed to the offspring, which are thus predisposed to developing cancer at an accelerated rate. Scientists study the interplay between oncogenes in the mice as a model for studying cancer in humans.

Currently, the Oncomouse is patented in the United States, Europe, and Japan but denied in Canada where the litigation went all the way to the Supreme Court.

17.10.7 Transgenic Plants

Unlike animal cells, plant cells have external cell wall that is difficult to penetrate when introducing genetic material. It is also difficult for the vector to move around in the cell because of the cellular environment. Novel techniques such as placing DNA molecules on the surface of micronized glass beads physically shot into cells are thus used. Once transformed, the plants can be bred in the normal process. The purpose of transgenic plants is to produce higher yields, improve nutritional quality, and lower cost of production. For example, one early product was a transgenic Flavr Savr tomato (Calgene, Davis, CA) that did not do well in the market. Insect and virus-resistant crops are one of the targets of plant transgenic research. Maize contains a gene from *Bacillus thuringiensis*, which produces a toxin harmful to insects but not to mammals; as a result, the larva of the corn borer is killed by eating the plant and insecticide treatment may be avoided.

17.11 PATENTING STRATEGIES

Pharmaceutical and biotechnology scientists face several major challenges in designing their research:

- Does the research create a product that is prohibited by statute to be patented: a thought process, a law of physics, an object of little utility, or another prohibited area of patentability? Obviously, the end goal is not always to secure a patent for a product; a proprietary process need not be patented if it is possible to keep it protected, something which is becoming very difficult to assure as the information flow becomes easier between individuals and around the world.

    Is the research likely to lead to a novel product or process meaning something that has never existed before? Novel is not necessarily patentable as we go through the legality of patenting process; this is, however, one of the fundamental requirement.

- Is the novel research unobvious to those with ordinary skill in the art; this aspect of patenting is most confusing and often leads to most rejections of patent applications. Researchers need to study existing art (what is called prior art) before designing experiments to assure that they can create sufficient features in the invention to take it out of the obviousness arena. What is needed here is a demonstration that there was an inventive step, or in ordinary words, something was actually discovered, and that it was not something that could have been easily discovered. A lot of experimentation goes into demonstrating unusual results to obviate the assertion of obviousness by the patent examiners.

- Can the claim made withstand court challenge? Even though these areas of interpretations are beyond what a scientist would be expected to have any expertise, a keen understanding of the scope of claims is essential; a patent with too broad a claim is not necessarily a good patent just as much as a patent with too narrow a claim. The patent disclosure must support the claim adequately.

    Does the disclosure in the patent meet the legal requirements of patent allowance. In the United States, the patentee must disclose the best mode, the best formula, and the best approach to use the research outcome. There is no need to disclose an industrial model but a workable model. Keeping the information out of a patent can a double-edge sword.

- Is it possible to create a sequel to a successful research product? It is not unusual for the companies to keep some portions of the research aside and out of a patent to be able to claim it later. This can be a dangerous practice. If prior art appears in the interim, then all research is lost, and even one's own patent can be taken as a prior art.

- Is it possible to continue the patent coverage by designing products around an issued patent. This is most critical to the pharmaceutical and biotechnology industry. Good examples of this practice include changes in the formulation to improve the product such as Abbott did when its patent on calcitriol came to expiry; the company changed the specification on the level of oxygen in the solution. What it meant was that there would be no generic equivalent to Abbott's calcitriol, though the generic forms may not be any less active. Smith Kline Beecham's remarkable patenting of amoxicillin and clavulanic combination is a good example of intelligent patenting; you will find patents not only for specific combination of the two antibiotics but for a score of different dosage forms; one patent is based only on the hardness of the tablet. This type of research requires a keen understanding of the patenting process.

- Is it possible to invent around a patent or a publication? Once sildenafil citrate became a success or once statins became the choice treatment for lowering cholesterol, the drug companies rushed to make similar products; obviously, there were problems in prior art. What is already disclosed cannot be obviated. The researchers are then faced with a challenge to find solutions novel enough to be patented; some degree of reverse engineering is required. However, as we see the results, they did succeed. With each patent issuing, the field gets narrower, as to what can be patented. Scientists often get bogged down with the science and do not realize that to receive a patent on an invention there is no need to explain how it works. In fact, there need not even be an explanation how it came into existence or how it worked. Just the fact that there is a working example is sufficient. In many instances, even a working example is not required. A new drug may be subject to the Food and Drug Administration comments before the U.S. Patent Office allows the claims; however, it is not required of the patent office. On the other hand, the Patent Office need not accept the approval by the regulatory authorities as a proof of the utility, a key requirement for patentability.

Obviously, a good research in an industrial environment is a research that yields good profits, and to achieve marketability and profitability from the research, the product must be either patentable or of a type that could not be reverse-engineered if proprietary techniques are relied on. The challenges to scientists are great with expanding technology and stiffer competition to produce new products. One way to take these challenges head-on is to understand the art of patenting as well as the science. Keeping abreast with the knowledge is critical, and the scientists are strongly urged to hone their skills in the use of computers to search the literature.

Questions

1. What benefit does filing a provisional application afford the inventors?
   Answer: Protection for the idea for 1 year while further preparations are made to file the patent.

2. Does having a U.S. patent protect the right to make the product all over the world?
3. What three requirements under the European patent law and generally patent law in other countries are needed to make something patentable?
4. What two trade organizations are heavily considered in patent law in terms of establishing patentability in the United States and other countries?
Answer: World Trade Organization and North American Free Trade Agreement.
5. While a person of ordinary skill in the art might have been considered a worker who does not have an established inventive spirit in the times when patents were primarily for machines, in the biotechnology sector what might be the "person or ordinary skill in the art"?
6. When determining the information available to someone with skill in the art, does a patent examiner consider the information available at present or at the time of invention?
7. The Internet makes finding patent information and doing prior literature searches much quicker if reliable sources are used. Visit and describe some of the sources that are listed in this chapter.
8. Before the claims section of the patent specification, the utility statement is given. What is not recommended to include here even though it may seem natural to speculate on?
Answer: The hypothesis for the mechanism of action.
9. Why do some think the patent term for pharmaceuticals should be extended?
Answer: Much of the 20-year term of the patent is spent preparing the product for market, so the window to earn revenue for the company is small.
10. How can a substance that occurs in nature be the subject of a patent? Consider the example of adrenaline.

BIBLIOGRAPHY

CHAPTER 1

Achuthsankar, S.N. January 2007. *Computational Biology & Bioinformatics: A Gentle Overview.* Communications of Computer Society of India.

Adomas, A., Heller, G., Olson, A. et al. 2008. Comparative analysis of transcript abundance in *Pinus sylvestris* after challenge with a saprotrophic, pathogenic or mutualistic fungus. *Tree Physiol.* 28(6): 885–897.

Allhoff, F., Lin, P., and Moore, D. 2010. *What Is Nanotechnology and Why Does It Matter? From Science to Ethics.* Hoboken, NJ: John Wiley & Sons, pp. 3–5.

Alsberg, B.K., and Sonnleitner, B. 2000. Bioanalysis and biosensors for bioprocess monitoring. *Adv. Biochem. Eng./Biotechnol.* 66: 1–231.

Aluru, S., ed. 2006. *Handbook of Computational Molecular Biology.* West Sussex, UK: Chapman & Hall/ CRC Press. (Chapman & Hall/CRC Computer and Information Science Series).

Anisfeld, M.H. 2002. *International Biotechnology, Bulk Chemical, and Pharmaceutical GMPS* (5th Ed.). Englewood, CO: Interpharm Press.

Atkinson, B., and Mavituna, F. 1991. *Biochemical Engineering and Biotechnology Handbook* (2nd Ed.). London: Macmillan

Attwood, T.K., Gisel, A., Eriksson, N.-E., and Bongcam-Rudloff, E. 2011. Concepts, historical milestones and the central place of bioinformatics in modern biology: A European perspective. In: *Bioinformatics—Trends and Methodologies.* InTech. Retrieved January 8, 2012. http://www.intechopen.com/books/bioinformatics-trends-and-methodologies/concepts-historical-milestones-and-the-central-place-of-bioinformatics-in-modern-biology-a-european-.

Augenlicht, L.H., and Kobrin, D. 1982. Cloning and screening of sequences expressed in a mouse colon tumor. *Cancer Res.* 42(3): 1088–1093.

Augenlicht, L.H., Taylor, J., Anderson, L., and Lipkin, M. 1991. Patterns of gene expression that characterize the colonic mucosa in patients at genetic risk for colonic cancer. *Proc. Natl. Acad. Sci. USA* 88(8): 3286–3289.

Augenlicht, L.H., Wahrman, M.Z., Halsey, H. et al. 1987. Expression of cloned sequences in biopsies of human colonic tissue and in colonic carcinoma cells induced to differentiate in vitro. *Cancer Res.* 47(22): 6017–6021.

Austin, M. 2008. *Business Development for the Biotechnology and Pharmaceutical Industry.* Hampshire, England: Gower

Balbas, P., and Lorence, A. 2004. *Recombinant Gene Expression: Reviews and Protocols* (2nd Ed.) Vol. 267. Methods in Molecular Biology. Totowa, NJ: Humana Press.

Baldi, P., and Brunak, S. 2001. *Bioinformatics: The Machine Learning Approach* (2nd Ed.). Cambridge, MA: MIT Press.

Bammler, T., Beyer, R.P., Bhattacharya, S. et al. 2005. Standardizing global gene expression analysis between laboratories and across platforms. *Nat. Methods* 2(5): 351–356.

Barnes, M.R., and Gray, I.C., eds. 2003. *Bioinformatics for Geneticists* (1st Ed.). West Sussex, UK: Wiley.

Baxevanis, A.D., and Ouellette, B.F.F., eds. 2005. *Bioinformatics: A Practical Guide to the Analysis of Genes and Proteins* (3rd Ed.). Hoboken, NJ: Wiley.

Baxevanis, A.D., Petsko, G.A., Stein, L.D., and Stormo, G.D., eds. 2007. *Current Protocols in Bioinformatics.* Hoboken, NJ: Wiley.

Becker, J.M., Caldwell, G.A., and Zachgo, E.A. 1996. *Biotechnology: A Laboratory Course* (2nd Ed.) New York: Academic Press.

Becker, T., Breithaupt, D., Doelle, H.W. et al. 2007. Biotechnology. In: Barbara, E. (ed.). *Ullmann's Encyclopedia of Industrial Chemistry*. Weinheim, Germany: Wiley-VCH.

Ben-Gal, I., Shani, A., Gohr, A. et al. 2005. Identification of transcription factor binding sites with variable-order Bayesian networks. *Bioinformatics* 21(11): 2657–2666.

Benson, D.A., Karsch-Mizrachi, I., Lipman, D.J., Ostell, J., and Wheeler, D.L. January 2008. GenBank. *Nucleic Acids Res.* 36(Database issue): D25–D30.

Berger, R.G. 2007. *Flavours and Fragrances: Chemistry, Bioprocessing and Sustainability*. Berlin, Germany: Springer.

Bhatt, S.M. *Enzymology and Enzyme Technology*. Amity University. Uttar Pradesh, India.

Biwer, A.P., Cooney, C.L., and Heinzle, E. 2006. *Development of Sustainable Bioprocesses: Modeling and Assessment*. Chichester, England: John Wiley & Sons.

Brauer, D. 1995. *Legal, Economic and Ethical Dimensions* (2nd Ed.). Vol. 12. Biotechnology. New York: VCH.

Brown, R.H., ed. 1988. *CRC Handbook of Engineering in Agriculture* (3 vols.). Boca Raton, FL: CRC Press

Burgess, J.G., Osinga, R., Tramper, J., and Wijffels, R.H. 1999. *Marine Bioprocess Engineering*. Vol. 35. Progress in Industrial Microbiology. Amsterdam, the Netherlands: Elsevier.

Butler, M. 2007. *Cell Culture and Upstream Processing*. New York: Taylor & Francis.

Carvajal-Rodríguez, A. 2012. Simulation of genes and genomes forward in time. *Curr. Genomics* 11(1): 58–61.

Chapanis, A. 1996. *Human Factors in Systems Engineering*. Hoboken, NJ: Wiley.

Chen, H.H., and Chen, W.H. 2007. *Orchid Biotechnology*. Singapore: World Scientific.

Churchill, G.A. 2002. Fundamentals of experimental design for cDNA microarrays. *Nat. Genet.* 32(Suppl.): 490–495.

Claverie, J.M., and Notredame, C. 2003. *Bioinformatics for Dummies*. NY: Wiley.

Corbitt, R.A., ed. 1990. *Standard Handbook of Environmental Engineering*. New York.

Cristianini, N., and Hahn, M. 2006. *Introduction to Computational Genomics*. Cambridge, UK: Cambridge University Press.

Cunningham, C., and Porter, A.J.R. 1998. *Recombinant Proteins from Plants: Production and Isolation of Clinically Useful Compounds*. Vol. 3. Methods in Biotechnology. Totowa, NJ: Humana Press.

Currell, B.R., and van Dam-Mieras, M.C.E. 1997. *Biotechnological Innovations in Chemical Synthesis*. Amsterdam, the Netherlands: Elsevier.

Cutler, P. 2003. *Purification Protocols* (2nd Ed.): Vol. 244. Methods in Molecular Biology. Totowa, NJ: Humana Press.

Datta, A.K., Mujumdar, A.S., Rahman, M.S., and Sablani, S.S. 2007. *Handbook of Food and Bioprocess Modeling Techniques*. Vol. 166. Food Science and Technology. Boca Raton, FL: CRC Press.

Daubert, C.R., and Steffe, J.F. 2006. *Bioprocessing Pipelines: Rheology and Analysis*. East Lansing, MI: Freeman Press.

Doran, P.M. 1995. *Bioprocess Engineering Principles*. San Diego, CA: Academic Press.

Doran, P.M. 1997. *Bioprocess Engineering Principles: Solutions Manual*. San Diego, CA: Academic Press.

Drew, S.W., and Flickinger, M.C. 1999. *Encyclopedia of Bioprocess Technology: Fermentation, Biocatalysis and Bioseparation* (Vols. 1–5). New York: John Wiley & Sons.

Durbin, R., Eddy, S., Krogh, A., and Mitchison, G. 1998. *Biological Sequence Analysis*. Cambridge, UK: Cambridge University Press.

Dutta, R. 2008. *Fundamentals of Biochemical Engineering*. New Delhi, India: Ane Books India.

Dutta, N.N., Hammar, F., Haralampidis, D. et al. 2001. *History and Trends in Bioprocessing and Biotransformation*. Vol. 75. Advances in Biochemical Engineering/Biotechnology. Berlin, Germany: Springer.

Elnashar, M. 2011. *Biotechnology of Biopolymers*. Rijeka, Croatia: InTech.

Emmert-Streib, F., and Dehmer, M. 2008. *Analysis of Microarray Data A Network-Based Approach*. Weinheim, Germany: Wiley-VCH.

Etzel, M.R., Gadam, S., and Shukla, A.A. 2007. *Process Scale Bioseparations for the Biopharmaceutical Industry*. New York: CRC Press.

Faye, L., and Gomord, V. 2009. *Recombinant Proteins from Plants: Methods and Protocols*. Vol. 483. Methods in Molecular Biology. New York: Humana Press.

Fleischmann, R.D., Adams, M.D., White, O. et al. July 1995. Whole-genome random sequencing and assembly of Haemophilus influenzae Rd. *Science* 269(5223): 496–512.

Gad, S.C. 2007. *Handbook of Pharmaceutical Biotechnology*. Hoboken, NJ: John Wiley & Sons.

Galaev, I., and Mattiasson, B. 2002. *Smart Polymers for Bioseparation and Bioprocessing*. New York Taylor & Francis.

Gellissen, G. 2005. *Production of Recombinant Proteins: Novel Microbial and Eukaryotic Expression Systems*. Weinheim, Germany: Wiley-VCH.

Gilbert, D. 2004. Bioinformatics software resources. *Brief. Bioinform.* 5(3): 300–304.

Goldmann, T., and Gonzalez, J.S. 2000. DNA-printing: Utilization of a standard inkjet printer for the transfer of nucleic acids to solid supports. *J. Biochem. Biophys. Methods* 42(3): 105–110.

Griensven, M.V., Kasper, C., and Portner, R. 2009. Bioreactor systems for tissue engineering. *Adv. Biochem. Eng./Biotechnol.* 112: 1–271.

Groves, M.J. 2006. *Pharmaceutical Biotechnology* (2nd Ed.). Boca Raton, FL: CRC Press.

Guilford-Blake, R., and Strickland, D. 2008. *Guide to Biotechnology*. Washington, DC: Biotechnology Industry Organization.

Hacia, J.G., Fan, J.B., Ryder, O. et al. 1999. Determination of ancestral alleles for human single-nucleotide polymorphisms using high-density oligonucleotide arrays. *Nat. Genet.* 22(2): 164–167.

Hesper, B., and Hogeweg, P. 1970. Bioinformatica: een werkconcept. *Kameleon* 1(6): 28–29.

Hofman, M., and Thonart, P. 2002. *Engineering and Manufacturing for Biotechnology*. Vol. 4. Focus on Technology. Dordrecht, the Netherlands: Kluwer.

Hogeweg, P. 1978. Simulating the growth of cellular forms. *Simulation* 31(3): 90–96. doi:10.1177/003754977803100305.

Hogeweg, P. and Searls, D.B., ed. 2011. The roots of bioinformatics in theoretical biology. *PLoS Comput. Biol.* 7(3).

Holst, O., and Mattiasson, B. 1991. *Extractive Bioconversions. Vol. 11*. Bioprocess Technology. New York: Marcel Dekker.

Hondermarck, H. 2004. *Proteomics: Biomedical and Pharmaceutical Applications*. Dordrecht, the Netherlands: Kluwer.

Jain, N., Thatte, J., Braciale, T., Ley, K., O'Connell, M., and Lee, J.K. 2003. Local-pooled-error test for identifying differentially expressed genes with a small number of replicated microarrays. *Bioinformatics* 19(15): 1945–1951.

Kar, A., and Sambamurthy, K. 2006. *Pharmaceutical Biotechnology*. New Delhi, India: New Age International.

Kayser, O., and Muller, R.H. 2004. *Pharmaceutical Biotechnology: Drug Discovery and Clinical Applications*. Weinheim, Germany: Wiley-VCH.

Keedwell, E. 2005. *Intelligent Bioinformatics: The Application of Artificial Intelligence Techniques to Bioinformatics Problems*. New York: Wiley.

Kelly, D.R. 1998. *Biotransformations* I (2nd Ed.). Vol. 8a. Biotechnology. Weinheim, Germany: Wiley-VCH.

Kelly, D.R. 2000. *Biotransformations* II (2nd Ed.). Vol. 8b. Biotechnology. Weinheim, Germany: Wiley-VCH.

Kiil, S., Vigild, M.E., and Wesselingh, J.A. 2007. *Design and Development of Biological, Chemical, Food and Pharmaceutical Products*. Chichester, England: John Wiley & Sons.

Klefenz, H. 2002. *Industrial Pharmaceutical Biotechnology*. Weinheim, Germany: Wiley-VCH.

Klein, J. 2000. *Environmental Processes II: Soil Decontamination* (2nd Ed.). Vol. 11b. Biotechnology. Weinheim, Germany: Wiley-VCH.

Klein, J., and Winter, J. 2000. *Environmental Processes III: Solid Waste and Waste Gas Treatment, Preparation of Drinking Water* (2nd Ed.). Vol. 11c. Biotechnology. Weinheim, Germany: Wiley-VCH.

Kleinkauf, H., and von Döhren, H. 1997. *Products of Secondary Metabolism* (2nd Ed.). Vol. 7. Biotechnology. Weinheim, Germany: Wiley-VCH.

Kline, J., ed. 1988. *Handbook of Biomedical Engineering*. San Diego, CA: Academic Press.

Kohane, I.S., Kho, A.T., and Butte, A.J. 2002. *Microarrays for an Integrative Genomics*. Cambridge, MA: MIT Press.

Kragl, U. 2005. Technology transfers in biotechnology. *Adv. Biochem. Eng./Biotechnol.* 92: 1–335.

Kristiansen, B., and Ratledge, C. 2001. *Basic Biotechnology* (2nd Ed.). Cambridge: Cambridge University Press.

Kulesh, D.A., Clive, D.R., Zarlenga, D.S., and Greene, J.J. 1987. Identification of interferon-modulated proliferation-related cDNA sequences. *Proc. Natl. Acad. Sci. USA* 84(23): 8453–8457.

Lad, R. 2006. *Biotechnology in Personal Care*. New York: Taylor & Francis.

Lahann, J. 2009. *Click Chemistry for Biotechnology and Materials Science*. Chichester, England: John Wiley & Sons.

Lashkari, D.A., DeRisi, J.L., McCusker, J.H. et al. 1997. Yeast microarrays for genome wide parallel genetic and gene expression analysis. *Proc. Natl. Acad. Sci. USA* 94(24): 13057–13062.

Lausted, C., Dahl, T., Warren, C. et al. 2004. POSaM: A fast, flexible, open-source, inkjet oligonucleotide synthesizer and microarrayer. *Genome Biol.* 5(8): R58.

Lawrence, E. 2005. *Henderson's Dictionary of Biology* (13th Ed.). Harlow, England: Pearson.

Leung, Y.F., and Cavalieri, D. 2003. Fundamentals of cDNA microarray data analysis. *Trends Genet.* 19(11) : 649–659.

Liese, A., Lin, G., and Tao, J. 2009. *Biocatalysis for the Pharmaceutical Industry: Discovery, Development and Manufacturing*. Singapore: John Wiley & Sons.

Little, M.A., and Jones, N.S. 2011. Generalized methods and solvers for piecewise constant signals: Part I. *Proc. Roy. Soc. A.* 1–26.

Lund, O., Nielsen, M., Lundegaard, C., Kesmir, C., and Brunak, S. 2005. *Immunological Bioinformatics*. Cambridge, MA: MIT Press.

Maggon, K. 2010. *Top Ten Monoclonal Antibodies*. Available: http://knol.google.com/k/krishan-maggon/top-ten-monoclonal-antibodies.

Maskos, U., and Southern, E.M. 1992. Oligonucleotide hybridizations on glass supports: A novel linker for oligonucleotide synthesis and hybridization properties of oligonucleotides synthesized in situ. *Nucleic Acids Res.* 20(7): 1679–1684.

McNally, E.J. 2000. *Protein Formulation and Delivery*. Vol. 99. Drugs and the Pharmaceutical Sciences. New York: Marcel Dekker.

Moran, G., Stokes, C., Thewes, S., Hube, B., Coleman, D.C., and Sullivan, D. 2004. Comparative genomics using *Candida albicans* DNA microarrays reveals absence and divergence of virulence-associated genes in *Candida dubliniensis*. *Microbiology* 150(Pt 10): 3363–3382.

Morris, J. 2006. *The Ethics of Biotechnology. Biotechnology in the 21st Century*. New York: Chelsea House.

Morris, P.C., and Bryce, J.H. 2000. *Cereal Biotechnology*. Cambridge, England: Woodhead Publishing.

Mosier, N.S., and Ladisch, M.R. 2009. *Modern Biotechnology: Connecting Innovations in Microbiology and Biochemistry to Engineering Fundamentals*. Hoboken, NJ: John Wiley & Sons.

Mount, D.W. May 2002. *Bioinformatics: Sequence and Genome Analysis*. Cold Spring Harbor, NY: Harbor Press.

Mountain, A., Ney, U.M., and Schomburg, D. 1999. *Recombinant Proteins, Monoclonal Antibodies and Therapeutic Genes* (2nd Ed.). Vol. 5a. Biotechnology. *Weinheim*, Germany: Wiley VCH.

Nagodawithana, T.W., and Reed, G. 1995. *Enzymes, Biomass, Food and Feed* (2nd Ed.). Vol. 9. Biotechnology. Weinheim, Germany: VCH.

Nair, A.J. 2007. *Introduction to Biotechnology and Genetic Engineering*. Hingham, MA: Infinity Science Press.

Najafpour, G.D. 2007. *Biochemical Engineering and Biotechnology*. Amsterdam, the Netherlands: Elsevier.

Nanoscience and Nanotechnologies: Opportunities and Uncertainties. July 2004. Royal Society and Royal Academy of Engineering. London, Retrieved May 13, 2011. Available: http://www.nanotec.org.uk/finalReport.htm.

Nanotechnology Information Center: Properties, Applications, Research, and Safety Guidelines. American Elements. Available: https://www.americanelements.com/nanomaterials-nanoparticles-nanotechnology.html. Retrieved May 13, 2011.

Nanotechnology: Drexler and Smalley make the case for and against 'molecular assemblers.' 2003. *Chem. Eng. News (Am. Chem. Soc.)* 81(48): 37–42. doi:10.1021/cen-v081n036.p037. Retrieved May 9, 2010.

Narula, A., Srivastava, P.S., and Srivastava, S. 2005. *Plant Biotechnology and Molecular Markers.* New York: Springer.

National Research Council, Committee on Bioprocess Engineering. 2002. *Putting Biotechnology to Work: Bioprocess Engineering.* Washington, DC: National Academies Press.

New Zealand Ministry of Research, Science and Technology. 2005. *Biotechnologies to 2025.* Wellington, New Zealand : The Royal Society of New Zealand.

Newell-McGloughlin, M., and Re, E. 2006. *The Evolution of Biotechnology: From Natufians to Nanotechnology.* Dordrecht, the Netherlands: Springer.

Niazi, S.K. 2009. *Handbook of Biogeneric Recombinant Protein Manufacturing.* Boca Raton, FL: CRC Press.

Niazi, S.K. 2012. *Disposable Bioprocessing Systems.* New York: Informa.

Nielsen, J. 2005. Biotechnology for the future. *Adv. Biochem. Eng./Biotechnol.* 100: 1–203.

Nuwaysir, E.F., Huang, W., Albert, T.J. et al. 2002. Gene expression analysis using oligonucleotide arrays produced by maskless photolithography. *Genome Res.* 12(11): 1749–1755.

OECD. 2006. *Innovation in Pharmaceutical Biotechnology: Comparing National Innovation Systems at the Sectoral Level.* Paris, France: OECD.

Oliver, A.L. 2009. *Networks for Learning and Knowledge Creation in Biotechnology.* Cambridge: Cambridge University Press.

Olson, S. 1986. *Biotechnology: An Industry Comes of Age.* Washington, DC: National Academy Press.

Pachter, L., and Sturmfels, B. 2005. *Algebraic Statistics for Computational Biology.* New York: Cambridge University Press.

Parekh, S.R., and Vinci, V.V. 2003. *Handbook of Industrial Cell Culture: Mammalian, Microbial and Plant Cells.* Totowa, NJ: Humana Press.

Pease, A.C., Solas, D., Sullivan, E.J. et al. 1994. Light-generated oligonucleotide arrays for rapid DNA sequence analysis. *PNAS* 91(11): 5022–5026.

Petrides, D. 2000. *Bioprocess Design and Economics.* Scotch Plains, NJ: Demetri Petrides.

Pevzner, P.A. 2000. *Computational Molecular Biology: An Algorithmic Approach.* Cambridge, MA: MIT Press.

Pfafflin, J.A., and Ziegler, E.N., eds. 1992. *Encyclopedia of Environmental Science and Engineering* (3rd Ed., rev. and updated, 2 vol.). Baton Raton, FL: CRC Press.

Placzek, M.R., Chung, I.M., Macedo, H.M. et al. 2009. Stem cell bioprocessing: Fundamentals and principles. *J. R. Soc. Interface* 6(32): 209–232.

Pollack, J.R., Perou, C.M., Alizadeh, A.A., Eisen, M.B., Pergamenschikov, A., Williams, C.F., Jeffrey, S.S., Botstein, D., and Brown, P.O. 1999. Genome-wide analysis of DNA copy-number changes using cDNA microarrays. *Nat. Genet.* 23(1): 41–46.

Portner, R. 2007. *Animal Cell Biotechnology: Methods and Protocols* (2nd Ed). Vol. 24. Methods in Biotechnology. Totowa, NJ: Humana Press, pp. 1–509.

Princss, I., Maimon, O., and Ben-Gal, I. 2007. Evaluation of gene-expression clustering via mutual information distance measure. *BMC Bioinform.* 8(1): 111.

Profio, E. 1993. *Biomedical Engineering.* Wiley, New York.

Puhler, A. 1993. *Genetic Fundamentals and Genetic Engineering* (2nd Ed.). Vol. 2. Biotechnology. Weinheim, Germany: VCH.

Rao, T.V.S.R. 2007. *Economics of Biotechnology.* New Delhi, India: New Age International.

Rathore, A.S., and Soter, G. 2005. *Process Validation In Manufacturing of Biopharmaceuticals: Guidelines, Current Practices, and Industrial Case Studies.* Boca Raton, FL: CRC Press.

Rehm, H.J. 2001. *Special Processes* (2nd Ed.). Vol. 10. Biotechnology. Weinheim, Germany: Wiley-VCH.

Riet, K.V., and Tramper, J. 1991. *Basic Bioreactor Design.* New York: Marcel Dekker.

Roehr, M. 1996. *Products of Primary Metabolism* (2nd Ed.). Vol. 6. Biotechnology. Weinheim, Germany: VCH.

Rosenthal, S.J., and Wright, D.W. 2005. *NanoBiotechnology Protocols.* Vol. 303. Methods in Molecular Biology. Totowa, NJ: Humana Press.

Saha, B.C. 2003. *Fermentation Biotechnology.* Vol. 862. American Chemical Society Symposium Series. Washington, DC: Oxford University Press.

Sahm, H. 1993. *Biological Fundamentals* (2nd Ed.). Vol. 1. Biotechnology. Weinheim, Germany: VCH.

Sanders, M.S., and Mccormick, E.J. 1993. *Human Factors in Engineering and Design* (7th Ed.). New York: McGraw Hill.

Sanger, F., Air, G.M., Barrell, B.G. et al. February 1977. Nucleotide sequence of bacteriophage phi × 174 DNA. *Nature* 265(5596): 687–695.

Schena, M., Shalon, D., Davis, R.W., and Brown, P.O. 1995. Quantitative monitoring of gene expression patterns with a complementary DNA microarray. *Science* 270(5235): 467–470.

Scheper, T. 1997. Biotreatment, downstream processing and modelling. *Adv. Biochem. Eng. Biotechnol.* 56: 1–205.

Scheper, T. 2000. New products and New areas of bioprocess engineering. *Adv. Biochem. Eng./ Biotechnol.* 68: 1–233.

Schugerl, K. 1991. *Measuring, Modelling, and Control* (2nd Ed.). Vol. 4. Biotechnology. Weinheim, Germany: VCH.

Sensen, C.W. 2001. *Genomics and Bioinformatics* (2nd Ed.). Vol. 5b. Biotechnology. Weinheim, Germany: Wiley-VCH.

Shalon, D., Smith, S.J., and Brown, P.O. 1996. A DNA microarray system for analyzing complex DNA samples using two-color fluorescent probe hybridization. *Genome Res.* 6(7): 639–645.

Shmaefsky, B.R. 2006. *Biotechnology 101.* Science 101. West Port, CT: Greenwood Press.

Sinha, R.K., and Sinha, R. 2008. *Environmental Biotechnology.* Jaipur, India: Aavishkar Publishers.

Skalak, R., and Chieun, S., eds. 1987. *Handbook of Bioengineering.* New York: McGraw Hill.

Smith, A. 1995. *Gene Expression in Recombinant Microorganisms.* New York: Marcel Dekker.

Smith, J.E. 2009. *Biotechnology* (5th Ed.). New York: Cambridge University Press.

Soinov, L. 2006. Bioinformatics and pattern recognition come together. *JPRR* 1(1): 37–41.

Spencer, A.L.R., and Spencer, J.F.T. 2004. Environmental microbiology: Methods and protocols. *Methods Biotechnol.* 16: 1–417.

Srinivas, T. 2008. *Environmental Biotechnology.* New Delhi, India: New Age International.

Stephanopoulos, G. *Bioprocessing* (2nd Ed.). Vol. 3. Biotechnology. Weinheim, Germany: VCH.

Swarbrick, J. 2007. *Encyclopedia of Pharmaceutical Technology* (3rd Ed., Vol. 1). New York: Informa.

Tang, T., François, N., Glatigny, A. et al. 2007. Expression ratio evaluation in two-colour microarray experiments is significantly improved by correcting image misalignment. *Bioinformatics* 23(20): 2686–2691.

Tisdall, J. 2001. *Beginning Perl for Bioinformatics.* Beijing, China: O'Reilly.

Tsai, W.-L., Autsen, J.L., Ma, J. et al. January 2012. Noninvasive optical sensor technology in shake flasks for mammalian cell cultures. *Bioprocess Int.* 10(1): 50–56.

Tuan, R.S. 1997. *Recombinant Gene Expression Protocols.* Vol. 62. Methods in Molecular Biology. Totowa, NJ: Humana Press.

Tuan, R.S. 1997. *Recombinant Protein Protocols: Detection and Isolation.* Vol. 63. Methods in Molecular Biology. Totowa, NJ: Humana Press.

Vesilind, P.A., Pierce, J.J., and Weiner, R.F. 1994. *Environmental Engineering* (3rd Ed.). Boston, MA: Butterworth-Heinemann.

Walsh, G. 2007. *Pharmaceutical Biotechnology: Concepts and Applications*. Chichester, England: John Wiley & Sons.

Waterman, M.S. 1995. *Introduction to Computational Biology: Sequences, Maps and Genomes*. Boca Raton, FL: CRC Press.

Wei, C., Li, J., and Bumgarner, R.E. 2004. Sample size for detecting differentially expressed genes in microarray experiments. *BMC Genomics* 5: 87.

Winter, J. 1999. *Environmental Processes I: Wastewater Treatment* (2nd Ed.). Vol. 11a. Biotechnology. Weinheim, Germany: Wiley-VCH.

Woodson, W.E., Tillman, B., and Tillman, P. 1992. *Human Factors Design Handbook: Information and Guidelines for the Design of Systems, Facilities, Equipment, and Products for Human Use* (2nd Ed.) New York: McGraw-Hill.

Wouters, L., Gōhlmann, H.W., Bijnens, L. et al. 2003. Graphical exploration of gene expression data: a comparative study of three multivariate methods. *Biometrics* 59(4): 1131–1139.

CHAPTER 2

Alberts, B., Johnson, A., Lewis, J., Raff, M., Roberts, K., and Walter, P. *Molecular Biology of the Cell*. New York: Taylor & Francis, 2007.

Karp, G. *Cell and Molecular Biology: Concepts and Experiments*. Hoboken, NJ: Wiley, 2013.

List of Sources

http://www.wikilectures.eu/index.php/File:06_chart_pu3.png.

http://commons.wikimedia.org/wiki/File:Gene_structure.svg.

CHAPTER 3

Baynes, J.W. and Dominiczak, M.H. 2005. *Medicinal Biochemistry* (2nd Ed.). Edinburgh: Elsevier, p. 18.

Black, J.G. 2013. *Principles and Explorations* (8th Ed.). Hoboken, NJ: John Wiley & Sons.

Buchholz, K., Kasche, V., and Bronscheur, U.T. 2013. *Biocatalysts and Enzyme Technology*. Hoboken, NJ: Wiley-Blackwell.

Karp, G. 2013. *Cell and Molecular Biology: Concepts and Experiments*. Hoboken, NJ: Wiley.

Willey, J., Sherwood, L., and Woolverton, C. 2013. *Prescott's Microbiology*. New York. McGraw-Hill.

List of Sources

http://www.biologycs.com/alpha-helix.htm.

https://sallyarjoon.wordpress.com/2013/03/22/proteins/.

http://en.wikipedia.org/wiki/Polysaccharide#/media/File:Amylose_3Dprojection.corrected.png.

http://commons.wikimedia.org/wiki/File:Phospholipids_aqueous_solution_structures.svg.

CHAPTER 4

Black, J.G. 2013. *Principles and Explorations* (8th Ed.). Hoboken, NJ: John Wiley & Sons.

Buchholz, K., Kasche, V., and Bronscheur, U.T. 2013. *Biocatalysts and Enzyme Technology*. Hoboken, NJ: Wiley-Blackwell.

Karp, G. 2013. *Cell and Molecular Biology: Concepts and Experiments*. Hoboken, NJ: Wiley.

Prescott et al. 1996. Microbiology (3rd ed.). McGraw-Hill.

Willey, J., Sherwood, L., and Woolverton, C. 2013. *Prescott's Microbiology*. New York: McGraw-Hill.

List of Sources

http://commons.wikimedia.org/wiki/File:Relative_scale.svg.
http://commons.wikimedia.org/wiki/File:Average_prokaryote_cell_pt.svg?uselang=en.
http://commons.wikimedia.org/wiki/File:Gram-Cell-wall.svg.
http://commons.wikimedia.org/wiki/File:Phylogenetic_Tree_of_Life.png.
http://commons.wikimedia.org/wiki/File:Virus_Replication_large.svg.

CHAPTER 5

House, J.E. 2007. *Principles of Chemical Kinetics* (2nd Ed.). San Diego, CA: Academic Press.

CHAPTER 6

Alberts, B., Johnson, A., Lewis, J., Raff, M., Roberts, K., and Walter, P. 2007. *Molecular Biology of the Cell*. New York: Taylor & Francis.
Chen, W.W.; Neipel, M.; Sorger, P.K. (2010). "Classic and contemporary approaches to modeling biochemical reactions". Genes Dev 24 (17): 1861–1875.
Karp, G. 2013. *Cell and Molecular Biology: Concepts and Experiments*. Hoboken, NJ: Wiley.
Lehninger, A.L.; Nelson, D.L.; Cox, M.M. (2005). Lehninger principles of biochemistry. New York: W.H. Freeman.
Michaelis, L.; Menten, M.L. (1913). "Die Kinetik der Invertinwirkung". Biochem Z 49: 333–369.

CHAPTER 7

Baird, D.C. 1988. *Experimentation: An Introduction to Measurement Theory and Experiment Design* (2nd Ed.). Englewood Cliffs, NJ: Prentice Hall.
Barry, B.A. 1978. *Errors in Practical Measurement in Science, Engineering, and Technology 7*. New York: John Wiley & Sons.
Comparison Chart of FDA and EPA Good Laboratory Practice (GLP). 2004. Available: http://www.fda.gov/ICECI/EnforcementActions/BioresearchMonitoring/ucm135197.htm.
Cooney, C.L., Wang, D.I.C., and Mateles, R.I. 1968. Measurement of heat evolution and correlation with oxygen consumption during microbial growth. *Biotechnol. Bioeng.* 11: 269–281.
General Principles of Software Validation; Final Guidance for Industry and FDA Staff. 2002. FDA, Center for Devices and Radiological Health, Center for Biologics Evaluation and Research. White Oak, MD. Available: http://www.fda.gov/cdrh/comp/guidance/938.html.
Glossary of Computerized System and Software Development Terminology. 1995. Division of Field Investigations, Office of Regional Operations, Office of Regulatory Affairs, FDA. White Oak, MD. Available: http://www.fda.gov/ora/inspect_ref/igs/gloss.html.
Guidance for Industry, FDA Reviewers, and Compliance on Off-the-Shelf Software Use in Medical Devices. 1999. FDA, Center for Devices and Radiological Health, 1999. White Oak, MD. Available: http://www.fda.gov/cdrh/ode/guidance/585.html.
Handbook Good Laboratory Practice (GLP). World Health Organization. Available: http://www.who.int/entity/tdr/publications/documents/glp-handbook.pdf.
ISO 14971:2002 Medical Devices—Application of Risk Management to Medical Devices. 2001. ISO.
ISO/IEC 17799:2000 (BS 7799:2000) Information Technology—Code of Practice for Information Security Management. 2000. ISO/IEC.
Massey, B.S. 1986. *Measures in Science and Engineering: Their Expression, Relation and Interpretation*. Chichester, England: Ellis Horwood.

Pharmaceutical CGMPs for the 21st Century: A Risk-Based Approach; A Science and Risk-Based Approach to Product Quality Regulation Incorporating an Integrated Quality Systems Approach. 2002. FDA. White Oak, MD. Available: http://www.fda.gov/oc/guidance/gmp.html.

Popper, K.R. 1972. *Conjectures and Refutations: The Growth of Scientific Knowledge.* London, England: Routledge and Kegan Paul.

Popper, K.R. 1972. *The Logic of Scientific Discovery.* London, England: Hutchinson.

The Good Automated Manufacturing Practice (GAMP) Guide for Validation of Automated Systems, GAMP 4. 2001. ISPE/GAMP Forum. Tampa, FL. Available: http://www.ispe.org/gamp/.

Walpole, R.E., and Myers, R.H. 1972. *Probability and Statistics for Engineers and Scientists.* New York: Macmillan.

Youden, W.J. 1962. Systematic errors in physical constants. *Technometrics* 4: 111–123.

List of Sources

http://commons.wikimedia.org/wiki/File:Accuracy_and_precision.svg.

CHAPTER 9

Makrides, S.C. 1996. Strategies for achieving high-level expression of genes in *Escherichia coli.* *Microbiol. Rev.* 60(3): 512–538.

Nilsson B, Moks T, Jansson B, Abrahmsen L, Elmblad A, Homgren E, Henrichson C, Jones TA and Uhlen M. A synthetic IgG-binding domain based on staphylococcal protein A. Protein Eng. 1987 Feb-Mar;1(2):107–13.

List of Sources

http://commons.wikimedia.org/wiki/File:Proinsulin_to_insulin.svg.
http://commons.wikimedia.org/wiki/File:DNA_chemical_structure.svg.
http://commons.wikimedia.org/wiki/File:PBR322.svg.

CHAPTER 11

Adam, E., Sarrazin, S., Landolfi, C. et al. 2008. Efficient long-term and high-yielded production of a recombinant proteoglycan in eukaryotic HEK293 cells using a membrane-based bioreactor. *Biochem. Biophys. Res. Commun.* 369: 297–302.

Aldington, S., and Bonnerjea, J. 2007. Scale-up of monoclonal antibody purification processes. *J. Chromatogr. B* 848: 64–78.

American Chemistry Council. *Information on Plastics and the Environment.* PlasticsResource.com. Available: http://www.plasticsresource.com/s_plasticsresource/index.asp.

Anders, K.D., Akhnoukh, R., Scheper, T., and Kretzmer, G. 1992. Culture fluorescence measurements for the monitoring and characterization of insect cell cultivation in bioreactors. *Chemie Ingenieur Technik* 64(6): 572–573.

Anders, K.D., Wehnert, G., Thordsen, O., Scheper, T., Rehr, B., and Sahm, H. 1993. Biotechnological applications of fiber-optic sensing—Multiple uses of a fiber-optic fluorometer. *Sens. Actuators B Chem.* 11(1–3): 395–403.

Anicetti, V. 2009. Biopharmaceutical processes: A glance into the 21st century. *BioProcess Int.* 7(4): S4–S11.

Arunakumari, A., Wang, J., and Ferreira, G. 2007. Improved downstream process design for human monoclonal antibody production. *BioPharm Int.* 20: 36–40.

Bail, P., Crawford, B., and Lindström, K. 2009. 21st century vaccine manufacturing. *BioProcess Int.* 4. 18 28.

Barbaroux, M., and Sette, A. 2006. *Properties of Materials Used in Single-Use Flexible Containers: Requirements and Analysis.* Available: http://biopharminternational.findpharma.com/biopharm/article/articleDetail.jsp?id=423541&sk=&date=&pageID=7.

Barnoon, B., and Bader, B. 2008. *Lifecycle Cost Analysis for Single-Use Systems.* BioPharm Int. 30–43.

Bender, J., and Wolk, B. 1998. Putting a spin on CHO harvest. Centrifuge technology development. In: *ACS Meeting*, Boston, MA.

Bernard, F., Chevalier, E., Cappia, J.-M. et al. 2009. Disposable pH sensors. *BioProcess Int.* 7(1): S32–S36.

Bestwick, D., and Colton, R. 2009. Extractables and leachables from single-use disposables. *BioProcess Int.* 7(1): S88–S94.

BioProcess Systems Alliance (BPSA) Disposal Subcommittee. 2008. Guide to disposal of single-use bioprocess systems. *BioProcess Int.* 6(5): S24–S27.

BioWorld Snapshots. 2009. Biotechnology products on the markets since 1982. *BioWorld Today*, Atlanta, GA.

Boehm, J., and Bushnell, B. 2007. Providing sterility assurance between stainless steel and single-use systems. *BioProcess Int.* 5(4): S66–S71.

Brecht, R. 2009. Maturation into pharmaceutical glycoprotein manufacturing. In: Eibl, D., and Eibl, R. (eds.), *Disposable Bioreactors*. Vol. 115. Advances in Biochemical Engineering/Biotechnology. Berlin, Germany: Springer, pp. 1–31.

Brorson, K. 2006. CDER/FDA. Virus filter validation and performance. In: *Recovery of Biological Products XII*, Phoenix, AZ.

Büchs, J., Maier, U., Milbradt, C., and Zoels, B. 2000. Power consumption in shaking flasks on rotary shaking machines: I. Power consumption measurements in unbaffled flask at low viscosity. *Biotechnol. Bioeng.* 68: 589–593.

Bush, L. 2008. Disposal of disposables. *BioPharm Int.* 7: 12.

Cappia, J.-M., and Holman, N.B.T. 2004. Integrating single-use disposable processes into critical aseptic processing operations. *BioProcess Int.* 2(4). Available: http://www.bioprocessintl.com/multimedia/archive/00078/0209su12_78577a.pdf.

Cardona, M., and Allen, B. 2006. Incorporating single-use systems in biopharmaceutical manufacturing. *BioProcess Int.* 4(Suppl. 4): 10–14.

Chapter <87> Biological Reactivity Tests, In Vitro, USP 30. 2007. Rockville, MD: United States Pharmacopeial Convention.

Chapter <88> Biological Reactivity Tests, In Vivo, USP 30. 2007. Rockville, MD: United States Pharmacopeial Convention.

Chmiel, H. 2006. Bioreaktoren. In: Chmiel, H (ed.), *Bioprozesstechnik*. München, Germany: Elsevier, pp. 195–215.

CHMP/CVMP. 2005. *Guideline on Plastic Immediate Packaging Materials*. European London, England: Medicines Evaluation Agency. Available: http://www.emea.europa.eu/pdfs/human/qwp/435903en.pdf.

Clutterbuck, A., Kenworthy, J., and Lidell, J. 2007. Endotoxin reduction using disposable membrane adsorption technology in cGMP manufacturing. *BioPharm Int.* 20: 24–31.

Colder Products. 2010. *Steam-Thru Connections—Product Description*. Available: http://www.colder.com/Products/SteamThruConnections/tabid/740/Default.aspx.

Cole, G. 1998. *Pharmaceutical Production Facilities: Design and Applications*. Pharmaceutical Science Series. London, England: Taylor & Francis.

Colton, R. 2007a. Recommendations for extractables and leachables testing—Part 1. *BioProcess Int.* 11: 36–44.

Colton, R. 2007b. The extractables and leachables subcommittee of the bio-process systems alliance. Recommendations for extractables and leachables testing, part 1: Introduction, regulatory issues and risk assessment. *BioProcess Int.* 12: 36–44.

Colton, R. 2008a. Recommendations for extractables and leachables testing—Part 2. *BioProcess Int.* 1: 44–52.

Colton, R. 2008b. The extractables and leachables subcommittee of the bio-process systems alliance. Recommendations for extractables and leachables testing, part 2: Executing a program. *BioProcess Int.* 1: 44–52.

CPT Consolidated Polymer Technologies. 2002. *Material Comparison.* Brochure. Available: http://www.stiflow.com/CFIex-Tubing-Material-Comparison.pdf.

Croughan, G. 2010. Beyond just high titers: The future of cell line engineering. In: *IBC Cell Line Development and Engineering Conference.* San Francisco, CA.

Curling, J., and Gottschal, U. 2007. Process chromatography: Five decades of innovation. *BioPharm Int.* 21: 70–94.

Curtis, W.R. 2004. Growing cells in a reservoir formed of a flexible sterile plastic liner. United States Patent 6709862B2.

De Jesus, M.J., Girard, P., Bourgeois, M. et al. 2004. TubeSpin satellites: A fast track approach for process development with animal cells using shaking technology. *Biochem. Eng. J.* 17: 217–223.

De Jesus, M.J., and Wurm, F.M. 2009. Medium and process optimization for high yield, high density suspension cultures: From low throughput spinner flasks to high throughput millilitre reactors. *BioProcess Int.* 7(Suppl. 1): 12–17.

De Wilde, D., Noack, U., Kahlert, W., Barbaroux, M., and Greller, G. 2009. Bridging the gap from reusable to single-use manufacturing with stirred, single-use bioreactors. *BioProcess Int.* 7(Suppl. 4): 36–41.

DeGrazio, F.L. 2006. *The Importance of Leachables and Extractables Testing for a Successful Product Launch.* Available: http://pharmtech.fmdpharma.com/pharmtech/Article/The-Importance-of-Leachables-and-Extractables-Test/ArticleStandard/Article/detail/482447.

Denton, A., Jones, C., and Tarrach, K. 2009. Integration of large-scale chromatography with nanofiltration for an ovine polyclonal product. *Pharm. Technol.* 1: 62–70.

DePalma, A. 2002. Options for anchorage-dependent cell culture. *Genet. Eng. Biotechnol. N.* 22: 58–62.

DePalma, A. 2004. Bioprocessing on the way to total-disposability manufacture. *Genet. Eng. Biotechnol. N.* 24(3): 40–41.

DePalma, A. 2006. Bright sky for single-use bioprocess products. *Genet. Eng. Biotechnol. N.* 26(3): 50–57.

Desai, M.A., Rayner, M., Burns, M., and Bermingham, D. 2000. Application of chromatography in the downstream processing of biomolecules. *Methods Biotechnol.* 9: 73–94.

DeWilde, D., Noack, U., Kahlert, W., Barbaroux, M., and Greller, G. 2009. Bridging the gap from reusable to single-use manufacturing with stirred, single-use bioreactors. *BioProcess Int.* 7(Suppl. 4): 36–41.

DiBlasi, K., Jornitz, M.W., Gottschalk, U., and Priebe, P.M. 2006. Disposable biopharmaceutical processes—Myth or reality? *BioPharm Int.* 11: 2–10.

Diehl, T. 2006. *Application of Membrane Chromatography in the Purification of Humanly Monoclonal Antibodies.* King of Prussia, PA: Downstream Technology Forum.

DiMasi, J.A., and Grabowski, H.G. 2007. The cost of biopharmaceutical R&D: Is biotech different? *Manage. Decis. Econ.* 28: 469–479.

Ding, W., and Martin, J. 2008. Implementing single-use technology in biopharmaceutical manufacturing: An approach to extractables/leachables studies, part one—Connections and filters. *BioProcess Int.* 6(9): 34–42.

Dremel, B.A.A., and Schmid, R.D. 1992. Optical sensors for bio-process control. *Chemie Ingenieur Technik* 64(6): 510–517.

Ducos, J.P., Terrier, B., and Courtois, D. 2009. Disposable bioreactors for plant micropropagation and cell cultures. In: Eibl, D., and Eibl, R. (eds.), *Disposable Bioreactors.* Vol. 115. Advances in Biochemical Engineering/Biotechnology. Berlin, Germany: Springer, pp. 89–115.

Ducos, J.P., Terrier, B., Courtois, D., and Pétiard, V. 2008. Improvement of plastic based disposable bioreactors for plant science needs. *Phytochem. Rev.* 7: 607–613.

Eibl, R., and Eibl, D. 2006a. Design and use of the wave bioreactor for plant cell culture. In: Dutta Gupta, S., and Ibaraki, Y. (eds.), *Plant Tissue Culture Engineering.* Vol. 6. Focus on Biotechnology. Dordrecht, the Netherlands: Springer, pp. 203–227.

Eibl, R., and Eibl, D. 2006b. Design and use of the wave bioreactor for plant cell culture. In: Dutta Gupta, S., and Ibaraki, Y. (eds.), *Plant Tissue Culture Engineering.* Dordrecht, the Netherlands: Springer, pp. 203–227.

Eibl, R., and Eibl, D. 2007a. Disposable Bioreactors for Cell Culture-Based Bioprocessing. *ACHEMA Worldwide News* 2: 8–10.

Eibl, R., and Eibl, D. 2007b. Disposable bioreactors for inoculum production and protein expression. In: Pörtner, R. (ed.), *Animal Cell Biotechnology: Methods and Protocols.* Vol. 24. Methods in Biotechnology. Totowa, NJ: Humana Press, pp. 321–335.

Eibl, R., and Eibl, D. 2008a. Application of disposable bag bioreactors in tissue engineering and for the production of therapeutic agents. In: Kasper, C., van Griensven, M., and Pörtner, R. (eds.), *Bioreactor Systems for Tissue Engineering.* Vol. 112. Berlin, Germany: Springer, pp. 183–207.

Eibl, R., and Eibl, D. 2008b. Bioreactors for mammalian cells: General overview. In: Eibl, R., Eibl, D., Pörtner, R., Catapano, G., and Czermak, P. (eds.), *Cell and Tissue Reaction Engineering.* Heidelberg, Germany: Springer, pp.55–82.

Eibl, R., and Eibl, D. 2008c. Design of bioreactors suitable for plant cell and tissue cultures. *Phytochem. Rev.* 7: 593–598.

Eibl, R., and Eibl, D. 2009a. Disposable bioreactors in cell culture-based upstream processing. *BioProcess Int.* 7(Suppl. 1): 18–23.

Eibl, D., and Eibl, R. (eds.), 2009b. *Disposable Bioreactors, Series: Advances in Biochemical Engineering/ Biotechnology.* Vol. 115. Berlin, Germany: Springer.

Eibl, R., Rutschmann, K., Lisica, L., and Eibl, D. 2003. Kosten reduzieren durch Einwegbioreaktoren? *BioWorld* 5: 22–23.

Eibl, R., Werner, S., and Eibl, D. 2009a. Bag bioreactor based on wave-induced motion: Characteristics and applications. In: Eibl, D., and Eibl, R. (eds.), *Disposable Bioreactors.* Vol. 115. Advances in Biochemical Engineering/Biotechnology. Berlin, Germany: Springer, pp. 55–87.

Eibl, R., Werner, S., and Eibl, D. 2009b. Bag bioreactor based on wave-induced motion: Characteristics and applications. In: Eibl, R., and Eibl, D. (eds.), *Disposable Bioreactors.* Vol. 115. Advances in Biochemical Engineering/Biotechnology. Heidelberg, Germany: Springer, pp. 55–87.

Eibl, R., Werner, S., and Eibl, D. 2009c. Disposable bioreactors for plant liquid cultures at litre-scale: Review. *Eng. Life Sci.* 9: 156–164.

Eibl, R., Kaiser, S., Lombriser, R., and Eibl, D. 2010. Disposable bioreactors: The current state-of-the-art and recommended applications in biotechnology. *Appl. Microbiol. Biotech.* 86(1): 41–49.

Ernst & Young Global Ltd. 2007. *Beyond Borders Global Biotechnology Report 2007.* Boston, MA: Ernst & Young Global Ltd.

Etzel, M., and Riordan, W. 2006. Membrane chromatography: Analysis of breakthrough curves and viral clearance. In: Shukla, A., Etzel, M., and Gadam, S. (eds.), *Process Scale Bioseparations for the Biopharmaceutical Industry.* Boca Raton, FL: Taylor & Francis, pp. 277–296.

Falkenberg, F.W. 1998. Production of monoclonal antibodies in the miniPerm bioreactor: Comparison with other hybridoma culture methods. *Res. Immunol.* 6: 560–570.

Farid, S.S. 2009. Process economic drivers in industrial monoclonal antibody manufacture. In: Gottschalk, U. (ed.), *Process Scale Purification of Antibodies.* New York: Wiley, pp. 239–262.

Farid, S.S., Washbrook, J., and Titchener-Hooker, N.J. 2005. Decision-support tool for assessing bio-manufacturing strategies under uncertainty: Stainless steel versus disposable equipment for clinical trial material preparation. *Biotechnol. Prog.* 21(2): 486–497.

Foulon, A., Trach, F., Pralong, A., Proctor, M., and Lim, J. 2008. Using disposables in an antibody production process. *BioProcess Int.* 6(6): 12–18.

Foulon, A., Trach, F., Pralong, A., Proctor, M., and Lim, J. 2008. Using disposables in an antibody production process: A cost-effectiveness study of technology transfer between two production sites. *BioProcess Int.* 6(Suppl. 3): 12–18.

Fox, S. 2005. Disposable processing: The impact of disposable bioreactors on the CMO industry. *Contract Pharma* 6: 62–74.

Fraud, N., Kuczewski, M., Zarbis-Papastoitsis, G., and Hirai, M. 2009. Hydrophobic membrane adsorbers for large-scale downstream processing. *BioPharm Int.* 23: 24–27.

Fries, S., Glazomitsky, K., Woods, A. et al. 2005. Evaluation of disposable bioreactors. *BioProcess Int.* 3(Suppl. 6). 36–44.

Fuller, M., and Pora, H. 2008. Introducing disposable systems into biomanufacturing: A CMO case study. *BioProcess Int.* 6(10): 30–36.

Galliher, P. 2008. Achieving high-efficiency production with microbial technology in a single-use bioreactor platform. *BioProcess Int.* 11:60–65.

Ganzlin, M., Marose, S., Lu, X., Hitzmann, B., Scheper, T., and Rinas, U. 2007. In situ multi-wavelength fluorescence spectroscopy as effective tool to simultaneously monitor spore germination, metabolic activity and quantitative protein production in recombinant *Aspergillus niger* fed-batch cultures. *J. Biotechnol.* 132(4): 461–468.

GE. 2009. *NPC-100 Pressure Sensor.* Available: http://www.gesensing.com/products/npc_100_series.htm?bc=bc_indust+bc_med_fluid.

GE Healthcare. 2006. *CHO Cell Supernatant Concentration with Kvick Lab Cassettes.* Application note 11-0013 62. Buckinghamshire, UK: GE Healthcare.

GE Healthcare. 2007. *Purification of a Monoclonal Antibody Using ReadyToProcess Columns.* Application Note 28–9198–56 AA. Buckinghamshire, UK: GE Healthcare.

GE Healthcare. 2008. *Rapid Production of Clinical Grade T Lymphocytes in the Wave Bioreactor.* Buckinghamshire, UK: GE Healthcare. Available: http://www.5.gelifesciences.com/aptrix/upp0091.nsf./Content/F7AD616DACC22171C125747400812B51/$file/28933149AA.pdf.

GE Healthcare. 2009a. *A Flexible Antibody Purification Process Based on Ready To Process Products.* Application note 28-9403-48 AA. Buckinghamshire, UK: GE Healthcare.

GE Healthcare. 2009b. *High-Throughput Screening and Optimization of a Multi Modal Polishing Step in a Monoclonal Antibody Purification Process.* Application note 28-9509-60. Buckinghamshire, UK: GE Healthcare.

GE Healthcare. 2009c. *High-Throughput Screening and Optimization of a Protein A Capture Step in a Monoclonal Antibody Purification Process.* Application note 28-9468-58. Buckinghamshire, UK: GE Healthcare.

GE Healthcare. 2009d. *Scale-Up of a Downstream Monoclonal Antibody Purification Process Using HiScreen and AxiChrom Columns.* Application note 28-9409-49. Buckinghamshire, UK: GE Healthcare.

GE Healthcare. 2010a. *Hot Lips Tube Sealer—Product Description.* Buckinghamshire, UK: GE Healthcare. Available: http://www.gelifesciences.com/aptrix/upp01077.nsf/Content/wave_bioreactor_home~wave_fluid_transfer~hot_lips_tube_sealer.

GE Healthcare. 2010b. *ReadyMate DAC—Product Description.* Buckinghamshire, UK: GE Healthcare. Available: http://www5.gelifesciences.com/aptrix/upp00919.nsf/Content/692F8252BA8B1477C125763C00827AEI/$file/28937902+ AC+.pdf.

GE Healthcare. 2010c. *Sterile Tube Fuser—Technical Information.* Buckinghamshire, UK: GE Healthcare. Available: http://www5.gelifesciences.com/aptrix/upp01077.nsf/Content/Products?OpenDocument&parentid=986919&moduleid=167710&zone=.

GE Healthcare. 2010d. *Wave Mixer Concept.* Buckinghamshire, UK: GE Healthcare. Available: http://www1.gelifesciences.com/aptrix/upp01077.nsf/Content/wave_bioreactor_home~how_it_works~how_it_works_wave_mixer.

Gebauer, K., Thommes, J., and Kula, M. 1997. Plasma protein fractionation with advanced membrane adsorbents. *Biotechnol. Bioeng.* 54: 181–189.

Genzel, Y., Olmer, R.M., Schaefer, B., and Reichl, U. 2006. Wave microcarrier cultivation of MDCK cells for influenza virus production in serum containing and serum-free media. *Vaccine*. 24: 6074–6087.

Georgiev, M.I., Weber, J., and Maciuk A. 2009. Bioprocessing of plant cell cultures for mass propagation of targeted compounds. *Appl. Microbiol. Biotechnol.* 83: 809–823.

Ghosh, R. 2004. Protein separation using membrane chromatography: Opportunities and challenges. *Chromatogr. A* 952: 13–27.

Glaser, V. 2005. Disposable bioreactors become standard fare. *Genet. Eng. Biotechnol. News* 25(14): 80–81.

Glaser, V. 2009. Bioreactor and fermentor trends. *Genet Eng. Biotechnol. News*. Available: http://www.genengnews.com/issues/item.aspx.

Gold, L.S. 2007. *Carcinogenic Potency Database (CPDB)*. Berkeley, CA: University of California. Available: http://www.potency.berkeley.edu/cpdb.html.

Goldstein, A., Loesch, J., Mazzarella, K., Matthews, T., Luchsinger, G., and Javier, D.S. 2009. *Freeze Bulk Bags: A Case Study in Disposables Implementation: Genentech's Evaluation of Single-Use Technologies for Bulk Freeze-Thaw, Storage, and Transportation*. Available: http://biopharminternational.findpharma.com/biopharm/Disposables+Articles/Freeze-Bulk-Bags-A-Case-Study-in-Disposables-lmple/ArticleStandard/Article/detail/637583.

Gorter, A., van de Griend, R.J., van Eendenburg, J.D., Haasnot, W.H., and Fleuren, G.J. 1993. Production of bi-specific monoclonal antibodies in a hollow-fibre bioreactor. *J. Immunol. Methods* 161: 145–150.

Gottschaik, U. 2005. Downstream processing of monoclonal antibodies: From high dilution to high purity. *BioPharm Int.* 19: 42–58.

Gottschaik, U. 2008. Bioseparation in antibody manufacturing: The good, the bad and the ugly. *Biotechnol. Prog.* 24: 496–503.

Gottschalk, U. 2005. New and unknown challenges facing biomanufacturing. *BioPharm Int.* 19: 24–28.

Gottschalk, U. 2009. Disposables in downstream processing. In: Eibl, R., and Eibl, D. (eds.), *Disposable Bioreactors*. Vol. 115. Advances in Biochemical Engineering/Biotechnology. Berlin, Germany: Springer, pp. 172–183.

Gottschalk, U., Fischer-Fruehholz, S., and Reif, O.W. 2004. Membrane adsorbers: A cutting-edge process technology at the threshold. *BioProcess Int.* 2:56–65.

Guth, U., Gerlach, F., Decker, M., Oelßner, W., Vonau, W. 2009. Solid-state reference electrodes for potentiometric sensors. *J. Solid State Electrochem.* 13(1): 27–39.

Hagedorn, A., Levadoux, W., Groleau, D., and Tartakovsky, B. 2004. Evaluation of multiwavelength culture fluorescence for monitoring the aroma compound 4-hydroxy-2(or 5)-ethyl-5 (or 2)-methyl-3(2H)-furanone (HEMF) production. *Biotechnol. Prog.* 20(1): 361–367.

Haughney, H., and Hutchinson, J. 2004a. A disposable option for bovine serum filtration and packaging. *BioProcess Int.* Suppl. 4(9): 2–5.

Haughney, H., and Hutchinson, J. 2004b. Single-use systems reduce production timelines. *Gen. Eng. News* 24(8). Available: www.hyclone.com/pdf/bp_single_use24gen8.pdf.

Heath, C., and Kiss, R. 2007. Cell culture process development: Advances in process engineering. *Biotechnol. Prog.* 23: 46–51.

Heller, A., and Feldmann, B. 2008. Electrochemical glucose sensors and their applications in diabetes management. *Chem. Rev.* 108: 2482–2505.

Henning, B., and Rautenberg, J. 2006. Process monitoring using ultrasonic sensor systems. *Ultrasonics* 44: e1395–e1399.

Hilmer, J.-M., and Scheper, T. 1996. A New version of an in situ sampling system for bioprocess analysis. *Acta Biotechnol.* 16(2–3): 185–192.

Hitchcock, T. 2009. Production of recombinant whole-cell vaccines with disposable manufacturing systems. *BioProcess Int.* 5: 36–43.

Hitzmann, B., Broxtermann, O., Cha, Y.L., Sobieh, O., Stark, E., and Scheper, T. 2000. The control of glucose concentration during yeast fed-batch cultivation using a fast measurement complemented by an extended Kalman filter. *Bioprocess Eng.* 23(4): 337–341.

Hopkinson, J. 1985. Hollow fibre cell culture systems for economical cell-product manufacturing. *Biotechnology* 3: 225–230.

Horowitz, B., Lazo, A., Grossberg, H., Page, G., Lippin, A., and Swan, G. 1998. Virus inactivation by solvent/detergent treatment and the manufacture of SD-plasma. *Vox Song.* 74(Suppl. I): 203–206.

Hou, K., and Mandaro, R. 1986. Bioseparation by ion exchange cartridge chromatography. *Biotechniques* 4: 358–366.

Houtzager, E., van der Linden, R., de Roo, G., Huurman, S., Priem, P., and Sijmons, P.C. 2005. Linear scale-up of cell cultures. The next level in disposable bioreactor design. *BioProcess Int.* 6: 60–66.

Hsiao, T.Y., Bacani, F.T., Carvalho, E.B., and Curtis, W.R. 1999. Development of a low capital investment reactor system: Application for plant cell suspension culture. *Biotechnol Prog.* 15: 114–122.

Hynetics Co. 2010. *Description of the HyNetics Disposable Mixing System.* Available: http://www.hynetics.com/default/WhatWeOffer.htm.

Jagschies, G. 2009. Flexible manufacturing: Driving monoclonal antibody process economics. *GIT BIOprocessing* 1: 30–31.

Jain, E., and Kumar A. 2008. Upstream processes in antibody production: Evaluation of critical parameters. *Biotechnol. Adv.* 26: 46–72.

Jenke, D. 2007a. An extractables/leachables strategy facilitated by collaboration between drug product vendors and plastic material/system suppliers. *PDA J. Pharm. Sci. Technol.* 61: 17–23.

Jenke, D. 2007b. Evaluation of the chemical compatibility of plastic contact materials and pharmaceutical products; safety considerations related to extractables and leachables. *J. Pharm. Sci.* 96: 2566–2581.

Jenke, D., Story, J., and Lalani, R. 2006. Extractables/leachables from plastic tubing used in product manufacturing. *Int. J. Pharm.* 315: 75–92.

Jia, Q., Li, H., Hui, M. et al. 2008. A bioreactor system based on a novel oxygen transfer method. *BioProcess Int.* 6: 66–78.

Joo, S., and Brown, R.B. 2008. Chemical sensors with integrated electronics. *Chem. Rev.* 108(2): 638–651.

Jornitz, M.W., and Meltzer, T.H. 2004. *Filtration Handbook Liquids.* River Grove, IL: PDA, DHI LLC.

Karlsson, E., Ryden, L., and Brewer, J. 1989. Ion exchange chromatography. In: Janson, J.C., and Ryden, L. (eds.), *Protein Purification: Principles, High-Resolution Methods and Applications.* New York: VCH, pp. 107–115.

Kelley, K. 2007. Very large scale monoclonal antibody purification: The case for conventional unit operations. *Biotechnol. Prog.* 23: 995–1008.

Kelley, B. 2009. Industrialization of mAb production technology. The bioprocessing industry at a crossroads. *MAbs* 1(5): 443–452.

Kemplen, R., Preissmann, A., and Berthold, W. 1995. Assessment of a disc stack centrifuge for use in mammalian cell separation. *Biotechnol. Bioeng.* 46: 132–138.

Kermis, H.R., Kostov, Y., and Rao, G. 2003. Rapid method for the preparation of a robust optical pH sensor. *Analyst* 128(9): 1181–1186.

Khanna, V. 2008. ISFET (ion-sensitive field-effect transistor)-based enzymatic biosensors for clinical diagnostics and their signal conditioning instrumentation. *IETE J. Res.* 54(3): 193–202.

Kliment, I., Kuhl, M., Glud, R.N., and Holst, G. 1997. Optical measurement of oxygen and temperature in microscale. Strategies and biological applications. *Sens. Actuat. D Chem.* 38(1–3): 29–37.

Knazek, R.A., Gullino, P.M., Kohler, P.O., and Dedrick, R.L. 1972. Cell culture on artificial capillaries: An approach to tissue growth in vitro. *Science* 178: 65–67.

Knudsen, H.L., Fahrner, R.L., Xu, Y., Morling, L.A., and Blank, G.S. 2001. Membrane ion-exchange chromatography for process-scale antibody purification. *J. Chromatogr. A* 907: 145–154.

Kranjac, D. 2004. Validation of bioreactors: Disposable vs. reusable. *BioProcess Int.* Industry Yearbook: 86.

Langer, E.S. 2009. Trends in single-use bioproduction. What Users Are Saying. *BioProcess Int.* 7(3) 2009:S6–S8.

Langer, E.S., and Ranck, J. 2005. The ROI case: Economic justification for disposables in biopharmaceutical manufacturing. *BioProcess Int.* 27(Suppl. 1): 46–50.

Leventis, H.C., Streeter, I., Wildgoose, G.G., Lawrence, N.S., Jiang, L., Jones, T.G.J., and Compton, R.G. 2004. Derivatised carbon powder electrodes: Reagentless pH sensors. *Talanta* 63(4): 1039–1051.

Levine, B. 2007. *Making Waves in Cell Therapy: The Wave Bioreactor for the Generation of Adherent and Non-Adherent Cells for Clinical Use.* Available: http://www.wavebiotech.com/pdf/literature/ISCT_2007_Levine_Final.pdf.

Li, C.Y., Zhang, X.B., Han, Z.X. et al. 2006. A wide pH range optical sensing system based on a sol-gel encapsulated amino-functionalised corrole. *Analyst* 131(3): 388–393.

Lim, J.A.C., and Sinclair, A. 2007. Process economy of disposable manufacturing: Process models to minimize upfront investment. *Am. Pharm. Rev.* 10: 114–121.

Lim, J.A.C., Sinclair, A., Kim, D.S., and Gottschalk, U. 2007. Economic benefits of single-use membrane chromatography in polishing. A cost of goods model. *BioProcess Int.* 5: 60–64.

Limke, T. 2009. Comparability between the Mobius CellReady 3 L bioreactor and 3 L glass bioreactors. *BioProcess Int.* 7: 122–123.

Liu, C.M., and Hong, L.N. 2001. Development of a shaking bio-reactor system for animal cell cultures. *Biochem. Eng. J.* 2: 121–125.

Liu, P. 2005a. Strategies for optimizing today's increasing disposable processing environments. *BioProcess Int.* 9: 10–15.

Liu, P. 2005b. Strategies for optimizing today's increasing disposable processing environments. *BioProcess Int.* 3(9): S10–S15.

Liu, P. 2005c. Strategies for optimizing today's increasingly disposable processing environments. *BioProcess Int.* 3(Suppl. 6): 10–15.

Lloyd-Evans, P., Phillips, D.A., Wright, A.C.C., and Williams, R.K. 2007. Disposable process for cGMP manufacture of plasmid DNA. *BioPharm Int.* 1: 18–24.

Lok, M., and Blumenblat, S. 2007. Critical design aspects of single-use systems: Some points to consider for successful implementation. *BioProcess Int.* Suppl. 5 (5): 28–31.

Lonza. 2008. *CELL-Tainer Single-Use Bioreactors.* Walkersville, MD: Lonza.

Lorenz, C.M., Wolk, B.M., Quan, C.P. et al. 2009. The effect of low intensity ultraviolet C light on monoclonal antibodies. *Biotechnol. Prog.* 25: 476–482.

Lorenzelli, L., Margesin, B., Martinoia, S., Tedesco, M.T., and Valle, M. 2003. Bioelectrochemical signal monitoring of in-vitro cultured cells by means of an automated microsystem based on solid state sensor-array. *Biosens. Bioelectron.* 18(5–6): 621–626.

Lu, J.Z., and Rosenzweig, Z. 2000. Nanoscale fluorescent sensors for intracellular analysis. *Fresenius J. Anal. Chem.* 366(6–7): 569–575.

Marose, S., Lindemann, C., Ulber, R., and Scheper, T. 1999. Optical sensor systems for bioprocess monitoring. *Trends Biotechnol.* 17(1): 30–34.

Menzel, C., Lerch, T., Scheper, T., and Schugerl, K. 1995. Development of biosensors based on an electrolyte isolator semiconductor (EIS)-capacitor structure and their application for process monitoring. Part I. Development of the biosensors and their characterization. *Anal. Chim. Acta* 317(1–3): 259–264.

Meyeroltmanns, F., Schmitz, J., and Nazlee, M. 2005. Disposable bioprocess components and single-use concepts for optimized process economy in biopharmaceutical production. *BioProcess Int.* 3: 60–66.

Migita, S., Ozasa, K., Tanaka, T., and Haruyama, T. 2007. Enzyme-based field-effect transistor for adenosine triphosphate (ATP) sensing. *Anal. Sci.* 23(1): 45–48.

Mikola, M., Seto. J., and Amanullah, A. 2007. Evaluation of a novel wave bioreactor cellbag for aerobic yeast cultivation. *Bioprocess Biosyst. Eng.* 30: 231–241.

Millipore. 2005. Lit. No. DS1002 EN00. Available: http://www.millipore.com/catalogue/module/c9423.

Millipore. 2008. *Mobius MIX500 Disposable Mixing System Characterization*. Billerica, MA: Millipore.

Millipore. 2009a. *Datasheet Mobius® CellReady 3 L Bioreactor*. Available: http://www.millipore.com/publications.nsf/a73664f9f981af8c852569b9005b4eee/228eeedd2285ebe1852575de00570375/$FILE/DS26770000.pdf.

Millipore. 2009b. *Mobius Disposable Mixing Systems*. Billerica, MA: Millipore.

Millipore. 2010a. *Lynx S2S—Product Description*. Available: http://www.millipore.com/catalogue/module/c9502.

Millipore. 2010b. *Lynx ST Connectors—Data Sheet*. Available: http://www.millipore.com/publications.nsf/a73664f9f981af8c852569b9005b4eee/402ffe097a6bIdca85256d510043ba64/$FILE/DS1750EN00.pdf.

Millipore. 2010c. *NovaSeptum Sampling System—Product Description*. Available: http://www.millipore.com/catalogue/module/c10713.

Monge, M. 2008. Disposables: Process economics—Selection, supply chain, and purchasing strategies. In: *BioProcess International Conference*. Anaheim, CA.

Mora, J., Sinclair, A., Delmdahl, N., and Gottschalk, U. 2006. Disposable membrane chromatography. Performance analysis and economic cost model. *BioProcess Int.* 4(Suppl. 4): 38–43.

Morrow, K. 2006. Disposable bioreactors gaining favor. *Genet Eng. Biotechnol. News* 26(12): 42–45.

Mukherjee, J., Lindemann, C., and Scheper, T. 1999. Fluorescence monitoring during cultivation of enterobacter aerogenes at different oxygen levels. *Appl. Microbiol. Biotechnol.* 52(4): 489–494.

Muller, C., Hitzmann, B., Schubert, F., and Scheper, T. 1997. Optical chemo- and biosensors for use in clinical applications. *Sens. Actuat. B Chem.* 40(1): 71–77.

Muller, N., Girard, P., Hacker, D., Jordan, M., and Wurm, F.M. 2004. Orbital shaker technology for the cultivation of mammalian cells in suspension. *Biotechnol. Bioeng.* 89: 400–406.

Munkholm, C., Walt, D.R., and Milanovich, F.P. 1988. A fiberoptic sensor for CO_2 measurement. *Talanta* 35(2): 109–112.

Niazi, S. 2012. *Disposable Bioprocessing Systems*. Boca Raton, FL: CRC Press.

Novais, J.L., Titchener-Hooker, N.J., and Hoare, M. 2001. Economic comparison between conventional and disposables-based technology for the production of biopharmaceuticals. *Biotechnol. Bioeng.* 75(2): 143–153.

Ozturk, S.S. 2007. Comparison of product quality: Disposable and stainless steel bioreactor. In: *BioProduction 2007*, Berlin, Germany.

Sandstrom, C., and Schmidt, B. 2005. Facility-design considerations for the use of disposable bags. *BioProcess Int.* (Suppl. 4): 56–60.

Sartorius Stedim Biotech. 2000. *Sacova Valve—Technical Information*. Gottingen, Germany: Sartoriu Stedim Biotech. Available: http://sartorius.or.kr/B_Braun_Biotech/Fermenters_and_Bioreactors/pdf/TI_SACOVAe_02-00.pdf.

Sartorius Stedim Biotech. 2009a. *Flexel 3D LevMix system for Palletank*. Göttingen, Germany: Sartoriu Stedim Biotech.

Sartorius Stedim Biotech. 2009b. *Flexel 3D System for Recirculation Mixing*. Göttingen, Germany: Sartoriu Stedim Biotech.

Sartorius Stedim Biotech. 2009c. *White Paper: Evolving Toward Single Use Bioprocessing: From Solutions to Holistic Value Creation*. Bioresearch Online. Sartoriu Stedim Biotech, Göttingen, Germany. Available: http://www.bioresearchonline.com/download.mvc/Evolving-Toward-Single-Use-Bioprocessing-From-0001.

Sartorius Stedim Biotech. 2010a. *Aseptic Transfer System—Definition of the Technology*. Göttingen, Germany: Sartoriu Stedim Biotech. Available: http://microsite.sartorius.com/fileadmin/Image_Archive/microsite/BB_sPort/White_Paper_Sterility_Assurance_in_%20Stopper_Processing_SBT4001-e.pdf.

Sartorius Stedim Biotech. 2010b. *Opta SFT-I—Product Description*. Göttingen, Germany: Sartoriu Stedim Biotech. Available: http://www.sartorius.com/fileadmin/sartorius_pdf/alle/biotech/Data_Opta_SFT-l_SLO2000-e.pdf.

Scheper, T., and Buckmann, A.F. 1990. A fiber optic biosensor based on fluorometric detection using confined macromolecular nicotinamide adenine-dinucleotide derivatives. *Biosens. Bioelectron.* 5(2): 125–135.

Scheper, T., Hitzmann, B., Stark, E. et al. 1999. Bioanalytics: Detailed insight into bioprocesses. *Anal. Chim. Acta* 400: 121–134.

Scheper, T., Lorenz, T., Schmidt, W., and Schugerl, K. 1987. Online measurement of culture fluorescence for process monitoring and control of biotechnological processes. *Ann. N. Y. Acad. Sci.* 506: 431–445.

Sinclair, A. October 12, 2009. *Biological Products Manufacturing: Cost Challenges and Opportunities Now and in the Future*. Raleigh, NC: BPI.

Sinclair, A., and Monge, M. 2002. Quantitative economic evaluation of single use disposables in bioprocessing. *Pharm. Eng.* 22: 20–34.

Sinclair, A., and Monge, M. 2004. Biomanufacturing for the 21st century: Designing a concept facility based on single-use systems. *BioProcess Int.* 2: 26–31.

Sinclair, A., and Monge, M. 2005a. Concept facility based on single antibody manufacture. *J. Chromatogr. B* 8–18: 848.

Sinclair, A., and Monge, M. 2005b. Concept facility based on single-use systems: Part 2. *BioProcess Int.* 3(9): S51–S55.

Sinclair, A., and Monge, M. 2009a. Evaluating disposable mixing systems. *Biopharm Int.* 22(2): 24–29.

Singh, S.K., Kolhe, P., Wang, W., and Nema, S. 2009a. Large-scale freezing of biologics: A practitioner's review, part 1: Fundamental aspects. *BioProcess Int.* 7(9): 32–44.

Singh, S.K., Kolhe, P., Wang, W., and Nema, S. 2009b. Urge-scale freezing of biologics: A practitioner's review, part 2: Practical advice. *BioProcess Int.* 7(10): 34–42.

Singh, V. 1999. Disposable bioreactor for cell culture using wave-induced motion. *Cytotechnology* 30: 149–158.

Singh, V. 2004. Bioprocessing tutorial: Mixing in large disposable containers. *Genet. Eng. Biotechnol. News* 24(3): 42–43.

Singh, V. 2005. *The Wave Bioreactor Story*, Wave Biotech LLC, Somerset.

Smith, M. January 2004. An evaluation of Protein A and non-Protein A methods for the recovery of monoclonal antibodies and considerations for process scale-up. In: *Scaling-Up of Biopharmaceutical Products*. Amsterdam, the Netherlands: The Grand.

Smith, M. April 2005. Strategies for the purification of high titer, high volume mammalian cell culture batches. In: *BioProcess International European Conference and Exhibition*. Berlin, Germany: Lonza Biologics.

Tartakovsky, B., Sheintuch, M., Hilmer, J.M., and Scheper, T. 1996. Application of scanning fluorometry for monitoring of a fermentation process. *Biotechnol. Prog.* 12(1): 126–131.

CHAPTER 12

List of Sources

http://www.bds-cy.com/GeneralLabEquipment/Fermentors.html. GE Life Sciences.

CHAPTER 13

List of Sources

Amersham Biotech Pharmacia. *Expanded Bed Adsorption Principles and Methods*. www.gelifesciences .com.

CHAPTER 14

List of Sources

Gel Filtration Principles and Methods, GE Healthcare (www.gelifesciences.com).

CHAPTER 15

Kaelin, W.G. Jr, Krek, W., Sellers, W.R. et al.1992. Expression cloning of a cDNA encoding a retinoblastoma-binding protein with E2F-like properties. *Cell* 70: 351.

Studier, F.W. and Moffatt, B.A. 1986. Use of bacteriophage T7 RNA polymerase to direct selective high-level expression of cloned genes. *J. Mol. Biol.* 189(1): 113–130.

CHAPTER 16

List of Sources

http://lexamed.com/New_Lex_Home_QualityManagementSystems.html.

CHAPTER 17

Niazi, S.K. 2003. *Filing Patents Online: A Professional Guide*. CRC Press.

INDEX